D1758349

THE COMPLETE SPLEEN

THE COMPLETE SPLEEN

STRUCTURE, FUNCTION, AND CLINICAL DISORDERS

Second Edition

EDITED BY

ANTHONY J. BOWDLER, MD, PhD

*EMERITUS PROFESSOR OF MEDICINE,
MARSHALL UNIVERSITY SCHOOL OF MEDICINE,
HUNTINGTON, WV*

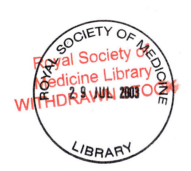
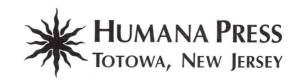

HUMANA PRESS
TOTOWA, NEW JERSEY

© 2002 Humana Press Inc.
999 Riverview Drive, Suite 208
Totowa, New Jersey 07512
humanapress.com

For additional copies, pricing for bulk purchases, and/or information about other Humana titles, contact Humana at the above address or at any of the following numbers: Tel.: 973-256-1699; Fax: 973-256-8341; E-mail:humana@humanapr.com; Website: humanapress.com

Production Editor: Mark J. Breaugh.

Cover Illustration: The spleen and pancreas, showing the major branches of the splenic artery and vein. *See* Fig. 1.7 on page 8.

Cover design by Patricia F. Cleary.

This publication is printed on acid-free paper. ∞
ANSI Z39.48-1984 (American National Standards Institute) Permanence of Paper for Printed Library Materials.

Printed in the United States of America.   10 9 8 7 6 5 4 3 2 1

Library of Congress Cataloging-in-Publication Data

The complete spleen : structure, function, and clinical disorders / edited by Anthony J.
Bowdler.--2nd ed.
     p. ; cm.
  Includes bibliographical references and index.
  ISBN 0-89603-555-7 (alk. paper)
  1. Spleen--Diseases. 2. Spleen. I. Bowdler, Anthony J. II. Spleen.
  [DNLM: 1. Spleen--anatomy & histology. 2. Spleen--physiology. 3. Splenic Diseases.
WH 600 C737 2002]
RC645 .S69 2002
616.4'1--dc21
                                                    2001039716

Dedications

To

Madeleine,

without whom this revision

would not have been possible,

and to the late professors

Auge Videbaek,
Jack Chamberlain,
and *Eric Schmidt,*

whose expertise is an intrinsic part of this book.

Preface to the Second Edition

The human spleen is an organ of very special and in some respects unique clinicopathological significance, and has emerged from a centuries-old scientific and medical obscurity only within living memory. Understanding of the biological functions and structure of the spleen has progressed through several phases: classical speculation, comparative studies confounded by profound differences between species, empirical studies of the disordered, and usually enlarged, spleen, and the outcome of splenectomy.

Each of these sources has left lingering fingerprints, often as widely accepted and persistent concepts at the clinical level, including those of (1) hypersplenism as a process or mechanism, (2) that there is no exclusive function of the spleen that cannot be performed by elements of the immune system everywhere, and (3) that the spleen acts as a useful reservoir of blood cells. The inherent errors of these concepts have proved limiting to the development of the rational interpretation of splenic disorder.

In the clinical context, the spleen long appeared as a silent, almost anonymous organ, presenting for notice principally when enlarged, or when peripheral blood cytopenias suggested the possibility of a splenic disorder. The discrete structural entity of the organ permitted surgical removal of the spleen (splenectomy) as a therapeutic intervention, which was long believed to carry no long-term penalties.

The first edition of this book, published in 1990 by Chapman and Hall Medical of London under the title *The Spleen: Structure, Function, and Clinical Significance* principally addressed the wealth of new information on the microscopic structure of the spleen, its immune functions, the mechanisms of related cytopenias, and the clinical sequelae of splenic disorders.

In the interval since that time there has been increasing recognition of the adverse consequences of absent or impaired splenic function, not only following splenectomy, but in a surprisingly wide range of diseases and disorders. This has led to a broad range of new surgical techniques designed to preserve sufficient splenic tissue to maintain the protective function of the organ. Related to this has been an increasing clinical interest, especially with respect to the investigation of the spleen radiologically, that has greatly improved the recognition of splenomegaly, atrophy, and intrasplenic pathology. In addition there has been a significant improvement in the sensitivity of techniques providing quantitative estimates of the various functions that are impaired in hyposplenism.

The changes appearing in this edition have therefore increased the clinical emphasis of the work, although some significant revisions and additions that focus on the supporting basic sciences related to the organ are also widely distributed throughout the chapters.

It is with great regret that I record the untimely passing of three distinguished contributors to the first edition. First, Professor Aage Videbaek of the Gentofte University Hospital, Copenhagen, Denmark, whose rigorous and insightful contributions to hematology ably represented the discipline in Scandinavia. He was the editor of the *Scandinavian Journal of Haematology*, and established the standards for critical research and clinical application for which the journal and its successor, the *European Journal*, are well known. He will be greatly missed. Second, Dr. Jack Chamberlain, a former student of Professor Leon Weiss, and a man whose hematological research in the field of scanning electron microscopy at the Universities of Rochester and East Carolina contributed greatly to an understanding of the structure of the spleen. I am grateful to Mrs. Chamberlain for her permission to consolidate elements of his first edition chapter into Chapter 2 of this edition. Last, I regretfully record the passing of Eric Schmidt who taught in the Department of Medical Biophysics at the University of Western Ontario. In the words of his colleague and chief, Professor Alan Groom, "Eric was a gifted experimentalist and electron microscopist, a shrewd observer, whose scientific observations have been of enormous value." Fortunately, one of his last collaborative contributions to the science of the spleen is incorporated into this edition.

I am grateful to those former authors who, while unable to complete revisions of their former work, nevertheless provided the framework for the contributions in this Edition. I also wish to thank Mr. Thomas Lanigan of the Humana Press for his interest and encouragement in the preparation of *The Complete Spleen: Structure, Function, and Clinical Disorders*, and also to Chapman and Hall of London, who were most helpful in making the transition to a new publisher practicable. I am also indebted to Ms. Lisa Watts and Ms. Sherry Puckett of the Department of Medicine at Marshall University, WV, and Ms. Katherine Carolan of the Department of Surgery at the University of Iowa, for their secretarial expertise and dedication. I am also grateful to the Huntington Clinical Foundation for support with respect to the editorial resources required, to Dr. F. G. Renshaw of Michigan State University and Dr. N. C. Bowdler of the University of Iowa for invaluable assistance in the preparation of this edition, to Mr. William Arnold for his valuable expertise with the illustrations, and to Mr. Jonathan Bowdler, whose communication skills were used to great advantage.

Anthony J. Bowdler, MD, PhD

Preface to the First Edition

INTRODUCTION

The last several years have seen a remarkable improvement in our understanding of the spleen, especially with respect to structure, and how this is related functionally to the many formed elements which perfuse the spleen from the general circulation. To this must be added the very considerable body of knowledge which has evolved from clinical experience. This book is the work of many authors of diverse expertise; each has provided an overview of his own area of interest, sometimes as a summary of the present state of the field, and sometimes with new information which has yet to be integrated into a more global understanding of the organ.

The spleen as yet belongs to no single discipline, and interest is shared among anatomists, immunologists, infectious disease physicians, surgeons, and many others. It is our intent that this book will present an overview of current understanding of the spleen, and provide a stimulus to continuing interest in the organ across many specialties. Several areas of considerable interest have had to be addressed in the context of other primary subjects, in order to keep the book within a moderate compass. However, individual authors have not been prevented from discussing some aspects of subjects which are given in greater detail in other chapters, when these have been relevant to their principal theme. In an expanding field of interest it is to be expected that specific concepts and data will be perceived differently from various specialized viewpoints. Consequently, I have not rigorously excluded some overlap in the subject matter, where this has been important to the development of the themes of more than one contributor.

THE STUDY OF THE SPLEEN

CLASSICAL STUDIES OF SPLEEN STRUCTURE AND FUNCTION

Of all the formed organs studied in the fields of medicine and mammalian biology, the spleen has until recently been the most difficult to place within the economy of the organism. Speculation concerning the spleen in the classical period commonly ascribed a digestive function to the organ: Hippocrates, Aristotle, and, subsequently, Galen supported the concept of an interchange of humors between the spleen and the stomach, probably through the short gastric vessels. However, there was later considerable doubt as to the mechanism of such a process, and for centuries the spleen remained Galen's "organ of mystery." It was for Vesalius (1514–1564 AD) to demonstrate that the postulated transfer was untenable on anatomical grounds. Nevertheless, the concept of a secretory function for the spleen died slowly, and even Malphighi inclined to the view that the lymphoid follicles of the spleen were minute secretory glands.

An insight into the special relationship between circulating blood and the spleen was evident in the suggestion by van Leeuwenhoeck (1632–1723 AD) that the spleen plays a role in the elaboration and "purification" of the blood. Stukely, in his Goulstonian lecture of 1722, showed remarkable prescience when, relying essentially on macroscopic structure, he rejected a secretory function for the organ, and proposed that it was a "diverticulum of the systemic circulation, filling and emptying with blood and acting as a controller of blood volume." This idea, with modifications, was supported by investigators such as Cooper, Winslow, Heister, and Hodgkin. In 1854 Gray, of Gray's *Textbook of Anatomy*, described his extensive researches into the comparative anatomy of the spleen, and concluded that its function "is to regulate the quantity and quality of the blood." He was especially impressed by the variable size of the equine spleen, and was also aware of the reservoir function of the spleen in diving mammals. Subsequently, the control of the quantity of circulating red cells by the spleen received much more attention than the control of quality, and researches by Barcroft and his colleagues in the period between 1923 and 1932 clarified many of the factors influencing this control in small mammals. Other studies relevant to this function were performed by Scheunert, Cannon and Cruickshank. Unfortunately it was many years before it was recognized that the physiological storage of blood cells is not a significant feature of the human spleen: indeed, with an average red cell content of 30–50 mL, there is no potential for augmenting the circulating red cell mass by the human spleen.

CLINICAL CONCEPTS: AN INTERMEDIATE PERIOD

One of the principal barriers to developing an understanding of the physiology of the human spleen has been the considerable interspecies variability of both functions and structure. Among these are the variable degree of smooth muscle development in the capsule and trabeculae, the structural differences between sinusal and non-sinusal spleens, and the relative development of arteriolar sheaths. These all suggest variations in function, which has made more complex the interpretation of animal studies and their relevance to human pathophysiology.

Uncertainty with respect to the validity of available animal models led clinicians to organize their clinical experiences conceptually in terms of postulated or apparently necessary splenic functions. Once the operation of splenectomy had been shown to be a reasonably safe procedure, and experience had been gained in the context of trauma to the organ, it was applied to the treatment of various disorders showing cell deficits in the blood. Conditions now identified as hereditary spherocytosis and idiopathic thrombocytopenic purpura were treated successfully by removal of the spleen, and later the procedure was applied to a heterogeneous group of disorders showing blood cell deficits under the rubric of "hypersplenism."

The original concept of "hypersplenism" was that of a pathogenic process whereby the spleen affected the hemopoietic activity of the bone marrow by a process analogous to the excessive endocrine activity of hyperthyroidism. This concept, first put forward by Chauffard in relation to hereditary spherocytosis in 1907, later culminated in a prolonged debate in the literature, between Dameshek as the proponent of a humoral influence on the bone marrow, and those such as Doan, who proposed that cell deficits such as thrombocytopenia are due to cell destruction mediated by the spleen.

The concept of "hypersplenism" has proved useful in a strictly clinical context, in that it describes a situation commonly found with one or more cell deficits in the peripheral blood, usually associated with enlargement of the spleen, and with a normal or excessive representation of the relevant cell precursors in the bone marrow. The term also carries the implication that the deficit will be corrected by splenectomy. It is important, however, to recognize that this is purely a syndromatic connotation, and does not imply a specific mechanism for the deficit. Indeed, the cause of a cytopenia is often multifactorial,

and it is of interest that the early debates on mechanism did not recognize the possibility of a dilutional form of anemia, which is probably the commonest factor in these circumstances. Nor did they recognize the "maldistribution thrombocytopenia" resulting from increased platelet pooling in the enlarged spleen.

Following this period, further clinical studies were made of hereditary spherocytosis, in which splenectomy corrects anemia without affecting the underlying membrane disorder of the spherocytes. The work of Lawrence Young, T. A. J. Prankerd, Robert Weed, and others showed that the spleen responds to the abnormal shape of red cells by impeding their flow through the organ, conditioning them to hemolysis both in the spleen and elsewhere, and disposing of a proportion of the damaged red cells in the organ itself.

Study of the mechanisms affecting the survival of red cells in conditions such as hereditary spherocytosis, in which the spleen plays so predominant a part, led to recognition of the importance of physical factors in the relationship of the spleen to blood cells. These gavepathophysiological meaning to concepts such as cell deformability, membrane rigidity, cell fragmentation, conditioning, and cell pooling. In one sense, such physical concepts have been a counterpoise to the assumptions made with respect to the special biological processes ascribed to the spleen, such as sequestration and hypersplenism, and have introduced a rigor into the investigation of the spleen that has been highly productive.

In a more general context, Crosby introduced the idea of the complete removal ("culling") and partial removal ("pitting") of red cells from the circulation. Such clinicopathological concepts were instrumental in leading to a search for the basic structures whereby the spleen could interact with red cells in this fashion.

CHANGING CONCEPTS OF THE SIGNIFICANCE OF THE SPLEEN

It is within the professional memory of many physicians still practicing that removal of the spleen by splenectomy was believed to carry no subsequent functional penalty, and indeed that there was no indispensable function of the spleen that could not be undertaken by organs and tissues elsewhere. Likewise it was commonly believed that the clinically enlarged spleen was invariably abnormal, and, conversely, that the abnormal spleen necessarily showed enlargement. Even though these clinical expectations have now been critically modified, it is of interest to look at the seminal concepts of the last 30 years, to identify those observations that have markedly changed the clinician's view of the significance of splenic disorders.

STUDIES WITH LABELED RED CELLS

The advent of radionuclide labeling for red cells, and later with more difficulty for platelets, radically changed the level of understanding of the relationship between the spleen and blood cells. In view of the red cell debris and liberated iron that remained in the spleen following the phagocytosis of red cells, it was anticipated that hemolysis would result in the accumulation of the labeling nuclide, usually chromium-51, in the organ responsible for destruction. Nuclide accumulation was detectable at the body surface, and patterns of increase in surface radioactivity were described; these were initially held to reflect a process of "sequestration." Sequestration was at first regarded as equivalent to destruction, but more careful analysis showed that radioactivity detectable at the body surface had several components, each of which varied individually with time. These consisted of the background radioactivity from red cells in the general circulation, that from a pool of red cells very slowly exchanging with the circulating red cells, and the subsequently slowly accumulated nuclide from cells destroyed in the organ. The processes of conditioning and spleen-dependent destruction at other sites were identified largely but not exclusively by inference.

The evidence of an enhancing red cell pool was especially important, as it implied that in pathological circumstances the circulation through the spleen might depart critically from normal. No other organ has been shown to have a comparable pooling component, and in some circumstances it appears to have an important effect on red cell life span. With respect to the red cell, pooling in man is essentially pathological; however, it was subsequently shown that platelets also pool in the spleen, and in this case the pool is present in normal circumstances, and expands when the spleen enlarges.

THE POSTSPLENECTOMY STATE

The recognition that splenectomy in infancy and early childhood could result in exceptional susceptibility to infection abruptly increased the clinical significance of the loss of splenic function. This has resulted in practical changes in clinical management, such as the deferring of elective splenectomy in young children, and has directed attention to the detailed consequences of impaired function of the spleen. The study of the hyposplenic state has, in fact, contributed extensively to the present understanding of the functions of the spleen, and indeed has proved to be much more informative than the investigation of "hypersplenism." It has also stimulated detailed investigation of the immune functions of the spleen, and has led to new surgical approaches to disorders involving the spleen, such as subtotal splenectomy, in order to reduce the disadvantages of the completely hyposplenic state.

The list of disorders that can contribute to the hyposplenic states continues to lengthen, and emphasizes the fact that the spleen has functions that are not readily matched by the compensatory activity of the immune system elsewhere. Recognition that the spleen has a very special role in defense against infection has given a special cogency to recent studies of the function of the red pulp, which are proceeding in both the ultrastructural

and clinical fields. In Chapter 3 (now revised as Chapter 2 by Professor Fern Tablin), Dr. Weiss describes his recent observations of the red pulp in experimental malaria, which demonstrate the mechanism by which the spleen can exclude intraerythrocytic parasites from infecting healthy red cells.

These observations illustrate well the importance of the spleen to human survival, and perhaps primate evolution. It has been estimated that more than half the deaths that have occurred since the emergence of the human species have been due to malaria, which emphasizes the very significant role which the organ must have played in protecting the survival and evolution of the species.

THE SIGNIFICANCE OF THE LYMPHOCYTE

If the spleen was at one time the classical "organ of mystery", it is equally true that until recently one of the most enigmatic of cells has been the lymphocyte. The extensive body of knowledge now available on the functions and identity of the lymphocyte has obscured how recent has been the elucidation of its functions, its complex taxonomy, and the subset interactions. It now appears that the spleen has a unique role in the immune system, and houses perhaps one-third of all the circulating lymphocytes. Of special interest to the hematologist is the significance of the spleen to the pathways of spread of the pathological cells in lymphomata, and the relationship of the surface characteristics of lymphocytes to the distribution of disease in these disorders.

DILUTION AND CELL-DISTRIBUTION AS MECHANISMS FOR BLOOD CELL DEFICITS

One mechanism contributing to anemia and other cell deficits, which has been recognized since the earlier discussion on "hypersplenism", has been the dilutional effect caused by the presence of an excess plasma volume in relation to the mass of circulating red cells. Frequently in the anemia accompanying the splenomegaly, the red cell mass is little changed from that which would be expected from the subject's height and weight. Anemia is then the result of an expansion of plasma volume, in circumstances in which a proportionate expansion of the red cell mass has not occurred despite an increase in total blood volume. This does not seem to be the consequence of control of plasma volume by the spleen, but to result from an expanded total blood volume without a proportionate increase in the number of red cells. It is of interest that such a phenomenon is unrelated to the principal functions of the spleen as presently understood; it appears to be the consequence of the additional vascularity of the organ, and its specific locus in the splanchnic pattern of blood vessels. An additional contributor to the blood cell deficits commonly present with splenomegaly is a maldistribution phenomenon: this is especially evident in the thrombocytopenia associated with the enlarged spleen, since the splenic pool of platelets enlarges in proportion to spleen volume. It is not yet clear why this does not produce a compensatory output of cells from the bone marrow, but a similar phenomenon also contributes in some cases to the anemia of splenomegaly.

PROSPECTS FOR THE CLINICAL MANAGEMENT OF DISORDERS OF THE SPLEEN

The study of the spleen has been passing through a particularly productive period, and this is reflected in changes in the surgical approach to the organ. These have yet to be proved effective empirically, but there has evolved a more flexible approach, and a willingness to review long-standing concepts of management in this field. One may reasonably hope that as the properties of the lymphoid system and pulp vasculature become increasingly well defined, there will be a basis for developing a new pharmacology for splenic disorders.

ACKNOWLEDGMENTS

This appears to be an especially appropriate time to summarize recent and current work, which has proceeded so far in many different fields. I am most grateful to many former colleagues and collaborators for their generous contributions to this work, and also to the publishers for encouraging this restatement of the clinical significance of the spleen, and of the basic biology which makes its understanding possible. I wish to thank the many con-tributors for their cooperation and high expertise, and to make clear that if there are deficiencies in this work then the responsibility is entirely mine. To any of the workers in this field who may have felt that their efforts have remained unrecognized, I offer my apologies and express the sincere hope that they will not be discouraged from continuing their efforts to unravel the enigmas of this fascinating organ.

Finally, I must acknowledge the influence of John Z. Young, FRS, Emeritus Professor of Anatomy at University College, London, who many years ago introduced me to the task of identifying the functional basis of perceived structure; and also to recall the late Robert I. Weed, MD, who personified the matching of intellectual insight by ingenuity in experiment. I also wish to thank Carolyn Endicott, Jennifer Long, and Patsy Dallas of the word Processing Unit of the Marshall University School of Medicine, for their unfailing patience and expertise. I am also grateful to my wife, Madeleine, who has contributed more than she knows to the completion of this work.

Anthony J. Bowdler, MD, PhD
Huntington, West Virginia
(August 1990)

A BIBLIOGRAPHY OF THE SPLEEN

Gray, H. (1854) *On the Structure and Use of the Spleen.* Astley Cooper Prize Essay. J. W. Parker, London.

Moynihan, B. (1921) *The Spleen and Some of its Diseases.* W. B. Saunders, Philadelphia.

Prankerd, T. A. J. (1963) The spleen and anaemia. *Br. Med. J.* **2,** 517–524.

Lennerts, K. and Harms, D. [eds.] (1970) *DieMilz; Struktur, Funktion, Pathologie, Klinik, Therapie.* Springer-Verlag, Berlin and New York. (German, with summaries in English).

Macpherson, A. I. S., Richmond, J., and Stuart, A. E. (1973) *The Spleen.* American Lecture Series, No. 893. Charles C. Thomas, Springfield, Ill.

Lewis, S. M. (1983) The spleen-mysteries solved and unresolved. *Clin. Haematol.* **12,** 363–373.

McCuskey, R. S. (1985) New trends in spleen research. *Experientia* **41,** 143–284.

Pochedly, C., Sills, R., and Schwartz, A. (1989) *Disorders of the Spleen; Pathophysiology and Management.* W. B. Saunders, Philadelphia and London.

Rosse, W. F. (1987) The spleen as a filter. *N. Engl. J. Med.* **317,** 704–705.

Videbaek, A., Christensen, B. E., and Jonsson, V. (1982) *The Spleen in Health and Disease.* Yearbook Medical Publishers, Copenhagen and Chicago.

Weiss, L., Geduldig, U., and Weidanz, W. (1986) Mechanisms of splenic control of murine malaria: reticular cell activation and the development of a blood-spleen barrier. *Am. J. Anat.* **176,** 251–285.

Wolf, B. C. and Neiman, R. S. (1988) *Disorders of the Spleen.* W. B. Saunders, Philadelphia and London.

Contents

Contributors

DAVID R. ANDERSON, MD, *Division of Haematology, Dalhousie University, Halifax, Nova Scotia, Canada*

RONALD A. BERGMAN, PhD, *Department of Anatomy and Cell Biology, University of Iowa College of Medicine, Iowa City, IA, USA*

ANTHONY J. BOWDLER, MD, PhD, FRCPLOND, FRCPATH, FACP, *Marshall University School of Medicine, Huntington, WV, USA*

JACK K. CHAMBERLAIN, MD, FACP, *Deceased, Formerly of East Carolina School of Medicine, Greenville, NC, USA*

MORRIS O. DAILEY, MD, PhD, *Department of Pathology and Program in Immunology, University of Iowa College of Medicine, Iowa City, IA, USA*

W. JEAN DODDS, DVM, *Hemopet, Santa Monica, CA, USA*

PETER N. FOSTER, PhD, BM, FRCPLOND, *Macclesfield District General Hospital, Macclesfield, UK*

GEOFFREY J. GORSE, MD, FACP *Department of Internal Medicine, Department of Veterans Affairs Medical Center, St. Louis University School of Medicine, St. Louis, MO, USA*

ALAN C. GROOM, PhD, *Department of Medical Biophysics, University of Western Ontario, London, Ontario, Canada*

PAUL M. HEIDGER, JR., PhD, *Department of Anatomy and Cell Biology, University of Iowa College of Medicine, Iowa City, IA, USA*

JOHN G. KELTON, MD, *Department of Medicine, McMaster University Medical Centre, Hamilton, Ontario, Canada*

JOHN LAWRENCE, MD, *Department of Surgery, University of New Mexico College of Medicine, Albuquerque, NM, USA*

MONTY S. LOSOWSKY, MD, FRCP, *Department of Medicine, University of Leeds, Leeds, UK*

IAN C. MACDONALD, PhD, *Department of Medical Biophysics, University of Western Ontario, London, Ontario, Canada*

ANNE T. MANCINO, MD, *Department of Surgery, University of Mississippi College of Medicine, Jackson, MS, USA*

MARK R. PALEY, MD, FRCR, *Department of Radiology, Frimley Park Hospital, Camberley, Surrey, UK*

CHARLES E. PLATZ, MD, *Department of Pathology, University of Iowa Health Center, Iowa City, IA, USA*

PETER C. RAICH, MD, *AMC Cancer Research Center, Colorado Cancer Research Program, University of Colorado Health Sciences Center, Denver, CO, USA*

FRANK GARY RENSHAW, PhD, *Marshall University School of Medicine, Huntington, WV, USA*

PABLO R. ROS, MD, FACR, *Department of Radiology, Brigham and Women's Hospital, Boston, MA, USA*

THOMAS C. RUSHTON, MD, *Division of Infectious Diseases, Department of Medicine, Marshall University School of Medicine, Huntington, WV, USA*

ERIC E. SCHMIDT, BSC, MCS, *Deceased, Formerly of Department of Medical Biophysics, University of Western Ontario, London, Ontario, Canada*

CAROL E. H. SCOTT-CONNER, MD, PhD, *Department of Surgery, University of Iowa College of Medicine, Iowa City, IA, USA*

GRAHAM R. SERJEANT, MD, FRCP, *Sickle Cell Trust, Kingston, Jamaica*

MICHAEL T. SHAW, MD, FRCP, FACP, DCH, *Department of Medicine, Mariopa Medical Center, Phoenix, AZ, USA*

FERN TABLIN, VMD, PhD, *Department of Anatomy, Physiology, and Cell Biology, School of Veterinary Medicine, University of California at Davis, Davis, CA, USA*

MOHAMMAD A. VASEF, MD, *Department of Pathology, University of Iowa College of Medicine, Iowa City, IA, USA*

LEON WEISS, MD, *School of Veterinary Medicine, University of Pennsylvania, Philadelphia, PA, USA*

Acknowledgments

The editor and Dr. C. Scott-Conner wish to thank Lippincott-Williams & Wilkins publishers, for permission to republish Figures 1.3, 1.5, 17.1, and 17.2 from *Operative Anatomy* and Springer-Verlag for Figures 17.11 and 17.14 from *The Sages Manual*. Dr. Fern Tablin acknowledges permission by Dr. T. Fujita and *Scanning Microscopy* to publish Figure 2.7, by Dr. S. Sasou and *Scanning Microscopy International Inc.*, to publish Figure 2.10, by Dr. T. Fujita and Birkhaeuser Publishing Ltd., publisher of *Experientia*, to publish Figures 2.8 and 2.9, by Dr. T. Fujita and the *Archivum Histologicum Japonicum* for Figures 2.12, 2.13, and 2.15. Likewise Dr. Tablin had the permission of Wiley-Liss, Inc., a subsidiary of John Wiley & Sons, Inc. to publish Figure 2.16.

The editor and Dr. Groom wish to thank Dr. J. A. Bellanti and W. B. Saunders Co., for permission to publish Figure 3.1, the Academic Press, Inc. for Figures 3.2, 3.3, 3.25, 3.26, 3.27, 3.38, and 3.39 from various titles, the American Physiological Society for 3.4 and 3.5, Dr. T. Fujita, the Japan Society of Histological Documentation and the *Archivum Histologicum Japonicum* for Figures 3.9, 3.13, 3.14, 3.15, 3.21, 3.31, 3.32, and 3.34, originally from the *American Journal of Anatomy*, and also Dr. Y. Hataba, the Center for Academic Publications, Japan and the *Journal of Electron Microscopy* for Figure 3.10, to Dr. T. Snook and Wiley-Liss Inc. (as cited above) for 3.11 from the *Anatomical Record*, and Scanning Microscopy International for Figure 3.19 from *Scanning Microscopy*, Dr. J. A. G. Rhodin and the Oxford University Press for Figure 3.24, Dr. A. de Boisfleury, the Academic Press, Inc. and *Blood Cells* for Figure 3.25, to Professor T. Suzuki, Springer-Verlag and *Cell and Tissue Research* for Figure 3.28, and also Springer-Verlag for Figures 3.36 and 3.37, the American Physiological Society and the *American Journal of Physiology* for 3.4, 3.5, 3.30, and 3.33, and W. B. Saunders Co. and *Blood* for Figures 3.40 and 3.41.

Dr. Groom also wishes to acknowledge research support provided by the Medical Research Council of Canada.

Dr. Peter Raich acknowledges the assistance of Ms. Jennifer Shaefer in the preparation of the manuscript for Chapter 14.

The editor and Dr. Renshaw wish to thank the American College of Physicians and the *Annals of Internal Medicine* for permission to publish Figure 7.3, W. B. Saunders, Co., and *Clinics in Haematology* for permission to publish Figure 7.3; also Blackwell Science Ltd. and the *British Journal of Haematology* for permission to publish Figures 7.4, 7.10, and 7.11. Likewise the permission of Blackwell Science Ltd. and Professor A. M. Peters is acknowledged for permission to publish Figure 7.6 from the *British Journal of Haematology*. Dr. A. Foss Abrahamsen, the *Scandinavian* (now *European*) *Journal of Haematology* and Munksgaard International are thanked for permission to reproduce Figures 7.8 and 7.9.

Drs. P. N. Foster and M. S. Losowsky acknowledge the permission granted by *Pediatrics* to reproduce Figure 10.3, originally published in *Pediatrics*, **76**, 392 (1985). Drs. David R. Anderson and John Kelton acknowledge with thanks the permission of Marcel Dekker, Inc., NY to republish Figure 3 from Pochedly, Sills, and Schwartz, *Disorders of the Spleen; Pathophysiology and Management* (1988) as Figure 12.1, and Margo Meyerhoff and the American Society of Hematology for permission to publish Figure 12.2 from *Blood*, **66**, 490–495 (1985). The editor and Dr. Michael T. Shaw thank Dr. P. Koeffler and Blackwell Science, Ltd. for permission to publish Figure 13.1 from the *British Journal of Haematology*, **43**, 69–77 (1977).

Dr. Graham Serjeant acknowledges the permission of the publishers to reproduce the following figures: Lancet Ltd for Figure 15.1; Harcourt Brace and Co., Ltd., Academic Press, W. B. Saunders Co., Ltd., and Churchill Livingstone for Figure 15.2, Blackwell Science, Ltd., and the *British Journal of Haematology* for Figure 15.3; Howard A. Pearson, M. D. and Mosby International, Ltd. for Figure 15.4, from the *New England Journal of Medicine*, **283** (1970); the BMJ Publishing Group for permission to publish Figures 15.5 and 15.8 from the *Archives of Disease in Childhood* and Figure 15.11 from the *British Medical Journal*; Mosby Inc. for Figure 15.7 from the *Journal of Pediatrics*, and the Oxford University Press for Figure 15.9.

The editor thanks Lippincott-Williams-Wilkins for permission to publish a composite table from Bowdler, A. J. (1970) *Transfusion* 10, 171–181 as Table 8.2.

Color Plates

Color plates 1–18 appear as an insert following page 78.

THE STRUCTURE AND FUNCTION OF THE SPLEEN

1 The Anatomy of the Spleen

RONALD A. BERGMAN, PhD, PAUL M. HEIDGER, JR., PhD,
AND CAROL E. H. SCOTT-CONNER, MD, PhD

1.1. INTRODUCTION

The spleen is a pulpy organ approximately the size of a fist, and contains the largest single aggregate of lymphoid tissue in the body. Despite its functional importance, the anatomy of the organ has not been studied as extensively as that of other organs, probably because its study presents intrinsic difficulties. Recent interest in the gross anatomy of the spleen has centered on the related topics of segmental anatomy, knowledge of which facilitates splenic repair and partial splenectomy; and the internal vascular structure, which remains a matter of considerable controversy. This chapter reviews the development, relationships, peritoneal attachments, vascular supply, lymphatic drainage, and nerve supply of the spleen, and concludes with a discussion of the surgical anatomy and some related surgical complications.

1.2. EMBRYOLOGIC DEVELOPMENT AND ANOMALIES

1.2.1. NORMAL EMBRYOLOGIC DEVELOPMENT
The spleen is derived from a group of mesenchymal cells that first appears during the fifth week of embryonic life as a thickening in the dorsal mesogastrium (Hamilton and Mossman, 1972; Moore, 1982). Lying along that portion of the stomach that will develop into the greater curvature, these cells aggregate and differentiate into the splenic anlage. During the second month of gestation a lobulated embryonic spleen forms. Primitive vessels grow into the developing spleen. As the lobules fuse during the third month, the spleen begins to assume a recognizable form. The occasional notches seen on the anterior border of the spleen, and segmentation of its internal vascular structures, reflect this fetal lobulation pattern (see Subheading 5.3.).

From the fourth to eighth month of gestation, the spleen has usually been considered to function as an hematopoietic organ, and this is a function that it may retain or regain, if the bone marrow is unable to provide adequate hematopoiesis (as in compensatory or pathological extramedullary hematopoiesis). This topic is discussed further in Chapters 9 and 13.

As the developing stomach elongates, the greater curvature grows faster than the lesser curvature. Subsequently, rotation places the greater curvature and the spleen to the left of the midline (Fig. 1). The developing pancreas, which grows simultaneously with rotation and fusion, becomes retroperitoneal. The tail of the pancreas retains a close anatomic relationship to the spleen in the region of the splenic hilum (Fig. 2).

1.2.2. DEVELOPMENTAL ANOMALIES
Accessory spleens are found in up to 35% of individuals, and are thus the most common anomaly of splenic development. They result from failure of fusion of the individual splenic anlagen, and usually appear as small nodules, located near the main organ (Fig. 3). Their size varies from 0.5 to 3.75 cm in diameter. In Halpert's autopsy series of 602 males with accessory spleens, 519 (86%) had a single accessory spleen, 65 (11%) had two, and 18 (3%) had three or more (Halpert and Eaton, 1951; Halpert and Gyorkey, 1959a,b). The most common locations are at the anterior aspect of the spleen and hilum, the greater omentum, the transverse mesocolon, the gastrolienal ligament, behind the left lobe of the liver, adjacent to the pancreas, and in the connective tissue surrounding the splenic vessels. On rare occasions, splenogonadal fusion (see below) allows splenic tissue to be pulled down into the presacral, pelvic, adnexal, or paratesticular region. Accessory spleens are principally of significance as a source of recurrent cytopenias, when splenectomy is performed for hematologic indications (Settle, 1940; Curtis and Movitz, 1946; Appel and Bart, 1976).

Splenogonadal fusion is a rare anomaly usually affecting males. On occasion, it may lead to a nodule of splenic tissue in proximity to the testis, and may be confused with a testicular tumor (Sneath 1913; Bennett-Jones and St. Hill, 1952; Wick and Rife, 1981). In one variation, splenogonadal fusion may result in a band of fibrous tissue, often containing nodules of splenic tissue, joining the spleen and the left testis, and is presumed to be caused by adherence of splenic anlagen to the developing mesonephros (Putschar and Marion, 1956; Hines and Eggum, 1961; Scholtmeijer, 1966).

Heterotopic islands of pancreatic tissue have been found in the spleen (Barbosa, Dockerty, and Waugh, 1946).

Splenic lobulation is frequently exaggerated, with prominent notches along the free anterosuperior border (Fig. 2). These lobulations and notches are the residual evidence of the primitive anlagen. In one series, only 8/113 specimens were completely free of

From: *The Complete Spleen: A Handbook of Structure, Function, and Clinical Disorders* Edited by: A. J. Bowdler © Humana Press Inc., Totowa, NJ

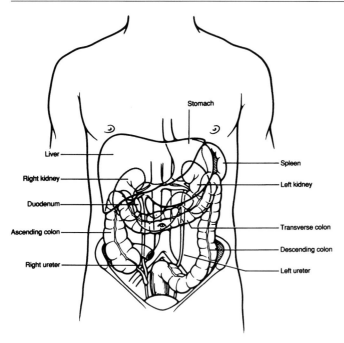

Fig. 1.1.   An outline diagram of the abdominal viscera, to show the approximate relations of the spleen to other major abdominal viscera.

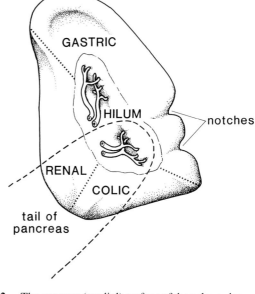

Fig. 1.2.   The concave (medial) surface of the spleen, demonstrating the three major impressions, notches, hilum with splenic vessels, and the relationship to the tail of the pancreas. A reflection of peritoneum surrounds the hilum.

notches. Most commonly, two notches were present, but as many as seven have been recorded. These notches give a hint of the internal vascular segmentation. Deep incisions may also be found on the diaphragmatic surface and posterior border, so that at times the entire organ appears to be completely divided into lobes.

Rarely, the spleen may appear to be reduplicated or broken up into its fundamental vascular units (Calori, 1862; Bergman et al., 1988). True polysplenia is rare, and is sometimes associated with severe congenital cardiac defects.

The term "situs inversus" encompasses several rare clinical presentations. When visceral situs inversus occurs, the spleen may be on the right side (Halff, 1904). From 18 to 26% of patients with complete situs inversus have Kartagener's syndrome (total situs inversus, bronchiectasis, and abnormal paranasal sinuses). In general, the situs inversus causes no problems *per se*, other than causing diagnostic and/or therapeutic confusion until the condition is recognized (e.g., the pain of appendicitis may localize to either side). The associated anomalies usually dominate the clinical picture.

Splenic agenesis, or asplenia, is rare, and is frequently associated with severe cardiac malformations, often of uncommon type, and with other congenital anomalies. In these cases, the splenic artery terminates in the pancreas (Robert, 1842; Arnold, 1868; Hodenpyl, 1898; Sternberg, 1903; Boggs and Reed, 1953; Murphy and Mitchell, 1957; Polhemus and Schafer, 1952).

1.3.   ANATOMIC RELATIONSHIPS

1.3.1. LOCATION   The spleen lies obliquely in the left hypochondrium. Its cranial pole may reach the epigastric region, and its caudal pole often extends into the lumbar region. It is located in a shallow pocket formed dorsally by the kidney and suprarenal gland, laterally by the costal part of the diaphragm, cranially by the dome of the diaphragm, caudally by the left colic flexure and the phrenicocolic ligament, and ventromedially by the stomach (Figs. 1, 2,

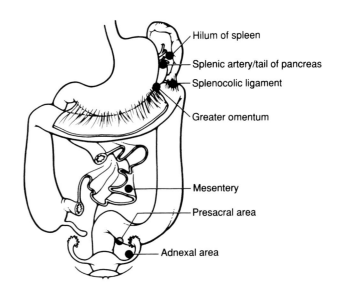

Fig. 1.3.   The common sites of accessory spleens. (Reproduced with permission from Scott-Conner and Dawson).

and 4). The long axis of the organ runs approximately in line with the tenth rib, with the projection of its margins reaching one rib width above and below this (Fig. 4). The spleen lies lateral to a line drawn from the left sternoclavicular articulation to the tip of the eleventh rib (Anson, 1966). Although the spleen is normally protected from trauma by the left lower rib cage (Fig. 4), injury to the spleen should be suspected with fractures of the left lower ribs (Hollinshead, 1971; Seufert and Mitrou, 1986).

1.3.2. PERITONEAL REFLECTIONS   The spleen has a complete peritoneal covering, except at the hilum (Fig. 2), and where there are peritoneal reflections to adjacent organs; these peritoneal attachments are termed "ligaments" (Fig. 5), and exert a mechanical function in tethering the spleen. Traction on adjacent organs

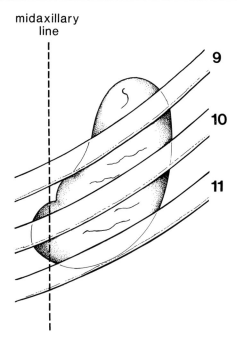

midaxillary
line

9

10

11

Fig. 1.4. The diaphragmatic surface of the normal spleen, showing its relationship to the ninth, tenth, and eleventh ribs. Note the presence of fissures on the convex surface.

(e.g., a downward pull on the splenic flexure of the colon, during colon resection) may tear the splenic capsule near the point of attachment of one of the ligaments, causing troublesome bleeding (Cioffiro et al., 1976; Lord and Gourevitch, 1965). The ligaments are named for the structures they connect. Thus, the gastrolienal, phrenicolienal, lienorenal, phrenicocolic, and lienocolic ligaments are recognized.

The gastrolienal ligament forms part of the wall of the omental bursa (lesser sac), and carries the vasa brevia (or short gastric vessels) from the splenic artery and vein to the stomach. An avascular presplenic fold may be found superficial to the lienogastric ligament. The ligament is generally triangular in shape, with the apex cephalad and the broad base inferior. For this reason, the highest vasa brevia tend to be the shortest. The phrenicolienal ligament tethers the spleen to the inferior aspect of the diaphragm, and is generally avascular.

Surgically, dividing both the phrenicolienal and the gastrolienal ligaments is necessary, to mobilize the spleen into the midline and recreate the embryonic situation. The peritoneum lateral to the spleen, which is a continuation of the phrenicolienal ligament, is incised, and an avascular plane posterior to the spleen is developed.

The lienorenal ligament covers the splenic hilar vessels and pancreas, then fuses posteriorly with the peritoneum of the abdominal wall.

The phrenicocolic and, when present, lienocolic ligaments tether the splenic flexure of the colon (van der Zypen and Revesz, 1984). These ligaments are generally avascular, and become continuous with the greater omentum. (Latarjet, 1908; Anson, 1966).

1.4. GROSS ANATOMY

1.4.1. GROSS APPEARANCE The shape of the spleen varies considerably in different individuals, no two being exactly alike. In general, it has the shape of an elongated, flattened, but curved,

ovoid body. The shape may also vary as the organ accommodates itself to contraction or distention of adjacent viscera. When the stomach is empty and the colon distended, a more tetrahedral shape may become pronounced. When the stomach is full and the colon empty, the colic surface of the spleen may disappear completely (Anson, 1966; Henle, 1868; Kopsch, 1908; Latarjet, 1908; Schaefer et al., 1915).

With these caveats, the spleen is usually seen to have 3–4 surfaces, and three rounded edges. The most extensive surface is the diaphragmatic aspect, facing the concavity of the diaphragm posterolaterally (Fig. 4). The visceral surface includes a gastric portion and a renal portion. The concavity of the gastric surface is deep, and rests ventromedially against the fundus of the stomach (Fig. 2). This gastric surface includes the hilus, which receives the splenic vessels, and, behind this, the spleen is in contact with the tail of the pancreas. The concavity of the renal surface is shallow, and rests posteromedially against the convex anterior surface of the left kidney and suprarenal gland. The most caudal part of this renal surface approaches, and may touch, the left colic flexure. If the colic or basal surface is enlarged, an additional surface is created, and the spleen may take the tetrahedral shape described above.

The spleen has superior and inferior borders. The superior border forms a sharp convex line, on which slight lobulations may be seen. The notches producing the lobulations expand in enlarged spleens. These lobulations are of clinical significance, because they distinguish the enlarged spleen from other enlarged organs, such as, e.g., gastric neoplasm, lymphoma of upper abdominal nodes, and the kidney in hypernephroma and other conditions (Anson, 1966). The inferior border is relatively straight, and less prominent than the superior border. The superior border contacts the fundus of the stomach, and the inferior border contacts the lumbar part of the diaphragm. In the tetrahedral-shaped spleen, the inferior border also separates the colic surface from the diaphragmatic surface (Cunningham, 1895).

The spleen also shows a posterior and an anterior extremity, the latter occupying the more ventral position. Between the gastric and renal surfaces of the spleen, but usually on the gastric surface, an elevated ridge, the so-called "intermediate border," may present a distinct tubercle. Along the edges of this ridge, the visceral layer of the peritoneum is attached. The visceral peritoneum surrounds the entire organ, from which it is reflected as the gastrolienal and phrenicolienal ligaments (Shepard, 1903; Anson, 1966).

The spleen, in life, normally has a dark, reddish-brown color, but develops a purplish tint soon after death. The organ has a soft consistency, but is covered by a tough, fibrous capsule composed of elastic and smooth muscle fibers, which permit considerable expansion. Smooth muscle fibers extend for a short distance into the trabeculae of the organ (Anson, 1966). The peritoneum is attached to the splenic capsule. The size of the spleen is subject to great variation, both within and between individuals. Normally, the spleen cannot be palpated, except when it is significantly enlarged (*see also* Chapter 9). In such cases, the lower pole extends downward and forward, following the line of the lower ribs, as shown in Fig. 6, toward the umbilicus, and subsequently below the costal margin. An early clinical manifestation of this is extension of the area of splenic dullness to percussion anterior to the midaxillary line, and thence to the costal margin, beyond which the organ becomes palpable (*see also* Chapter 9).

1.4.2. DIMENSIONS When examined after death, the length of the spleen varies from 10 to 14 cm, the width from 6 to 10 cm,

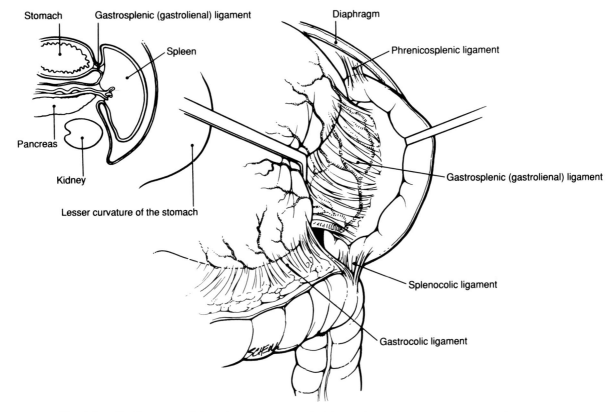

Fig. 1.5. The ligaments of the spleen. (Reproduced with permission from Scott-Conner and Dawson).

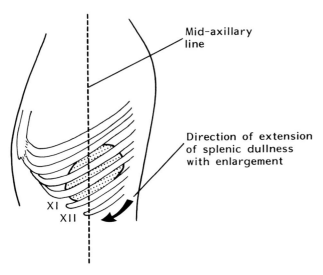

Fig. 1.6. A left lateral projection of the spleen on the body wall and lower ribs: This shows the common direction of splenic enlargement, and shows that an early sign of splenic enlargement is the extension of splenic dullness to percussion anterior to the midaxillary line along the line of the tenth rib.

and the thickness from 3 to 4 cm. The organ may weigh from 80 to 300 g or more (Krumbhaar and Lippincott, 1939; McCormick and Kashgarian, 1965). In subjects over the age of about 60 yr, the spleen undergoes some visible involution (Barcroft and Stephens, 1936; Anson, 1966), although the lymphoid tissue diminishes steadily after the first decade of life. The organ readily enlarges under increased venous pressure. After a meal, and during exer-

cise, the organ enlarges temporarily, but subsequently returns to its resting size.

Radiographic studies of the spleen, in living, healthy young males, demonstrate that the shadow of the spleen varies in size in the erect posture, the length of the shadow varying from 11 to 15 cm, and the width from 6 to 7 cm. The values for young females, who are usually smaller in stature than males, were only slightly less (Barcroft and Stephens, 1936; Mainland and Gordon, 1941). The spleen may extend from the upper half of the first lumbar to the upper half of the fifth lumbar vertebra. On changing from the standing to the recumbent position, there is a craniad shift of the spleen, on average, of about the length of one vertebra (approx 2.5 cm). Splenic volume can be estimated by computed tomography or ultrasound (Watanabe et al., 1997).

The normal adult spleen weighs between 100 and 175 g. Males have generally larger spleens (mean weight 180 g for males, 140 g for females). At birth, the weight of the spleen is relatively similar in males and females, at 10.5 and 10.4 g, respectively (Sprogoe-Jakobsen and Sprogoe-Jakobsen, 1997).

1.4.3. TOPOGRAPHIC CONFIGURATION The surface of the spleen is composed of a 1–2-mm-thick fibrous capsule, surrounding a pulpy interior spanned by fibrous trabeculae. Its shape is somewhat plastic, generally assumes the shape of the space it occupies, being convex on the surface facing the diaphragm and lateral abdominal wall, and concave (with indentations) on the surface facing the stomach, pancreas, kidney, and colon (Fig. 2).

The presence of deep notches on the anterior edge of the spleen has been shown to correlate with early branching of the splenic artery, which fans out into multiple hilar branches (Skandalakis et al., 1983; Skandalakis, 1990). In contrast, spleens with smooth borders are associated with late branching of the splenic artery.

Table 1.1
Reported Variations
in the Celiac Axis, with Approximate Frequency

Origin	Vessels	%
Hepatosplenogastric	Usual	90
Hepatosplenic trunk	Hepatic, splenic	3.5
Hepatosplenomesenteric	Hepatic, splenic, superior mesenteric	0.5
Hepatogastric trunk	Hepatic, left gastric	1.5
Splenogastric	Splenic, left gastric	5.5
Celiacomesenteric trunk	Superior mesenteric in conjunction with hepatosplenogastric	1.2–2.5

These variations are of importance to the performance of partial or total splenectomy.

1.5. VASCULAR ANATOMY

Unlike lymph nodes, which lie along major lymphatic trunks and filter lymph, the spleen filters blood. Inflow comes predominantly from the splenic artery, and the major outflow is through the splenic vein. In an arrangement similar to that in lymph nodes, the major artery and vein enter and leave through a defined hilum. The hilum of the spleen faces medially, and the splenic artery and vein as described above, are covered by the lienorenal ligament (Soson-Jaroschewitsch, 1927). The internal vascular anatomy is segmental, and reflects the embryonic origin of fused anlagen, giving a pattern of organization that facilitates partial splenectomy.

Within the spleen, the arteries branch to pass into the trabeculae. As these trabecular arteries further branch and leave the trabeculae for the splenic pulp, they form vessels termed "central arteries," which further ramify and become surrounded by lymphoid tissue. When an artery has decreased in size to a diameter of 50 µm, it emerges from its coat of lymphatic tissue, to ramify in the red pulp as a penicillary artery (see Chapter 2).

1.5.1. ARTERIES The splenic (lienal) artery provides the major blood supply to the spleen. It is the largest of the three major branches of the celiac artery, but anomalies are frequent (Michels, 1942; Poynter, 1922). The celiac trunk may lack one or more of its branches (Adachi, 1928, Chadzypanagiotis and Amerski, 1978; Lipshutz, 1917; Piquard, 1910; Tischendorf, 1973). In such cases, the missing branch may arise from the aorta or the superior mesenteric artery, either independently or in conjunction with another branch (Clausen, 1955; Henle, 1868; Kostinovitch, 1937; Tanigawa, 1963). Variations in pattern have been reported (Tischendorf, 1973), as detailed in Table 1.

The splenic and hepatic arteries may arise from a common trunk, or directly from the superior mesenteric artery (Henle, 1868).

Regardless of its site of origin, the splenic artery then follows the superior border of the pancreas in a horizontal plane, to enter the spleen at the hilum. With advancing age, the splenic artery becomes increasingly tortuous. It varies in length from 8 to 32 cm. In the most common arrangement, the splenic artery lies above the splenic vein (Abadia-Fenoll, 1964; Carmell, 1925; Waizer et al., 1989). It may, on occasion, lie posteriorly around the splenic vein, or divide, then recombine, forming a loop penetrated by the splenic vein. Although the splenic artery only rarely runs through the pancreas, it is closely applied to the pancreas, and tethered to it by a variable number of small, short arterial twigs.

As the splenic artery progresses toward the spleen, it sends branches to the stomach (via the left gastroepiploic artery, the posterior gastric artery, which is present in 48–68% of individuals, and the vasa brevia), and the pancreas.

The splenic artery branches a variable number of times (between 6 and 36) into vessels divisible into superior, inferior, and, occasionally, intermediate groups, before reaching the hilum (Anson, 1966; Garcia-Porrero and Lemes, 1988; Vandamme and Bonte, 1986, 1990; Machalek et al., 1998). As described previously, prominent notches on the anterior surface of the spleen correlate with early branching of the splenic artery. It is not unusual to find several smaller intermediate branches that supply the poles of the spleen.

The vasa brevia, and, to a lesser extent, the left gastroepiploic artery (if it anastomoses with the right gastroepiploic artery), form potential collaterals, which may protect the spleen if the splenic artery is ligated or thrombosed (Anson, 1966). In the event of ligation of the splenic artery, the fate of the spleen or splenic segment depends on the level of ligation: ligation of the segmental branches is generally followed by segmental infarction, a fact that is exploited during segmental splenic resection (Anson, 1966; see also Chapter 17).

1.5.2. VEINS The venous drainage of the spleen begins in the sinusoids of the red pulp. Trabecular veins accompany trabecular arteries, to terminate in approximately nine branches, uniting at the hilum, and leaving as tributaries of the splenic vein. In general, these branches accompany the corresponding branches of the splenic artery, so that internal venous segmentation lies parallel to the internal arterial segmentation. The spleen can thus be divided into segments separated by relatively avascular planes (Dawson et al., 1986).

The large-diameter splenic vein runs posterior to the pancreas (Fig. 7). The left gastroepiploic vein drains into the most inferior segmental splenic vein or directly into the splenic vein, and may provide collateral venous drainage in splenic vein thrombosis.

Multiple, small, short venous twigs tether the pancreas to the splenic vein (Dawson et al., 1986). Anastomoses between the splenic and left renal veins are not unusual, and the left spermatic vein has been reported draining into a splenic vein (MacAlister, 1868).

The splenic vein and superior mesenteric vein combine behind the pancreas, to form the portal vein (Douglas et al., 1950; Gerber et al., 1951). The inferior mesenteric vein enters the splenic vein at a variable distance from the juncture of the splenic vein and the superior mesenteric vein. Although the course of the splenic vein roughly approximates that of the splenic artery, the vein lacks the tortuosity of the artery.

The veins of the vasa brevia accompany the arteries, and drain directly into the substance of the spleen. These collaterals dilate and produce varices, in cases of splenic vein thrombosis.

1.5.3. SEGMENTAL ANATOMY The internal vascular anatomy is segmentally ordered in the manner described above, with venous distribution in parallel with the arterial segments (Dixon et al., 1980; Whitesell, 1960). Major segments tend to be oriented transversely, and to correspond to the external notches or visible branches of the splenic artery and vein (Gupta et al., 1976a,b; Parry, 1988; Trooskin et al., 1989). Minor segments are randomly oriented (Dawson et al., 1986).

1.6. LYMPHATICS

The issue of the extent and depth of penetration of lymphatic vessels within the lymphoid tissue of the human spleen remains

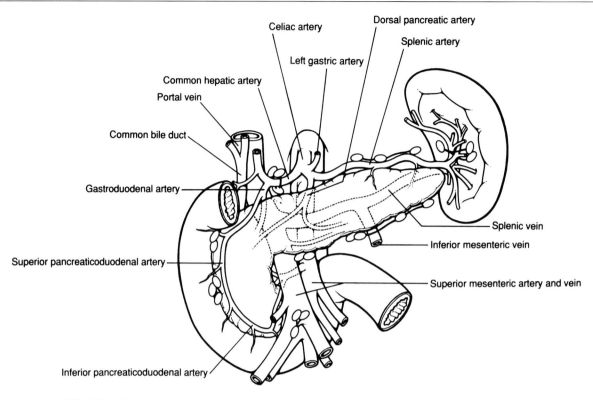

Fig. 1.7.   The spleen and pancreas, showing the major branches of the splenic artery and vein.

controversial (Milicevic et al., 1996). Lymphatic capillaries appear to originate in the large trabeculae and capsule. These drain into 8–10 small lymph nodes at the splenic hilum, which also receive drainage from the greater curvature of the stomach and the pancreas. Splenic nodes also lie within the layers of the gastrolienal ligament. Additional lymphatic drainage is to the pancreaticosplenic nodes along the superior border of the pancreas (Anson, 1966) and, to some extent, to the pancreaticoduodenal nodes. Efferent vessels from these nodes drain into the celiac and preaortic nodes, along with lymphatics from the stomach and pancreas.

1.7. INNERVATION

Sympathetic nerve fibers, from the median and anterior parts of the celiac plexus, form a dense network, the splenic plexus, associated with the splenic artery and its branches. These postganglionic sympathetic fibers are principally vasomotor, supplying the musculature of the branching vessels. Fibers from the right vagus have also been traced entering the spleen. The few myelinated fibers are believed to be sensory.

1.8. SURGICAL CONSIDERATIONS

Surgical exposure and mobilization of the spleen requires division of the phrenicolienal, lienocolic, and lienogastric ligaments (Fig. 5). Generally, full mobilization will also require division of the vasa brevia. Because the vasa brevia are potential collaterals in the event of splenic artery ligation, it may be advisable to preserve at least some of these, if splenic salvage (e.g., for trauma) is planned. Care must be taken not to injure the greater curvature of the stomach during ligation of the vasa brevia (Harrison et al., 1977).

The hilar vessels are best approached from behind, and must be carefully separated from the tail of the pancreas. The operative techniques of open and laparoscopic splenectomy, as well as splenic repair, are detailed in Chapter 17.

Careful search for, and removal of, accessory spleens is an important part of splenectomy for hematologic problems, such as idiopathic thrombocytopenic purpura.

REFERENCES

Abadia-Fenoll, F. (1964) Uber eine aussert stark geschlangelte und verlangerte Arteria lienalis. *Anat. Anz.* **115,** 339–344.

Adachi, B. (1928) *Das Arteriensystem der Japaner.* Kenkyusha, Kyoto.

Anson, B. J., ed. (1966) Morris' *Human Anatomy*, 12th ed. McGraw-Hill, New York.

Appel, M. F. and Bart, J. B. (1976) The surgical and hematologic significance of accessory spleens. *Surg. Gynecol. Obstet.* **143,** 191–192.

Arnold, J. (1868) Ein Fall von Cor triloculare biatriatum, Communication der Lungenvenen mit der Pfortader und Mangel der milz. *Arch. Pathol. Anat. Physiol. Klin. Med.* **42,** 449–472.

Barbosa, J. J., Dockerty, M. B., Waugh, J. M., et al. (1946) Pancreatic heterotopia: review of literature and report of 41 authenticated surgical cases, of which 25 were clinically significant. *Surg. Gynecol. Obstet.* **82,** 527–542.

Barcroft, J. and Stephens, J. G. (1936) Observations on the size of the spleen. *J. Physiol.* **64,** 1–22.

Bennett-Jones, M. J. and St. Hill, C. A. (1952) Accessory spleen in the scrotum. *Br. J. Surg.* **40,** 259–262.

Bergman, R. A., Thompson, S. A., Afifi, A. K., and Saadeh, F. A. (1988) *Compendium of Human Anatomic Variation. Text, Atlas, and World Literature.* Urban & Schwarzenberg, New York.

Boggs, J. D. and Reed, W. (1953) Congenital absence of the spleen. *Q. Bull. Northwestern Univ. Med. School* **27,** 289–293.

Calori, L. (1862) Sulla dupilicita congenita della milza. *Mem. Accad. Sci. Istituto di Bologna* **2,** 243–360.

Carmel, A. G. (1925) The tortuous splenic artery. *Anat. Rec.* **29,** 352.

Chadzypanagiotis, D. and Amerski, L. (1978) A rare case of the celiac trunk anomaly. *Folia Morphol. (Warsaw)* **37,** 401–405.

Cioffiro, W., Schein, C. H., and Gliedman, M. L. (1976) Splenic injury during abdominal surgery. *Arch Surg.* **111,** 167–171.

Clausen, H. J. (1955) An unusual variation in origin of hepatic and splenic arteries. *Anat. Rec.* **123,** 335–340.

Cunningham, D. J. (1895) The form of the spleen and the kidneys. *J. Anat. Physiol.* **29**, 501–517.

Curtis, G. M. and Movitz, D. (1946) The surgical significance of the accessory spleen. *Ann. Surg.* **123**, 276–298.

Dawson, D. L., Molina, M. E., and Scott-Conner, C. E. H. (1986) Venous segmentation of the human spleen: a corrosion cast study. *Am. Surg.* **52**, 253–256.

Dixon, J. A., Miller, F., McCloskey, D., and Siddoway, J. (1980) Anatomy and techniques in segmental splenectomy. *Surg. Gynecol. Obstet.* **150**, 516–520.

Douglas, B. E., Baggenstoss, A. H., and Hollinshead, W. H. (1950) The anatomy of the portal vein and its tributaries. *Surg. Gynecol. Obstet.* **91**, 562.

Garcia-Porrero, J. A. and Lemes, A. (1988) Arterial segmentation in the human spleen. *Acta Anat.* **131**, 276–283.

Gerber, A. B., Lev, M., and Goldberg, S. L. (1951) The surgical anatomy of the splenic vein. *Am. J. Surg.* **82**, 339.

Gupta, C. D., Gupta, S. C., Arora, A. K., and Singh, P. J. (1976a) Vascular segments of the human spleen by post-mortem angiograms and corrosion casts. *Angiology* **33**, 720–727.

Gupta, C. D., Gupta, S. C., Arora, A. K., and Singh, P. (1976b) Vascular segments in the human spleen. *J. Anat.* **121**, 613.

Halff, J. (1904) Ein Fall von Situs inversus des Magens, des Duodenums und der Milz bei einem 63jahrigen, weiblichen Individuum. *Munchener Med. Wochenschrift* **2**, 2287–2289.

Halpert, B. and Eaton, W. L. (1951) Accessory spleens: a pilot study of 600 necropsies. *Anat. Rec.* **109**, 371.

Halpert, B. and Gyorkey, F. (1959a) Lesions observed in the accessory spleens of 311 patients. *Am. J. Clin. Pathol.* **32**, 165–168.

Halpert, B. and Gyorkey, F. (1959b) Accessory spleens: a survey of 3000 necropsies. *Anat. Rec.* **133**, 389.

Hamilton, W. J. and Mossman, H. W. (1972) *Human Embryology*. 4th ed., W. Heffer, Cambridge, W Heffer.

Harrison, B. F., Glanges, E., and Sparkman, R. S. (1977) Gastric fistula following splenectomy: its cause and prevention. *Ann. Surg.* **185**, 210–213.

Henle, J. (1868) *Handbuch der Systematischen Anatomie des Menschen.* Von Friedrich Vieweg, Braunschweig, Germany.

Hines, J. R. and Eggum, P. R. (1961) Splenogonal fusion causing bowel obstruction. *Arch. Surg.* **83**, 109–111.

Hodenpyl, E. (1898) Case of apparent absence of the spleen, with general compensatory lymphatic hyperplasia. *Med. Rec.* **54**, 695–698.

Hollinshead, W. H. (1971) *Anatomy for Surgeons,* vol. 2, ed. 2. Harper and Row, New York.

Kopsch, F. (1908) Rauber's *Lehrbuch und Atlas der Anatomie des Menschen.* Georg Thieme, Leipzig.

Kostinovitch, L. I. (1937) A case of simultaneous occurrence of a number of variations of the visceral branches of the abdominal aorta. *Anat. Rec.* **67**, 399–403.

Krumbhaar, E. B. and Lippincot, S. W. (1939) Postmortem, weight of the "normal" human spleen of different ages. *Am. J. Med. Sci.* **197**, 344–358.

Latarjet, A. (1908) Testut's *Traite d'Anatomie Humaine*, 9th ed. G. Doin & Cie., Paris.

Lipschutz, B. (1917) A composite study of the coeliac axis artery. *Ann. Surg.* **65**, 159–169.

Lord, M. D. and Gourevitch, A. (1965) The peritoneal anatomy of the spleen, with special reference to the operation of partial gastrectomy. *Br. J. Surg.* **52**, 202–204.

MacAlister, A. (1868) Irregularity of the spermatic vein. *Med. Press Circular* **5**, 404–405.

Machalek, L., Holibkova, A., Tuma, J., and Houserkova, D. (1998) The size of the splenic hilus, diameter of the splenic artery and its branches in the human spleen. *Acta Univ. Palackianae Olomucensis Fac. Med.* **141**, 45–48.

Mainland, D. and Gordon, E. J. (1941) The position of organs determined from thoracic radiographs of young adult males with a study of the cardiac apex beat. *Am. J. Anat.* **68**, 397–456.

McCormick, W. F. and Kashgarian, M. (1965) The weight of the adult human spleen. *Am. J. Clin. Pathol.* **43**, 332,333.

Michels, N. A. (1942) The variational anatomy of the spleen and splenic artery. *Am. J. Anat.* **70**, 21–72.

Milicevic, Z., Cuschieri, A., Xuereb, A., and Milicevic, N. M. (1996) Stereological study of tissue compartments of the human spleen. *Histol. Histopathol.* **11**, 833–836.

Moore, K. L. (1982) *The Developing Human: Clinically Oriented Embryology.* 3rd ed. Saunders, Philadelphia.

Murphy, J. W. and Mitchell, W. A. (1957) Congenital absence of the spleen. *Pediatrics* **20**, 253–256.

Parry, J. F., Jr. (1988) Injuries of the spleen. *Curr. Problems Surg.* **25**, 759–819.

Piquand, G. (1910) Recherches sur l'anatomie du tronc coeliaque et de ses branches. *Bibl. Anat.* **19**, 159–201.

Polhemus, D. W. and Schafer, W. B. (1952) Congenital absence of the spleen: syndrome with atrioventricularis communis and situs inversus. *Pediatrics* **9**, 696–718.

Poynter, C. W. M. (1922) Congenital anomalies of the arteries and veins of the human body with bibliography. *Univ. Stud. Univ. Nebr.* **24**, 1–106.

Putschar, W. G. J. and Marion, W. C. (1956) Congenital absence of the spleen and associated anomalies. *Am. J. Clin. Pathol.* **26**, 429–470.

Robert, H. L. F. (1842) Hemmungsbildung des magens, Mangel der Milz und des Netzes. *Arch. Anat. Physiol. Wissen Med.* **1842**, 57–60.

Schaefer, E. A., Symington, J., and Bryce, T. H., eds. (1915) Quain's *Anatomy*, 11th ed., Longmans, Green, London.

Scholtmeijer, R. J. (1966) An accessory spleen in the scrotum. *Ned. T. Geneesk.* **110**, 90–92.

Settle, E. B. (1940) The surgical importance of accessory spleens with report of two cases. *Am. J. Surg.* **50**, 22–26.

Seufert, R. and Mitrou, P. (1986) The healthy spleen. In: *Surgery of the Spleen* (Reber, H. A., ed.), Thieme, New York, pp. 1–13.

Shepard, R. K. (1903) The form of the human spleen. *J. Anat. Physiol.* **37**, 50–69.

Skandalakis, J. E., Colborn, G. L., Pemberton, L. B., Skandalakis, T. N., Skandalakis, L. J., and Gray, S. W. (1990) The surgical anatomy of the spleen. *Problems Gen. Surg.* **7**, 1–17.

Skandalakis, J. E., Gray, S. W., and Rowe, J. S., Jr. (1983) *Anatomical Complications in General Surgery.* McGraw Hill, New York.

Sneath, W. A. (1913) An apparent third testicle consisting of a scrotal spleen. *J. Anat. Physiol.* **47**, 340–342.

Soson-Jaroschewitsch, A. J. (1927) Zur Chirurgischen Anatomie der Milzhilus. *Z. Anat. Entwicklungsges.* **84**, 218–237.

Sprogoe-Jakobsen, S. and Sprogoe-Jakobsen, U. (1997) The weight of the normal spleen. *Forensic Sci. Int.* **88**, 215–223.

Sternberg, C. (1903) Ein Fall von Agenesie der Milz. *Arch. Path. Anat. Physiol. Klin. Med.* **173**, 571–575.

Tanigawa, K. (1963) Ihidomyaku ni Kansuru kenkyu (On the arteria gastrolienalis branching from the lienal artery). *Fukuoka igaku zasshi (Fukuoka Acta Med.)* **54**, 592.

Tischendorf, F. (1973) Zum Problem der Milzarterie, ll. Eine abnorm stark und unregelmassig geschlangelte A. Iienalis mit zweiteiligem Truncus coeliacus. *Anat. Anz.* **134**, 108–119.

Trooskin, S. Z., Flancbaum, L., Boyarsky, A. H., and Greco, R. S. (1989) A simplified approach to techniques of splenic salvage. *Surg. Gynecol. Obstet.* **168**, 546–548.

Vandamme, J. P. and Bonte, J. (1986) Systematisation of the arteries in the splenic hilus. *Acta Anat.* **125**, 217–224.

Vandamme, J. P. and Bonte, J. (1990) Arteria splenica and the blood supply of the spleen. *Problems Gen. Surg.* **7**, 18–27.

van der Zypen, E. and Revesz, E. (1984) Investigation of development, structure and function of the phrenicocolic and duodenal suspensory ligaments. *Acta Anat. (Basel)* **119**, 142.

Waizer, A., Baniel, J., Zin, Y., and Dintsman, M. (1989) Clinical implications of anatomic variations of the splenic artery. *Surg. Gynecol. Obstet.* **168**, 57.

Watanabe, Y., Todani, T., Noda, T., and Yamamoto, S. (1997) Standard splenic volume in children and young adults measured from CT images. *Surg. Today* **27**, 726–728.

Whitesell, F. B. (1960) A clinical and surgical anatomic study of rupture of the spleen due to blunt trauma. *Surg. Gynecol. Obstet.* **110**, 750.

Wick, M. R. and Rife, C. C. (1981) Paratesticular accessory spleen. *Mayo Clin Proc.* **56**, 455–456.

2 The Microanatomy of the Mammalian Spleen

Mechanisms of Splenic Clearance

FERN TABLIN, VMD, PhD, JACK K. CHAMBERLAIN, MD, FACP, AND LEON WEISS, MD

2.1. INTRODUCTION

The spleen is a uniquely adapted lymphoid organ that is dedicated to the clearance of blood cells, microorganisms, and other particles from the blood. This chapter deals with the microanatomy of the spleen, its highly specialized extracellular matrix components, distinctive vascular endothelial cell receptors, and the extraordinary organization of the venous vasculature. We also address the cellular mechanisms of splenic clearance, which are typified by the vascular organization of the spleen; mechanisms and regulation of clearance, and the development of a unique component; specialized barrier cells, which may be essential to the spleen's clearance functions in stress.

2.2. ANATOMICAL ORGANIZATION OF THE SPLEEN

The mammalian spleen consists of an encapsulated, trabeculated pulp, made up of stroma and vasculature supporting a large population of circulating, migrating, and differentiating blood and hematopoietic cells (Figs. 1–6). The vascular layout of the spleen is as follows: arteries enter the capsule and move into the splenic parenchyma within the trabeculae. From there, they enter the white pulp (WP), where they are surrounded by lymphocytes. The white pulp selectively clears lymphocytes and their accessory cells from the blood. They equip the spleen to engage in immunological reactions. Arteries continue into the adjacent marginal zones (MZs), which consist of shells of tissue surrounding the white pulp, and are interposed between white pulp centrally and red pulp (RP) peripherally. Marginal zones are heavily trafficked, receiving blood from many arterial terminals, and selectively distribute its components to other parts of the spleen. The marginal zone also stores erythrocytes, platelets, and monocyte-macrophages, and initiates their processing. The red pulp is that large part of the pulp that extends outward from the marginal zone. It too receives arterial terminals, clears, tests, and stores erythrocytes, and is primed for erythroclasia and erythropoiesis. Blood deposited in the marginal zone and red pulp moves through the filtration beds, and is drained by a system of venous vessels in both the marginal zone and red pulp.

From: *The Complete Spleen: A Handbook of Structure, Function, and Clinical Disorders* Edited by: A. J. Bowdler © Humana Press Inc., Totowa, NJ

2.2.1. CAPSULE AND TRABECULAE

The human spleen weighs approx 150 g, in adults, and is enclosed by a capsule composed of dense connective tissue, with little smooth muscle (Faller, 1985; Weiss, 1983, 1985). This arrangement reflects the minimal contractile role of the capsule and trabeculae in altering the blood volume of the human spleen, under normal circumstances. The capsule measures 1.1–1.5 mm thick, and is covered by a serosa, except at the hilus, where blood vessels, nerves, and lymphatics enter the organ. There are two layers of the capsule: This can be determined by the orientation of collagen fibers (Faller, 1985), which are moderately thick and uniform, but which become finer in the deeper regions, where the transition to pulp fibers occurs. There are also elastic fibers present in the capsule. The capsule is continuous on its inner surface, with a richly ramified system of trabeculae, which penetrates and supports the pulp.

In most mammalian spleens, the capsule is sympathetically innervated, and there is a species-dependent blend of smooth muscle and collagenous tissue. In certain species, the capsule and trabeculae are rich in smooth muscle. These spleens, of which the equine and feline are examples, are termed "storage spleens." Sympathetic stimulation results in the contraction of the capsule and trabeculae, causing delivery of large reserves of blood into the circulation. The horse has a huge spleen, and its outstanding athletic prowess is dependent on the spleen's capacity to increase the hematocrit, and, thus, the oxygen-carrying capacity of the circulation (Persson et al., 1973a,b). In fact, splenic reserves of mature erythrocytes are so large and readily mobilized that the reticulocytes are rarely present in the circulation, although they are produced in the bone marrow, which holds them in reserve and releases them only under conditions of severe chronic anemia. Thus, the splenic store of mature erythrocytes can be used to compensate for all but the most persistent, long-term blood loss. In contrast, in the spleen of humans, rabbits, dogs, and mice, erythrocyte reserves are quite small. These spleens do retain some significant storage capacity, however, holding large numbers of platelets in ready reserve. Because these less-contractile spleens have been thought to have greater immunological and other antimicrobial capacity, they have been termed "defense spleens."

2.2.2. SPLENIC PARENCHYMA

The splenic parenchyma, or pulp, consists of white pulp, the intermediate marginal zone, and

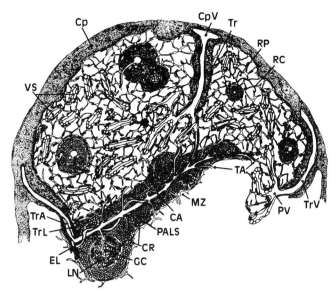

Fig. 2.1. Schematic drawing of a sinusal spleen. The spleen is enclosed by a capsule (Cp) and, from its internal surface, trabeculae (Tr) branch to compartmentalize the pulp. The splenic artery pierces the capsule and branches into trabecular arteries (TrA). The trabecular artery enters the pulp as the central artery (CA), which runs in the central axis of the periarteriolar lymphatic sheath (PALS). This is the component of the white pulp (WP) in which T-cells are concentrated. The second major component of the white pulp consists of the lymphatic nodules (LNs), which occur as nodules within the PALS, where their presence forces the central artery into an eccentric position. LNs are sites of concentration of B-cells, and may contain germinal centers (GCs), when there is a high level of antibody formation. Branches of the central artery supply LNs, and pass laterally through the white pulp to terminate in the marginal zone (MZ), which closely surrounds the WP. In addition to its arterial vessels, efferent lymphatic vessels (EL) drain the white pulp, entering the trabeculae as trabecular lymphatics (TrL). In this schema, the lymphocytes of the WP are shown, and, with the vasculature, dominate the picture. Note, however, that there is a circumferential reticulum (CR) limiting the periphery of WP. The MZ and red pulp (RP), which occupy the bulk of the spleen, are schematized, and show no free cells. The red pulp consists of terminating arterial vessels (TA), a meshwork, or filtration bed, consisting of reticular cells (RCs) and associated reticular fibers, and a system of venous vessels. The proximal venous vessel, which receives blood from the filtration beds, is the venous sinus (VS). These distinctive vessels end blindly, anastomosing richly, deeply penetrating the filtration beds of RP, supported by the reticular network. VSs receive blood through their interendothelial slits, which then drains into pulp veins (PVs), trabecular veins (TrVs), and capsular veins (CpVs).

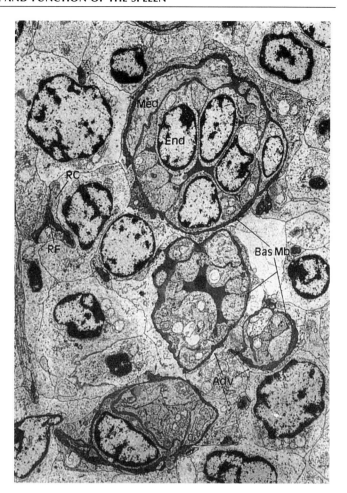

Fig. 2.2. White pulp, human spleen. Four cross-sections of an arteriole and its smaller branches lie in white pulp. Each of the vessels may possess an endothelium (End), basement membrane (Bas Mb), media (Med), and adventitia (Adv). Especially in the smaller vessels, the media and adventitial layers are rather incomplete. Lymphocytes occupy much of the rest of this field, held in a meshwork of reticular cells (RCs) and reticular fibers (RFs) (×6250).

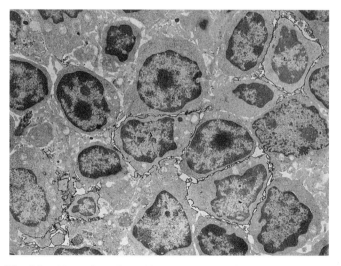

Fig. 2.3. Normal murine white pulp stained for T-cells. The field consists mostly of T-cells, the surfaces of some of which are stained by immunocytochemistry for the T-cell marker, Thy 1.2. Note the short cell processes of many of the lymphocytes, establishing transient junctional complexes with vicinal cells (×2500).

the red pulp (Fig. 7; Kashimura and Fujita, 1987; Sasou et al., 1986; van Krieken and te Velde, 1988).

2.2.2.1. White Pulp The white pulp consists predominantly of lymphocytes, antigen-presenting cells, and macrophages, lying on a specialized reticular meshwork composed of concentric layers of stromal cells, now recognized to be specialized fibroblasts (Borrello and Phipps, 1996; Van Vliet et al., 1986; Fujita et al., 1982, 1985). The reticular meshwork is most dense in association with the periarterial lymphatic sheath (PALS) and marginal zone. Matrix proteins produced by these fibroblasts include: type III collagen, laminin, fibronectin, vitronectin, and tenascin (Liakka et al., 1995). These proteins may play an important role in the migration of lymphocytes during fetal development of lymphatic tissue, as well as

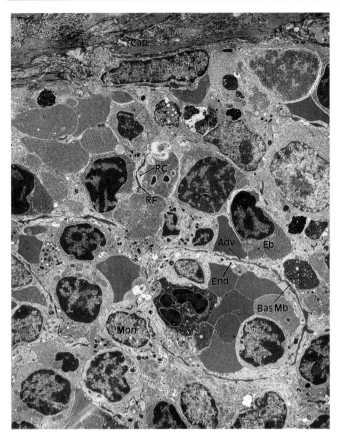

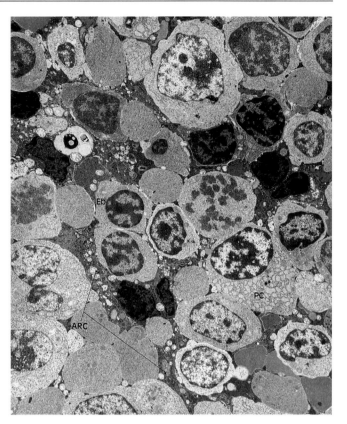

Fig. 2.4.   Subcapsular red pulp mouse spleen. The capsule is rich in muscle and collagen. The subjacent red pulp contains a bifurcating pulp vein. The right limb has endothelium (End), basement membrane (Bas Mb), and adventitia labeled. A mononuclear cell (Mon) sends delicate cytoplasmic processes into the vascular wall, penetrating adventitia and basement membrane (*). The perivascular red pulp is pervaded by a reticular meshwork consisting of reticular cells (RCs), which branch from the adventitial layer of pulp veins, and reticular fibers (RFs). The reticular meshwork of mouse red pulp is, however, typically scanty. The red pulp contains many reticulocytes and some erythroblasts (Eb) (×5000).

Fig. 2.5.   Red pulp, murine spleen in malaria. This field of red pulp, in precrisis *Plasmodium yoelii* malaria, consists of many erythroblasts (Eb), some in mitosis, and a few plasma cells (PCs). Note the dark, syncytially fused stromal cells, forming a complex, extensive membrane, which constitutes a barrier surrounding many free cells. These stromal cells are barrier cells (ARC) (×5000).

during the normal adult immune response. Fibroblasts in the white pulp and marginal zone may express the lymphoid marker, Thy-1 (Borrello and Phipps, 1996), thus forming a distinct microenvironment for T-cell interaction (Van Vliet et al., 1986).

The organization of the white pulp is closely associated with its arterial supply (Fig. 2). Those lymphocytes immediately adjacent to the central arteries constitute the PALS. The lymphocytes in the PALS are predominantly T-cells; B-cells are concentrated in the lymphatic nodules, most often situated at the periphery, or at points of arterial branching (Fig. 3).

The central artery supplies radial branches to the white pulp, marginal zone, and red pulp, and terminates in an attenuated vessel of variable structure supplying the red pulp (Fig. 8). The distal portion of the vessel may be surrounded by a loose macrophage arrangement known as the "periarterial macrophage sheath" (PAMS), which is usually not prominent in humans (Fig. 9; Blue and Weiss, 1981; Biussens et al., 1984; Weiss, 1983; Weiss et al., 1985). It is, however, more obvious in younger subjects. PAMS are also found in mouse and rabbit spleens; however, in canine, feline, herbivore, and avian spleens, the macrophages are organized in a tight cuff or sheath, also referred to as an "ellipsoid."

Deep efferent lymphatic vessels are also present in white pulp, where they are entwined with arterial vessels. These lymphatics run from the white pulp into the trabeculae, then leave the spleen at the hilus. The splenic lymphatic vessels are mostly well-developed, but inconspicuous, because, running in lymphocyte-crowded beds and possessing a lymphocyte-crowded lumen surrounded by the thinnest of vascular walls, they are difficult to discern from their background. These lymphatic vessels carry lymph countercurrent to the flow of blood in their adjacent arterial vessels. They provide splenic lymphocytes with a major efferent pathway for the migration of immunologically competent lymphocytes of the recirculating lymphocyte pool. Venous vessels are notably absent from the white pulp, and are discussed further in the Subheading 2.2.3.

2.2.2.2. Marginal Zone   The marginal zone, as its name implies, lies at the periphery of the white pulp and its outer surface blends with the structure of the red pulp. In the human spleen, the reticular meshwork is fine; and the zone is the site of termination of many arterioles, which frequently bifurcate just before their termination (Fig. 10). The marginal zone receives a disproportionately large number of terminal arterial vessels. Blood entering the marginal zone is directed selectively to other arterial beds: Lymphocytes and their accessory cells pass to the white pulp (van Ewij and Nieuwenhuis, 1985); platelets and erythrocytes pass into the red pulp. Studies on the kinetics of splenic cell migration have shown that 25% of the cells that transit through the spleen stay in the marginal

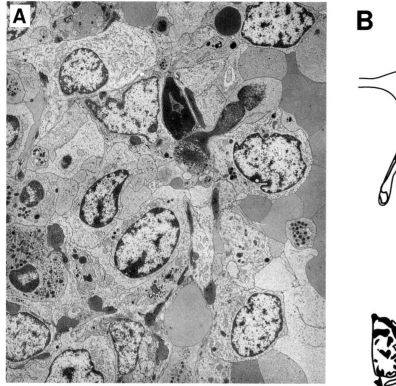

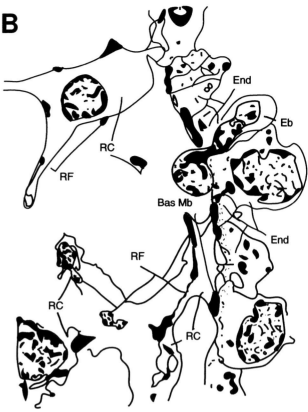

Fig. 2.6.   (**A**) Transmission micrograph; (**B**) key to part (**A**). Red pulp, human spleen, thalassemia. Human spleen is a sinusal spleen, and this field contains a venous sinus. Its wall runs vertically, its luminal surface to the right lined by cross-sections of the rod-shaped endothelial cells. Nuclei are present in three of these endothelial cells. The basal portion of the endothelial cell is rich in longitudinally running filaments, which stipple the cell, and, when interwoven, present as dense plaques. The fenestrated basement membrane (Bas Mb) appears in short segments at the base of the endothelium. Red blood cells in thalassemia vary considerably in appearance, and are floppy, tending to fold flexibly on one another. Many reticulocytes are present, and erythroblasts (Ebs) circulate. An Eb, with its nucleus deeply constricted in two places, is passing through the endothelium in an interendothelial slit (the erythroblast itself is deeply constricted in the interendothelial slit at the lower nuclear constriction). The cord on the left is fully packed with leukocytes and reticular cells (RCs). The latter serve as the fibroblastic stroma of the cord, and ensheathe reticular fibers (RFs) (×8000).

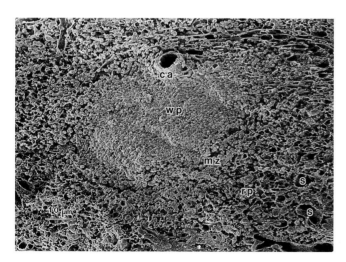

Fig. 2.7.   Scanning electron micrograph of the human spleen at low power. Central artery (CA), white pulp (WP), marginal zone (MZ), red pulp (RP) and sinuses (S) in a freeze-cracked surface of the splenic pulp. (Reproduced with permission from Kashimura, M. and Fujita, T. [1987]).

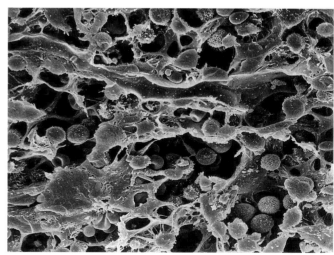

Fig. 2.8.   Scanning electron micrograph of the human spleen. A longitudinally fractured arterial capillary terminates in the cordal spaces of the red pulp. The arterial capillary fans out to the right-hand side, where fenestrations provide openings to the cordal spaces (×1350). (Adapted with permission from Fujita, T., et al. [1985]).

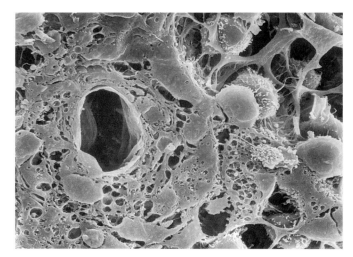

Fig. 2.9. Scanning electron micrograph of the human spleen, to show a sheathed artery enveloped by macrophages and reticular cells. The specimen is taken from the spleen of a patient with immune thrombocytopenia: The honeycombing of the cytoplasm of the macrophages results from the phagocytosis of platelets (×4000). (Reproduced with permission from Fujita, T., et al. [1985]).

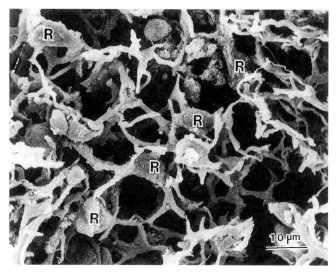

Fig. 2.11. Scanning electron micrograph of the red pulp of the human spleen. The meshwork is formed by reticular cells (RCs), their processes and reticular fibers. Critical point drying has produced cell retraction, so that the cells shrink against the reticular fibers they surround (×1500).

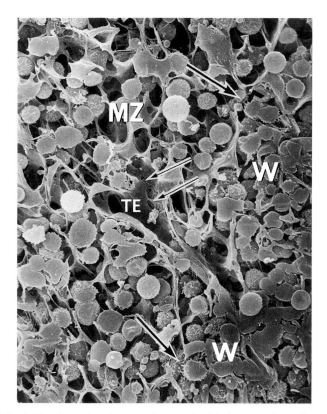

Fig. 2.10. Scanning electron micrograph of the human spleen, showing the terminal end (TE) of a follicular artery in the marginal zone (MZ). The thin arrows show openings in the flat reticular cells, which demarcate the MZ from the white pulp (W). (Reproduced with permission from Sasou, S., et al. [1986]).

zone for approx 50 min; 10% of the lymphocytes will migrate to white pulp, and stay an average of 4–5 h. The majority of the cells rapidly pass through the spleen via the venous vasculature of the red pulp (Hammond, 1975; Ford, 1968; Pabst, 1988; *see also* Chapter 7). An enormous number of lymphocytes migrate through

the spleen at any given time, and it has been calculated to surpass the combined traffic of all lymph nodes in the body (Ford, 1969). Numerous studies clearly demonstrate that entrance and retention of T- and B-cells into white pulp is not a random process, but requires a selective interaction between lymphocytes and endothelial cells. This interaction may be mediated by the mucosal adressin adhesion molecule, MAdCAM-1, which has previously been shown to be involved in lymphocyte homing to mucosal sites, and is expressed on the high endothelial venules of Peyer's patches and mesenteric lymph nodes. MAdCAM-1 has been shown to be present on endothelial cells of marginal zone terminal arterioles closest to the white pulp of the mouse spleen (Kraal et al., 1995), and may serve to regulate lymphocyte traffic to the white pulp. Additionally, marginal zone macrophages have been suggested to play a similar role in the migration of lymphocytes to white pulp (Buckley et al., 1987; Lyons and Parish, 1995). In the alymphoplastic *aly* mutant mouse, which is affected by a spontaneous autosomal-recessive mutation, there is a deficiency in systemic lymph nodes, Peyer's patches, and the splenic marginal zone. This phenotype can be rescued by bone marrow transplantation, and provides further evidence for the role of the marginal zone in lymphatic development and its relationship to sites of lymphocyte-mucosal homing (Koike et al., 1996).

2.2.2.3. Red Pulp Three-fourths of the volume of the human spleen consists of the red pulp, which comprises four vascular structures in sequence: slender nonanastomosing arterial vessels (penicilli), the splenic cords, or cords of Bilroth; the venous sinuses; and the pulp veins. All of these vessels are supported by a reticular meshwork (Fig. 11), provided by fibroblasts and their various extracellular matrix proteins, similar to those noted for the white pulp: fibronectin, laminin, vitronectin, tenascin, type III collagen, as well as type IV collagen (Liakka et al., 1995). Macrophages are also found in the splenic cords, both as single cells associated with the reticular fibroblasts and as constituents of the PAMS associated with arterioles of the red pulp.

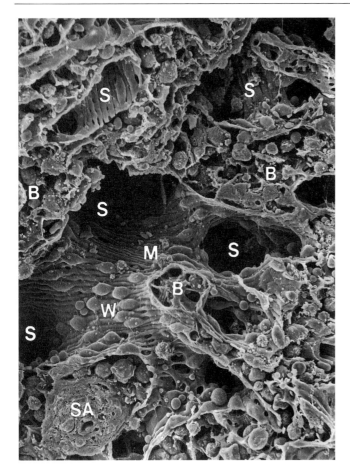

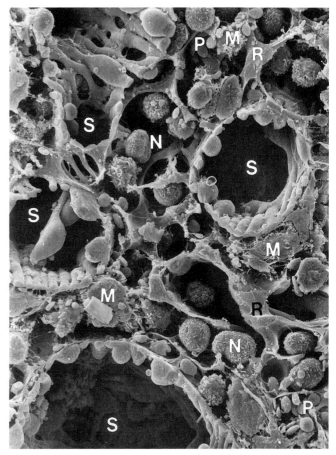

Fig. 2.12.   Scanning electron micrograph of the red pulp of the human spleen at low power. The splenic cords (B) are fractured, and the sinuses (S) are seen mostly from the surface. The endothelial cells (or "rod cells of Weidenreich," W) are arranged in parallel, and show enlarged nuclear portions, which project into the lumen of the sinus. Red blood cells can be seen protruding into the sinuses through the junctions of the endothelial cells. MP, macrophages. SA, sheathed artery (×875). (Reproduced, with modification, with permission from Fujita, T. [1974]).

Fig. 2.13.   Scanning electron micrograph of the red pulp of the human spleen, at higher power than in Fig. 12. The splenic cords are seen to be supported by reticulum cells (RCs), and the cord meshwork contains macrophages, leukocytes, mainly neutrophils (N), and blood platelets (P). The endothelial pattern of the sinuses (S) is demonstrated; the sinuses in the upper part of the micrograph suggest a perforated structure (×1800). (Reproduced by permission from Fujita, T. [1974]).

The human, rat, and dog spleens are of the sinusal type. In the human spleen, the splenic sinuses comprise approx one-third of the volume of the red pulp (van Krieken and te Velde, 1988); they consist of long anastomosing vascular channels, which ultimately drain into the pulp veins. The sinuses have a unique endothelium, in which the cells are arranged longitudinally, like the staves of a barrel, and run parallel to the long axis of the sinus. Tight junctional complexes are present at regular intervals along their lateral and basolateral surfaces (Uehara and Miyoshi, 1997), and, in the rat spleen, macula occludens are also present at irregular intervals.

Sinusal endothelial cells have two sets of cytoplasmic filaments: The intermediate filaments (vimentin) are loosely arranged; thin filaments are tightly organized into dense actin bands in the basal cytoplasm (Drenckhahn and Wagner, 1986). These stress fibers arch between attachments to circumferential components of the basement membrane, and contain nonmuscle myosin, and probably contract, to vary the tension in the endothelial cell. Endothelial cell-signaling, via adherens junctions, can result in contraction of adjacent endothelial cells resulting in the production of inter-endothelial slits. Potential slit-like spaces, which can be penetrated by cells flowing from the pulp spaces (Fig. 12–16), are a critical

point in the flow pathway of particulates through the spleen, and represent an important regulator of selective particulate flow (Fig. 6).

A fenestrated basement membrane is present on the abluminal surface of the endothelial cells; its transverse ring-like component reinforces the sinus structure, like the hoops of a barrel (Fig. 15; Groom, 1987; Weiss, 1983). Immunoelectron microscopic studies have shown that these ring-like fibers are predominantly composed of type IV collagen and laminin, with sparser components of type III collagen and tenascin (Liakka et al., 1995), produced both by the adventitial reticular cells and by endothelial cells which probably associate with this matrix through the β-1 integrins on their basolateral surfaces.

In the human spleen, the basement membrane of the venous sinuses has well-marked circumferential components and a lesser longitudinal component. It is continuous with the reticular meshwork of the surrounding cords, and is overlaid with fibroblasts. The junction of the venous sinuses with the pulp veins is obvious, because there is a transition from rod-like endothelial cells with a fenestrated basement membrane, to the flattened endothelium of the pulp veins and a continuous basement membrane. This transition is most easily seen as the pulp veins enter the trabeculae, and

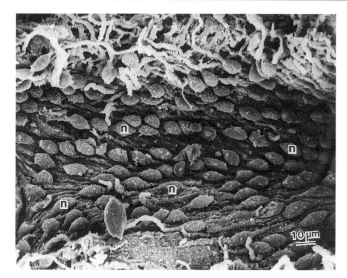

Fig. 2,14. Scanning electron micrograph of the human spleen, showing the luminal surface of a vascular sinus. The endothelial cells are arranged in parallel rows. The portions of the cells containing nuclei (n) bulge into the lumen; there are no visible gaps between the endothelial cells (×3000).

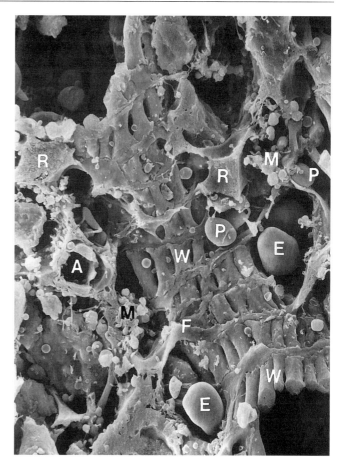

Fig. 2.15. Scanning electron micrograph of the human spleen, showing the abluminal surface of a vascular sinus. The rod-like endothelial cells are crossed by the encircling hoops of basement membrane. Sinus endothelial cells (W). Reticular cell foot processes (F). Artery (A). Erythrocytes (E). Macrophage (MP). Platelets (P). Reticulum cells (Rs) (×3700). (Reproduced by permission from Fujita, T. [1974]).

can be abrupt and without an intermediate structural organization (Weiss, 1983).

Nonsinusal spleens lack venous sinuses, and efferent blood is received initially by pulp veins. In the mouse, cat, and horse, pulp veins are thin-walled, large-lumened vessels with squamous endothelium, and a thin, intermittent basement membrane (Fig. 4). They typically display transmural apertures, which may be large. Pulp veins often lie close to trabeculae, and enter them, becoming trabecular veins. The walls of pulp veins, unlike venous sinuses, offer little impedance to the passage of blood cells, because of their large transmural apertures.

2.3. PATHWAYS OF BLOOD FLOW

The afferent arterial vessels course through the white pulp as central arteries, and their radial branches supply the marginal zone or red pulp. The attenuated main stem of a central artery drains, in most instances, into the reticular meshwork of the red pulp. In humans, the majority of the arterial terminations have no endothelial continuity with venous structures, and the circulation is predominantly "open" in form, with the pathway of blood flow crossing a connective tissue space. This does not mean that, in normal circumstances, there is a random process of flow in the intermediate circulation, since the orientation of the arterial terminations to the splenic sinus walls, and of the reticular cell stroma intervening between arterial termination and sinus wall, effectively produces an unimpeded pathway. As a consequence, the greater part of the blood flow through the human spleen passes through a functional "fast pathway," in contrast to the small fraction of flow that traverses the slow pathway (Groom, 1987). However, the volume of blood is greater in the "slow pathway," because of its slow turnover; this occupies part of the pulp cords, where they are both physiologically and structurally open. Groom et al. and Levesque and Groom (1981) have demonstrated vascular pathways in the marginal zone, which have the potential for bypassing the red pulp; these are discussed in more detail in Chapter 3.

The regulation of volume and distribution of blood flow is critical to the effective functioning of the spleen. A high proportion of a bolus of abnormal red blood cells entering the spleen is retained on initial passage through the organ, indicating that the filtration process is dependent on the structures of the afferent circulation, and does not require adaptive changes and prolonged flow (Groom, 1987). The arterial structures appear to direct plasma to the marginal zone, marginated cells to the white pulp, and marginal zone; the axial flow (especially erythrocytes and platelets) is directed to the red pulp. The marginal zone receives an overly large number of terminal arterial vessels, and blood entering this area is selectively channeled to either the white or red pulp.

The arteries of the human spleen appear to have sympathetic innervation, but parasympathetic innervation remains to be demonstrated (Reilly, 1985). Plasma skimming appears to require an intact nerve supply; pooling and concentration of red blood cells are inhibited by sympathomimetic drugs.

The reticular stroma of the human marginal zone and the PALS contains numerous reticular cells, which have smooth muscle actin and myosin (Toccanier-Pelte et al., 1987), which are not present in red pulp. These "myoid" cells have long, slender processes, which are intimately associated with reticular fibers. Similar contractile

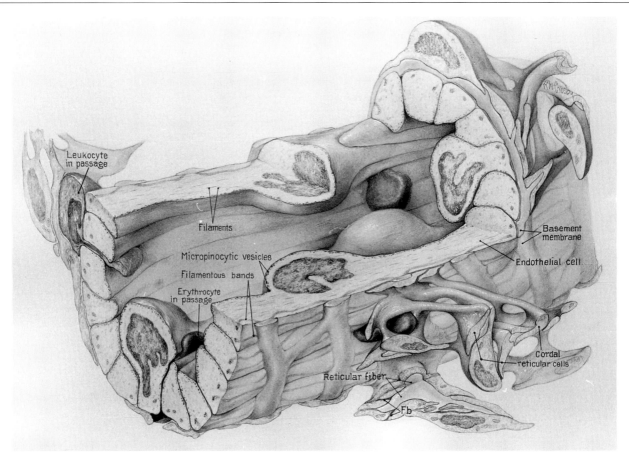

Fig. 2.16. Schematic diagram of a red pulp sinus. The parallel orientation of the sinus endothelial cells is shown, with endothelial nuclei caus-ing protrusion into the sinus lumen. On the abluminal surface of the sinus is the fenestrated basement membrane, to which the cordal macro-phages are attached. A blood cell, in this case a leukocyte, is passing between adjacent endothelial cells, to enter the lumen from the pulp cord. (Reproduced with permission from Chen, L. T. and Weiss, L. [1972]).

reticular cells have been shown to be present throughout horse and dog spleen, and are associated with sympathetic nerve terminals (Tablin and Weiss, 1983; Blue and Weiss, 1981). Smooth muscle cells and fibroblasts are closely related, and many fibroblastic cells are contractile. This group includes reticular cells of the spleen, as discussed previously, barrier cells discussed in Subheading 3.3., the myofibroblasts of wound healing, and the myoepithelial cells encircling epithelial structures, notably the ducts and acini of glands. This arrangement, in addition to the smooth muscle cells associated with PAMS, may regulate cellular traffic in areas of high blood flow.

Blood that enters the red pulp is in an open anatomical system, in which significant filtration can occur. This blood continues through the pulp sinuses, pulp veins, and trabecular veins, and sub-sequently the splenic veins at the hilus. Because the splenic vein enters the portal vein, any increase in portal pressure increases the blood contained in the spleen, and consequently the blood volume of the spleen. When this volume increase is long-standing, it may result in congestive splenomegaly. The myoelastic structure of the splenic vein suggests that the diameter of the vein can be actively varied to modify both intrasplenic pressure and venous flow (Reis and Ferraz de Carvalho, 1988). Secondary splenic distention could in turn modify the relationship of the arterial terminations to the sinus walls, increasing the length and duration of the flow path-way, and improving the filtration efficacy of the red pulp.

2.3.1. FILTRATION PATHWAY   The tissues between the ter-minal arterial vessels and the initial venous vessels comprise a retic-ulum or reticular meshwork, composed of reticular cells and their associated extracellular matrix "reticular" fibers. In the human spleen, and indeed in spleens in general, the pulp consists of a reticular meshwork in which arterial and venous vessels are sup-ported by adventitial reticular cells, which branch out perivascu-larly and contribute to the reticular meshwork. If the meshwork is extensive enough, it will contain reticular cells that are entirely confined to it, without an adventitial relationship to blood vessels. In the human spleen, as well as rat, dog, and horse spleens, the reticular meshwork is well-developed. These cells form a system of thin-walled domains reinforced by extracellular matrix fibers. These domains communicate with one another and, as a system, are open, directly or indirectly, to the blood that enters the spleen. Variation in the location and arrangement of the reticular cells, and their matrix components, occurs in a variety of meshworks, termed, by Weiss (1985), "filtration beds."

Two types of filtration beds make up the white pulp, which serve to direct T-cells to the PALS, and hold them there for a period of hours, and B-cells to lymphatic nodules or their mantles, and, for a somewhat longer time than T-cells, hold them there. Reticular cells, dendritic cells, and macrophages probably regulate this traf-fic. Lymphocytes that do not immunologically react in the white pulp, are cleared by the deep efferent lymphatics. In pathologic states, filtration beds, through which lymphocytes normally flow rather rapidly, may hold them for long periods, as in the parasinusal red pulp (i.e., splenic cords) in malaria.

In sinusal spleens, the filtration beds comprising the marginal zone are unusually fine-meshed, and are associated with the large number of terminal arterioles present in this region. These extensive arterial terminal vessels deposit large volumes of blood into the marginal zone, making it one of the most highly trafficked parts of the spleen. Blood cells entering the marginal zone may migrate selectively to other filtration beds, e.g., lymphocytes, may go to the white pulp, to be sorted into T- and B-cell zones. In addition, blood cells may be held in the marginal zone and processed there. Damaged erythrocytes are pooled and phagocytosed, monocytes are sequestered and differentiate into macrophages, and platelets may be stored in the marginal zone, in ready reserve for quick release into the circulation.

The reticular meshwork of the red pulp consists of additional terminal arterial vessels, which empty into this specialized domain, and venous vessels, which drain it. Red pulp filtration beds are known as "pulp spaces," and are especially extensive in non-sinusal spleens, because of their role as storage spaces. In sinusal spleens, this meshwork is more limited, because of the vast anastomosing system of venous sinuses. Macrophages present in this domain may quickly increase in number, as a result of trapping and differentiation of circulating monocytes. In addition, the resident macrophage population in the PAMS also participates in cellular surveillance. Red pulp filtration beds contain reticulocytes, which undergo final maturation to erythrocytes before their release into the circulation, and, at the end of their life-span, lead to their phagocytosis. In murine spleens, these filtration beds regularly support extramedullary hematopoiesis, particularly, erythroid stem cell pro-liferation and differentiation (colony-forming unit, burst-forming unit, erythrocytes). This diverse filtration bed also is the site of lymphocyte sequestration and plasma cell proliferation, as well as antibody production in infectious disease, as in malaria, cited previously.

2.3.2. CLEARANCE OF BLOOD BY THE SPLEEN   The spleen possesses a remarkable capacity for clearance of blood cells, infectious organisms, particles, and macromolecules. This clearance is dependent on the splenic filtration beds, which provide the appropriate microenvironment for phagocytosis, as well as cell proliferation and differentiation. Under normal conditions, aged erythrocytes and platelets are cleared from the blood by the filtration beds of the marginal zone and red pulp, and, in sinusal spleens, inclusion-containing erythrocytes, such as those containing Heinz bodies, may be pitted of their inclusions, as they squeeze through the interendothelial slits of venous sinuses in their passage out of the spleen, and return to the circulation (Fig. 16; *see also* Chapter 12). Lymphocytes and their accessory cells are sequestered in the filtration beds of the white pulp, and are arranged so as to be able to undergo immune stimulation and responses, or to leave the spleen via deep efferent lymphatics. Monocytes are cleared from the circulation in all beds of the spleen and readily differentiate into macrophages. Bacteria and other infectious particles, such as the plasmodial-parasitized erythrocytes of malaria, are cleared from the circulation by the spleen. Slightly to moderately damaged erythrocytes, such as occur in such congenital hemolytic diseases as hereditary spherocytosis, and erythrocytes damaged by such extrinsic factors as autoantibodies, parasites, and heat, are cleared by the spleen, and are phagocytosed or repaired.

2.3.3. BARRIER-FORMING SYSTEMS   Reticular cells constitute a large, stable component of the filtration beds of hematopoietic tissues. Like many fibroblastic cell types, notably the myofibroblast of wound healing, they appear to be contractile, as shown by the significant numbers of actin filaments they contain. Indeed, extracellular matrix formation and contractility are common properties of these cells. Smooth muscle cells are girdled by a sleeve of reticular fibers and the elastic fibers they synthesize. Curiously, reticular fibers (preponderantly collagen type III) lie on the reticular cell cytoplasm, as closely as the elastic fibers on their smooth muscle cells. Myoepithelial cells, whose contractile tentacles squeeze down upon acini and ducts of mammary and other glands, forcing out secretion, and which, by secretion of extracellular matrix of their basal lamina, illustrate the combination of extracellular matrix formation and contractility.

Splenic filtration beds do not normally show a high level of filtration, since more than 90% of the blood circulates through the spleen as rapidly as through tissues with a conventional vasculature. Yet splenic behavior may change rapidly in stress, and the organ can become hypersplenic. We have documented the presence of contractile fibroblasts that are capable of dynamically altering the responsive nature of this filtration domain. These contractile cells, or one or more of their subsets, are capable of fusing with one another in the filtration beds, to form complex, branching, syncytial sheets that form a variety of barriers. These cells have been termed "activated reticular cells" (Weiss et al., 1986), but, on the basis of continued studies, we now define them as "barrier cells" (Weiss, 1991), recognizing their remarkable capacity for diverse structural and functional barrier formation. Barrier cells are present in large numbers in murine and human spleens, under conditions in which splenic clearance appears heightened, pathologically (including sickle cell disease, spectrin deficiency, congenital spherocytic anemia, thalassemia, malaria, and Hodgkin's disease). They may well be evolutionarily conserved, because they are present in the spleen of stressed teleosts. They occur in small numbers in the normal mammalian spleen. Barrier cells proliferate and show morphological signs associated with intense protein synthesis: large nucleoli, dense cytoplasm, and widened perinuclear cisternae continuous with endoplasmic reticulum, so branched and expanded that it imparts a lacy appearance to the cytoplasm.

Splenic barrier cells originate by activation of fibroblasts on the surface of trabeculae and the adventitial aspect of blood vessels; activation is signaled by increased cytoplasmic density, accompanied by increases in rough endoplasmic reticulum, as well as dilated mitochondria. Parallel changes occur in bone marrow, the barrier cells differentiating from the bone-lining layer covering trabeculae and myeloid diaphyseal bone. Barrier cells also originate from circulating precursors; circulating blood contains fibroblast stem cells (colony-forming unit, fibroblastoid), as determined in tissue culture assays. Barrier cells initially accumulate in the spleen, perivascularly, as dense, round cells with relatively short cell processes. Fusing with one another, they migrate from their initial perivascular location, and, in many instances, adhere to existing extracellular matrix, and associate with established reticular cells. They move apart, remaining associated with the resident reticular meshwork, and attached to one another by extended cell processes. Barrier cells thereby augment the functions and structure of the basic reticular cell filtration beds.

Barrier cells enclose blood vessels, providing or enhancing an adventitial layer. They tightly surround single blood cells and multicellular hematopoietic colonies, isolating and protecting them. Such barrier cell enclosures form a blood–tissue barrier in the spleen, in the precrisis phase of reticulocyte-prone plasmodia (as with *Plasmodium berghei* in murine malaria), preventing bloodborne parasites from parasitizing reticulocytes and their precursors. A remarkable splenic synchrony occurs at crisis. At the same time, the moment of crisis, barrier cell–cell associations are disrupted, relieving the isolation of the hematopoietic, notably erythroid, colonies. The colonies reach the precise point of maturity that permits their erythroid cells, no longer confined by barrier cells, to be released into the circulation, and the parasite (contained in parasitized erythrocytes), excluded precrisis from the splenic filtration beds by the intact barrier-cell barrier, enters these beds, readily crossing the now-disrupted barrier-cell barrier. The post-crisis filtration beds of the spleen are open to the circulation, in contrast to the precrisis spleen, in which they are shut off from the circulation by the intact barrier-cell barriers.

The precrisis spleen accordingly embodies a paradox: It is a large spleen exhibiting splenomegaly, yet it is not hypersplenic, because, with the spleen blood barrier intact, its level of clearance is reduced. It is hyposplenic, or "asplenic," rather than, as would be more characteristic of a large spleen, hypersplenic. These changes are marked and evident in malaria. Yet, on close evaluation of other splenomegalies, such as those of sickle cell disease and thalassemia, they too display hyposplenia in the course of splenomegaly. It may well be, moreover, that the splenic fibrosis in chronic sickle cell disease is not caused, as has been inferred, by cumulative, successive small infarcts, but by the accumulation of barrier cells, which, with chronicity, become fibroblastic, resulting in the fibrotic splenic nubbin that had been the spleen. Examination of the spleen in murine malaria, and the spleen in human sickle cell anemia, moreover, reveals that fibrosis is not figured as a flame-shaped fibroblastic aggregate at the end of a splenic vessel, as would occur in infarction, but rather as a perivascular cuff, where barrier cells lay.

Barrier cells infiltrate existing circumferential matrix reticulum, and adhere to its marginal zone surface, thus transforming the circumferential reticulum into a more effective barrier surrounding and protecting the white pulp. This change may occur after an immune response is initiated in the white pulp, thereby causing that white pulp, already engaged in antibody production, to be refractory to further stimulation by antigen. In the marginal zone and the cords of red pulp of human and other sinusal spleens, where filtration beds are best-developed, barrier cells intercalate into these domains, and may help to regulate their cellular traffic. In contrast, in murine (nonsinusal) spleen, the matrix reticulum composing the filtration domains in red pulp and marginal zone is scanty and less well developed. Yet, in these spleens, as in the sinusal spleens, barrier cells are present as extensive, branched, syncytial arrays, but, with relatively little reticulum to infiltrate, barrier cells appear to be tethered to nonfibrillar matrix components, as well as to the adventitial reticular cells present on the abluminal surface of blood vessels. We believe that barrier cells augment the basal filtration activity of the filtration beds, and serve to regulate their traffic.

Barrier cells provide dynamic, diverse blood–spleen barriers, which, acting in coordination with macrophages and other stromal cells, regulate splenic filtration and its intrasplenic consequences, including blood flow, cell homing and migration, hematopoietic and immune responses, and the clearance of infectious organisms. Barrier cells trap circulating infectious organisms and monocytes on their cell surfaces, clearing them from the blood, providing a selective environment for monocyte differentiation into macrophages and subsequent phagocytosis of the microorganisms. Barrier cells enclosing hematopoietic colonies are positioned to confine factors controlling colony growth and differentiation. They may protect colonies from parasitism, e.g., as erythroblastic colonies in malaria. Activated barrier cells and their associated matrix molecules may effectively close off white pulp. An initial antigen stimulus is thereby met by a complete response, which confines the lymphokines, cytokines, and other regulatory substances, to the white pulp, and prevents secondarily derived antigen from dissipating immunological resources. Closing off the white pulp, in the presence of contagious cellular damage, would reduce autoimmune responses. As barrier cells close off the selected filtration domains, they constitute a shunt, permitting an efficient closed circulation between arterial terminals and veins. The spleen, unlike the marrow, lacks a cellular barrier between hematopoietic tissues and the blood. These specialized cells provide such barriers, thereby conferring on the spleen certain attributes of the marrow.

2.4. CONCLUSION

In a normal spleen, the level of filtration activity may well be regulated by the degree of contraction of the filtration beds, the capsule and trabeculae; the placement of the terminating arterial vessels; and the capacity of the sheet-like processes of the reticular cells to establish tubular connections between arterial and venous vessels. The normal spleen does not appear to depend heavily upon its barrier cells, although they are present in the circumferential reticulum of white pulp, and, in sinusal spleens, they may also be found in the marginal zone and red pulp. In pathological spleens in which the locules of the filtration bed come tightly crowded, as a result of heightened filtration, the spleen becomes firm and enlarged; consequently, the mechanisms regulating blood flow under normal circumstances cannot function, since the spleen is distended and becomes incapable of contraction. The syncytial membrane and meshworks produced by the fusion of barrier cells become the means by which the character of the blood flow is determined. The character of blood flow, in turn, determines whether or not the filtration beds are perfused, whether the circulation is open or closed, and whether or not the blood is cleared.

REFERENCES

Blue, J. and Weiss, L. (1981a) Periarterial macrophage sheaths (ellipsoids) in cat spleen: an electron microscope study. *Am. J. Anat.* **161,** 115–134.

Blue, J. and Weiss, L. (1981b) Electron microscopy of the red pulp of the dog spleen including vascular arrangements, perarterial macrophage sheaths (ellipsoids) and the contractile innervated reticular meshwork. *Am. J. Anat.* **161,** 189–281.

Borrello, M. A. and Phipps, R. P. (1996) Differential Thy-1 expression by splenic fibroblasts defines functionally distinct subsets. *Cell. Immunol.* **173,** 198–206.

Buckley, P. J., Smith, M. R., Braverman, M. F., and Dickson, S. A. (1987) Human spleen contains phenotypic subsets of macrophage and dendritic cells that occupy discrete microanatomic locations. *Am. J. Pathol.* **128,** 505–520.

Drenckhahn, D. and Wagner, J. (1986) Stress fibers in the splenic sinus endothelium in situ: molecular structure, relationship to the extracellular matrix and contractility. *J. Cell Biol.* **102,** 1738–1747.

Faller, A. (1985) Splenic architecture as reflected in the connective tissue structure of the human spleen. *Experientia* **41,** 164–167.

Ford, W. L. (1969) Immunological and migratory properties of lymphocytes recirculating through the rat spleen. *Br. J. Exp. Pathol.* **50,** 257–269.

Ford, W. L. (1968) The mechanism of lymphopenia produced by chronic irradiation of the rat spleen. *Br. J. Exp. Pathol.* **49,** 502–513.

Fujita, T., Kashimura, M., and Adachi, K. (1982) Scanning electron microscopy studies of the spleen: normal and pathological. *Scan. Electron Microsc.* **1,** 435–444.

Fujita, T., Kashimura, M., and Adachi, K. (1985) Scanning electron microscopy and terminal circulation. *Experientia* **41,** 167–179.

Groom, A. C. (1987) Microcirculation of the spleen: new concepts, new challenges. *Microvasc. Res.* **34,** 269–289.

Hammond, B. J. (1975) A compartmental analysis of circulatory lymphocytes in the spleen. *Cell Tissue Kinet,* **8,** 153–169.

Kashimura, M. and Fujita, K. (1987) A scanning electron microscope study of human spleen: relationship between microcirculation and functions. *Scan. Microsc.* **1,** 841–851.

Koike, R., Nishimura, T., Yasumizu, R., Tanaka, H., Hataba, Y., Hataba, Y., et al. (1996) The splenic marginal zone is absent in alymphoplastic *aly* mutant mice. *Eur. J. Immunol.* **26,** 669–675.

Kraal, G., Schornagel, K., Streeter, P. R., Holzmann, B., and Butcher, E. C. (1995) Expression of the mucosal vascular addressin, MadCAM-1, on sinus-lining cells in the spleen. *Am. J. Pathol.* **147,** 763–771.

Levesque, M. J. and Groom, A. C. (1981) Fast transit of red cells and plasma in contracted versus relaxed spleens. *Can. J. Phys. Pharm.* **59,** 53–58.

Liakka, A., Apaja-Sarkkinen, M., Karttunen, T., and Autio-Harmainen, H. (1991) Distribution of laminin and types IV and III collagen in fetal, infant and adult human spleens. *Cell Tissue Res.* **263,** 245–252.

Liakka, A. and Autio-Harmainen, H. (1992) Distribution of extracellular matrix proteins tenascin, fibronectin, and vitronectin in fetal, infant and adult human spleens. *J. Histochem. Cytochem.* **40,** 1203–1210.

Liakka, A., Karjalainen, H., Virtanen, I., and Autio-Harmainen, H. (1995) Immuno-electron-microscopic localization of types III pN- collagen and IV collagen, laminin and tenascin in developing and adult human spleen. *Cell Tissue Res.* **282,** 117–127.

Lyons, A. B. and Parish, C. R. (1995) Are murine marginal-zone macrophages the splenic white pulp analog of high endothelial venules? *Eur. J. Immunol.* **25,** 3165–3172.

Pabst, R. (1988) The spleen in lymphocyte migration. *Immunol. Today* **9,** 43–45.

Persson, S. G., Ekman, L., Lydin, G., and Tufvesson, G. (1973a) Circulatory effects of splenectomy in the horse. I. Effect on red cell distribution and variability of haematocrit in the peripheral blood. *Zentralbl. Veterinarmed.[A]* **20,** 441–455.

Persson, S. G., Ekman, L., Lydin, G., and Tufvesson, G. (1973b) Circulatory effects of splenectomy in the horse. II. Effect of plasma volume and total and circulating red cell volume. *Zentralbl. Veterinarmed.[A]* **20,** 456–468.

Reilly, F. D. (1985) Innervation and vascular pharmacodynamics of the mammalian spleen. *Experientia* **41,** 187–192.

Reis, F. P. and Ferraz de Carvalho, C. A. (1988) Functional architecture of the splenic vein in the adult human. *Acta. Anat.* **132,** 109–113.

Sasou, S., Satodate, R., Masuda, T., and Takayama, K. (1986) Scanning electron microscopic features of the spleen in the rat and human: a comparative study. *Scan Electron Microsc.* **3,** 1063–1069.

Tablin, F. and Weiss, L. (1983) The equine spleen: an electron microscopic analysis. *Am. J. Anat.* **166,** 393–416.

Toccanier-Pelte, M. F., Skalli, O., Kapanci, Y., and Gabbiani, G. (1987) Characterization of stromal cells with myoid features in lymph nodes and spleen in normal and pathologic conditions. *Am. J. Pathol.* **129,** 109–118.

Uehara, K. and Miyoshi, M. (1997) Junctions between the sinus endothelial cells of rat spleen. *Cell Tissue Res.* **287,** 187–192.

Van Ewijk, W. and Nieuwenhuis, P. (1985) Compartments, domains, and migration pathways of lymphoid cells in the splenic pulp. *Experientia* **41,** 199–208.

van Krieken, J. H. J. M. and te Velde, J. (1988) Normal histology of the human spleen. *Am. J. Surg. Pathol.* **12,** 777–785.

Van Vliet, E., Melis, M., Foidart, J. M., and Van Ewijk, W. (1986) Reticular fibroblasts in peripheral lymphoid organs identified by a monoclonal antibody. *J. Histochem. Cytochem.* **34,** 883–890.

Weiss, L. (1983) The red pulp of the spleen: structural basis of blood flow. *Clin. Haematol.* **12,** 375–393.

Weiss, L. (1985) New trends in spleen research: conclusion. *Experientia* **41,** 243–248.

Weiss, L., Powell, R., and Schiffman, F. J. (1985) Terminating arterial vessels in red pulp of the spleen. *Experientia* **40,** 233–242.

Weiss, L., Geduldig, U., and Weidanz, W. (1986) Mechanisms of splenic control of murine malaria: reticular cell activation and the development of a blood-spleen barrier. *Am. J. Anat.* **176,** 251–285.

Weiss, L. (1991) Barrier cells in the spleen. *Immunol. Today* **12,** 24–29.

3 Splenic Microcirculatory Blood Flow and Function with Respect to Red Blood Cells

ALAN C. GROOM, PhD, IAN C. MACDONALD, PhD, AND ERIC E. SCHMIDT, BSc, MCS*

3.1. INTRODUCTION

The microcirculation of the spleen is perhaps the most complex of any organ in the body: Splenic arterioles lead to capillaries, most of which do not lead to venules, but discharge blood into a labyrinthine reticular meshwork. The spleen contains blood with a packed cell volume twice that of arterial blood, and a long-standing question is why this high hematocrit is necessary and how it is achieved. Red blood cell (RBC) transit times through some microcirculatory routes are as short as through skeletal muscle, but transit times through other routes can be up to 1000× longer. The distribution of the total flow among these various routes can change dramatically under neural or hormonal stimulation, and as a result of increased portal venous pressure. Unlike most other organs and tissues studied from a microcirculatory viewpoint, the spleen is not concerned with transcapillary exchange in relation to metabolism, but constitutes the only lymphatic organ specialized for the filtration of blood. The unique structure of the microvascular pathways in the spleen must be understood as a reflection of this function.

For humans and a group of common laboratory animals, splenic weight, expressed as a proportion of body weight, is variable (Davies and Withrington, 1973). Approximate values are given as 1% (cat, dog), 0.7% (mouse), 0.25% (human, rat), 0.15% (monkey, guinea pig), and 0.05% (rabbit). The highest values are found in species with an abundance of smooth muscle in the splenic capsule and trabeculae, and in which the organ is known to be contractile. Conversely, the intermediate and low values occur in species with little capsular and trabecular smooth muscle, and in which active contraction probably does not occur: The spleens with lower weights are probably those that lack the reservoir function. Resting splenic blood flow in all species studied lies in the range of 40–100 mL/min/100 g tissue: This corresponds to 1–10% of the cardiac output, depending on the species (Davies and Withrington, 1973).

The blood-filled space in the spleen is a large fraction of the total volume of the organ; in the relaxed spleen of the cat, this amounts to 50%. When the high hematocrit is taken into consideration, this

*Deceased August 19, 1999.

From: *The Complete Spleen: A Handbook of Structure, Function, and Clinical Disorders* Edited by: A. J. Bowdler © Humana Press Inc., Totowa, NJ

means that stored red blood cells represent about 40% of the total volume of the organ. In species with contractile spleens, a large proportion of these stored cells can be released promptly into the general circulation when needed. It is possible that this happens to a lesser extent in species such as humans, in which the spleen is noncontractile. Because the compliance of the spleen is so great, elevated portal venous pressure can cause a considerable increase in the splenic blood volume, and in the overall size of the organ.

Blood vessels enter the spleen along the hilus of its concave surface, and are conveyed within trabeculae into the interior of the organ. Suspended within the trabecular network is an open three-dimensional (3-D) web of reticular tissue housing white pulp and red pulp (Fig. 1). The white pulp forms a sheath of lymphatic tissue surrounding the arteries after they leave the trabeculae (periarterial lymphatic sheath [PALS]), and it is thickened in places to form lymphatic nodules. The red pulp, in which the filtration function of the spleen is carried out, occupies most of the parenchyma, and amounts to 75% of the normal human spleen (Van Krieken et al., 1985a). Its basic structure, a meshwork of reticular cells and fibers (reticular meshwork), appears honeycombed by an anastomosing system of venous sinuses in ~50% of mammalian species examined (Snook, 1950); in other species, the venous system begins, instead, as small, fenestrated pulp venules. Spleens are referred to as "sinusal" and "nonsinusal," the human spleen being of the sinusal type.

The red pulp occupies most of the space not taken up by trabeculae and white pulp, and its interstices are lined with both fixed and free phagocytes, which remove abnormal particulate material from the blood passing through. Because cellular components of the blood are concentrated within the spleen, the reticular meshwork is filled with blood of very high hematocrit. Figure 1 shows that blood flows through the white pulp, and then the red pulp, in series. The white pulp is intimately associated with the arterial tree; red pulp is similarly associated with the venous system draining the spleen. Most capillaries empty into the reticular meshwork (open circulation), to drain into the venous system. Thus, the reticular meshwork constitutes an intermediate circulation between the capillaries and venous channels. Whether direct vascular connections also exist (closed circulation), bypassing the intermediate circulation, has been controversial.

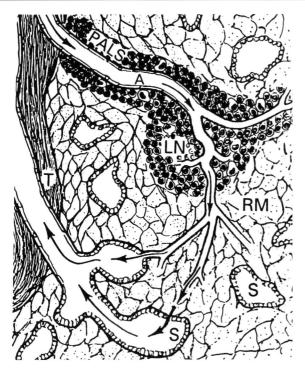

Fig. 3.1. Schematic diagram showing structure of sinusal spleen. A, central artery; PALS, periarterial lymphatic sheath; LN, lymphatic nodule; RM, reticular meshwork of red pulp; S, venous sinus; T, trabecula. (Adapted with permission from J. A. Bellanti, 1979).

The microcirculatory pathways bordering the white pulp have received little attention, and are not included in Fig. 1, or in most standard histology texts. However, most of the inflowing blood passes through the marginal sinus (MS) and marginal zone (MZ), which lie between the white pulp and red pulp. The circumferential arrangement of the MS immediately adjacent to the white pulp causes blood to be distributed over the outer surface of the white pulp, before passing on to the MZ and red pulp. The MZ is now recognized as a region distinct from the reticular meshwork of the red pulp, and in some species it is the largest B-lymphocyte compartment within the spleen (rat: Kumararatne et al., 1981). Our research has served to elucidate these pathways bordering the white pulp, and Subheading 3.8. presents a revised schematic diagram (Fig. 19), which summarizes the current state of knowledge.

The filtration of blood by the spleen, with the removal of blood cells unsuitable for continued circulation, has been studied principally with respect to red blood cells. Reticulocytes released from bone marrow are retained in the organ (Wade, 1973), perhaps for destruction (Sorbie and Valberg, 1970), maturation (Song and Groom, 1971c, 1972), or remodeling (Crosby, 1977). Inclusion bodies, such as Heinz bodies, are removed from red blood cells in the spleen (pitting function: Chen and Weiss, 1973; Matsumoto et al., 1977). The selective retention (culling) of abnormal red blood cells has been demonstrated for pathological red blood cells (Schnitzer et al., 1973), and for normal red blood cells altered in various ways (Levesque and Groom, 1977, 1980a). The extent to which the spleen culls normally senescent red blood cells remains unclear.

Little is known of the mechanisms underlying the sequestration and treatment of red blood cells in the spleen, in terms of properties of the cells or morphology of the splenic red pulp areas involved.

Red blood cell trapping may be based on size restriction (Chen and Weiss, 1973; Boisfleury and Mohandas, 1977) or cell-to-cell adhesion (Song and Groom, 1971b,c, 1972, 1974). Phagocytosis of aged red blood cells may occur because of reduced surface electrical charge (Skutelsky and Danon, 1970a,b), which unmasks immunoglobulins and leads to recognition and degradation by macrophages (Kay et al., 1982). Whether permanent sequestration occurs on the first or subsequent passages of a cell through the splenic pulp appears to depend on the transit time through the pulp. In many diseases in which splenic enlargement occurs, there is marked retention of blood within the organ (Witte et al., 1974; Bowdler and Videbaek, 1990; *see also* Chapter 7), and the stay of red blood cells is greatly prolonged. If, on the other hand, the spleen is atrophied, it will fail to filter effete red blood cells from the circulation. Such atrophy (auto-splenectomy) may occur in sickle cell anemia, thrombocythemia, malabsorption, and other diseases (Nordy, 1974; Foster and Losowsky, 1990). The consequences of damaged red blood cells remaining in the general circulation, e.g., microcirculatory obstruction, have yet to be assessed adequately.

Of course, the role of the spleen with respect to blood cells also includes platelets and leukocytes. As many as 30% of all platelets in the body are normally found in the spleen (Shulman and Jordan, 1987), but why this should be so is unknown. In immune thrombocytopenia, the spleen produces antiplatelet antibodies, and becomes the major site of platelet destruction (McMillan, 1981; Bussel, 1990). Changes in splenic microcirculatory pathways in ITP, and possibly other diseases, have been demonstrated (Schmidt et al., 1991). Much work has been done recently on the immune functions of the spleen (e.g., Van Rooijen et al., 1989; Yednock and Rosen, 1989; Kopp, 1990; Kraal et al., 1995; Westermann and Pabst, 1997; *see also* Chapter 4). A continuous traffic of lymphocytes throughout the body is the basis for their contact with antigens and their interaction with other immunocompetent cells in lymphoid organs (Jalkanen et al., 1986). On a quantitative basis, the spleen is the most important single organ in lymphocyte recirculation (Pabst, 1988), with T- and B-cells migrating between blood and the white pulp compartments. Studies on lymphocyte migration have been carried out using autoradiography or immunohistochemistry (Ford, 1969; Pabst, 1988; Pellas and Weiss, 1990; Kraal et al., 1995; Tanaka, Hataba, Saito et al., 1996). Lymphocyte interactions with vessel walls, and other cells within the spleen in vivo, have been studied by high-resolution videomicroscopy (Schmidt, 1990), which presents a potential opportunity for direct observation of lymphocyte homing within the spleen.

3.2. METHODS FOR STUDYING SPLENIC MICROCIRCULATORY PATHWAYS AND BLOOD FLOW

3.2.1. THE BLACK BOX APPROACH
One can learn a great deal about intrasplenic blood flow under different conditions, and about splenic retention of abnormal red blood cells, by considering the organ as a "black box," and studying input/output relationships. For example, total splenic blood flow has been measured by washout of radioactive gas (^{133}Xe, ^{85}Kr); the presence of both fast and slow pathways for flow was shown by biexponential washout curves (Sandberg, 1972; Vaupel et al., 1977). Because the spleen is a filter for blood, red blood cells may be treated differently from plasma during passage through this organ; therefore, there is the

need for washout studies of red blood cells and plasma to be performed separately. Three black box approaches to the study of microcirculatory blood flow through the spleen will now be described.

3.2.1.1. Red Blood Cell and Plasma Washout During Ringer Perfusion
One simple way to study the storage and transit of red blood cells in this organ is to perfuse an isolated spleen preparation with cell-free Ringer's solution, sampling the outflow as a function of time (Song and Groom, 1971a). This system has the advantage that the red blood cells are not processed first, as with radiolabeling; the red blood cells collected at the outflow are those that were contained in the spleen in vivo at the time of cannulation, and are now simply being washed out by Ringer perfusion. Moreover, since this is a nonrecirculating system, and the perfusate entering the organ is cell-free, slow as well as fast clearance of red blood cells from the spleen may be quantitated. Cell concentrations in successive samples of the outflow may be measured precisely, over several orders of magnitude, by means of an electronic particle counter. If a small quantity of radioiodinated (^{125}I) serum albumin is injected into the general circulation and allowed to equilibrate intravascularly, prior to isolating the spleen, then the washout of both red blood cells and plasma from the organ may be studied simultaneously (Levesque and Groom, 1976a). Red blood cell and plasma concentrations are plotted semilogarithmically against the sequential volumes of perfusing fluid per gram splenic weight.

3.2.1.2. Splenic Drainage with Inflow Occluded
This procedure consists of anaerobic collection of blood drained from the organ, during contraction with inflow occluded, as successive discrete samples (Levesque and Groom, 1976b). It provides a means of selectively sampling blood from the reticular meshwork, because expulsion of blood from the fast-transit pathways is completed ahead of expulsion of blood from the slower-transit pathways of the reticular meshwork. The increase in hematocrit of the venous outflow during this procedure, from an initial value comparable to that of arterial blood to a final value of almost 80%, suggests that the last samples are indeed representative of blood from the reticular meshwork. This conclusion is also reinforced by the progressive changes in gas tensions and glucose concentrations that are found during drainage.

3.2.1.3. Bolus Injections of Abnormal Red Blood Cells into Ringer-Perfused Spleens
The isolated perfused spleen preparation offers a number of advantages, compared to the use of intact animals, for studying the sequestration of abnormal red blood cells. The results do not depend on the ratio of splenic blood flow to cardiac output. They are not complicated by the simultaneous activities of other organs of the mononuclear phagocyte system, such as bone marrow or liver, which, in the intact animal, can make the interpretation of splenic function difficult. The technique allows for the accurate quantitative assessment of the efficiency of trapping abnormal red blood cells during a single passage through the spleen. The use of two or three serial injections of red blood cells offers the means of assessing whether it is possible to saturate the splenic trapping mechanism.

The spleen is isolated and perfused at constant pressure with oxygenated, buffered Ringer's solution, to wash out most of the contained red blood cells. Samples of the outflow are then collected for measurement of the background, or preinjection, red blood cell concentration. A small bolus of a red blood cell suspension, containing a known number of cells (approx 2×10^6 red blood cells for a 30-g spleen of cat) is then injected quickly into the arterial cannula close to the spleen itself. At the same time, rapid sequential sampling of the venous outflow is begun, and is continued until the red blood cell concentration has returned to its preinjection level. Red blood cell concentrations are determined by an electronic cell counter, and the cumulative outflows of red blood cells (expressed as percentages of the number injected) are then used to derive plots of percentage red blood cell recovery vs outflowing volume of perfusate (Levesque and Groom, 1980a).

3.2.2. FIXED SECTIONS OF SPLENIC TISSUE, INCLUDING HISTOLOGICAL STUDIES DURING RED BLOOD CELL WASHOUT
Much has been learned about microcirculatory pathways from examination of sections of splenic tissue, using either the light microscope or transmission electron microscopy (TEM). For example, the classic study by Snook (1950) used serial histological sections to provide schematic diagrams of microcirculatory routes in spleens of several mammalian species. Greater detail is shown in TEM photographs, especially concerning the cells lining venous sinuses and blood cells in transit through interendothelial slits (IESs) (e.g., Blue and Weiss, 1981d). The study of fixed sections by means of light microscopy or TEM is limited by the very small depth of focus, leading to problems in tracing vascular pathways over long distances. The greater depth of focus of the scanning electron microscope (SEM) has allowed 3-D views of such pathways to be obtained (e.g., Fujita, 1974). However, little information about the dynamics of flow through the complex pathways of the spleen can be obtained from fixed tissue.

Information regarding flow has been obtained by preparing histological sections at serial intervals from the start of splenic perfusion with Ringer's solution (Song and Groom, 1971b). Perfusion by only 1–2 mL solution/g spleen weight is sufficient to eliminate virtually all red blood cells comprising the fast compartment. Perfusion by a larger volume (up to 15 mL/g) will reduce, by a factor of 10, the red blood cells of the intermediate compartment. If the volume of solution perfused is increased to 50–150 mL/g, the red blood cells comprising the intermediate compartment are reduced to zero; the red blood cells of the slow compartment remain at roughly one-half the value of the normal blood-perfused spleen. This technique has helped to identify the morphological counterparts to the fast, intermediate, and slow compartments identified by the study of red blood cell washout kinetics.

3.2.3. MICROCORROSION CASTING STUDIES
In this technique, a methyl-methacrylate resin of low viscosity, e.g., modified Batson's compound (Nopanitaya et al., 1979) or Mercox (Dainippon Ink and Chemicals, Tokyo), is injected into the splenic artery or vein. After polymerization of the resin, the tissue is corroded away using concentrated KOH at 60°C, which leaves a rigid cast that faithfully reproduces the morphology of the blood pathways, including fine details of vascular luminal surfaces. Examination of vascular corrosion casts by SEM offers a way of studying circulatory pathways and their interconnections over a considerable length, with the view unobstructed by surrounding tissue. The black box studies of red blood cell washout showed that, in the relaxed spleen, 90% of the inflow travels to the splenic vein via the fast pathways that occupy only 18% of the total blood space. This suggested that microcorrosion casting could offer a unique opportunity to study the morphology of the fast arteriovenous pathways, provided that small quantities of material were injected. Under these conditions, extensive filling of slower routes through the reticular meshwork is avoided. By varying the volume of material injected in successive experiments, other red blood cell compartments of the splenic microcirculation can also be studied.

Red blood cell washout studies also showed that, in dilated spleens, the customary fast component of flow appears to be absent; in contracted spleens, the fast pathways carry almost the entire blood flow. Therefore, in order to demonstrate the morphology of the fast pathways, preferentially, one injects minimal amounts of casting material into spleens contracted by norepinephrine. In order to view the slow pathways, minimal injections are used in spleens dilated by perfusion against a high venous pressure. In all cases, clearer views of pathways in the interior of the organ can be obtained by making use of the natural dissection occurring at a boundary between a perfused segment of the spleen and adjacent unperfused tissue. This can be achieved by injection of casting material into an arterial branch supplying only a limited segment of the organ. Fragmentation of the cast, which occurs inevitably at cut faces, may thereby be avoided.

3,2.4. VIDEOMICROSCOPIC STUDIES OF TRANSILLU-MINATED SPLEENS IN VIVO
In vivo microscopy of the spleen was begun more than 50 years ago, but the quality of recorded images was not adequate for quantitative analysis of red blood cell flow within the organ. In addition, the interpretation of in vivo observations has been difficult, because of lack of a 3-D map of the diverse pathways available for flow, and this led to contradictory conclusions (Knisely, 1936; MacKenzie et al., 1941). Use of in vivo microscopy is restricted to animal spleens that are sufficiently thin to be transilluminated (e.g., rat, mouse). With the aid of microcorrosion casts of spleens from these same species (Schmidt et al., 1985a,b), positive identification can be made of the channels through which the red blood cells are seen to flow. In vivo microscopy permits the direction and kinetics of blood flow to be determined, so that one can visualize and describe quantitatively the movement of blood through the various pathways elucidated by other techniques. In addition, in vivo microscopy of Ringer-perfused spleens, injected with a bolus of abnormal or senescent red blood cells, promises to give valuable information on the sites and mechanisms of red blood cell trapping during a single passage through the spleen.

Successful in vivo microscopy of the spleen requires a method by which the position of the organ can be completely stabilized for long periods, with minimal application of pressure to the capsule. A standard upright microscope requires constant adjustment as the organ moves with respiration and varies in volume spontaneously; in addition, the surface being viewed is often at an angle to the plane of focus. However, if an inverted microscope is used, the viewed tissue rests on a stationary cover slip, and problems associated with respiratory movement are minimized. A transparent Saran film can be used to hold the spleen gently against the cover slip, restricting lateral and vertical motion at the plane of focus. Objective lenses of high magnification (up to ×100, dry) and short working distance can then be used over a large working area.

The high blood content of the spleen presents a problem, in that virtually all the transilluminated light must pass through red blood cells, and thus color contrast is poor. However, image contrast can be enhanced considerably by using oblique lighting, rather than conventional illumination. If a fiberoptic source is positioned at about 45 degrees to the optical axis of the microscope, more light is reflected from one side of each structure than the other, which results in shadowing that imparts a 3-D quality to the image (Fig. 2). Use of a black and white videocamera with extended red sensitivity (Panasonic WV-1550) results in image contrast far superior to that obtained by eye, viewing through the eyepieces of the

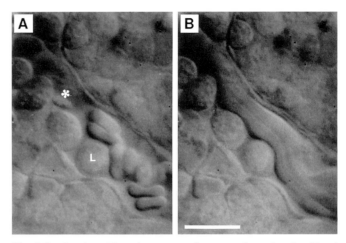

Fig. 3.2. In vivo videomicroscopy of mouse spleen showing blood cells, including marginated lymphocytes, within a venule. Shadowing effect produced by oblique transillumination imparts a 3-D quality to the images. (**A**) Individual red blood cells and a platelet (*) can be distinguished when the flow is momentarily zero. Four lymphocytes (L) adhere to the vessel wall. (**B**) Blood flow has resumed, giving blurred images, except for the marginated lymphocytes, which are stationary. The endothelial wall of the venule may be seen clearly in both views. Bar = 10 μm. (Reproduced with permission from Schmidt et al., 1990).

microscope. By combining the use of an inverted microscope and oblique lighting with slow-motion video playback, one can obtain sequential images of individual blood cells flowing within the spleen, which are of sufficient quality for still-frame viewing and quantitative analysis (MacDonald et al., 1987; Schmidt et al., 1990).

3.3. KEY ISSUES CONCERNING SPLENIC MICROCIRCULATORY BLOOD FLOW

3.3.1. FAST VS SLOW PATHWAYS FOR BLOOD FLOW
Studies of red blood cell washout from cat spleen during Ringer perfusion (Subheading 2.1.1.) have shown that the red blood cells leaving the organ do so as three distinct groups, traveling with very different mean velocities (Song and Groom, 1971a; Levesque and Groom, 1976a). These groups are designated fast, intermediate, and slow, based on the volumes of the perfusate required to reduce their concentrations by one-half ($V_{1/2}$: 0.067, 4.7, and 97 mL/g splenic weight, respectively). By histological examination of spleens in which Ringer perfusion was terminated after different volumes of perfusate had passed through (Subheading 2.2.), the locations of red blood cells have been compared before perfusion and after cells, comprising the fast and intermediate components, respectively, have been almost completely washed out. These experiments (Song and Groom, 1971b) showed that the fast component corresponded to red blood cells in splenic vessels, the intermediate component to free red blood cells in the interstices of the reticular meshwork, and the slow component to red blood cells adhering to fine structures of the reticular meshwork (bound red blood cells).

Because the sum of the three exponential terms can completely describe the red blood cell washout curve, a simple model, consisting of three compartments in parallel, is sufficient to approximate the washout processes from the spleen. However, histological evidence showed that the bound red blood cells (slow compartment) are accumulated from blood flowing through the reticular meshwork (Song, 1972; Song and Groom, 1971b); when released

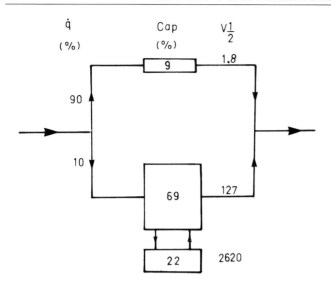

Fig. 3.3. Three-compartment model, derived from cell washout kinetics and morphological studies, for distribution of red blood cells in cat spleen. Cap, capacity of compartment (% of total); q, flow to compartment (% of total flow); $V_{1/2}$, desaturation half-volume of compartment (mL perfusate). (Reproduced with permission from Groom, 1987).

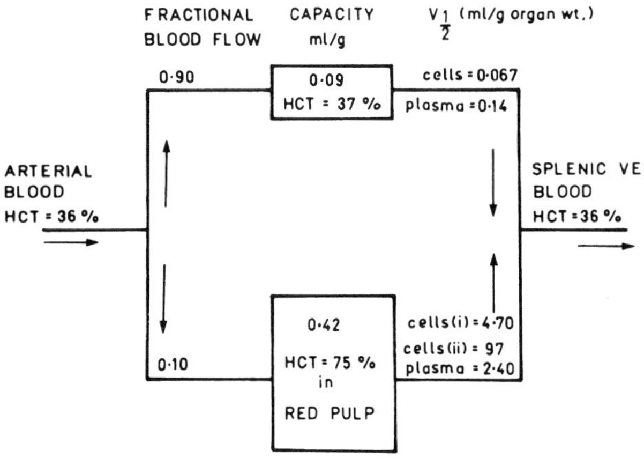

Fig. 3.4. Compartmental model for distribution of whole blood in cat spleen (see text). Nine-tenths of splenic arterial blood passes through the smaller compartment, which contains blood of similar hematocrit (37%). One-tenth of total blood flow passes through red pulp (the major compartment) that contains blood of hematocrit 75%. (Reproduced with permission from Levesque and Groom, 1976a).

from their bound state, they must rejoin the free red blood cells flowing through. These findings suggest that there are only two vascular compartments within the spleen, namely, the vessels constituting the fast pathway, and the reticular spaces of the red pulp. The distinction between the intermediate and slow compartments is entirely the result of a cellular factor. For this reason, the compartment model (Levesque and Groom, 1976a) presented in Fig. 3 shows the slow and intermediate red blood cell compartments in a mamillary arrangement, rather than in parallel. Because of the great differences in $V_{1/2}$ values, it is not possible to distinguish between these two arrangements on the basis of washout kinetics alone. The model shows that 90% of the flow passes through a small (fast) compartment containing only 9% of the total red blood cells, the remaining flow passing to the other two compartments (Fig. 3). The intermediate compartment is perfused by 9.6% of the total inflow, and contains 69% of all splenic red blood cells; the slow compartment is perfused by only 0.15% of the inflow, and represents 22% of the total red blood cells. Results qualitatively similar to the above have also been obtained from red blood cell washout studies in rats (Cilento et al., 1980; Stock et al., 1983).

Black box studies of the washout of both red blood cells and plasma simultaneously have provided measurements of the total volume and hematocrit of blood in the fast and slow pathways, respectively (cat spleen: Levesque and Groom, 1976a). The plasma washout curve consisted of only two exponential components, the $V_{1/2}$ values corresponding closely to those of the fast and intermediate components of red blood cell washout. There existed no counterpart to the slow component of red blood cell washout, indicating that the latter must have been caused by a process peculiar to the red blood cells. By combining the data of both plasma and red blood cell washout, a single model for the morphological distribution of blood within the spleen was derived (Fig. 4). This is a two-compartment model, in which the red blood cells of the intermediate and slow compartments are combined. From the volumes of red blood

cells and plasma in each vascular compartment, the hematocrits were calculated to be 37% (fast pathways) and 75% (slow pathways). The total blood volume was 0.51 mL/g splenic weight, of which more than 80% was located in the slow pathways of the red pulp. Confirmation of the hematocrit values determined by the washout method was obtained by means of the splenic drainage procedure (Subheading 1.2.). Figure 5B shows that the initial hematocrit (representing blood from the fast pathways) was 33.5%, and comparable to that of peripheral blood; the final hematocrit, reflecting the blood from the slow pathways, was 78.5%. For discussion of the mechanisms of red blood cell concentration that give rise to such a high hematocrit in the red pulp, *see* Subheading 3.12.

From microcorrosion casts prepared by the minimal-injection technique, the microcirculatory pathways corresponding to the two vascular compartments, fast and slow, have been identified. Photomicrographs of these pathways are presented in Subheadings 7–11), but a brief summary of the conclusions is given here.

The fast pathways in sinusal spleens we have studied (dog, rat, human) (Schmidt et al., 1982, 1983a, 1985a, 1988) include:

1. Venous sinuses originating as open-ended tubes continuous with the MS or the MZ surrounding the white pulp (this pathway carries a large proportion of the flow).

2. Direct connections of arterial capillaries to venous sinuses (which are more plentiful in some species than in others).

3. Flow from arterial capillaries, radially outward through ellipsoid sheaths, and into closely adjacent venous sinuses, via IESs in sinus walls (in some species, such as the rat, ellipsoids are absent).

4. The perimarginal cavernous sinus (PMCS) bordering lymphatic nodules. Flow into the PMCS occurs via direct connections with arterial capillaries, via connections with ellipsoid sheaths, and via connections with the MZ. Drainage from the PMCS occurs directly into venous sinuses.

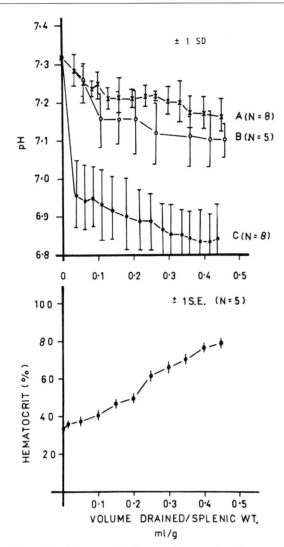

Fig. 3.5. pH and hematocrit of successive samples of venous blood drained from cat spleen with inflow occluded (*see* Subheading 2.1.2.) (**A**) With no stasis, pH fell to 7.16 (group A); with stasis during cannulation procedures (8–10 min), pH fell to 7.10 (group B); and, after stasis for 60 min, the pH fell to 6.83 (group C). (**B**) Initial hematocrit represents that of blood from the fast pathways through the spleen; final hematocrit represents that of blood in the slow pathways through the reticular meshwork of the red pulp. (Reproduced with permission from Levesque and Groom, 1976b).

The fast pathways in nonsinusal spleens we have studied (cat, mouse; Schmidt et al., 1983b, 1985b) include:

1. Short routes through the reticular meshwork of the red pulp, from arterial capillary terminations to nearby pulp venules (for details regarding the distinction between pulp venules and venous sinuses, *see* Subheading 7.) The authors have found no direct arteriovenous connections in nonsinusal spleens.
2. Short routes through the reticular meshwork, from MS or MZ to pulp venules.
3. Short routes through the reticular meshwork, from ellipsoid sheaths (when present, as in the cat) to pulp venules.

The slow pathways, in both sinusal and nonsinusal spleens, all involve longer distances through the labyrinthine reticular mesh-

work of the red pulp, where filtration of abnormal red blood cells takes place. Blood flows into the reticular meshwork from arterial capillary terminations, from the MZ, and from ellipsoid sheaths. From the reticular meshwork, blood enters the venous system by passing through IESs in walls of venous sinuses, or, in the case of nonsinusal spleens, by passing into pulp venules via their open ends or fenestrated walls.

3.3.2. IMMATURE RED BLOOD CELLS AND THE SPLEEN
Histological studies at different stages of red blood cell washout indicated that the slow component consisted of red blood cells adhering to the reticular meshwork (Song and Groom, 1971b; Song, 1972). What was different about these red blood cells that became trapped in the reticular meshwork? At different stages of the washout, fairly pure (>85%) samples of red blood cells from each compartment could be collected at the outflow. The specific gravity and cell volume of red blood cells from the three compartments showed that the cells from the slow compartment differed significantly from those of arterial blood, being larger and lighter (Groom et al., 1971), and suggesting that these were younger cells (Piomelli et al., 1967). Supravital staining of blood smears confirmed that they were indeed reticulocytes (Song and Groom, 1972), and measurements showed that the reticulocyte washout curve was almost identical to that of red blood cells from the slow compartment. These reticulocytes amounted to 8% of all splenic red blood cells, and were equal to 1.5× the total daily production.

Counts of red blood cell precursors in histological sections (Song and Groom, 1972) showed that the reticulocytes could not have arisen by splenic erythropoiesis, for proerythroblasts were never found, and the ratio of reticulocytes to rubricytes was 75× the number that would have been expected, if they had been derived from red blood cell precursors in the spleen. These results suggest that reticulocytes released from bone marrow are retained in the spleen for a 1–2-d period of maturation, then returned to the circulation (Song and Groom, 1971c, 1972). It is hardly conceivable that such large numbers of reticulocytes would undergo destruction simultaneously in normal animals. Instead, the spleen appears to function as a "finishing school," with maturation of reticulocytes proceeding within the organ (Song, 1972). Moreover, there is evidence that splenic macrophages serve as nurse cells, assisting in the maturation of immature red blood cells (Pictet et al., 1969).

3.3.3. NONSPECIFICITY OF SPLENIC FILTRATION OF ABNORMAL RED BLOOD CELLS
The role of the spleen in re-moving abnormal red blood cells from the circulation has long been recognized (Weisman et al., 1955; Wennberg and Weiss, 1969; Schnitzer et al., 1973). Red blood cells containing inclusion bodies are remodeled at the IESs, and probably also by contact with macrophages in the reticular meshwork. Those with impaired deformability, such as the sickle cell, may be subjected to mechanical trauma and lysis before phagocytosis of the cellular fragments. Other abnormal red blood cells that adhere to the reticular meshwork and macrophages in the red pulp may be phagocytosed. The factors that determine whether there is maturation of young red blood cells or destruction of old red blood cells, when these cells adhere to macrophages, are apparently the characteristics of the cells themselves, rather than of the macrophages (Pictet et al., 1969). Grossly damaged red blood cells are taken up in vivo, primarily by the liver, which has a much higher mass and blood flow than the spleen (Jacob and Jandl, 1962; Wagner et al., 1962; Kimber and Lander, 1964; Ultmann and Gordon, 1965). However, the spleen has a remarkable ability to remove, selectively from the blood, those red

blood cells that are so slightly damaged that they would escape retention elsewhere.

What are the key cellular or membrane properties that, when modified, determine whether the initial trapping event will occur? The percentage of altered red blood cells retained during a single transit through the isolated, Ringer-perfused spleen of the cat has been measured (Levesque and Groom, 1980a). A variety of altered red blood cells (autologous red blood cells damaged with glutaraldehyde, heat, neuraminidase, or N-ethylmaleimide; autologous, bound red blood cells drained previously from the spleen; and foreign red blood cells from a human donor) was used to explore the effects of changes in bulk properties (deformability, shape, and size) and surface properties (adhesiveness) on trapping in the spleen. In every case, extensive sequestration occurred. The results showed that no single cellular property uniquely determines whether red blood cells will be retained in the spleen: The degree of injury is more important than type. Thus, red blood cells are retained because of loss of deformability, increased sphericity, loss of surface charge, inhibition of membrane sulfhydryl groups, immaturity, or incompatibility.

Although the most obvious effect of treating red blood cells with heat or glutaraldehyde is a reduction in cellular deformability, concomitant changes in membrane properties also occur. Thus, all types of abnormal red blood cells used in this study would have had membrane properties differing in various ways from those of mature autologous cells; significantly, splenic sequestration occurred in every case. What happens to red blood cells after initial trapping will depend on the precise way in which their properties differ from those of normal mature cells. Immature red blood cells are retained for maturation; most other abnormal cells will ultimately be phagocytosed.

By observing the spleen filtering abnormal red blood cells from the blood, it should be possible to determine which cellular properties are important for them to function appropriately in the general circulation (Groom, 1980). The unequivocal answer from such experiments seems to be that deformability and suitable surface properties are both important; therefore, it was surprising to find that cellular deformability alone seems to matter when red blood cells are in transit through skeletal muscle. In an isolated, perfused, cat gastrocnemius muscle, recovery of glutaraldehyde-treated red blood cells from the venous outflow, after intra-arterial injection, was only 21%, but that of every other type of abnormal red blood cell studied was not significantly different from 100% (Bowden, 1978). This may indicate that the surface properties of red blood cells are not as important for safe transit in the general microcirculation; however, it has been shown that reticulocytes are cleared from skeletal muscle much more slowly than mature red blood cells, and this was attributed to cell adherence to vessel walls (Groom et al., 1973). Why then should the spleen sequester autologous red blood cells with altered surface properties? It is probable that the basic mechanism of filtration of pathological red blood cells in the reticular meshwork in vivo is not mechanical, but physicochemical. Alteration of red blood cell surface properties may deceive the spleen, so that it treats functionally adequate red blood cells as abnormal and filters them out of the circulating blood.

3.3.4. SITES OF TRAPPING OF ABNORMAL RED BLOOD CELLS
Where and how is red blood cell filtration carried out? The traditional view is that this occurs solely at IESs in the walls of venous sinuses. The IES is known to impede or prevent the movement of abnormal red blood cells from the reticular mesh-

work into venous sinuses; a well-studied example is that of red blood cells containing Heinz bodies induced by phenylhydrazine (Koyama et al., 1964; Chen and Weiss, 1973; Leblond, 1973; Chen, 1980). Although such retention occurs at the IES, for remodeling (pitting) or subsequent phagocytosis, the spleens of many mammalian species lack venous sinuses (see Subheading 3.7.). Moreover, our research has shown that retention of immature or abnormal red blood cells takes place on a large scale within the reticular meshwork itself. Since the interstices of the reticular meshwork are larger than the red blood cells, and do not constitute a test of cell deformability (as do the IES), factors other than bulk properties of the red blood cells must necessarily be involved. It appears that immature or abnormal cells develop altered surface properties, in addition to whatever internal changes may have occurred. Histological evidence demonstrates that these red blood cells adhere to fine structures of the reticular meshwork (Song, 1972; Song and Groom, 1971b, 1974).

Thus, there are two distinct mechanisms that can form the basis for trapping abnormal red blood cells: altered surface properties of the red blood cell membrane, giving rise to adhesion at low shear rates to structures and macrophages within the MZ and reticular meshwork; and changes in the bulk properties of the cell, such as reduced cellular deformability, which can cause cell retention at the IES. Sinusal spleens appear to have an advantage over non-sinusal spleens, in that IES provide a second means of filtering out abnormal red blood cells from the blood.

Selective retention of abnormal or immature red blood cells probably occurs wherever circulatory paths have an open configuration. Such sites include the reticular meshwork of the MZ and red pulp, and possibly the ellipsoid sheaths (Blue and Weiss, 1981a), which are present in many species, including humans. This means that red blood cell filtration is primarily a function of the slow pathways in the spleen (see Subheading 3.1.). In contrast, the fast pathways bypass the sites for trapping abnormal red blood cells in the reticular meshwork of the red pulp, as well as in the IES of sinusal spleens (see Subheading 3.9.).

3.3.5. SATURATION OF THE SPLENIC RED BLOOD CELL TRAPPING MECHANISM
Under conditions of constant-pressure perfusion, more than one-third of injected, heat-treated red blood cells become entrapped in the cat spleen during a single transit (Levesque and Groom, 1977), which raises a series of important questions about splenic sequestration of abnormal red blood cells in vivo. Do such cells reduce the total splenic blood flow in vivo and change intrasplenic flow distribution? Are normal red blood cells immobilized behind the sequestered red blood cells? To what extent does saturation of the splenic trapping mechanism occur?

A study of these questions was carried out in cat spleen (Levesque and Groom, 1977). Heat-treated red blood cells were injected into the splenic artery in vivo, followed 1 h later by red blood cell washout during Ringer perfusion. The number of red blood cells injected (1.6×10^9 cells) was equivalent to only 0.8% of the splenic red blood cell volume, yet this caused immobilization of 50% of the red blood cells in the red pulp. Such spleens remained deep red throughout the perfusion; control spleens became very pale. Adhesion of abnormal red blood cells to the reticular meshwork would retard flow, promoting further sequestration (Holzbach et al., 1964). This could explain extensive clogging of the red pulp, as a result of the trapping of only a small volume of heat-treated red blood cells. Nevertheless, all the plasma remained free to circulate, although much of it did so slowly. In sinusal spleens, blocking of IESs in the walls of venous sinuses by heat-treated red blood cells (Vaupel et al., 1977) or red blood cells containing Heinz bodies (Chen, 1980) further contributes to clogging of the red pulp.

Saturation of the sequestration mechanism can occur, even leading to functional asplenia, in the case of trapped sickle cells (Pearson et al., 1969), although some authors have thought this to be a consequence of the limited capacity of splenic phagocytes for phagocytosis (Miescher, 1957; Mollison, 1962). The authors' results suggest that this explanation may not be correct, since, for both neuraminidase- and NEM-treated red blood cells, the percentage of red blood cells trapped in the spleen decreased significantly with each repeated bolus injection into Ringer-perfused spleens (Levesque and Groom, 1980a). By the third injection of NEM-treated red blood cells, all the injected cells reached the venous outflow, which suggests that all the slow pathways through the red pulp had been blocked, but a sufficient number of the fast pathways remained open. Thus, the reduced removal of nonviable red blood cells by the spleen, when larger quantities are injected, primarily results from reduced red blood cell flow through the red pulp. In clinical investigations, therefore, the dose of heat-treated red blood cells employed is an important consideration when clearance half-lives from the blood are to be measured.

3.3.6. HOSTILE METABOLIC ENVIRONMENT FOR RED BLOOD CELLS?

Red blood cells in the reticular meshwork are exposed to the local splenic environment for long periods, because of their slow transit. It is known that splenic red blood cells exhibit increased mechanical and osmotic fragility (Emerson et al., 1956), and have a lower sodium: potassium ratio (Prankerd, 1960). It has been hypothesized that the metabolic environment for cells in the red pulp may be similar to that which develops in blood incubated at 37°C in vitro, including low pH, O_2 tension, and glucose concentration. The red blood cell membrane loses its deformability at O_2 tensions below 30 torr (LaCelle, 1970). At a pH < 6.8, red blood cells show increased mean cellular volume, rigidity, blood viscosity at low shear rate, and osmotic fragility (Dintenfass and Burnard, 1966; Murphy, 1967, 1969; LaCelle, 1970). Such physical changes might predispose red blood cells, especially when abnormal, to destruction in the circulation. The term "conditioning" has been used to describe the modification of red blood cells that makes them more susceptible to further challenge within spleen or peripheral circulation (Griggs et al., 1960).

The hypothesis of low intrasplenic pH, O_2 tension, and glucose concentration has been difficult to test, because blood samples from the splenic pulp (either from the cut surface of the spleen, or withdrawn by tissue aspiration) are always contaminated with blood from the fast circulation. Use of the splenic drainage procedure permitted selective sampling of blood from the reticular meshwork of the red pulp, as described in Subheading 2.1.2.), and shown in Fig. 5B. The measurements showed that the pH in the reticular meshwork is normally 7.2 (Fig. 5A, group A) (Levesque and Groom, 1976b). Further experiments showed that intrasplenic pH results from the interplay of two separate factors: pH-determining elements of the splenic tissue that buffer at 6.8, and buffering provided by red blood cells passing through the reticular meshwork. Stasis for 10 min (Fig. 5A, group B) or 60 min (Fig. 5A, group C) reduced the pH to 7.16 and 6.83, respectively. Measurements of O_2 tension (approx 54 torr) and glucose concentration (60% of that in venous blood), in the reticular meshwork, showed them to be well above critical values, unless arterial inflow was occluded completely for 20 min or more (Groom et al., 1977). Thus, the notion

of a hostile environment for red blood cells in the reticular meshwork, simply because of very low values of pH, O_2 tension, and glucose concentration, is incorrect. Other explanations must be sought for deleterious changes observed in red blood cells sequestered in the spleen.

Unfavorable metabolic conditions develop rapidly within the spleen when blood flow is occluded, the principal stress being substrate deprivation, which raises the question: Do such unfavorable conditions also develop when red blood cell stasis occurs following trapping of abnormal cells? (see Subheading 3.5.). If so, these conditions would promote further deterioration and destruction of trapped cells. When this hypothesis was tested by injecting heat-treated red blood cells, then repeating the splenic drainage experiments (Groom et al., 1985), the results showed unequivocally that hostile metabolic conditions did not develop in the red pulp. Inasmuch as red blood cell stasis was known to be present, presumably, there must have been sufficient residual flow of plasma through the reticular meshwork to prevent serious deterioration of the environment.

There is no question that red blood cells, incubated within the splenic pulp, show deleterious changes, and these changes may indeed represent direct damage by the spleen in preparation for their eventual destruction (Motulsky et al., 1958). However, clearly, the levels of pH, O_2 tension, and glucose concentration in the splenic red pulp are not as low as had been thought previously, and additional explanations must be sought for the deleterious changes observed in red blood cells sequestered within the spleen.

3.3.7. SINUSAL VS NONSINUSAL SPLEENS

Although the main features of the arterial circulation are similar in all mammalian spleens (with the exception of the ellipsoid sheaths, which are well-developed in some species and absent in others), two different types of venous circulation are found, namely, those with and those without venous sinuses in the red pulp. In ~50% of mammalian species examined by Snook (1950), venous sinuses were absent (nonsinusal type). Instead, the venous origins in the reticular meshwork consisted of "primordial veins" (or "pulp venules") (Blue and Weiss, 1981b). The sinusal group includes humans, dog, and rat; cat and mouse belong to the nonsinusal group.

Venous sinuses can be distinguished from pulp venules by their larger size, greater abundance, arrangement into a richly anastomosing plexus, and the characteristic structure of their walls, which are encircled by rings of argyrophilic fibers (Snook, 1950). By means of transmission and scanning electron microscopy (TEM and SEM), a more detailed description of the contrasting arrangements of elements in the walls of venous sinuses and pulp venules has been obtained (Blue and Weiss, 1981b,c; Fujita, 1974; Hataba et al., 1981). The walls of venous sinuses consist of long, spindle-shaped endothelial cells aligned parallel to the axis of the vessel (Fig. 6). These cells are held in position by the processes of reticular cells, which fit into transverse grooves in the endothelial cells, and thus form hoops around the abluminal surface of the sinus (Fig. 7). Slit-like gaps exist between the endothelial cells (interendothelial slits [IESs]); in vivo, the IESs may be very narrow (Weiss, 1974), or exist only as potential spaces (Cho and DeBruyn, 1975), but, in many SEM micrographs, the IESs appear widened into oval or rounded apertures, probably as a result of drying artefacts. Blood cells from the reticular meshwork penetrate the IESs into the lumens of venous sinuses (see Subheading 3.9.). A clear view of venous sinuses and their 3-D relationships is obtained by microcorrosion casts (Fig. 8), if only small amounts of material are injected. Venous

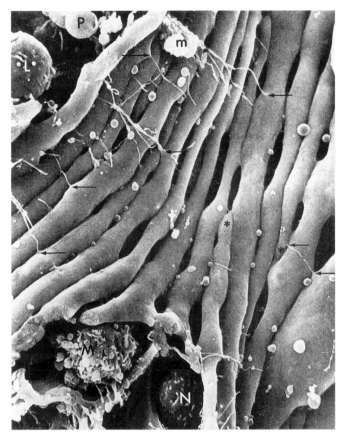

Fig. 3.6. SEM micrograph showing luminal surface of venous sinus in human spleen. Long, spindle-shaped endothelial cells lie side by side, with slit-like gaps between them; a few cells terminated in tapered end (*). Threadlike processes (→) extend from endothelial cells. Some threads may belong to macrophage (M) processes (m). L, lymphocyte; N, neutrophil; P, platelet (×3400). (Reproduced with permission from Fujita, 1974).

Fig. 3.7. SEM micrograph showing abluminal surface of venous sinus in human spleen. Footlike processes (r) of reticulum cells (R) fit into transverse grooves in endothelial cells (W), and thus form hoops around abluminal surface of sinus. P, platelet (×8200). (Reproduced with permission from Fujita, 1974).

sinuses are generally believed to originate in the red pulp or MZ as blind-ended sacs, and that inward passage of blood occurs exclusively through the IES; this view has now been shown to be incorrect (*see* Subheading 3.9.).

The pulp venules in nonsinusal spleens appear, in microcorrosion casts, either as short lateral twigs, branching individually from a collecting vein, or as a root system, with many fine rootlets merging into one trunk (Fig. 9). In contrast to the extensive system of interconnected venous sinuses in sinusal spleens, pulp venules are nonanastomosing, shorter and smaller in caliber, and all receive blood cells, which flow freely from the reticular meshwork through the open ends and fenestrations in their walls. SEM of tissue (Hataba et al., 1981) shows that the walls of pulp venules lack the characteristic "rod cells" aligned parallel to the long axis of the vessel; instead, they are lined with smooth, flattened, irregularly shaped endothelial cells and have relatively few and irregularly distributed fenestrations in their walls (Fig. 10).

The distinction between venous sinuses and pulp venules has important functional implications. The narrow IESs in the walls of venous sinuses serve to impede, or even prevent, entry of red blood cells into the sinus lumen (*see* Subheading 3.9.). Pulp venules lack such IESs, but receive flow freely through the open ends and rounded fenestrations in their walls; the sizes of the fenestrations are mostly

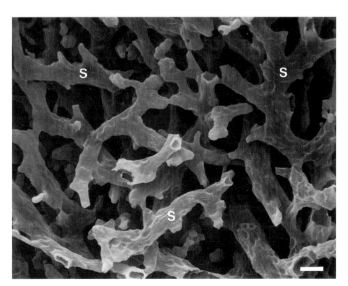

Fig. 3.8. Microcorrosion cast (viewed by SEM) of interconnected, 3-D network of venous sinuses (S) in normal human spleen. Since only a small amount of casting material was injected (*see* Subheading 2.3.), some sinuses are incompletely filled, and reticular meshwork is unfilled. Bar = 20 μm. (Reproduced with permission from Groom and Schmidt, 1990).

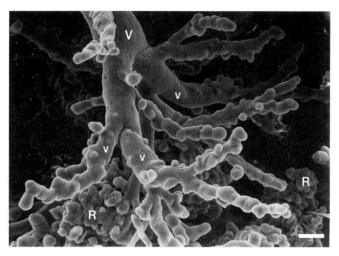

Fig. 3.9. Microcorrosion cast from cat spleen (nonsinusal). Rootlike system of nonanastomosing pulp venules (v) drains into collecting vein (V); knobby appearance results from emergence of material into reticular meshwork (R) via fenestrations in venular walls and via open ends. Bar = 50 μm. (Reproduced with permission from Schmidt et al., 1983b).

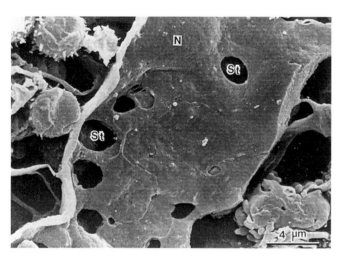

Fig. 3.10. SEM micrograph of luminal aspect of pulp venule from mouse spleen, showing flattened, irregularly shaped endothelial cells and relatively few, irregularly distributed fenestrations. St, stomata; N, nuclear region of endothelial cell which bulges slightly into lumen (×5700). (Reproduced with permission from Hataba et al., 1981).

large enough to allow unimpeded entry of red blood cells into the venule (Blue and Weiss, 1981b). Thus, in nonsinusal spleens, trapping of immature and abnormal red blood cells occurs by adhesion to the fine structures of the reticular meshwork; in sinusal spleens, the reticular meshwork must, presumably, serve a similar function, but the IESs provide an important second mechanism for trapping red blood cells.

3.3.8. FLOW PATHWAYS BORDERING THE WHITE PULP

The region bordering the white pulp has received little attention from investigators, and its importance for filtration and immunologic functions has not been sufficiently appreciated. However, microcorrosion casts prepared using minimal volumes of injected material, indicate that most of the splenic blood flow passes through this region. The microcirculatory routes bordering the white pulp constitute a major area of uncertainty, especially in the human

spleen. Van Krieken et al. (1985) have claimed that the human spleen lacks the MS found in many other species. Barnhart and Lusher (1979) referred to the MS as a "poorly delimited" component of the MZ, and stated that additional work is necessary to identify the precise vascular routes through this region. The existence of the MS as a distinct vascular space was first described in rat spleen (Andrew, 1946; Snook, 1950), and consists of a series of anastomosing vascular spaces lying between the white pulp and the MZ. Serial sections revealed that the MS is not a vessel, but a cleft-like space surrounding the white pulp (Fig. 11). Many follicular capillaries terminate in the MS, their endothelial walls being in continuity with the cells lining the MS. Red blood cells have direct access to the MZ through discontinuities in the outer wall of the MS (Fig. 11). Blood leaving the MS moves outward through the MZ, a well-defined and finely meshed region of reticular meshwork surrounding the white pulp, which contains a large population of lymphocytes and other blood cells. Blood then moves into the red pulp, and joins blood that has entered the red pulp directly from arterial capillaries.

A 3-D view of the interrelationships in the human spleen, among lymphatic nodules, MS, MZ, and venous sinus network in the red pulp, may be obtained from microcorrosion casts (Fig. 12). In this figure, the nodule appears hollow, because the white pulp has been corroded away, and an opening in the MS represents the site where the central artery entered the nodule (the casts of the artery and follicular capillaries were broken off during processing). The reticular meshwork of the red pulp is unfilled, because of the small amount of material injected, although the network of venous sinuses and part of a collecting vein can be seen; the thickness of the MZ is not uniform around each nodule, but varies from 200 μm down to a narrow band in the region where two nodules are in close approximation.

The schematic diagram in Fig. 1 shows clearly that, before reaching lymphatic nodules, the central artery travels down the axis of a cylindrical sheath of lymphoid tissue, the PALS. The microcorrosion cast in Fig. 13 gives a 3-D view of the relationship between the PALS, the central artery, and the surrounding MZ and venous sinuses, which are incompletely filled (dog spleen). The artery bifurcates several times, giving rise to arterioles, which extend laterally beyond the PALS, and branch repeatedly, before ending as capillaries, either in the MS/MZ or within the red pulp itself. Many of the casts of the smallest vessels end blindly (Fig. 13, top left), indicating incomplete filling.

A cast of a lymphatic nodule with intact central artery and follicular capillaries is shown in Fig. 14 (dog spleen). These follicular capillaries terminate in ampullary dilatations that are continuous with the MS. The major arterioles, arising from the central artery, pass intact through both the MS and MZ, into the red pulp. Many of these arterioles then curve back toward the nodule, and branch to form an array of smaller arterioles (penicilli), which terminate as capillaries in the MS or MZ; other arterioles terminate some distance away in the red pulp (again, many arterial and venous vessels are incompletely filled in Fig. 14). There is strong evidence that the whole MS is filled by circumferential spreading of the injected material, before radial spreading occurs outwardly into the MZ, through fenestrations in the outer surface of the MS. This is shown particularly well in casts from spleens of dog (Fig. 14) and cat (Fig. 15); it is also seen in rat, mouse, and, to a lesser extent, in humans (Schmidt et al., 1985a,b; 1988). When a suitably small volume of casting material is injected, each nodule is surrounded

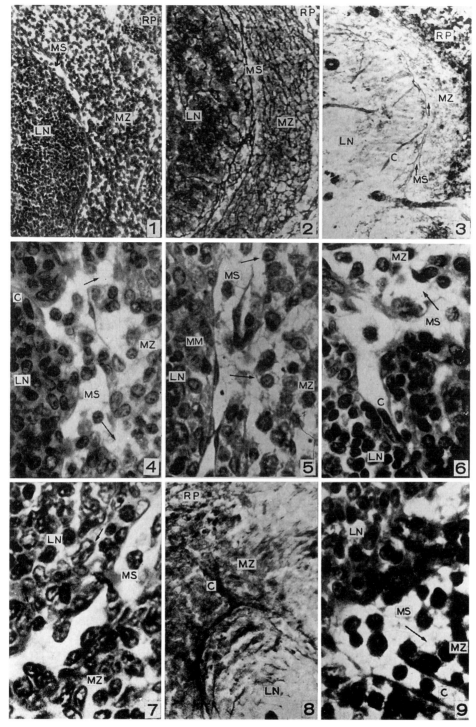

Fig. 3.11. Relationship among lymphatic nodule (LN), marginal sinus (MS), marginal zone (MZ), and red pulp (RP) in rat spleen, shown by histology. (**1**) Overview; hematoxylin and eosin stain (×160). (**2**) Reticular fiber network of MZ/MS; Snook's reticular stain (×240). (**3**) White pulp capillaries (C) emptying into MS (arrows); periodic acid-Schiff stain (×160). (**4**) MS showing pores (arrows) through which red blood cells pass into MZ; pyronin-methyl green stain (×650). (**5**) MS showing endothelial cells and pores (arrows); pyronin-methyl green stain (×650). (**6**) Ampullary ending of white pulp capillary. Pore (arrow) connects MS with interstices of MZ; pyronin-methyl green stain (×650). (**7**) Diapedesis of cell through inner lining of MS; arrows, nuclei of marginal metalophils; Giemsa stain (×700). (**8**) Capillary from white pulp traversing MZ; periodic acid-Schiff stain (×170). (**9**) Capillary from red pulp opening into MS; arrow, MS pore; H&E (×650). (Reproduced with permission from Snook, 1964).

by a thin, spherical annulus of material (<10 μm) sharply delineating the outer limits of the nodule, but not enclosing it completely (Fig. 15). In human spleen, the inner aspect of the MS casts adjoining the white pulp appears as a flattened, almost continuous system of anastomosing spaces (*see* Subheading 3.13.; Fig. 41A). We have consistently found that the MS is present in normal human spleens

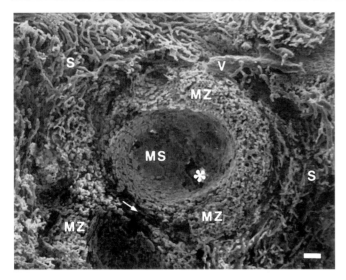

Fig. 3.12. Microcorrosion cast of normal human spleen showing relationship between lymphatic nodules (white pulp corroded away), marginal sinus (MS), marginal zone (MZ), and venous sinus network (S) in red pulp. Opening in MS (*) is site where central artery (cast accidentally broken off) entered nodule. In region where two nodules are close together, MZ is narrow (→). A collecting vein (V) has begun to fill. Bar = 100 μm. (Reproduced with permission from Schmidt et al., 1988).

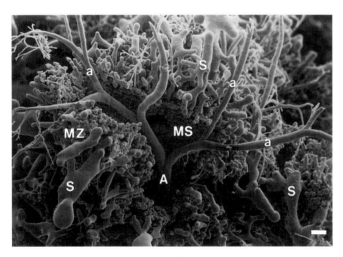

Fig. 3.13. Microcorrosion cast of dog spleen, showing central artery (A) passing down the axis of periarterial lymphatic sheath (with white pulp corroded away). Many arteriolar branches (a) extend through marginal sinus (MS) and marginal zone (MZ) into red pulp (incompletely filled). Many venous sinuses (S) originating in MS/MZ have begun to fill. Bar = 100 μm. (Reproduced with permission from Schmidt et al., 1983a).

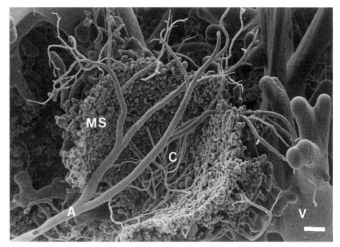

Fig. 3.14. Microcorrosion cast of dog spleen. Central artery (A) bifurcates repeatedly within lymphatic nodule, giving rise to follicular capillaries (C), ending in marginal sinus (MS), and to capillaries in red pulp (casts with blind ends, because of incomplete filling). Collecting veins (V) partially filled. Bar = 100 μm. (Reproduced with permission from Schmidt et al., 1983a).

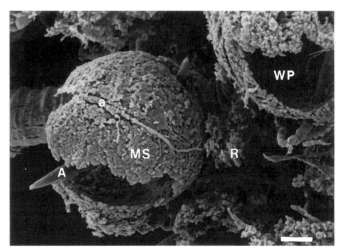

Fig. 3.15. Microcorrosion cast of cat spleen showing marginal sinus (MS) surrounding lymphatic nodule (white pulp [WP] corroded away). MS appears as a thin spherical annulus, because of circumferential spreading of injectate before outward radial spreading into marginal zone occurred. Arteriole (a) ramifies over convex surface of MS, before terminating there via capillaries. Branch of central artery (A) leaves the nodule. Reticular meshwork (R) has just begun to fill between the two nodules. Bar = 100 μm. (Reproduced with permission from Schmidt et al., 1983b).

obtained from organ transplant donors, but it is absent in certain diseases (*see* Subheading 3.13.; Fig. 41B). Few follicular capillaries terminate on the inner aspect of the MS: Perfusion occurs mainly through capillaries that terminate on the outer aspect facing the MZ.

Within some lymphatic nodules, the arteries are seen to branch many times over a very short distance, the branches remaining together as arteriolar–capillary bundles; after running parallel for some distance, these vessels fan out and terminate in the MZ (Snook, 1975; Schmidt et al., 1988). In many instances, however, the central artery continues to the margin of the nodule as a single vessel

and, at this point, branches repeatedly in the MZ, thereby giving rise to numerous circumferentially directed arterioles and capillaries, which terminate there (Fig. 16). From the MZ, blood enters the venous system through two routes: open-ended venous sinuses in continuity with the outer aspect of the MZ (*see* Subheading 3.9.), and a pathway of flow outward into the reticular meshwork of the red pulp, from where it enters venous sinuses through the IESs in sinus walls (*see* Subheading 3.9.).

An additional flow pathway bordering the white pulp is the perimarginal cavernous sinus (PMCS), discovered in the human spleen by Yamamoto et al. (1979), and in human, dog, and rat spleens by

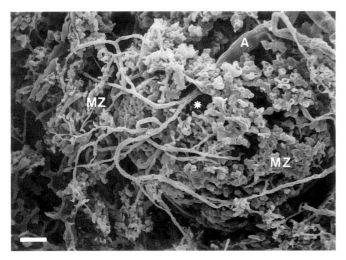

Fig. 3.16. Microcorrosion cast of normal human spleen. Central artery (A) passes to marginal zone (MZ) and, at this point (*), gives rise to numerous circumferentially directed arterioles and capillaries, most of which terminate there. Bar = 50 μm. (Reproduced with permission from Schmidt et al., 1988).

Schmidt et al. (1988, 1993). Using scanning electron microscopy of tissue, Yamamoto et al. showed the following:

1. The PMCS is a large blood space located between the MZ and the red pulp, except in areas where the MZ is not well developed, and the PMCS borders the white pulp directly.
2. The PMCS is lined by thin endothelial cells with flattened nuclei, in contrast to venous sinuses, in which the endothelial nuclei protrude into the lumen.
3. Sinuses of the PMCS plexus communicate with each other through narrow channels.
4. Many thin endothelial cells and their processes bridge opposite walls of the PMCS.
5. The PMCS communicates with the reticular meshwork of the MZ.

They were unable to elucidate the vascular connections between PMCS and other structures, but the microcorrosion casts obtained in our investigations (Schmidt et al., 1988, 1993) have provided 3-D views of the PMCS and its vascular connections. The following description is based on our findings in the human spleen.

The PMCS is different in appearance from any other structure in the casts. Large, flattened masses of casting material are seen, up to 300 × 1000 μm in area and 30–100 μm in thickness (Fig. 17A,B). The PMCS may be situated either outside the MZ or directly adjacent to the lymphatic nodule itself, in an area devoid of MS (Fig. 17A). The surface of the PMCS cast is smooth and flat, except for small pock-marks and shallow impressions (Fig. 17A–C). A considerable volume of casting material may reach the PMCS, even when minimal filling of adjacent reticular spaces is evident, as shown in Fig. 17A. Flow of material into the PMCS occurs through direct connections with arterial capillaries (Fig. 17C), via ellipsoid sheaths (Fig. 18A), and through points of continuity with the MZ (Fig. 18B). Drainage from the PMCS occurs directly into venous sinuses (Fig. 18C). Thus, the casts confirm Yamamoto's observations 1, 3, and 5 above, provide evidence consistent with 2 and 4, and furnish new information regarding the flow pathways into and out of the PMCS. The function of the PMCS is

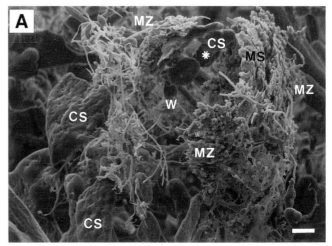

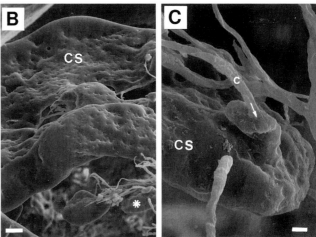

Fig. 3.17. Microcorrosion cast of normal human spleen. (**A**) Perimarginal cavernous sinus plexus (CS) appears as large, flattened masses, situated either directly adjacent to white pulp (*, in an area devoid of marginal sinus [MS]), or outside the marginal zone (MZ, at left of figure). W, white pulp corroded away; red pulp is unfilled. Bar = 10 μm. (**B**) Magnified view of perimarginal cavernous sinus (CS) from (a) (seen at different angle). Surface of CS is smooth and flat, except for small pockmarks and shallow impressions. (*, region shown at higher magnification in [c]). Bar = 50 μm. (**C**) Magnified view of perimarginal cavernous sinus (CS) from (B). Arterial capillary (C) connects directly to CS (→). A second capillary, at bottom of figure, is not continuous with CS cast. Bar = 10 μm. (Reproduced with permission from Schmidt et al., 1988.

not yet clear, but it may provide a route for lymphocyte migration into the white pulp. SEM micrographs of splenic tissue showed a great number of lymphocytes adhering to the wall of the PMCS, or in the process of passing through it into the white pulp (Yamamoto et al., 1979). The extension of PMCS into the white pulp, found in our microcorrosion casts, would presumably enhance this process.

We present a modified version of the schematic diagram shown at the start of this chapter (Fig. 1), which incorporates the new insights discussed above. The original schematic, although showing the general structure of the sinusal spleen, did not include any reference to microcirculatory pathways bordering the white pulp. It showed, incorrectly, that follicular capillaries terminate within the lymphatic nodule, and that all other vessels pass out substantial

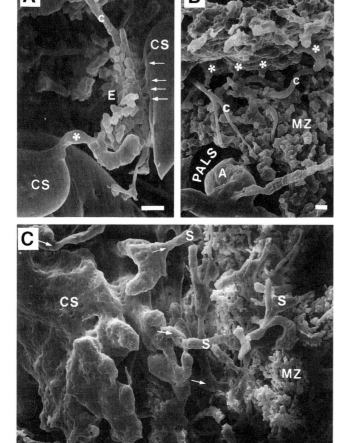

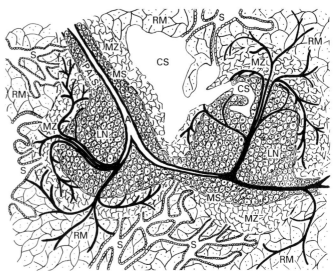

Fig. 3.18. Microcorrosion casts of normal human spleen. (**A**) Two separate areas of perimarginal cavernous sinus (CS) have begun to fill from an ellipsoid sheath (E), either via several small lateral channels (→) or via a larger channel continuous with one end of the CS (*). C, arterial capillary proximal to ellipsoid sheath. Bar = 20 μm. (**B**) Perimarginal cavernous sinus (CS) receives flow via numerous short, irregular channels (*) from the marginal zone (MZ) surrounding the periarterial lymphatic sheath (PALS). Several arterial capillaries (c) end in MZ. A, central artery. Bar = 20 μm. (**C**) Perimarginal cavernous sinus (CS) drains directly (→) into the interconnected system of venous sinuses (S) adjacent to marginal zone (MZ). Bar = 50 μm. (Reproduced with permission from Schmidt et al., 1988).

Fig. 3.19. Schematic diagram of microcirculatory pathways in and around the white pulp of normal human spleen, summarizing our findings. The central artery (A) passes through the periarterial lymphatic sheath (PALS) and lymphatic nodules (LN), giving rise to numerous arterioles and capillaries (shown in black). Directly bordering the white pulp is the marginal sinus (MS), consisting of a series of thin anastomosing vascular spaces. Surrounding the MS lies the marginal zone (MZ), in which the reticulum is more finely meshed than that of the reticular meshwork (RM) in the red pulp beyond. Abundant venous drainage is provided by anastomosing venous sinuses (S), most of which originate as open-ended vessels at the boundary between the MZ and RM. Some venous sinuses originate within the MZ itself, or at the MS. For simplicity, only a few representative regions of venous sinuses are shown, and capillary terminations in the RM are illustrated in separate areas of the figure. In reality, both the system of venous sinuses and the capillary terminations completely surround the MZ. The perimarginal cavernous sinus (CS), a plexus of large blood spaces, lies either between the MZ and RM or else adjacent to and extending into the white pulp. The CS receives flow principally from the MZ, and is drained by open-ended venous sinuses. After leaving the white pulp, numerous arterial capillaries curve circumferentially, and terminate at the outer aspect of the MS or within the MZ (or occasionally at the CS). Other capillaries extend out into the RM, and terminate in the meshwork itself; rarely, direct connections to venous sinuses are present. Many capillaries in the MZ and RM are surrounded by ellipsoid sheaths (not shown), before their terminations. (Reproduced with permission from Schmidt et al., 1993).

distances into the red pulp; the white pulp was shown as bordering directly on red pulp, and the venous drainage began some distance away in the red pulp. Current understanding of microcirculatory pathways bordering the white pulp in the normal human spleen is summarized in Fig. 19. Pathways in this region are of great importance, because animal studies have demonstrated that 90% of the arterial inflow to the spleen is distributed to the region bordering the white pulp (the fast pathway), whereas only ~10% passes through the reticular meshwork of the red pulp (the slow pathway) (Levesque and Groom, 1976a; Schmidt et al., 1993). This suggests that immunologic functions of the spleen take precedence over the filtration of blood cellular elements in the red pulp.

3.3.9. ENTRY OF BLOOD INTO VENOUS SINUSES Venous sinuses are widely believed to originate in the red pulp or MZ as

blind-ended sacs, and entry of blood into sinuses occurs exclusively through the IESs in their walls (Chen and Weiss, 1973; Leblond, 1973; Cho and DeBruyn, 1975; Barnhart and Lusher, 1976; Weiss et al., 1985; Fujita et al., 1985). This is represented schematically in Fig. 20. However, microcorrosion casts have revealed that there are two additional routes for blood flow into venous sinuses. First, many venous sinuses begin as open-ended tubes continuous with the MS or MZ, allowing free entry of blood into the venous system and bypassing the reticular meshwork of the red pulp. Such open-ended sinuses are abundant in all the sinusal spleens (dog, rat, and human) we have examined (Schmidt et al., 1983a, 1985a, 1988). Second, direct connections of arterial capillaries to venous sinuses exist (*see* Subheading 3.10.). Thus, blood enters the system of interconnected venous sinuses by three

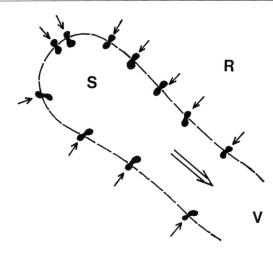

Fig. 3.20. Schematic diagram representing the traditional view that all venous sinuses originate in the marginal zone or red pulp as blind-ended sacs, and that entry of blood into sinuses occurs exclusively via interendothelial slits in their walls. R, reticular meshwork; S, venous sinus lumen; V, collecting vein; arrows indicate direction of flow. (Reproduced with permission from Groom and Schmidt, 1990).

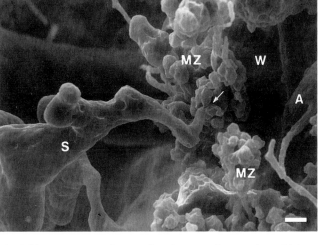

Fig. 3.22. Microcorrosion cast from human spleen (patient with lymphocytic leukemia) showing open-ended origin (→) of venous sinus (S) in marginal zone (MZ). Note lack of filling of reticular meshwork surrounding the sinus. A, central artery; W, white pulp corroded away. Bar = 20 μm. (Reproduced with permission from Schmidt et al., 1988).

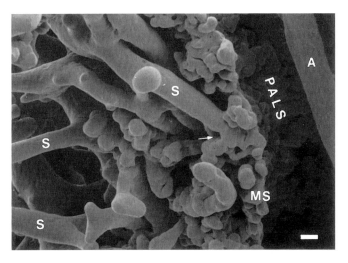

Fig. 3.21. Microcorrosion cast of dog spleen, showing interconnecting venous sinuses (S) originating in marginal sinus (MS) bordering periarterial lymphatic sheath (PALS). Note continuity (→) between MS and lumen of venous sinus, i.e., the sinus begins as an open-ended tube that has filled before any filling of the reticular meshwork occurred. A, central artery. Bar = 25 μm. (Reproduced with permission from Schmidt et al., 1983a).

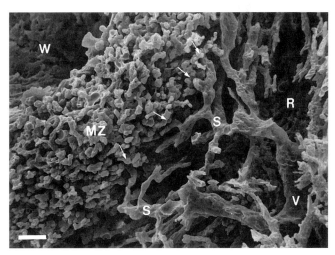

Fig. 3.23. Microcorrosion cast from normal human spleen, showing many venous sinuses (S) originating via open ends (→) in marginal zone (MZ). Note interconnected nature of venous sinus network, draining into collecting vein (V). W, white pulp corroded away; R, reticular meshwork of red pulp mostly unfilled. Bar = 50 μm. (Reproduced with permission from Schmidt et al., 1988).

different routes: open-ended sinuses, direct arteriovenous connections, and IES in sinus walls.

Many venous sinuses drain the region bordering the white pulp. In Fig. 21, open-ended venous sinuses, originating in the MS bordering the PALS are shown (dog spleen). The diameters of the regions of continuity are 20–25 μm, the same caliber as venous sinuses, and much larger than would be expected if flow into the sinuses were limited to channels the size of IES. In casts prepared by injection of only small amounts of material, there is no filling of reticular meshwork around most venous sinuses: The surfaces of the sinuses are bare and exposed. These sinuses could not have filled through the IESs in their walls. These same features in hu-

man spleen are shown in Fig. 22, where an open-ended venous sinus received its flow freely from the MZ surrounding a lymphatic nodule; this is demonstrated by the continuity that exists between the cast of the sinus (a cylinder at least 10 μm in diameter at its interface with the MZ) and the clusters of casting material representing the MZ. The abundance of such open-ended origins of venous sinuses is shown in Fig. 23 (human spleen). This particular cast demonstrates well the whole route for blood flow from the MS, through the meshwork of the MZ, into the interconnected system of venous sinuses by their open-ended origins, and from there into collecting veins. The quantity of material that has passed into the venous system indicates that the route provided by open-ended venous sinuses must be one of low resistance to flow, and represents a major part of the fast pathway through the spleen.

Demonstration of open-ended venous sinuses has been possible for the first time, because the modified microcorrosion casting technique selectively reveals the fast channels for flow, and allows them to be visualized three-dimensionally, in the absence of surrounding tissue. Based on SEM of tissue, Fujita and Kashimura (1983) showed the presence of a large window (approx 10 μm diameter) at the tapered end of a venous sinus in human spleen, which may correspond to the open-ended sinuses we have found. Microcorrosion casts also reveal that some venous sinuses do indeed originate as blind-ended sacs; casts made by venous retrograde injection of material show some well-filled sinuses with genuine blind ends completely covered with endothelial nuclear impressions, in contrast to the artifactual blind ends caused by incomplete filling with casting material (Fig. 21). The presence of open-ended venous sinuses explains how spleens injected with minimal quantities of casting material show filling of the venous system, without filling of the reticular meshwork surrounding venous sinuses.

That blood can enter venous sinuses by passing through the IES was demonstrated by earlier investigators using transmission and scanning electron microscopy: Fig. 24 is a TEM micrograph showing red blood cells caught in passage. Clearly, in this figure, the red blood cells are severely deformed in passing through the narrow IES. A comparable picture is presented in the SEM micrograph in Fig. 25, in which a 3-D view is obtained. The "heads" of the red blood cells are always on the luminal side of the sinus walls, and the "tails" on the side facing the reticular meshwork, which suggests that the direction of flow is into, not out of, the sinus. However, there has been no universal agreement about this (Chen and Weiss, 1973; Leblond, 1973; Cho and DeBruyn, 1975; Blue and Weiss, 1981a; Weiss et al., 1985; Fujita et al., 1985; compare also Pictet et al., 1969; Tischendorf, 1985). Studies of fixed splenic tissue cannot answer this question directly, nor can they address questions regarding the kinetics of red blood cell flow through the IES: For this, microscopy in vivo is necessary.

Videomicroscopy of transilluminated rat spleens in vivo (*see* Subheading 2.4.) has analyzed the kinetics of red blood cell passage through IES (MacDonald et al., 1987). The direction of red blood cell flow was invariably from reticular meshwork into venous sinuses, in normal spleens. Sequential photomicrographs of a red blood cell squeezing through an IES are shown in Fig. 26. The time-course can be seen from the stopwatch characters at the bottom left of each picture. The venous sinus (diameter 17 μm) runs vertically at the left of each micrograph, and is only partially shown (*see* schematic, Fig. 26C). Rapid flow of red blood cells within the lumen is seen only as a blur; to the right of the sinus wall are the reticular spaces of the red pulp, where numerous red blood cells are visible. Although the IES itself cannot be seen, the position and conformation of the red blood cell within it reveal its location. In Fig. 26A, one red blood cell has begun to emerge into the lumen of the venous sinus. Figure 26B shows it at the half-way point in its passage through the IES; in Fig. 26F, the red blood cell has passed into the lumen, but remains tethered by a long tail, which remains momentarily trapped by the IES, before the cell escapes completely, and is swept away by rapid flow in the lumen of the sinus.

The striking feature of the flow of red blood cells through the IES is that it occurs as a series of brief, discontinuous bursts separated by periods of zero, or near zero, flow (Fig. 27). Three factors could contribute to this pattern of flow: changes in pressure differ-

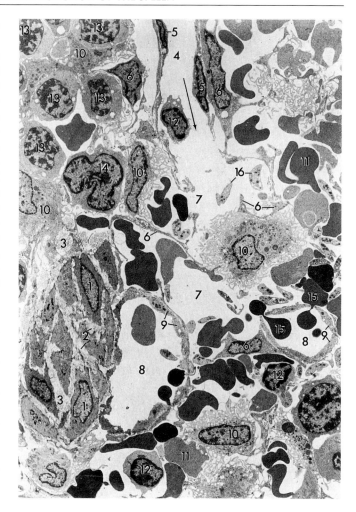

Fig. 3.24. TEM micrograph of rat spleen. 1, Smooth muscle cells of trabecula; 2, elastic fibers; 3, bundles of collagenous fibrils; 4, open termination of arterial capillary (→, direction of flow); 5, endothelial cells; 6, reticular cells; 7, interstitial space; 8, venous sinuses; 9, endothelial cells lining sinuses; 10, macrophages; 11, red blood cells; 12, small lymphocytes; 13, proerythroblasts; 14, lymphocyte; 15, red blood cells squeezing through interendothelial slits in sinus wall; 16, platelets, ×1650. (Reproduced with permission from Rhodin, 1974).

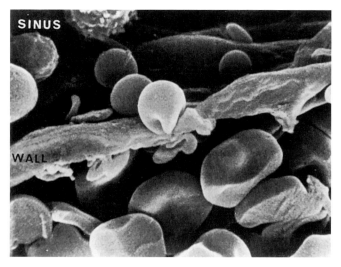

Fig. 3.25. SEM micrograph from rat spleen showing red blood cells squeezing through interendothelial slits in the wall of a venous sinus. (Reproduced with permission from Boisfleury and Mohandas, 1977).

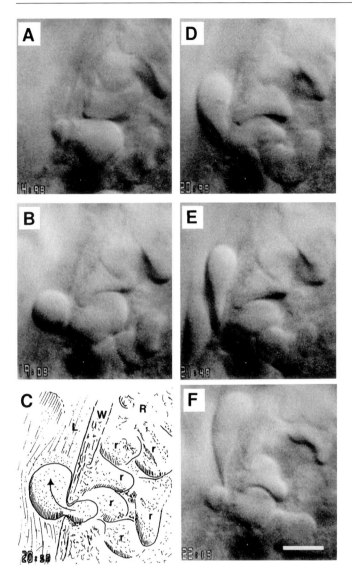

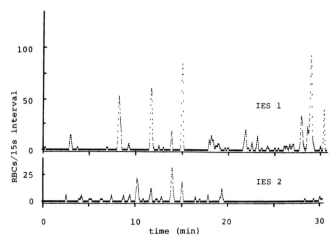

Fig. 3.27. Rate of red blood cell flow (red blood cells/15 s) through two closely adjacent interendothelial slits (IESs) in a venous sinus in rat spleen, measured simultaneously over a 30-min period by in vivo microscopy (*see* Fig. 26). Flow consisted of a series of brief, discontinuous bursts of red blood cells, separated by periods of zero, or near zero, flow (see text). (Reproduced with permission from MacDonald et al., 1987).

Fig. 3.26. Photomicrographs from videomicroscopy of transilluminated rat spleen in vivo. Sequential images of a red blood cell squeezing through an interendothelial slit in the wall of a venous sinus. Numbers in lower left corners give time in seconds and hundredths of a second. The venous sinus (diameter 17 μm) runs vertically at left of photos, and is only partially shown. The schematic (c) shows the locations of the sinus lumen (L), sinus wall (W), and numerous red blood cells (r) within the reticular spaces of the red pulp (R). Bar = 5 μm. (Reproduced with permission from MacDonald et al., 1987).

ence across the sinus wall, changes in supply of red blood cells to the reticular meshwork in the region of the IES, and changes in flow resistance at the IES itself. The first two factors would give rise to synchronous bursts of red blood cells through closely adjacent IES; the third would lead, in general, to asynchronous bursts of red blood cells. Analysis of red blood cell flow through two such IES, simultaneously, for 30 min, showed that most of the bursts were asynchronous (Fig. 27). Thus, changes in flow resistance of the IES itself were primarily responsible for the observed pattern of flow.

Examination of the videorecordings showed that temporary obstruction of IES by white cells or platelet aggregates was not a major cause of the changes in flow resistance, although such ob-

struction did occur occasionally. Therefore, the red blood cell bursts must have been caused by changes in the caliber of IESs themselves. Drenckhahn and Wagner (1986) demonstrated the contractility of microfilamentous bundles, running along either side of the IES, within the endothelial cells of the sinus wall, and suggested that such contractile activity might control the width of the IES. Our in vivo studies support this view: IES can be held closed for considerable periods of time, and only approx 20% of the total number of IES present anatomically allow passage of red blood cells during any 5-min period. The mean red blood cell flow rate per IES was 15 red blood cells/min for six active IES analyzed; the maximum instantaneous red blood cell flow rate was 10 red blood cells/s. The time required for a red blood cell to pass through an IES, varied greatly; even for a single IES it ranged from 0.02 to 60 s (MacDonald et al., 1987).

The view that all venous sinuses originate in the red pulp as blind sacs, into which blood enters solely through the IES in the sinus walls, is incorrect. Two additional routes for blood flow into venous sinuses exist, besides that involving IES: open-ended venous sinuses originating in the MS or MZ, which represent a major component of the fast pathway through the spleen; direct connections of arterial capillaries to venous sinuses, a route that is also part of the fast pathway (*see* Subheading 3.10.). The route for flow from the reticular meshwork into venous sinuses, through IESs in sinus walls, forms part of the slow pathway through the spleen.

3.3.10. SPLENIC MICROCIRCULATION: OPEN, OR BOTH OPEN AND CLOSED? The question of whether all blood passing through the spleen must flow through the reticular meshwork of the red pulp or MZ, in order to reach the venous system (open circulation), or whether some of the blood flows through direct connections of arterial capillaries to venous vessels, has been the subject of much controversy for almost a century (Weidenreich, 1901; Helly, 1902). The controversy came into sharp focus with the radically divergent results of Knisely (1936) and MacKenzie et al. (1941), both obtained by the same transillumination procedure. Similarly, studies of fixed splenic tissue or corrosion casts examined by light or electron microscopy have produced conflicting results. Most investigators, having failed to find evidence of direct arteriovenous pathways, have concluded that a closed circulation does not exist (human spleen: Irino et al., 1977; Suzuki et al., 1978; Weiss et al., 1985; Van Krieken et al., 1985; Fujita et al., 1985; sinusal spleens of dog, rat, rabbit: Snook, 1950; Lewis, 1957; Suzuki et al., 1977; Blue and Weiss, 1981d; nonsinusal spleens of cat, mouse: Snook, 1950; Lewis, 1957; Blue and Weiss, 1981b; Hataba et al., 1981). In contrast, Barnhart et al. (1976) found evidence of both open and closed pathways in human spleen; others have maintained that the circulation is entirely closed (human and other sinusal spleens: Tischendorf, 1969; Pictet et al., 1969; Miyamoto et al., 1980).

Why is there still controversy? The beautiful SEM micrographs of arterial capillary endings in the reticular meshwork (in dog), produced by Suzuki et al. (1977), and Irino et al. (1977) (in human) clearly demonstrate the existence of an open circulation. Such clear evidence has been lacking for closed circulation. Although many investigators have not found evidence for a closed circulation, one should not use the "argument from silence" to conclude that a closed circulation does not exist. Much of the evidence for a closed circulation has been unconvincing, often because of the rarity with which direct arteriovenous connections have been found. Recently, clear evidence of abundant connections of arterial capillaries to venous sinuses (as well as capillary endings in the reticular meshwork) was obtained (Schmidt et al., 1982) in dog spleen, by means of the microcorrosion casting procedure described in Subheading 2.3. Thus, in this species, both open and closed circulations exist. This is also the case in rat and human spleens (Schmidt et al., 1985a, 1988), although direct connections are less abundant than in the dog. In nonsinusal spleens, however, no direct connections of arterial capillaries to pulp venules were found (Schmidt et al., 1983b [cat]; 1985b [mouse]).

Evidence for open circulation is presented in Figs. 24 and 28–32. In TEM micrographs, arterial capillaries may sometimes be seen terminating in the reticular meshwork (Fig. 24), and 3-D views of such open terminations may be obtained by SEM. In Fig. 28, an arterial capillary terminates rather abruptly in the loose irregular meshwork of reticulum cells and their fibrous processes; such processes are fixed on the outer surface of the capillary, supporting the vessel. The transition from endothelial sheet to reticular meshwork is shown clearly in this figure. In microcorrosion casts, continuity of flow from capillary lumen to reticular meshwork may be seen. In the example from human spleen (Fig. 29) only a few of the interstices of the reticular meshwork have begun to fill; in Fig. 30 (cat spleen), entire pathways, from arterial capillary through the reticular meshwork to a pulp venule, are shown. The most direct route that we have found in a nonsinusal spleen, from arterial capillary to pulp venule, is shown in Fig. 31 (cat spleen); the distance through the reticular meshwork between the two vessels is merely 15–25 μm. Another part of the open circulation consists of flow through fenestrations in the capillary wall, radially outward into ellipsoid sheaths (the "periarterial macrophage sheaths" of Blue and Weiss, 1981a.) The interstices of ellipsoid sheaths are considerably smaller than those of the reticular meshwork, as may be seen from Fig. 32. Ellipsoid sheaths are usually found just before the termination of arterial capillaries, and they are thought to represent sites of filtration of particulate matter from the blood.

Evidence for a closed circulation is presented in Figs. 33–35. Abundant direct connections of arterial capillaries to venous sinuses

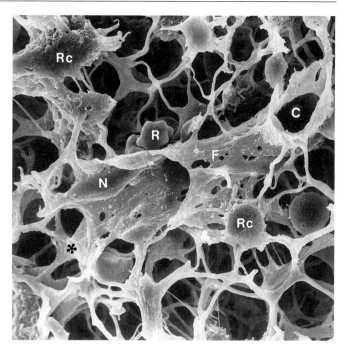

Fig. 3.28. SEM micrograph showing reticular meshwork in red pulp of dog spleen. Loose irregular 3-D network of reticulum cells (Rc) and their fibrous processes. Arterial capillary terminates abruptly in red pulp. Processes from reticulum cells are fixed on outer capillary surface supporting vessel. Note transition from endothelial sheet to reticular meshwork (*). C, capillary lumen; F, fenestration in capillary wall; N, nuclear elevation of endothelial cell; R, red blood cell. (×2850). (Reproduced with permission from Suzuki et al., 1977).

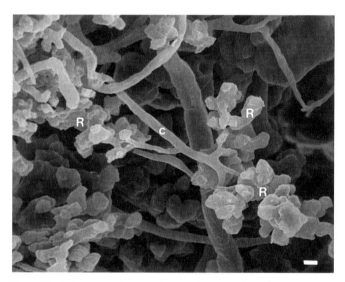

Fig. 3.29. Microcorrosion cast of normal human spleen showing arterial capillary (c) endings in reticular meshwork of the red pulp (R). Because of injection of only a small amount of material, the interstices of the reticular meshwork have barely begun to fill. Bar = 10 μm. (Reproduced with permission from Groom and Schmidt, 1990).

have been demonstrated in dog spleen, by means of the minimal-injection microcorrosion casting technique (*see* Subheading 2.3.). Typically, the terminal arteriole bifurcates repeatedly, to give rise to many short capillaries, each of which leads to one end of a venous sinus. This is shown in Fig. 33, in which at least 10 venous sinuses are fed from the same terminal arteriole. In this particular

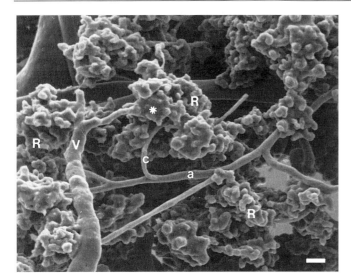

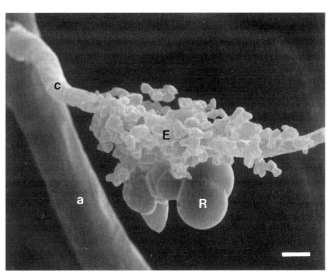

Fig. 3.30. Microcorrosion cast of cat spleen (nonsinusal). Large, slender arterial vessels (a) branch, forming capillaries (c), which end in reticular meshwork of the red pulp (R). Short pathway (*) through reticular meshwork connects capillary with pulp venule (V). Longer routes through reticular meshwork are unfilled (because of small amount of injectate). Bar = 50 μm. (Reproduced with permission from Goresky and Groom, 1984).

Fig. 3.32. Microcorrosion cast of dog spleen. Capillary branch (c) from arteriole (a) shows leakage pattern of casting material into ellipsoid sheath (E), and thence into surrounding reticular meshwork (R). Note that interstices of the ellipsoid sheath are considerably smaller than those of the reticular meshwork. Bar = 10 μm. (Reproduced with permission from Schmidt et al., 1983a).

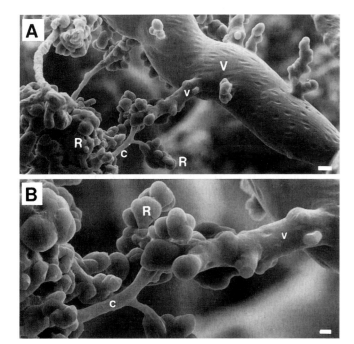

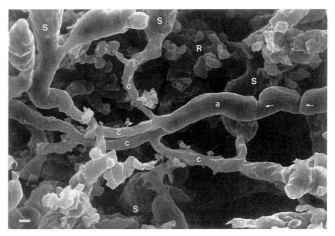

Fig. 3.33. Microcorrosion cast of dog spleen showing direct connections of arterial capillaries (c) to venous sinuses (S), i.e., closed circulation. Arteriole (a) entering from right is constricted in two places (arrows): Note endothelial nuclear impressions on this vessel. Vessel bifurcates repeatedly in quick succession, giving rise to many very short capillaries, each of which leads to one end of a venous sinus. Sinuses are only partially filled, because of very small amount of casting material injected; nevertheless, 10 venous sinuses are fed from this one terminal arteriole. Between sinuses, areas show start of reticular meshwork filling (R). Bar = 10 μm. (Reproduced with permission from Goresky and Groom, 1984).

Fig. 3.31. Microcorrosion cast of cat spleen (nonsinusal). (**A**) Arterial capillary (c) terminates in reticular meshwork (R), closely adjacent to pulp venule (v), which drains into collecting vein (V). Because of retrograde flow, material is beginning to emerge from fenestrations in pulp venule into reticular meshwork. Bar = 25 μm. (**B**) Close-up of area from (A) shows shortest route found between capillary ending and pulp venule. The forward (capillary, c) and retrograde (venular, v) flows have reached adjacent reticular spaces (R), but have not quite merged. Bar = 10 μm. (Reproduced with permission from Schmidt et al., 1983b).

example, the venous sinuses have just begun to fill; in Fig. 34, more extensive filling of some venous sinuses has occurred. In human spleen, direct connections of arterial capillaries to venous sinuses are fewer than in dog spleen (Schmidt et al., 1988). The overview in Fig. 35A shows several long capillaries, one giving off two short branches that terminate in adjacent venous sinuses, after approaching them from a radial direction. At higher magnification, it may be seen that the two short branches are indeed continuous with the sinuses (Fig. 35B,C). Direct connections also occur to the perimarginal cavernous sinus (*see* Subheading 3.8.). Although microcorrosion casts cannot demonstrate endothelial continuity between

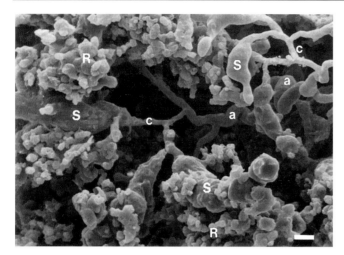

Fig. 3.34. Microcorrosion cast of dog spleen. More extensive filling of some venous sinuses has occurred in this cast than that shown in Fig. 33. Arterioles (a) connect via short capillary segments (c) directly to several venous sinuses (S). Little filling of the reticular meshwork of the red pulp (R) has occurred. Bar = 25 μm. (Reproduced with permission from Schmidt et al., 1983a).

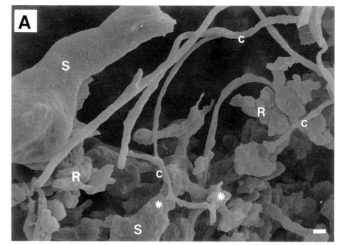

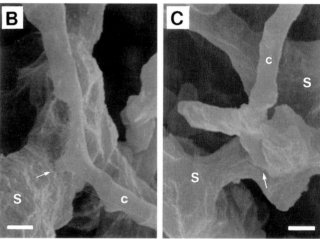

Fig. 3.35. Microcorrosion cast of normal human spleen. (**A**) Overview shows several long capillaries (c), one giving off two short branches that connect directly (*) to adjacent venous sinuses (S). Some filling of reticular meshwork (R) is seen. Bar = 10 μm. (**B** and **C**) Magnified views from (A) show continuity between capillary branches (C) and venous sinuses (→). Incomplete filling of capillary resulted from injection of only small amounts of casting material. Bars = 5 μm. (Reproduced with permission from Schmidt, 1988).

capillary and sinus, these results provide convincing evidence of direct connections. Furthermore, endothelial continuity has been demonstrated in chicken spleen by Miyamoto et al. (1980), and by Olah and Glick (1982).

The circulation in sinusal spleens appears to be primarily open, but a closed circulation also exists: The frequency of closed pathways differs among species. In nonsinusal spleens, closed pathways have not yet been demonstrated, and the circulation appears to be exclusively open.

3.3.11. SWITCHING OF MICROCIRCULATORY FLOW PATHS Studies of red blood cell washout from the spleen during Ringer perfusion (*see* Subheading 2.1.1.) have shown that, in the relaxed spleen, 90% of the inflowing blood travels to the splenic vein by fast pathways (cat: Song and Groom, 1971a), in the norepinephrine-contracted spleen, the proportion of the flow carried by fast pathways rises to 98.7% (Groom and Song, 1971). By contrast, when the spleen is dilated by perfusion against an elevated venous outflow pressure of 25 cm H₂O, the flow fraction carried by the fast pathways falls to zero (Levesque and Groom, 1980b). These results suggest that switching of flow between alternate paths can occur. Application of the microcorrosion casting technique (*see* Subheading 2.3.) under each of these conditions has allowed the morphology of the different pathways to be studied selectively.

In the contracted spleen of cat, the casts showed that flow occurred through short routes through the reticular meshwork, from capillary terminations to nearby venous vessels, as well as by short routes from MS or MZ to venous vessels. In addition, direct connections of arterial capillaries to venous sinuses were found in contracted spleens of dog. In dilated spleens, many more capillary terminations in the reticular meshwork of the red pulp were filled with casting material, but direct connections to venous sinuses were not filled. The picture that emerges is that flow through the reticular meshwork of the red pulp is minimized in contracted spleens, but predominates in dilated spleens.

What control mechanisms are responsible for this switching of flow pathways? One factor would be contraction of arteriolar smooth muscle, and, in spleens injected with norepinephrine, abun-

dant evidence of this is present. In the region where an arteriole becomes reduced to an arterial capillary, the contraction of discontinuous bands of vascular smooth muscle produces a series of constrictions, some of which appear as particularly narrow, deep impressions on the cast (Fig. 36A). An example of extreme arteriolar constriction is seen in Fig. 36B, in which the lumen is almost completely closed, and a fine thread of casting material, 4–5 μm in diameter, precariously supports the weight of the cast downstream. Because of the increased resistance to flow, the capillaries distal to the constrictions (Fig. 36A,B) are incompletely filled, and therefore appear to end blindly. Taken together with the minimal filling of the reticular meshwork in these casts, the results suggest a shunting of flow to the fast pathway.

Further control of blood flow could be mediated by strategically placed sphincters at the level of the venous sinuses. Knisely's (1936) transillumination studies suggested the presence of such sphincters at both the entrances and exits of venous sinuses, but conclusive morphological evidence of their existence has yet to be

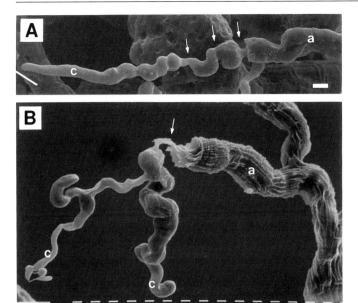

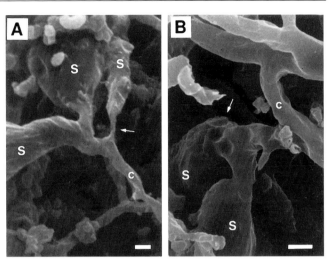

Fig. 3.36. (A) Microcorrosion cast of dog spleen contracted by injection of norepinephrine. In the region where an arteriole (a) becomes reduced to an arterial capillary (c), the contraction of discontinuous bands of vascular smooth muscle (corroded away) produces a series of constrictions, some of which appear as particularly narrow, deep impressions on the cast (→). Bar = 15 μm. (B) Microcorrosion cast of cat spleen contracted by norepinephrine, showing extremely constricted region (→) in an arteriole (a), just before it branches into two capillaries (c). Only a fine thread of material supports the cast downstream. Casts of capillaries end blindly, because of incomplete filling due to the increased resistance to flow at the constriction. Bar = 10 μm. (Reproduced with permission from Schmidt et al., 1983c).

Fig. 3.37. Microcorrosion casts of dog spleen, showing possible sites for control of flow from arterial capillaries (c) directly into venous sinuses (S). (A) Extreme narrowing of the neck (→) leading to one venous sinus is seen; the entrances to two adjacent sinuses are more widely open. Bar = 10 μm. (B) A ring of impressions (→), possibly made by endothelial cell nuclei, is seen around the entrance to a venous sinus (i.e., where the localized constriction was found in [A]). This figure is a high magnification view of a region in Fig. 33. Bar = 10 μm. (Reproduced with permission from Schmidt et al., 1982).

obtained. Several observations from microcorrosion casts also suggest that constrictions (perhaps temporary) at the two ends of the venous sinuses may play a part in controlling flow. An extreme narrowing of the neck leading to a venous sinus is sometimes seen (Fig. 37A), and a ring of impressions, probably made by endothelial cell nuclei, often occurs around the entrance to a sinus (Fig. 37B). Such narrowings and impressions could conceivably be the result of the contraction of specialized endothelial cells, as seen in other tissues (Lubbers et al., 1979; Weigelt, 1982), as well as in spleen (Drenckhahn and Wagner, 1986). Recent evidence, obtained by in vivo microscopy suggests that endothelial contractility may also modify red blood cell flow at the arterial capillary level in the spleen (Ragan et al., 1988). Spontaneous cyclic contractions of the capillary wall (Fig. 38) were quantitatively analyzed in relaxed spleens (rat, mouse), and it was found that during 50% of the contractions luminal diameter was reduced to less than 1 μm, stopping red blood cell flow in that capillary. Regression analysis showed that the vessel narrowing primarily resulted from bulging of endothelial cells into the lumen, and not from bulging of pericytes or closure caused by changes in transmural pressure. Reduction of flow in such arterial capillaries would decrease red blood cell supply to the reticular meshwork.

Results from kinetic and morphological studies show that redistribution of intrasplenic blood flow can occur, away from the slow pathways of the reticular meshwork, to the fast pathways described earlier (*see* Subheading 3.1.), and vice versa. The functional significance of this switching of microcirculatory flow paths is not yet

clear, but a reduction in flow through the reticular meshwork would presumably reduce the filtration of abnormal red blood cells by the spleen.

3.3.12. MECHANISMS OF RED BLOOD CELL CONCENTRATION IN SPLEEN

In dogs, the hemoglobin concentration of splenic blood is much higher than that of peripheral blood (Barcroft and Poole, 1927; Kramer and Luft, 1951). More recently, measurements on blood drained from excised dog spleens, contracting under electrical stimulation, have shown the hematocrit to be as high as 90% (Opdyke and Apostolico, 1966). These observations confirm the impression gained from histological sections, that the red pulp is packed with red blood cells in all species studied.

What is the mechanism of red blood cell concentration that gives rise to such a high hematocrit in the red pulp? From in vivo studies of the transilluminated spleens of mouse, rat, and cat, Knisely (1936) suggested that hemoconcentration was a function of venous sinuses. He claimed that the actions of afferent and efferent sinus sphincters caused the sinuses to fill with blood, then allowed plasma to drain out through fenestrations in their walls: This resulted in sinuses filled with packed red blood cells, which could be discharged into the venous outflow. However, other investigators were unable to confirm this mechanism (MacKenzie et al., 1941; McCuskey and McCuskey, 1977). Furthermore, the spleens of cat and mouse are nonsinusal (Snook, 1950): Their pulp venules are different from venous sinuses (*see* Subheading 3.7.). Yet, despite the absence of venous sinuses, such spleens as those of cat, mouse, and many other mammalian species also develop hematocrits of twice the arterial value. Consequently, the primary mechanism of red blood cell concentration must be independent of the presence of venous sinuses.

Other explanations for the red blood cell concentration mechanism have been proposed. The earliest of all was that filtration of fluid occurs from blood into splenic lymphatic vessels, the red blood cells remaining in the pulp spaces: This separation was thought to require splenic innervation (Barcroft and Poole, 1927; Barcroft

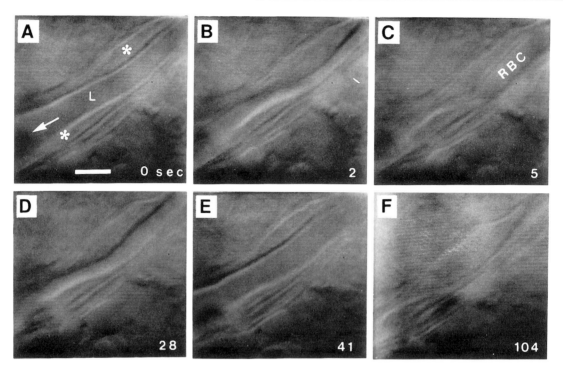

Fig. 3.38. Sequential photomicrographs of a capillary wall contracting spontaneously in rat spleen, viewed by in vivo videomicroscopy. L, lumen; ←, direction of flow; *, endothelial cells. Photos (**A–E**) were taken during a single cycle of contraction/relaxation; (**F**) came from a subsequent cycle. Elapsed time intervals (s) from view (A) are shown in each lower right corner. In (C), bulging of both endothelial cells into the lumen is seen, impeding red blood cell flow; a red blood cell (RBC) became trapped at the constriction for >20 s. In (F) the luminal width was reduced to zero. In (A,B,D, and E) the velocity of blood flow was so high that the images of red blood cells are blurred, and individual cells are not seen. Bar = 5 μm. (Reproduced with permission from Ragan et al., 1988).

and Florey, 1928). However, Greenway (1979) showed that red blood cell concentration could occur in the absence of splenic innervation, and that plasma was separated from red blood cells, even when the lymphatic outflow was occluded. Another explanation was that, in terminal arterioles and arterial capillaries, narrowing of the lumen, resulting from slight constriction in the presence of a high endothelium, causes plasma to be passed on, but red blood cells are retained (Weiss, 1962). However, the total volume of the splenic arterial circulation is undoubtedly too small to accommodate the volume of red blood cells known to be sequestered. Weiss (1962) has also suggested that plasma skimming, because of the large branching angles in the splenic arterial tree, may contribute to red blood cell concentration. This mechanism suffers from the same drawback as the previous explanation. None of the above mechanisms has been adequate to explain red blood cell concentration in the spleen.

The key microcirculatory feature, which is the common denominator of both sinusal and nonsinusal spleens, is the reticular meshwork, which is interposed between the capillary endings and the start of the venous channels, forming an intermediate circulation. This arrangement, which is unique to the spleen, is shown schematically in Fig. 39. The high intrasplenic hematocrit has recently been demonstrated to be a rheological consequence of red blood cell flow through the reticular meshwork, and is merely a side effect of the mechanisms for filtration of abnormal red blood cells (MacDonald et al., 1991). The meshwork of reticular cells and fibers gives rise to an interconnected system of short irregular

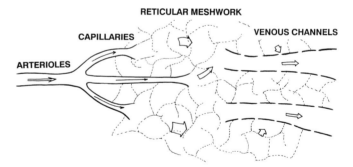

Fig. 3.39. Schematic diagram showing unique arrangement of the splenic microcirculation. Much of the blood percolates through a reticular meshwork interposed between capillary endings and the start of venous channels (fenestrated). This meshwork presents an enormous contact surface area for red blood cells, and its large total cross-sectional area for flow results in very low blood velocities. (Reproduced with permission from MacDonald et al., 1991).

channels, different from the usual arrangement of walled vessels present in other organs (analogous to the gas filter in an automobile). The pore size of the reticular meshwork is several red blood cell diameters, too large to impede flow on the basis of cell deformability. However, the meshwork presents an enormous contact surface area for blood cells, and its large cross-sectional area for flow results in low red blood cell velocities (mean: 7 μm/s). As a consequence of the resulting low shear rates, immature and abnormal red blood cells adhere to the meshwork, and no longer circulate. Normal red blood cells adhere repeatedly, but transiently, analogous to the repeated adsorptions of gas molecules, which take place when a gas mixture flows through a gas chromatograph column. Thus, the mean red blood cell velocity through the reticular meshwork falls below that of plasma, and the hematocrit must rise, in consequence. This follows from the law of conservation of mass, and is the inverse of the Fahraeus-Lindqvist effect, whereby red blood cells move toward the axis of flow when blood flows through narrow tubes, and, with the mean velocity of red blood cells greater than that of plasma, the tube hematocrit falls below that of the inflowing and outflowing blood. In vivo videomicroscopic analysis of the movements of individual red blood cells through the splenic reticular meshwork has confirmed that mean red blood cell velocities are only 20–40% of the corresponding plasma velocities (MacDonald et al., 1991). As a biophysical consequence, intrasplenic hematocrit rises up to twice that of arterial blood.

IESs in venous sinus walls provide an additional mechanism of red blood cell filtration, by sequestering cells that have reduced deformability. However, since such slits are present in spleens of only 50% of mammalian species, and the high hematocrit exists in all species examined, the role of IESs in red blood cell filtration appears to be secondary to the role of the reticular meshwork. The presence of ellipsoid sheaths in some species provides yet another site for filtration of the blood. The human spleen possesses both venous sinuses and ellipsoids, in addition to the reticular meshwork, giving it every advantage for its task of filtering the cellular elements of the blood.

Blood "doping" in athletes is a recent innovation, but, in some mammalian species, the expulsion of high hematocrit intrasplenic blood, in order to raise the O_2-carrying capacity of peripheral blood, is an effective physiological mechanism. Spleens of such species as horse, dog, cat, and diving seal are very contractile, and serve as a reservoir of blood at high hematocrit. In times of "fight or flight," splenic contraction transfers blood from the reservoir into the circulation, and the splenic filtration function is put on hold, since all blood flows via the fast pathways in contracted spleens, until the organ relaxes again. In the human spleen, this reservoir function appears to be lacking, and the high intrasplenic hematocrit remains unexploited.

Pooling of platelets occurs in the spleen. Intravenous injection of epinephrine in dogs causes an immediate, but transient, increase in the platelet count of peripheral blood, which does not occur following splenectomy (Binet and Kaplan, 1923). In humans, platelet pooling also occurs (Branehog et al., 1973), and young platelets are preferentially retained in the spleen (Watson and Ludlam, 1986), probably undergoing late maturation, analogous to that shown to occur for reticulocytes (Song and Groom, 1972). The exchangeable platelet pool in the human spleen has been estimated as one-third of the total number of circulating platelets in the body (Shulman and Jordan, 1987), but how this comes about is unknown. Based on our findings regarding the mechanism of red blood cell concentration in the spleen, we hypothesize that normal platelets also adhere transiently to the reticular meshwork, giving rise to an inverse Fahraeus effect and a massive concentration of platelets in the spleen.

3.3.13. DIFFERENCES BETWEEN MICROCIRCULATORY PATHWAYS IN NORMAL HUMAN SPLEEN AND THOSE IN OTHER SPECIES: CHANGES IN DISEASE Confusion regarding microcirculatory pathways in normal human spleen has arisen in the past, because of extrapolations from pathological samples and from spleens of other mammalian species. In addition, it has been difficult to trace 3-D routes for blood flow simply from the study of thin sections or cut surfaces of tissue. More recently, however, flow pathways have been studied in normal human spleens from organ transplant donors (Schmidt et al., 1988), using the minimal-injection microcorrosion casting technique described in Subheading 2.3., and compared with results from other species (Schmidt et al., 1982; 1983a,b; 1985a,b; 1993). These studies show that, in mammals, there appears to be a basic common pattern of splenic microcirculatory pathways; however, many species differences are found, in terms of the pattern of arterial branching, the configuration of the MS, the presence or absence of ellipsoid sheaths or perimarginal cavernous sinus, the presence of venous sinuses or pulp venules, and the frequency of direct arteriovenous connections. A brief summary of some of the differences between microcirculatory pathways in normal spleens of humans and other species is therefore presented next.

The degree of arterial branching in human spleen is much greater than that found in other species, and the peculiar branching that forms arteriolar-capillary bundles within lymphatic nodules has been reported only for human and monkey spleens. Other characteristics of the arterial branching in human spleen are the presence of many arterioles curving within the MZ around lymphatic nodules, like fingers grasping a ball: This is similar to the arrangement in dog spleen, but differs from that of the rat and mouse. In addition, most follicular capillaries do not originate from branches of the central artery within the nodule, but from arterioles in the MZ. Ellipsoid sheaths, which are not present in all species (such as rat and mouse) are present in human spleen. These may be sites where filtration of the blood occurs, but they are certainly not the primary site, although this was implied by Van Krieken et al. (1985a).

The existence of the MS around lymphatic nodules has been confirmed in normal human spleens (*see* Subheading 3.8.); however, species differences exist with respect to its 3-D configuration. In human spleen, the inner aspect of the MS adjoining the white pulp appears in microcorrosion casts as a flattened, almost continuous system of anastomosing spaces, similar to those in the dog spleen, but different from the small discontinuous spaces found in spleens of rat and mouse. The blood supply to the MS in humans comes primarily from capillaries that end on its outer aspect facing the MZ; in many other species, the blood supply comes from follicular capillaries terminating on the inner aspect of the MS. The perimarginal cavernous sinus plexus (PMCS), a large blood space, usually bordering the white pulp, has been identified only in human, dog, and rat spleens, to date (Yamamoto et al., 1979; Schmidt et al., 1988, 1993). At present, the role of the PMCS is poorly understood.

The rarity with which direct connections of arterial capillaries to venous sinuses occur in human spleen (*see* Subheading 3.10.) is in marked contrast to the abundance of such connections in dog spleen. Direct arteriovenous connections appear to be absent from nonsinusal spleens. Thus, there exists great variability among species with respect to the closed circulation, and extrapolations from animals to man are not valid. A major component of the fast pathway for blood flow through sinusal spleens is abundant, open-ended venous sinuses beginning in the MZ. Such open-ended sinuses are a prominent feature in microcorrosion casts of human spleens, as well as those of dog and rat. Flow by this route bypasses the reticular meshwork of the red pulp and IESs in sinus walls, where filtration of red blood cells occurs.

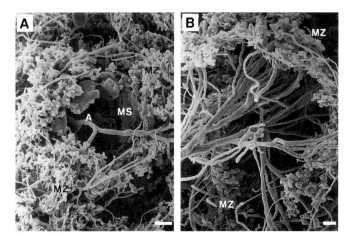

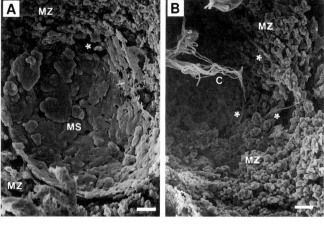

Fig. 3.40. (**A**) Microcorrosion cast from normal human spleen, showing 3-D relationship between the arterial tree (A), a lymphatic nodule (white pulp corroded away), and the surrounding MS and MZ. Note sparcity of vessels within the nodule, typical of normal spleens. Bar = 50 μm. (**B**) Splenic cast from patient with idiopathic thrombocytopenia, showing great proliferation of arterioles and capillaries within lymphatic nodule. Most of these vessels pass out into the surrounding MZ. MS is absent. Bar = 50 μm. (Reproduced with permission from Schmidt et al., 1991).

Fig. 3.41. (**A**) Microcorrosion cast from normal human spleen. MS consists of flattened, anastomosing vascular spaces between lymphatic nodule and MZ. Note sheetlike appearance of MS vs knobbly configuration of MZ. One region of MS is fragmented (→) as a result of incomplete filling. The opening in MS (*) is the site where the central artery (cast accidentally broken off) entered nodule. Bar = 50 μm. (**B**) Splenic cast from patient with idiopathic thrombocytopenia. Note absence of MS; the MZ borders lymphatic nodule. Several capillaries (*) terminate in MZ. C, follicular capillaries, incompletely filled. Bar = 50 μm. (Reproduced with permission from Schmidt et al., 1991).

In order to explore whether changes in splenic microcirculatory pathways occur with disease, microcorrosion casts of spleens surgically removed from patients with idiopathic thrombocytopenic purpura (ITP) have been compared with those of normal human spleens from transplant donors. Two changes were found consistently (Schmidt et al., 1991). First, a striking proliferation of arterioles and capillaries was found in the white pulp and MZ. The cast in Fig. 40A shows a sparcity of vessels within a lymphatic nodule, typical of normal spleens. In contrast, a cast from a patient with ITP (Fig. 40B) shows a profusion of small vessels branching from the central artery within the nodule, and passing outward into the surrounding MZ. Second, the MS was absent in ITP. Casts from normal spleens show the MS as a very distinct entity, consisting of a series of flattened, anastomosing vascular spaces lying between the white pulp and the MZ (Fig. 41A). In contrast, casts from ITP spleens consistently lacked an MS, except for small isolated patches found infrequently. In Fig. 41B, the cast bordering the region formerly occupied by a lymphatic nodule has the knobbly appearance characteristic of MZ filling. Comparison of 224 nodules from 8 normal spleens and 191 nodules from 7 ITP spleens showed that these changes occurred with remarkable consistency. Extensive proliferation of vessels was found in 92.3% of lymphatic nodules in ITP spleens, compared with 0.6% in normal spleens. The MS was absent in 89.4% of nodules in ITP spleens, compared with 4.9% in normal spleens (Schmidt et al., 1991).

The causes of these changes and their functional implications are not yet understood. However, the absence of the MS could have significant consequences. Distribution of blood flow to the MZ would become less uniform, producing areas of low flow, and causing platelets and other blood cells to spend increased time in the proximity of splenic macrophages. This change, along with the presence of high concentrations of antiplatelet antibody, could

lead to the accelerated destruction of platelets that is characteristic of ITP. In addition, preliminary evidence indicates that similar vascular hyperplasia and loss of the MS also occur in hypersplenism and chronic lymphocytic leukemia (Schmidt et al., 1991). Thus, these changes may not be specific to ITP, but could be a reflection of lymphoid hyperplasia, which occurs in several disorders. Clearly, conclusions regarding microcirculatory pathways in normal human spleen should not be based on material obtained from diseased subjects.

3.4. OVERVIEW OF CURRENT UNDERSTANDING OF MICROCIRCULATORY BLOOD FLOW IN THE HUMAN SPLEEN

Studies of the distribution of intrasplenic blood flow and the morphology of the microcirculatory pathways, using the methods described in Subheading 3.2., have provided much new information, which has led to a revision of some commonly accepted concepts of the splenic microcirculation in humans. A number of key issues have already been focused on in detail (*see* Subheading 3.3.), and at this point an overview is presented. The modified version (Fig. 19) of the schematic diagram shown at the start of this chapter (Fig. 1) incorporates the new insights obtained regarding the intermediate circulation between arterial capillaries and the venous channels.

In the normal human spleen, a MS, 5–10 μm thick, lies directly adjacent to the white pulp. It consists of a series of cleft-like, anastomosing, vascular spaces between the white pulp and the surrounding MZ, and receives a plentiful blood supply from capillaries terminating on its outer aspect. These vessels are derived from branches of the central artery, which curve circumferentially within the MZ. Microcorrosion casts show that the MS fills preferentially, before filling of the MZ and surrounding red pulp. A uniform distribution of blood from MS to MZ is provided, through discontinuities in the outer wall of the MS; in addition, the MZ receives a substantial blood supply from arterial capillaries that terminate within its reticular meshwork. In the white pulp, relatively few capillaries are found, and these originate either from the central artery or from vessels in the MZ. Capillaries do not terminate in an open fashion within the reticulum of the white pulp.

From the MZ, a large proportion of the blood flows into the perimarginal cavernous sinus, or into open-ended venous sinuses originating there; a small portion flows radially outward from the MZ into the reticular meshwork of the red pulp. The perimarginal cavernous sinus is a very large blood space situated either directly adjacent to the white pulp or between the MZ and the red pulp. It receives blood from direct connections with arterial capillaries, through ellipsoid sheaths, and via points of continuity with the MZ. Perimarginal cavernous sinus blood drains directly into open-ended venous sinuses.

The traditional view has been that venous sinuses begin in the red pulp as blind-ended sacs; blood can enter them, on its way from the reticular meshwork to venous outflow, only by passing through IESs in sinus walls. However, microcorrosion casts have revealed that many venous sinuses begin as open-ended tubes continuous with the MZ (or, in some instances, the MS), allowing free entry of blood into the venous system and bypassing both the reticular meshwork of the red pulp and the IESs in venous sinus walls. The extensive filling of venous sinuses, seen in microcorrosion casts prepared by injection of very small amounts of material, occurs even when the surrounding reticular meshwork is completely unfilled. This indicates that most of the flow enters the interconnected network of venous sinuses through their open ends in the MZ. This route forms a major component of the fast pathway for blood flow through the spleen.

Another component of the fast pathway is provided by direct connections of arterial capillaries to venous sinuses (closed circulation). Such routes seem to be rare in human spleen, where most of the arterial capillaries in the red pulp terminate in the reticular meshwork (open circulation). Ellipsoid sheaths surround many of these capillaries, as well as those ending in the MZ, a short distance before the vessel terminations. Flow can occur through fenestrations in the capillary wall, radiating outward into ellipsoid sheaths, and on into the reticular meshwork.

All blood entering the reticular meshwork of the red pulp, by the various routes just described, must pass through IESs in walls of venous sinuses, in order to reach the venous outflow. In vivo videomicroscopy of rat spleen showed that red blood cell flow through individual IESs occurs as a series of brief, discontinuous bursts separated by periods of zero, or near zero, flow. This behavior is caused primarily by changes in caliber of the IESs themselves, mediated by contraction of sinus endothelial cells. Contrary to the impression gained from SEM showing all IESs widely open, in vivo microscopy showed that only approx 20% of the total number of slits present anatomically allow passage of red blood cells during any particular 5-min period. Because of this, the weighted average flow rate per interendothelial slit is only three red blood cells/min. These results from rat spleen provide the only information presently available with respect to the flow rates that might be expected through IESs in human spleen.

The reticular meshwork of the red pulp gives rise to the slow pathways for flow through the spleen, and it is here that filtration

of immature and abnormal red blood cells and the concentration of normal red blood cells to a hematocrit of approx 80% take place. However, only 10% of the total splenic inflow travels through these slow pathways, during a single pass through the organ; 90% travels via fast pathways that bypass the reticular meshwork. This raises the question: Since the spleen represents the only lymphatic tissue specialized to filter the blood, why should 90% of the arterial inflow bypass the sites where filtration is carried out? The answer may lie in the fact that most of the blood in the fast pathways passes into the MS, where it is spread widely over the surface of the white pulp, before being evenly distributed to the MZ, and thereby, migration of lymphocytes and macrophages into lymphatic nodules would be facilitated, as well as immunological interactions within the MZ. The proportions of the inflowing blood, following the fast vs slow pathways (90 vs 10%), support the view that the spleen's primary function is immunologic, and that filtration in the red pulp is a secondary function.

ACKNOWLEDGMENTS

Our research was supported by a grant from the Medical Research Council of Canada.

REFERENCES

Andrew, W. (1946) Age changes in the vascular architecture and cell content in the spleens of 100 Wistar Institute rats, including comparison with human material. *Am. J. Anat.* **79**, 1–73.

Barcroft, J. and Florey, H.W. (1928) Some factors involved in the concentration of blood by the spleen. *J. Physiol. (London)* **60**, 231–234.

Barcroft, J. and Poole, L. T. (1927) The blood in the spleen pulp. *J. Physiol. (London)* **64**, 23–29.

Barnhart, M. I., Baechler, C. A., and Lusher, J. M. (1976) Arteriovenous shunts in the human spleen. *Am. J. Hematol.* **1**, 105–114.

Barnhart, M. I. and Lusher, J. M. (1976) The human spleen as revealed by scanning electron microscopy. *Am. J. Hematol.* **1**, 243–264.

Barnhart, M. I. and Lusher, J. M. (1979) Structural physiology of the human spleen. *Am. J. Pediatr. Hematol. Oncol.* **1**, 311–330.

Bellanti, J. A. (1979) *Immunology: Basic Processes*. Saunders, Philadelphia.

Binet, L. and Kaplan, M. (1923) Mobilisation des plaquettes par l'adrenaline. Plaquettose par spleno-contraction adrenalinique. *C.R. Soc. Biol.* **97**, 1659–1660.

Blue, J. and Weiss, L. (1981a) Periarterial macrophage sheaths (ellipsoids) in cat spleen—an electron microscope study. *Am. J. Anat.* **161**, 115–134.

Blue, J. and Weiss, L. (1981b) Vascular pathways in nonsinusal red pulp —an electron microscope study of the cat spleen. *Am. J. Anat.* **161**, 135–168.

Blue, J. and Weiss, L. (1981c) Species variation in the structure and function of the marginal zone: an electron microscope study of cat spleen. *Am. J. Anat.* **161**, 169–187.

Blue, J. and Weiss, L. (1981d) Electron microscopy of the red pulp of the dog spleen including vascular arrangements, periarterial macrophage sheaths (ellipsoids), and the contractile, innervated reticular meshwork. *Am. J. Anat.* **161**, 189–218.

Boisfleury, A. De, and Mohandas, N. (1977) Antibody-induced spherocytic anemia. II. Splenic passage and sequestration of red cells. *Blood Cells* **3**, 197–208.

Bowden, T. J. (1978) Storage and transit of red blood cells in skeletal muscle of the cat (PhD thesis). University of Western Ontario, London, ON.

Bowdler, A. J. and Videbaek, A. (1990) Splenic pooling and the survival of blood cells. In: *The Spleen: Structure, Function and Clinical Significance* (Bowdler, A. J., ed.), Chapman and Hall, London, pp. 167–190.

Branehög, I., Weinfeld, A., and Roos, B. (1973) The exchangeable splenic platelet pool studied with epinephrine infusion in idiopathic thrombocytopenic purpura and in patients with splenomegaly. *Br. J. Haematol.* **25,** 239–248.

Bussel, J. B. (1990) Autoimmune thrombocytopenic purpura. *Hematol. Oncol. Clin. North Am.* **4,** 179–191.

Chen, L. T. (1980) Intrasplenic microcirculation in rats with acute hemolytic anemia. *Blood* **56,** 737–740.

Chen, L. T. and Weiss, L. (1973) The role of the sinus wall in the passage of erythrocytes through the spleen. *Blood* **41,** 529–537.

Cho, Y. and DeBruyn, P. P. H. (1975) Passage of red blood cells through the sinusoidal wall of the spleen. *Am. J. Anat.* **142,** 91–106.

Cilento, E. V., McCuskey, R. S., Reilly, F. D., and Meineke, H. A. (1980) Compartmental analysis of circulation of erythrocytes through the rat spleen. *Am. J. Physiol.* **239,** (*Heart Circ. Physiol.* **8**), H272–H277.

Crosby, W. H. (1977) Splenic remodeling of red cell surfaces. *Blood* **50,** 643–645.

Davies, B. N. and Withrington, P. G. (1973) The action of drugs on the smooth muscle of the capsule and blood vessels of the spleen. *Pharmacol. Rev.* **25,** 373–412.

Dintenfass, L. and Burnard, E. (1966) Effect of hydrogen ion concentration on *in vitro* viscosity of packed red cells and blood at high hematocrits. *Med. J. Aust.* **1,** 1072–1074.

Drenckhahn, D. and Wagner, J. (1986) Stress fibers in the splenic sinus endothelium *in situ*: Molecular structure, relationship to the extracellular matrix, and contractility. *J. Cell Biol.* **102,** 1738–1747.

Emerson, C. P., Shen, S. C., Ham, T. H., Fleming, E. M., and Castle, W. B. (1956) Studies on the destruction of red blood cells. IX. Quantitative methods for determining the osmotic and mechanical fragility of red cells in the peripheral blood and splenic pulp; the mechanism of increased hemolysis in hereditary spherocytosis (congenital haemolytic jaundice) as related to the function of the spleen. *Arch. Intern. Med.* **97,** 1–38.

Ford, W. L. (1969) The immunological and migratory properties of the lymphocytes recirculating through the rat spleen. *Br. J. Exp. Pathol.* **50,** 257–269.

Foster, P. N. and Losowsky, M. S. (1990) Hyposplenism. In: *The Spleen: Structure, Function and Clinical Significance* (Bowdler, A. J. ed.), Chapman and Hall, London, pp. 233–259.

Fujita, T. A. (1974) A scanning electron microscopy study of the human spleen. *Arch. Histol. Jpn.* **37,** 187–216.

Fujita, T. and Kashimura, M. (1983) Scanning electron microscope studies of human spleen. *Surv. Immunol. Res.* **2,** 375–384.

Fujita, T., Kashimura, M., and Adachi, K. (1985) Scanning electron microscopy and terminal circulation. *Experientia* **41,** 167–179.

Goresky, C. A. and Groom, A. C. (1984) Microcirculatory events in the liver and spleen. In: *Handbook of Physiology*, Section 2, *The Cardiovascular System*, vol. IV, *Microcirculation*, Part 2, American Physiological Society, Washington, DC, pp. 689–780.

Greenway, C. V. (1979) Splenic erythrocyte concentration mechanism and its inhibition by isoproterenol. *Am. J. Physiol.* **236** (*Heart Circ. Physiol.* **5**) H238–H243.

Griggs, R. C., Weisman, R. Jr., and Harris, J. W. (1960) Alteration in osmotic and mechanical fragility related to *in vivo* erythrocyte aging and splenic sequestration in hereditary spherocytosis. *J. Clin. Invest.* **39,** 89–101.

Groom, A. C. (1980) Microvascular transit of normal, immature, and altered red blood cells in spleen versus skeletal muscle. In: *Erythrocyte Mechanics and Blood Flow* (Cokelet, G. R., Meiselman, H. J., and Brooks, D. E., eds.), Liss, New York, pp. 229–259.

Groom, A. C. (1987) The Microcirculatory Society Eugene M. Landis Award Lecture. Microcirculation of the spleen: new concepts, new challenges. *Microvasc. Res.* **34,** 269–289.

Groom, A. C., Levesque, M. J., and Bruckschweiger, D. (1977) Flow stasis, blood gases and glucose levels in the red pulp of the spleen. *Adv. Exp. Med. Biol.* **94,** 567–572.

Groom, A. C., Levesque, M. J., Nealon, S., and Basrur, S. (1985) Does an unfavorable metabolic environment for red cells develop within the cat spleen when abnormal cells become trapped? *J. Lab. Clin. Med.* **105,** 209–213.

Groom, A. C. and Schmidt, E. E. (1990) Microcirculatory blood flow through the spleen. In: *The Spleen: Structure, Function and Clinical Significance* (Bowdler, A. J., ed.), Chapman and Hall, London, pp. 45–102.

Groom, A. C. and Song, S. H. (1971) Effects of norepinephrine on washout of red cells from the spleen. *Am. J. Physiol.* **221,** 255–258.

Groom, A. C., Song, S. H., and Campling, B. (1973) Clearance of red blood cells from the vascular bed of skeletal muscle with particular reference to reticulocytes. *Microvasc. Res.* **6,** 51–62.

Groom, A. C., Song, S. H., Lim, P., and Campling, B. (1971) Physical characteristics of red cells collected from the spleen. *Can. J. Physiol. Pharmacol.* **49,** 1092–1099.

Hataba, Y., Kirino, Y., and Suzuki, T. (1981) Scanning electron microscopic study of the red pulp of mouse spleen. *J. Electron Microsc.* **30,** 46–56.

Helly, K. (1902) Zum Nachweise des geschlossenen Gefasssystem der Milz. *Arch. Mikrosk. Anat. Entwicklungsmech.* **59,** 93–105.

Holzbach, R. T., Shipley, R. A., Clark, R. E., and Chudzik, E. B. (1964) Influence of spleen size and portal pressure on erythrocyte sequestration. *J. Clin. Invest.* **43,** 1125–1135.

Irino, S. Murakami, T., and Fujita, T. (1977) Open circulation in the human spleen. Dissection scanning electron microscopy of conductive stained tissue and observation of resin vascular casts. *Arch. Histol. Jpn.* **40,** 297–304.

Jacob, H. S. and Jandl, J. H. (1962) Effects of sulfhydryl inhibition on red blood cells. II. Studies *in vivo*. *J. Clin. Invest.* **41,** 1514–1523.

Jalkanen, S., Reichert, R. A., Gallatin, W. M., Bargatze, R. F., Weissman, I. L., and Butcher, E. C. (1986) Homing receptors and the control of lymphocyte migration. *Immunol. Rev.* **91,** 39–60.

Kay, M. M., Sorensen, K., Wong, P., and Bolton, P. (1982) Antigenicity, storage, and aging: physiologic autoantibodies to cell membrane and serum proteins and the senescent cell antigen. *Mol. Cell Biochem.* **49,** 65–85.

Kimber, R. J. and Lander, H. (1964) The effect of heat on human red cell morphology, fragility, and subsequent survival *in vivo*. *J. Lab. Clin. Med.* **64,** 922–933.

Knisely, M. H. (1936) Spleen studies. I. Microscopic observations of the circulatory system of living, unstimulated mammalian spleens. *Anat. Rec.* **65,** 23–50.

Kopp, W. C. (1990) The immune functions of the spleen. In: *The Spleen: Structure, Functions and Clinical Significance* (Bowdler, A. J., ed.), Chapman and Hall, London, pp. 103–126.

Koyama, S., Aoki, S., and Deguchi, K. (1964) Electron microscopic observations of the splenic red pulp with special reference to the pitting function. *Mie Med. J.* **14,** 143–188.

Kraal, G., Schornagel, K., Streeter, P. R., Holzmann, B., and Butcher, E. C. (1995) Expression of the mucosal vascular addressin, MAdCAM-1, on sinus-lining cells in the spleen. *Am. J. Pathol.* **147,** 763–771.

Kramer, K. and Luft, U. C. (1951) Mobilization of red cells and oxygen from the spleen in severe hypoxia. *Am. J. Physiol.* **165,** 215–228.

Kumararatne, D. S., Bazin, H., and MacLennan, I. C. M. (1981) Marginal zones: the major B cell compartment of rat spleens. *Eur. J. Immunol.* **11,** 858–864.

LaCelle, P. L. (1970) Alteration of membrane deformability in hemolytic anemias. *Semin. Hematol.* **7,** 355–371.

Leblond, P. F. (1973) Etude, au microscope electronique à balayage, de la migration des cellules sanguines à travers les parois des sinusoides spleniques et medullaires chez le rat. *Nouv. Rev. Fr. Hematol.* **13,** 771–788.

Levesque, M. J. and Groom, A. C. (1976a) Washout kinetics of red cells and plasma from the spleen. *Am. J. Physiol.* **231,** 1665–1671.

Levesque, M. J. and Groom, A. C. (1976b) pH environment of red cells in the spleen. *Am. J. Physiol.* **231,** 1672–1678.

Levesque, M. J. and Groom, A. C. (1977) Sequestration of heat-treated autologous red cells in the spleen. *J. Lab. Clin. Med.* **90,** 666–679.

Levesque, M. J. and Groom, A. C. (1980a) A comparative study of the sequestration of 'abnormal' red cells by the spleen. *Can. J. Physiol. Pharmacol.* **58,** 1317–1325.

Levesque, M. J. and Groom, A. C. (1980b) Blood flow distribution within the spleen distended by perfusion at high venous pressure. *J. Lab. Clin. Med.* **96,** 606–615.

Lewis, O. J. (1957) The blood vessels of the adult mammalian spleen. *J. Anat.* **91**, 245–250.

Lubbers, D. W., Hauck, G., Weigelt, H., and Addicks, K. (1979) Contractile properties of frog capillaries tested by electrical stimulation. *Bibl. Anat.* **17**, 3–10.

MacDonald, I. C., Ragan, D. M., Schmidt, E. E., and Groom, A. C. (1987) Kinetics of red blood cell passage through interendothelial slits into venous sinuses in rat spleen, analyzed by *in vivo* microscopy. *Microvasc. Res.* **33**, 118–134.

MacDonald, I. C., Schmidt, E. E., and Groom, A. C. (1991) The high splenic hematocrit: a rheological consequence of red cell flow through the reticular meshwork. *Microvasc. Res.* **42**, 60–76.

MacKenzie, D. W., Whipple, A. O., and Wintersteiner, M. P. (1941) Studies on the microscopic anatomy and physiology of living transilluminated mammalian spleen. *Am. J. Anat.* **68**, 397–456.

Matsumoto, N., Ishihara, T., Adachi, H., Takahashi, M., and Miwa, S. (1977) An ultrastructural study of the red pulp of the spleen and the liver in unstable hemoglobin hemolytic anemia. *Virchows Arch. A. Pathol. Anat. Histol.* **374**, 339–351.

McCuskey, R. S. and McCuskey, P. A. (1977) *In vivo* microscopy of the spleen. *Bibl. Anat.* **16**, 121–125.

McMillan, R. (1981) Chronic idiopathic thrombocytopenic purpura. *N. Engl. J. Med.* **304**, 1135–1147.

Miescher, P. (1957) The role of the reticulo-endothelial system in haematoclasia. In: *Physiology of the Reticuloendothelial System.* Blackwell, Oxford, pp. 147–171.

Miyamoto, H., Seguchi, H., and Ogawa, K. (1980) Electron microscope studies of the Schweigger-Seidel sheath in hen spleen with special reference to the existence of a 'closed' microcirculation. *J. Electron Microsc.* **29**, 158–172.

Mollison, P. L. (1962) The reticulo-endothelial system and red cell destruction. *Proc. R. Soc. Med.* **55**, 915–920.

Motulsky, A. G., Casserd, F., Giblett, E. R., Broun, G. O., and Finch, C. A. (1958) Anemia and the spleen. *N. Engl. J. Med.* **259**, 1164–1169.

Murphy, J. R. (1967) The influence of pH and temperature on some physical properties of normal erythrocytes and erythrocytes from patients with hereditary spherocytes. *J. Lab. Clin. Med.* **69**, 758–775.

Murphy, J. R. (1969) Erythrocyte osmotic fragility and cell water: influence of pH and temperature. *J. Lab. Clin. Med.* **74**, 319–324.

Nopanitaya, W., Aghajanian, J. G., and Gray, L. D. (1979) An improved plastic mixture for corrosion casting of the gastrointestinal microvascular system. In: *Scanning Electron Microscopy*, Part III (Becker, R. P. and Johari, O., eds.), SEM, IL, pp. 751–755.

Nordy, A. (1974) Clinical and pathophysiological aspects of the asplenic state. *Ann. Chir. Gynaecol. Fenn.* **63**, 373–382.

Olah, I. and Glick, B. (1982) Splenic white pulp and associated vascular channels in chicken spleen. *Am. J. Anat.* **165**, 445–480.

Opdyke, D. F. and Apostolico, R. (1966) Splenic contraction and optical density of blood. *Am. J. Physiol.* **211**, 329–334.

Pabst, R. (1988) The role of the spleen in lymphocyte migration. In: *Migration and Homing of Lymphoid Cells*, vol. 1 (Husband, A. J., ed.), CRC, Boca Raton, FL, pp. 63–84.

Pearson, H. A., Spencer, R. P., and Cornelius, E. A. (1969) Functional asplenia in sickle-cell anemia. *N. Eng. J. Med.* **281**, 923–926.

Pellas, T. C. and Weiss, L. (1990) Migration pathways of recirculating murine B cells and CD4+ and CD8+ T lymphocytes. *Am. J. Anat.* **187**, 355–373.

Pictet, R., Orci, L., Forssmann, W. G., and Girardier, L. (1969) An electron microscopic study of the perfusion-fixed spleen. II. Nurse cells and erythrophagocytosis. *Z. Zellforsch. Mikrosk. Anat.* **96**, 400–417.

Piomelli, S., Lurinsky, G., and Wasserman, L. R. (1967) The mechanism of red cell aging. I. Relationship between cell age and specific gravity evaluated by ultracentrifugation in a discontinuous density gradient. *J. Lab. Clin. Med.* **69**, 659–674.

Prankerd, T. A. J. (1960) Studies on the pathogenesis of haemolysis in hereditary spherocytosis. *Q. J. Med.* **29**, 199–208.

Ragan, D. M., Schmidt, E. E., MacDonald, I. C., and Groom, A. C. (1988) Spontaneous cyclic contractions of the capillary wall *in vivo*, impeding red cell flow: a quantitative analysis. Evidence for endothelial contractility. *Microvasc. Res.* **36**, 13–30.

Rhodin, J. A. G. (1974) Spleen. In: *Histology: A Text and Atlas.* Oxford University, Press, New York, pp. 399–415.

Sandberg, G. (1972) Splenic blood flow in the guinea pig measured with ^{133}Xe and calculation of the venous output of lymphocytes from the spleen. *Acta. Physiol. Scand.* **84**, 208–216.

Schmidt, E. E., MacDonald, I. C., and Groom, A. C. (1982) Direct arteriovenous connections and the intermediate circulation in dog spleen, studied by scanning electron microscopy of microcorrosion casts. *Cell Tissue Res.* **225**, 543–555.

Schmidt, E. E., MacDonald, I. C., and Groom, A. C. (1983a) Circulatory pathways in the sinusal spleen of the dog, studied by scanning electron microscopy of microcorrosion casts. *J. Morphol.* **178**, 111–123.

Schmidt, E. E., MacDonald, I. C., and Groom, A. C. (1983b) The intermediate circulation in the nonsinusal spleen of the cat, studied by scanning electron microscopy of microcorrosion casts. *J. Morphol.* **178**, 125–138.

Schmidt, E. E., MacDonald, I. C., and Groom, A. C. (1983c) Luminal morphology of small arterial vessels in the contracted spleen, studied by scanning electron microscopy of microcorrosion casts. *Cell Tissue Res.* **228**, 33–41.

Schmidt, E. E., MacDonald, I. C., and Groom, A. C. (1985a) Microcirculation in rat spleen (sinusal), studied by means of corrosion casts, with particular reference to intermediate pathways. *J. Morphol.* **186**, 1–16.

Schmidt, E. E., MacDonald, I. C., and Groom, A. C. (1985b) Microcirculation in mouse spleen (nonsinusal) studied by means of corrosion casts. *J. Morphol.* **186**, 17–29.

Schmidt, E. E., MacDonald, I. C., and Groom, A. C. (1988) Microcirculatory pathways in normal human spleen, demonstrated by scanning electron microscopy of corrosion casts. *Am. J. Anat.* **181**, 253–266.

Schmidt, E. E., MacDonald, I. C., and Groom, A. C. (1990) Interactions of leukocytes with vessel walls and with other blood cells, studied by high-resolution intravital videomicroscopy of spleen. *Microvasc. Res.* **40**, 99–117.

Schmidt, E. E., MacDonald, I. C., and Groom, A. C. (1991) Changes in splenic microcirculatory pathways in chronic idiopathic thrombocytopenic purpura. *Blood* **78**, 1485–1489.

Schmidt, E. E., MacDonald, I. C., and Groom, A. C. (1993) Comparative aspects of splenic microcirculatory pathways in mammals: The region bordering the white pulp. *Scan. Microsc.* **7**, 613–628.

Schnitzer, B., Sodeman, T. M., Mead, M. L., and Contacos, P. G. (1973) An ultrastructural study of the red pulp of the spleen in malaria. *Blood* **41**, 207–218.

Shulman, N. R. and Jordan, J. V. Jr. (1987) Platelet kinetics. In: *Hemostasis and Thrombosis*, 2nd ed. (Colman, R. W., Hirsh, J., Marder, V. J., and Salzman, E. W. eds.), Lippincott, Philadelphia, pp. 431–451.

Skutelsky, E. and Danon, D. (1970a) Electron microscopical analysis of surface charge labeled density at various stages of the erythroid line. *J. Membr. Biol.* **2**, 173–179.

Skutelsky, E. and Danon, D. (1970b) Reduction in surface charge as an explanation of the recognition by macrophages of nuclei expelled from normoblasts. *J. Cell Biol.* **43**, 8–15.

Snook, T. (1950) A comparative study of the vascular arrangements in mammalian spleens. *Am. J. Anat.* **87**, 31–61.

Snook, T. (1964) Studies of the perifollicular region of the rat's spleen. *Anat. Rec.* **148**, 149–159.

Snook, T. (1975) The origin of the follicular capillaries in the human spleen. *Am. J. Anat.* **144**, 113–117.

Song, S. H. (1972) A study of splenic functions with respect to red blood cells (PhD Thesis), University of Western Ontario, London, ON.

Song, S. H. and Groom, A. C. (1971a) Storage of blood cells in spleen of the cat. *Am. J. Physiol.* **220**, 779–784.

Song, S. H. and Groom, A. C. (1971b) The distribution of red cells in the spleen. *Can. J. Physiol. Pharmacol.* **49**, 734–743.

Song, S. H. and Groom, A. C. (1971c) Immature and abnormal erythrocytes present in the normal, healthy spleen. *Scand. J. Haematol.* **8**, 487–493.

Song, S. H. and Groom, A. C. (1972) Sequestration and possible maturation of reticulocytes in the normal spleen. *Can. J. Physiol. Pharmacol.* **50**, 400–406.

Song, S. H. and Groom, A. C. (1974) Scanning electron microscope study of the splenic red pulp in relation to the sequestration of immature and abnormal red cells. *J. Morphol.* **144,** 439–452.

Sorbie, J. and Valberg, L. S. (1970) Splenic sequestration of stress erythrocytes in the rabbit. *Am. J. Physiol.* **218,** 647–653.

Stock, R. J., Cilento, E. V., Reilly, F. D., and McCuskey, R. S. (1983) A compartmental analysis of the splenic circulation in rat. *Am. J. Physiol.* **245** (*Heart Circ. Physiol.* **14**), H17–H21.

Suzuki, T., Furusato, M., Takasaki, S., Shimizu, S., and Hataba, Y. (1977) Stereoscopic scanning electron microscopy of the red pulp of dog spleen with special reference to the terminal structure of the cordal capillaries. *Cell Tissue Res.* **182,** 441–453.

Suzuki, T., Shimizu, S., Hataba, Y., et al. (1978) Three dimensional fine structure of the capillary terminals in the red pulp of the human spleen. In: *Electron Microscopy 1978. Ninth International Congress on Electron Microscopy* (vol. II) (Sturgess, J. M., ed.), Microscopical Society, Toronto, pp. 468–469.

Tanaka, H., Hataba, Y., Saito, S., Fukushima, O., and Miyasaka, M. (1996) Phenotypic characteristics and significance of reticular meshwork surrounding splenic white pulp of mice. *J. Electron Microsc.* **45,** 407–416.

Tischendorf, F. (1969) Die Milz. In: *Handbuch der mikroskopischen Anatomie des Menschen. Band VI, Blutgefass und Lymphgefassapparat, innersekretorische Drusen* (Mullendorff, W. and Bargmann, W., eds.), Springer-Verlag, Berlin, pp. 572–612.

Tischendorf, F. (1985) On the evolution of the spleen. *Experientia* **41,** 145–152.

Ultmann, J. E. and Gordon, C. S. (1965) The removal of *in vitro* damaged erythrocytes from the circulation of normal and splenectomized rats. *Blood* **26,** 49–62.

Van Krieken, J. H., Te Velde, J., Hermans, J., and Welvaart. K. (1985a) The splenic red pulp; a histomorphometrical study in splenectomy specimens embedded in methylmethacrylate. *Histopathol.* **9,** 401–416.

Van Krieken, J. H., Te Velde, J., Kleiverda, K., Leenheers-Binnendijk, L., and van de Velde, C. J. (1985b) The human spleen; a histological study in splenectomy specimens embedded in methylmethacrylate. *Histopathology* **9,** 571–585.

Van Rooijen, N., Claassen, E., Kraal, G., and Dijkstra, C. D. (1989) Cytological basis of immune functions of the spleen.Immunocytochemical characterization of lymphoid and non-lymphoid cells involved in the 'in situ' immune response. *Progr. Histochem. Cytochem.* **19,** 1–71.

Vaupel, P., Ruppert, H., and Hutten, H. (1977) Splenic blood flow and intrasplenic flow distribution in rats. *Pflugers Arch.* **369,** 193–201.

Wade, L. Jr. (1973) Splenic sequestration of young erythrocytes in sheep. *Am. J. Physiol.* **224,** 265–267.

Wagner, H. N. Jr., Razzak, M. A., Gaertner, R. A., et al. (1962) Removal of erythrocytes from the circulation. *Arch. Intern. Med.* **110,** 90–97.

Watson, H. H. K. and Ludlam, C. A. (1986) Survival of 111-Indium platelet subpopulations of varying density in normal and postsplenectomized subjects. *Br. J. Haematol.* **62,** 117–124.

Weidenreich, F. (1901) Das Gefasssystem der menschlichen Milz. *Arch. Mikrosk. Anat. Entwicklungsmech.* **58,** 247–376.

Weigelt, H. (1982) Die spezialisierte Endothelzelle erregbare Zelle und mechanischer Effektor der Mikrozirkulation. *Funkt. Biol. Med.* **1,** 53–60.

Weisman, R., Ham, T. H., Hing, C. F., et al. (1955) Studies on the role of the spleen in the destruction of erythrocytes. *Trans. Assoc. Am. Physicians* **68,** 131–140.

Weiss, L. (1962) The structure of fine splenic arterial vessels in relation to hemoconcentration and red cell destruction. *Am. J. Anat.* **111,** 131–179.

Weiss, L. (1974) A scanning electron microscopic study of the spleen. *Blood* **43,** 665–691.

Weiss, L., Powell, R., and Schiffman, F. J. (1985) Terminating arterial vessels in red pulp of human spleen: a transmission electron microscopic study. *Experientia* **41,** 233–242.

Wennberg, E. and Weiss, L. (1969) The structure of the spleen and hemolysis. *Ann. Rev. Med.* **20,** 29–40.

Westermann, J. and Pabst, R. (1997) Autotransplantation of the spleen in the rat: donor leukocytes of the splenic fragment survive implantation to migrate and proliferate in the host. *Cell Tissue Res.* **287,** 357–364.

Willführ, K. U., Westermann, J., and Pabst, R. (1990) Absolute numbers of lymphocyte subsets migrating through the compartments of the normal and transplanted rat spleen. *Eur. J. Immunol.* **20,** 903–911.

Witte, C. L., Witte, M. H., Renert, W., and Corrigan, J. J. Jr. (1974) Splenic circulatory dynamics in congestive splenomegaly. *Gastroenterology* **67,** 498–505.

Yamamoto, K., Arisma, N., Yamamoto, T., et al. (1979) Scanning electron microscopy of the perimarginal cavernous sinus plexus of the human spleen. In: *Scanning Electron Microscopy* (Part III) (Becker, R. P. and Johari, O., eds.), SEM, IL, pp. 763–768.

Yednock, T. A. and Rosen, S. D. (1989) Lymphocyte homing. *Adv. Immunol.* **44,** 313–378.

4 The Immune Functions of the Spleen*

MORRIS O. DAILEY, MD, PhD

4.1. INTRODUCTION

As the largest secondary lymphoid organ, the spleen has a number of important roles in the immune response, including the clearance of effete or damaged cells from the bloodstream and host resistance to infection. Other organs serve some functions similar to those of the spleen. The widely dispersed system of lymph nodes situated throughout the host responds vigorously with antibodies and T-cells to foreign antigens that gain access to peripheral tissues. Again, like the spleen, the liver, with its large mass of phagocytic Kupffer cells lining vascular sinusoids, is an important site of clearance of particulate antigens from the bloodstream and a major contributor to resistance to infection. The spleen, however, has a unique place in host defense, because it combines all of these functions in one organ. Thus, because of its anatomic location directly connected to the circulation, it responds promptly to bloodborne antigens with antigen-specific immune responses, much more effectively than can lymph nodes or other lymphoid tissues (Rowley, 1950a,b). It also has a major role in mediating the effects of the innate immune system, and under some circumstances is more effective in its role in the reticuloendothelial system than the liver.

This chapter reviews the functions of the spleen as an immunologic organ, but does not describe in depth general aspects of the immune system, for which there are other comprehensive textbooks and reviews. Rather, focus is primarily on those aspects of the immune system that are unique to the spleen, and which are therefore of particular importance in maintaining host defense. Although the anatomy of the human spleen has been described in detail (as in Chapters 1 and 2), much of what is known of splenic function has of necessity been learned from experiments in animals, particularly rats and mice. Nevertheless, the basic principles and mechanisms elucidated in such studies appear to hold true across species, as they do for most of the immune system, and are consistent with observations of patients with defects in splenic function and with studies of isolated human splenocytes in vitro. Thus, a clearer picture is emerging of the workings of this complex organ.

4.2. FUNCTIONAL ANATOMY OF THE SPLEEN

The spleen is a highly vascular organ, receiving approx 5% of the cardiac output in humans. Unlike the lymph nodes, through which flows a large volume of tissue-derived lymph, the spleen has no afferent lymphatics, although it is drained by a rich network of efferent lymphatic vessels. Thus, all cells and foreign material entering the spleen do so through the bloodstream. The major anatomic compartments of the spleen, described in detail in Chapter 2, are organized in such a way as to optimize the disparate functions of the organ. The white pulp (WP) consists of the periarteriolar lymphoid sheath (PALS), containing T-cells, together with the antigen-presenting cells (APCs) that are necessary for their activation. The PALS is atrophic in athymic (nude) mice and in neonatally thymectomized animals, demonstrating that its development is dependent on a functional thymus (Sprent, 1973). The PALS contains a specific type of stromal cell, the interdigitating reticulum cells (or interdigitating cells [IDCs]), which are characteristic of the T-cell zones of the spleen and lymph nodes. These cells, derived from circulating dendritic cells (DCs), have long, ramifying membrane processes and are strongly major histocompatibility complex (MHC) class II (MHC-II)-positive. They also express high levels of co-stimulatory molecules, such as B7, and are the most potent cells for the processing and presentation of antigens for activation of naïve T-lymphocytes (Stein et al., 1980; Dijkstra, 1982; Banchereau and Steinman, 1998). As discussed in Subheading 3.2., later, these cells also secrete factors that are important in the homeostatic regulation of the PALS architecture.

Peripheral to the PALS are the lymphoid follicles, which are cohesive nests of B-cells enmeshed in a framework of APCs highly specialized for capturing and presenting antigens to B-lymphocytes, known as the follicular dendritic cells (FDC). FDC strongly express receptors for complement fragments and for the Fc region of immunoglobulin (Ig) (Fc receptors [FcR]), and have numerous long, fine dendritic processes that are intimately associated with the surrounding B-cells. These are distinct from IDCs, which are present in the T-cell zone. During an immune response, primary follicles form germinal centers, in which the resting B-cells undergo blast transformation, proliferate rapidly, and subsequently give rise to small B-cell progeny. Germinal center B-cells can be recognized in tissue sections or isolated in vitro by their characteristic strong staining with the lectin PNA (Rose et al., 1980; Kraal et al., 1982). So-called tingible body macrophages, present in germinal centers, are readily observable phagocytic cells that have

*Developed from the chapter by Dr. William C. Kopp in the First Edition.

taken up the apoptotic B-cells that are generated in large numbers during the rapid proliferation of follicular B-lymphocytes. A small number of T-lymphocytes are also present within germinal centers. These cells are almost exclusively of the CD4 (helper) cell subset, with very few CD8 T-cells (Rouse et al., 1982). Germinal centers also contain a specialized DC that presents antigen to follicular T-cells, which probably plays a role in activating these T-cells to deliver help to the surrounding B-lymphocytes (Grouard et al., 1996).

The third major splenic compartment is the marginal zone (MZ), a collection of lymphocytes, highly phagocytic macrophages, and scattered DCs surrounding the periphery of the PALS and follicles, thus being at the interface between the red and white pulp (Kraal, 1992; Chadburn, 2000). Although the MZ contains a looser arrangement of cells, it nonetheless covers a larger area and contains more lymphocytes than either the PALS or B-cell follicles (Kumararatne et al., 1981). Much of the blood entering the spleen arrives in the MZ, which is therefore the initial site of localization of most antigens and of lymphocytes circulating through the organ. The MZ of the rat and mouse contains a prominent marginal sinus, which is lined by two distinct populations of macrophages, the MZ macrophages along the outer edge, near the red pulp, and the marginal metallophilic macrophages, which are situated adjacent to the PALS and follicles. MZ macrophages are extremely potent phagocytic cells, which can take up and phagocytose large foreign particles, such as bacteria. There is no distinct marginal sinus in humans, nor are there marginal metallophilic macrophages, and the exact circulation pattern in the MZ is less clearly defined than in experimental animals (Steiniger et al., 1997). Despite these differences in microanatomy, the various cells in the murine MZ nevertheless appear to have functional counterparts in the human, and the overall function of the MZ in the host response to antigens is well conserved among species.

The PALS and B-cell follicles in the spleen are analogous to the paracortical and cortical areas of lymph nodes, respectively, and serve similar functions in the immune response. The regulation of traffic of B- and T-cells into these two organs, however, is different. In lymph nodes, lymphocytes enter into the parenchyma by adhering to, then migrating through, the endothelium of the postcapillary venules in the paracortex, the so-called high endothelial venules (von Andrian and Mackay, 2000). Similar vessels, lined by thickened endothelial cells, are present in Peyer's patches and tonsils, and specialized site-specific adhesion molecules expressed on these endothelial cells regulate the influx of lymphocytes expressing complementary counter-receptors. In contrast, traffic into the spleen is thought to be mostly passive, lymphocytes simply entering as a component of the blood emptying into splenic sinusoids. However, once they are in the spleen, lymphocytes follow well-defined pathways of migration, and, as shown above, localize in an anatomically precise manner, indicating that cell traffic within the organ is highly regulated. Recirculating T- and B-cells isolated from thoracic duct lymph and injected into experimental animals localize in the recipient's MZ (Sprent, 1973; Nieuwenhuis and Ford, 1976). Lymphocyte localization occurs rapidly, within 15 min of the intravenous (iv) injection of labeled cells. Most of these cells enter the MZ through the branching arterioles that terminate in the MZ, although studies have not yet been reported that would demonstrate whether access is also gained by transmigration through vessels in the PALS, followed by migration into the MZ.

Although cells lining the sinusoids closest to the white pulp express mucosal addressin cell adhesion molecule 1 (MAdCAM-1), an adhesion molecule previously shown to mediate lymphocyte traffic to mucosa-associated lymphoid tissues (MALT), there is no evidence that it functions in an analogous manner in the spleen (Kraal et al., 1995). There is some evidence that interactions between circulating lymphocytes and MZ macrophages may regulate the entry of lymphocytes into the white pulp, which could be analogous to the function of high endothelial venules in lymph nodes (Kraal et al., 1989a; Lyons and Parish, 1995). Although the adhesion molecules involved in this intercompartmental cell sorting have not been elucidated, soluble molecules, such as chemokines, play a critical role in this process, as discussed in Subheading 3.2.

Most of the T- and B-cells in the spleen are part of the recirculating pool of lymphocytes that continuously migrate throughout all secondary lymphoid organs, and, at a lower level, traffic through most other tissues. In addition to the recirculating cells passing through the MZ, this compartment contains a separate nonrecirculating population of resident B-cells (Kumararatne et al., 1981; Gray et al., 1982). Unlike most B-cells in the primary follicles, which express both IgM and IgD on their surface, these nonrecirculating MZ B-cells are $\mu^+\delta^-$, i.e., they express little or no membrane IgD. These cells are larger than follicular B-cells, they are noncycling, and they express a high level of CD21, or complement receptor 2 (CR2), a receptor for the complement fragment, C3d, which has an important role in the immune response to thymus-independent antigens (Timens et al., 1989; Kraal, 1992; Peset Llopis et al., 1996). The MZ is also enriched for B-cells with hypermutated Ig V region genes, a hallmark of previously activated B-cells that have undergone affinity maturation (Dunn-Walters et al., 1995). Memory B-cells persisting long after the cessation of a primary immune response are also characterized by hypermutated Ig genes. In experiments examining the immune response to haptens, it was shown that antigen-specific memory B-cells reside in the MZ, and that these cells rapidly respond to secondary immunization (Liu et al., 1988; Zhang et al., 1988). The MZ therefore consists of a functionally heterogeneous mixture of memory B-cells and the $\mu^+\delta^-$ CD21^{hi} cells involved in the rapid primary response to carbohydrate antigens (see Subheading 5.1).

Approximately 90% of the blood entering the spleen passes through the red pulp. With its large number of macrophages, which are both produced locally and derived from circulating monocytes (van Furth and Diesselhoff-den Dulk, 1984), it is a major component of the effector arm of the immune response. Red pulp macrophages express MHC-II antigens and bear Fc receptors as well as receptors for complement, and hence are capable of removing IgG-coated (opsonized) particles from the bloodstream (Christensen et al., 1978). Because blood filters relatively slowly through the dense meshwork of the splenic cords, the red pulp macrophages and phagocytic sinus-lining endothelial cells (De Bruyn and Farr, 1980) are also able to remove even poorly opsonized organisms, moreso than are phagocytes present at other sites. As discussed later in this chapter, this ability to take up particulate antigens plays a unique role in host resistance to infection. Splenic red pulp is not considered to be a major site of initiation of the primary immune response, but the red pulp cords (the cords of Billroth) contain plasma cells that secrete Ig. The red pulp does contain lymphocytes, and there is evidence that red pulp macrophages can present antigen to T-lymphocytes (Ciavarra et al., 1997). In contrast to observations on T-cell subsets in the PALS, a relatively high proportion of CD8$^+$ cells has been observed in red pulp cords (Hsu et al., 1983). In addition, B-lymphocytes are often found situated about small vessels, and are positive for CD19, CD20, and CD21 (Timens and Poppema, 1985). At least some of these B- and T-cells are probably passing from the white pulp through the red pulp, on their way to returning to the systemic circulation.

4.3. DEVELOPMENT OF THE SPLEEN

The spleen appears early in fetal development, the initial rudiment appearing as a collection of mesenchymal cells on the coelomic epithelium adjacent to the developing stomach at wk 5 of human gestation (Langman, 1969). By wk 9, the vascular supply forms separate channels, which empty into sinusoids lined by endothelial cells (Jones, 1983). In the ensuing few weeks, lymphocytes, both B-cells and a lesser number of T-cells, and macrophages begin to appear, first appearing around wk 12–14 at the PALS, and forming the nascent white pulp (Hayward and Ezer, 1974; Chadburn, 2000). Surface Ig-positive B-cells are clearly apparent by wk 14 (Kamps and Cooper, 1982). Follicular dendritic cells (FDCs), the major stromal cell of B-cell follicles that trap antigen, are present by wk 24 (Bofill, Janossy, Janossa et al., 1985). Although B-cells and FDCs are organized into inactive primary lymphoid follicles *in utero*, no germinal centers are present until after birth.

4.3.1. DEVELOPMENT OF SPLENIC LYMPHOID COMPARTMENTS
Development of the B-lymphocyte lineage in the bone marrow involves heavy-chain gene rearrangement, bringing a single variable region gene segment into proximity to the short D and J segments close to the μ heavy-chain sequence. Transcription of this results in μ-chain synthesis and the formation of large, proliferating pre-B-cells. This is followed by light-chain gene rearrangement, and, if both rearrangements are productive, forming active Ig heavy- and light-chain polypeptides, the dimeric (μκ or μλ) IgM becomes expressed on the cell surface as the major component of the active B-cell antigen receptor complex. During this stage, the immature B-cell first undergoes selection against recognition of self-antigens, effectively killing or inactivating those clones of B-cells that recognize auto-antigens. This process of B-cell development, which begins during fetal life, continues throughout the life of the host, continuously seeding the periphery with immature B-lymphocytes.

Further maturation of these marrow-derived immature B-cells must occur before they can respond productively to exogenous antigen. This differentiation takes place after the IgM$^+$ B-cells migrate to the T-cell-rich PALS of the spleen (Allman et al., 1992; Chan and MacLennan, 1993; MacLennan, 1998), where they receive signals which promote further maturation. These μ$^+$δ$^-$ immature cells are excluded from the B-cell follicles. Although the exact nature of the stimuli that cause further maturation is unclear, this differentiation requires signals transduced through an intact B-cell receptor complex (Loder et al., 1999). The majority of immature B-lymphocytes, approx 70%, do not complete the transition to maturity, and Levine et al. (2000) have proposed that this reflects positive clonal selection based upon the specificity of the B-cell receptor, leading to a considerable skewing of the B-cell immune specificity repertoire. During the maturation process, alternative mRNA splicing results in the co-expression of both IgM and IgD on the cell surface, CR2 (CD21, both a complement receptor and an integral part of the B-cell co-receptor) upregulates, and the expression of the receptor for the chemokine B-lymphocyte chemoattractant (BLC) is induced. Completion of this differentiative program results in the production of mature naïve B-cells, which join the recirculating pool, can populate the B-cell regions of lymphoid tissue, and are capable of responding to foreign antigen. This requisite post-bone marrow development of B-lymphocytes, which has no counterpart for post-thymic T-lymphocytes, shows that the spleen functions as an important lymphopoietic organ.

B-cells of a separate lineage, so-called B-1 or CD5 B-cells, develop early in ontogeny, have a relatively restricted receptor repertoire, and frequently respond to carbohydrate antigens. These cells are first seen in the spleen at 22 wk gestation (Hayakawa and Hardy, 1988). A few of these cells populate the adult secondary lymphoid organs, including the spleen, but they form the major B-cell population in the abdominal and pleural cavities, in which they replicate autonomously without further input from the bone marrow. CD5 B-cells secrete much of the natural IgM and IgG3 antibody in normal mouse serum, and they appear to be responsible for autoantibody secretion in several model systems (Hayakawa and Hardy, 2000). Natural antibody can be secreted by B-1 B-cells in the absence of antigenic stimulation. B-1 B-cell-associated anti-phosphatidylcholine IgM antibody, as well as other natural antibodies, play a role in host innate resistance to bacterial infection (Briles et al., 1981; Boes et al., 1998).

The major structural and functional aspects of the spleen are well developed by the time of birth, and the white pulp is well-populated by both T- and B-lymphocytes (Namikawa et al., 1986). A major exception is the lack of development of the MZ until well after birth. In mice, the MZ is not fully developed until 1–4 wk of age, the exact time depending on the strain. Similarly, the spleens of normal children do not contain mature MZs, or B-cells with an adult MZ phenotype, until they are 2 yr old (Timens and Poppema, 1985; Timens et al., 1989). Given the unique anatomic structure and cell composition of this compartment, this delayed development has clinically significant consequences for the young host, as discussed later.

4.3.2. CYTOKINE REGULATION OF DEVELOPMENT AND MAINTENANCE OF SPLENIC ARCHITECTURE
4.3.2.1. Tumor Necrosis Factor/Lymphotoxin Family
Some of the molecular requirements for the development and maintenance of secondary lymphoid tissue have been elucidated in the last few years. Members of the tumor necrosis factor (TNF) family, in particular, have been shown to be required for such differentiation. In addition to TNF-α, this family includes two major forms of lymphotoxin (LT). LT-α, a homotrimer of α-subunits, is a soluble cytokine secreted by T- and B-lymphocytes. In general, it has been considered to be primarily a proinflammatory molecule. The predominant form of LT-β is a trimer of one α chain and two β chains (LTα$_1$β$_2$), and is a membrane-anchored protein. It exerts its action through binding to the LT-β receptor, which is expressed by stromal cells in lymphoid tissue, but not by either B- or T-lymphocytes (Murphy et al., 1998). The only known function of LT-β is in lymphoid organogenesis, and LT-α also appears to play a role in development (Chaplin and Fu, 1998): Both forms of LT are required for the normal development of secondary lymphoid organs, including the spleen. Mice rendered genetically deficient (by gene knockout) in LT-α do not develop LN or Peyer's patches. In the spleens of LT$^{-/-}$ mice, B- and T-cells fail to organize into discrete regions, there are no germinal centers, and the white pulp is small and blends into the surrounding red pulp (Matsumoto et al., 1997). The MZ is severely disrupted, with absence of MZ B-cells

and the marginal sinus with its MAdCAM-1-expressing lining cells and marginal metallophilic macrophages. These animals do not form clusters of FDCs, implying that LT is required for FDC differentiation and that this then results in the lack of follicular organization and inability to form germinal centers. LT-$\beta^{-/-}$ and LT-β receptor$^{-/-}$ mice have similarly disordered splenic development (Koni et al., 1997; Futterer et al., 1998). When the activity of the LT system is blocked in adult mice by injecting a soluble form of the LT-β receptor, or a blocking monoclonal antibody against LT-β, follicles in the spleen become disrupted, and the MZ is lost (Mackay et al., 1997). Thus, LT is necessary for initial spleen organogenesis during ontogeny, and is also required throughout life, to provide a trophic influence necessary for the continued maintenance of tissue organization. In several experiments involving the adoptive transfer of wild-type and knockout lymphocytes, it was shown that the cells that provide this trophic signal are LT-α-expressing B-lymphocytes (Matsumoto et al., 1996; Chaplin and Fu, 1998). Thus, the injection of wild-type bone marrow or B-cells into LT knockout mice induced the formation of normal FDC clusters, B-cells areas, and germinal centers (Fu et al., 1997; Matsumoto et al., 1997). LT-expressing T-cells are not necessary for the maintenance of tissue structure (Fu et al., 1998).

Genetic deficiency in TNF-α or its type I receptor (TNF-RI) do not affect fetal lymphoid organogenesis. However, such animals lack FDC networks and germinal centers, and, in the spleen, there is loss of discrete B-cell follicles around the PALS, these being replaced by a rim of B-cells (Matsumoto et al., 1997; Cook et al., 1998). TNF-α and TNF-RI knockout mice also exhibit defects in MZ macrophages and in the marginal sinus endothelial cells (Pasparakis et al., 2000). Therefore, TNF-α and its type I receptor appear to be are required for the maintenance of lymphoid structure, but, unlike LT, have little or no role in fetal organogenesis. FDC-like cells that stain for FDC-specific antigens are present in the disrupted MZ in these animals. This has led to the suggestion that, in the absence of the TNF-α signal, the FDC precursors remain in the MZ, and are unable to migrate to the white pulp. Then, in the absence of FDC in the correct location in the periphery of the white pulp, B-cell follicles and germinal centers are unable to form (Pasparakis et al., 2000).

4.3.2.2. Chemokines and Lymphoid Tissue Organization

Chemokines constitute a large group of low-mol-wt chemotactic proteins that serve diverse functions throughout the immune system (reviewed in Cyster, 1999; von Andrian and Mackay, 2000). Some chemokines are secreted by hematolymphoid cells; others are expressed by a variety of stromal cells. Chemokine signals are transduced into lymphocytes and other target cells through cell surface G-protein-coupled chemokine receptors, of which approx 15 are now known. A major function of chemokines is to regulate the migration and tissue localization of leukocytes, including both lymphocytes and myeloid cells. Chemokines regulate leukocyte–endothelial adhesion and motility, leading to leukocyte infiltration into inflamed tissues, as well as to the homing of T- and B-cells into lymphoid organs, and to specific compartments within those organs. Thus, chemokines are key regulators of the plastic environment in which immune responses are organized.

Secondary lymphoid-tissue chemokine (SLC) plays a major role in facilitating the traffic of lymphocytes from the bloodstream into lymph nodes (Cyster, 1999). The chemokines SLC and ELC act through the CCR7 chemokine receptor and are chemoattractant for naïve T-lymphocytes, with less activity for B-cells. SLC and the related chemokine, ELC, are secreted by stromal cells within the T-cell-rich areas of lymphoid organs, including IDCs within the PALS of the spleen (Willimann et al., 1998; Cyster, 1999). Mice with the natural *plt* mutation do not express SLC or ELC, and their T-cells exhibit markedly reduced homing to the T-cell zones of the spleen, lymph nodes, and gut-associated lymphoid tissue (Ansel et al., 1999). These findings have been confirmed in experiments with CCR7$^{-/-}$ mice (Forster et al., 1999), and show that the chemotactic proteins SLC and ELC, and their receptor, CCR7, are important in the organization of, and traffic of cells through, T-cell zones in all peripheral lymphoid tissue.

Immunohistochemical staining for the chemokine BLC shows that its expression is in a pattern precisely complementary to that of SLC and ELC (Cyster, 1999). The latter are secreted in the T-cell zones, but BLC is localized to the B-cell follicles, secreted by FDCs, and is strongly chemotactic for B-lymphocytes (Gunn et al., 1998; Cyster, 1999). Thus, B-cells recirculating through the spleen, which express the chemokine receptor for BLC (CCR5), are attracted to the B-cell zone. B-cells in CCR5 knockout mice cannot migrate into follicles, resulting in defective development of B-cell areas in the spleen and Peyer's patches and a lack of FDC clusters (Forster et al., 1999; Ansel et al., 2000). TNF-α and LT$\alpha_1\beta_2$ are necessary for the development of FDC, and both are also required for the expression of BLC in vivo (Ngo et al., 1999). Thus, one of the mechanisms by which LT deficiency causes defective white pulp organization is by blocking the secretion of BLC, resulting in the lack of chemoattraction of B-cells into nascent follicles. BLC also induces the upregulation of LT$\alpha_1\beta_2$ on the membrane of B-lymphocytes (Ansel et al., 2000). This then establishes a positive feedback loop that would progressively increase B-cell LT levels, BLC secretion by FDC, and increased recruitment of B-cells into follicles, perhaps being important in initiating the germinal center reaction (Forster et al., 1996; Ansel et al., 2000).

The precise localization of lymphocytes within the spleen, as well as in other lymphoid organs, and their routes of migration within the tissue, play an important role in the cell-to-cell interactions that must take place during the immune response to an antigen. Only by bringing together antigen-specific helper T-cells, specific B-cells, antigen, and corresponding antigen-presenting cells (APCs) in the appropriate microenvironment can the necessary signals be generated for inducing lymphocyte activation and differentiation. The mystery of how this microarchitecture is generated and maintained is not yet solved, but the evolving story of chemokine regulation of lymphocyte chemotaxis and compartmental homing is clearly a major contributor to understanding of this process.

4.4. THE ROLE OF THE SPLEEN IN HOST DEFENSE

The complex architecture of the various compartments of the spleen allows it to serve its two general functions as a filter in the bloodstream and as a site of generating immune responses to iv antigens. These two functions are interrelated in fundamentally important ways. Thus, the uptake, transport, and processing of antigens by phagocytes and other stromal cells is critically important for the induction of B- and T-cell immune responses and the secretion of specific Ig. Conversely, the clearance function of the spleen is markedly enhanced by products of the specific immune response, both T-cell-derived cytokines and, especially, B-cell-derived cytophilic antibody.

4.4.1. NONSPECIFIC UPTAKE OF PARTICULATE MATERIAL

Particulate materials are removed from the circulation by the phagocytic cells of the reticuloendothelial system, even in the absence of immune recognition. The spleen is an especially efficient nonspecific filter of bloodborne particles, a characteristic that has important implications for host resistance to the early stage of bacteremia. After the iv injection of colloidal carbon, phagocytic uptake can be observed rapidly in the red pulp (Nossal et al., 1966; Burke and Simon, 1970; Mitchell and Abbot, 1971). Within 20 s, electron microscopy demonstrates that macrophages in the red pulp cords have ingested carbon, the amount increasing over time. At 30 min after injection, carbon can be seen by light microscopy only in the red pulp, but MZ macrophages accumulate it by 1 h (Kotani et al., 1985; Kotani et al., 1986). Several other particulate materials of varying types, including sheep red blood cells (SRBCs), are also localized in the MZ within 2 h (van Ewijk et al., 1977; Van den Eertwegh et al., 1992), the amount after several hours being more than that seen in the red pulp. Only after several hours to days do they begin to accumulate in the white pulp (van Ewijk et al., 1977; Kotani et al., 1986). This type of uptake is a model for the antigen-nonspecific phagocytic clearance of bloodborne microorganisms, which occurs in hosts who have had no prior exposure to the organism, and hence no circulating antibody.

A special case of nonimmune clearance of particles from the circulation is the physiologic removal of effete or damaged erythrocytes. With a normal life-span of 120 d in humans, red blood cells are removed from the circulation at the rate of about $2 \times 10^{11}/d$*, mostly by being phagocytosed by macrophages in the splenic red pulp cords, with some removal by macrophages in the liver and other organs. The exact mechanism by which these red blood cells are targeted for destruction is unclear, but it involves the slowed circulation through the mesh-like splenic cords resulting from structural changes in the erythrocyte, followed by phagocytosis by red pulp macrophages. Red blood cells with defects in membrane structure or cell shape, such as those of sickle cell anemia or hereditary spherocytosis, have more difficulty passing through the cords, and are correspondingly destroyed at an increased rate (*see also* Chapter 3).

4.4.2. THE ROLE OF ANTIBODY AND COMPLEMENT IN ANTIGEN CLEARANCE

Although macrophages in the spleen and liver can remove particles from the blood nonspecifically, much less soluble antigen is taken up, and both soluble and particulate antigens are taken up much more efficiently in immune animals. The binding of circulating antibody to an antigen results in the formation of an immune complex, the size of which depends on the relative ratio of circulating antigen and antibody. These complexes interact with receptors on phagocytes (and some other stromal cells) for the Fc region of the Ig. Fc receptors interact at relatively low affinity with unbound antibody, but Ig that has been rendered polyvalent, either by heat aggregation or by interacting with a polyvalent antigen, is bound avidly. The increased uptake of antigen induced by antibody, the process of opsonization, involves many FcR-positive cell types, including neutrophils and splenic macrophages. In the absence of adjuvant, most soluble protein antigens are taken up in only small amounts in the lymphoid tissues of naïve animals. For example, after the injection of soluble monomeric serum albumins, little antigen is retained in the spleen or lymph nodes and there is little immune response (Coon and Hunter, 1973; Su and Van Rooijen, 1989). When this antigen is modified in such a way as to increase its interaction with macrophages and, perhaps, with DCs, antigen is retained in lymphoid tissue and a brisk immune response ensues (Coon and Hunter, 1973; Dailey et al., 1977; Su and Van Rooijen, 1989). Opsonization of circulating soluble antigen by preformed antibody in an immune host markedly increases its trapping in the spleen. This antigen can then be both destroyed, protecting the host from its ill effects, and also processed and presented to the immune system in an immunogenic form, resulting in an enhanced immune response. FcR-mediated uptake of antigens not only increases phagocytosis quantitatively, but some Fc receptors also transduce a signal that activates macrophages and thereby increases the breakdown of the foreign material. The binding of antigen–IgG$_1$ complexes to Fcγ receptor type I (FcγRI, or CD64), expressed by both macrophages and neutrophils, increases the rate of phagocytosis, and, at the same time, triggers the intracellular respiratory burst and the secretion of proinflammatory mediators (reviewed in McKenzie and Schreiber, 1998). Fc receptors on Langerhans cells, the DCs located in the skin, increase the ingestion of immune complexes, and thereby enhance the presentation of antigenic peptides to T-lymphocytes.

Opsonization also takes place through the activation of complement and deposition of fragment C3b in the immune complex. Thus, circulating antibody and complement cooperate in opsonization (Ehlenberger and Nussenzweig, 1977). Immune complexes containing C3b or some its derivative fragments, such as iC3b, bind to complement receptors on phagocytes in the red pulp of the spleen and on MZ macrophages, so that both of these areas are major sites of localization of opsonized antigen. Complement-mediated clearance of complexes is particularly important when the antibody involved is IgM, because there are no macrophage FcRs for this Ig class, and phagocytosis therefore must depend principally on binding to complement receptors. Antigen uptake can be enhanced, even in the absence of complement activation by antibody in the classical pathway. Thus, direct complement activation through binding to bacterial surfaces (the alternate pathway), with the resulting deposition of C3 fragments, can give rise to increased phagocytic clearance. A third mechanism of activating complement is through the lectin pathway in which mannan-binding lectin, a soluble protein secreted by the liver during the acute phase response, binds to carbohydrates on the surface of Gram-positive and Gram-negative bacteria and yeast. This initiates cleavage of C3 and thereby enhances phagocytic clearance (Fraser et al., 1998). In general, the most efficacious clearance of any antigen requires opsonization by both antibody and complement, with internalization then occurring after binding to macrophage receptors for both complement and the Ig Fc region.

The opsonization process is generally very effective in removing target antigens from the bloodstream, as well as enhancing pathogen removal by phagocytes in other lymphoid and nonlymphoid tissues. However, the efficiency of opsonization is all too often demonstrated clinically by the rapid splenic clearance of erythrocytes or platelets sensitized by Ig or complement, and the frequent alleviation of such a condition by splenectomy (*see also* Chapter 12). In such immune-mediated cytopenias, antibody-coated cells are phagocytosed by macrophages in the red pulp, which express FcγRs. This is discussed in further detail in Subheading 4.6.

*Note: There is considerable interspecies variation in red blood cell life-span and the proportion of effete red blood cells destroyed in the spleen. -Editor.

4.4.3. MICROANATOMICAL LOCALIZATION OF ANTIGEN IN APC

4.4.3.1. Role of APCs in Immune Response
The uptake of antigen by stromal cells in the spleen and other lymphoid tissues is important not only for the destruction of pathogenic antigens, but is also a critical first step in the induction of both primary and secondary (memory) immune responses. The various anatomic compartments of the spleen perform specific functions, and within each compartment there are distinct cells specialized for the local capture and processing of antigen and the activation of nearby lymphocytes. Antigen capture is important for concentrating antigen in areas rich in reactive B-cells. However, the interactions of antigen-containing cells with T-lymphocytes are considerably more complex. The activation of splenic T-cells in response to a protein requires that stromal cells capture and concentrate antigen from the circulating blood, transport the antigen to the appropriate microenvironment within the spleen, and process this antigen, breaking it down into antigenic peptides, which are then expressed on the cell surface within the peptide-binding grooves of MHC-I or MHC-II major histocompatibility complex molecules (MHC).

In general, macrophages are optimized for taking up antigen, particularly for degrading particulate antigens, this being enhanced by opsonization. Activated macrophages are induced to express cell adhesion molecules (e.g., CD11a/CD18) and co-stimulatory molecules (e.g., B7.1 and B7.2), which interact with stimulatory receptors (e.g., CD28) on T-cells, thereby facilitating T-cell activation and proliferation. B-lymphocytes can also present antigen to T-cells, but, unlike macrophages, they are unable to break down particulate structures. However, in the case of soluble foreign proteins, a B-cell can take up specific antigen through its surface B-cell receptor, then process it and present immunogenic peptide with MHC to T-cells with the corresponding specificity. This has important implications for the delivery of T-cell help to B-lymphocytes for inducing Ig synthesis. In addition, under conditions in which there is an increased proportion of B-cells with a given specificity, such as occurs late in a primary response or after a secondary encounter with antigen, there is a sufficient number of specific B-cells in the spleen or lymph nodes to be the major source of APCs for activation of the T-cells. Thus, when antigen-specific B- and T-cells come together in the presence of cognate antigen, the resulting T–B interaction leads to the bidirectional exchange of activation signals.

4.4.3.2. Antigen Trapping and Transport in Spleen Compartments
Much of the blood entering the spleen empties into the MZ, and both particulate and soluble antigens therefore localize rapidly in the spleen MZ after iv injection (Kotani et al., 1985; Van den Eertwegh et al., 1992). Some antigens are also localized in red pulp macrophages early after injection (van Ewijk et al., 1977; Van den Eertwegh et al., 1992). Particulate antigens are taken up rapidly by macrophages in the MZ, which are highly phagocytic (Van den Eertwegh et al., 1992). As occurs with macrophages elsewhere, the uptake of soluble protein antigen, as well as particulates, by macrophages in the MZ is increased in the presence of opsonizing antibody, and a large proportion of injected immune complexes become trapped in the MZ (van Rooijen, 1977; Van den Berg et al., 1992). Antigen in the MZ is localized to both macrophages and B-lymphocytes (Mitchell and Abbot, 1971; Veerman and van Rooijen, 1975). Although MZ macrophages are generally thought to be relatively fixed in location, some appear to migrate from the MZ into the adjacent white pulp, transporting any associated antigen in the process (Kotani et al., 1985; Matsuno et al., 1985). In addition, some of the macrophages traversing the MZ may in fact originate in the red pulp or may be derived from circulating monocytes, thus transporting antigen from more distant sites (Kotani et al., 1986).

There is one highly specialized characteristic of MZ macrophages: They are particularly efficient in taking up from the circulation neutral polysaccharide antigens, such as the model antigens fluorescein- or DNP-conjugated Ficoll and hydroxyethyl starch, and some bacterial polysaccharides (Humphrey and Grennan, 1981; Kraal et al., 1989b). Intact encapsulated bacteria and *Candida* yeast are also taken up by MZ macrophages (Van den Eertwegh, 1992; Qian et al., 1994). The selective localization of such antigens in the MZ is of considerable interest, because this region is important in the immune response to thymus-independent (TI) antigens. TI type 2 (TI-2) antigens have regularly repeating antigenic determinants, commonly polysaccharide in nature, which can directly crosslink the Ig B-cell receptor and thereby activate B-cells without the aid of T-cell help. Many bacterial antigens, such as capsular polysaccharides or polymerized flagellar proteins, are strong TI-2 antigens. In addition to binding to MZ macrophages, bacterial polysaccharides also bind directly to the surface of MZ B-lymphocytes. This interaction is thought to result from the ability of these antigens to directly activate the alternate pathway of complement, fixing fragment C3d to the surface, and binding this complex to complement receptor 2 (CD21), which is expressed at particularly high levels on these B-cells.

Peset Llopis et al. (1996) showed that injected pneumococcal capsular polysaccharide, a prototypical TI-2 antigen, co-localized with C3 fragments on strongly CD21$^+$ B-cells in the MZ. Localization of pneumococcal polysaccharides on these B-cells preceded their later appearance in lymphoid follicles (Harms et al., 1996). The trapping of some polysaccharides is also enhanced by the recognition of mannose moieties mediated by a mannan recognition receptor, which is expressed by MZ macrophages (Chao and MacPherson, 1990). This receptor is distinct from the classical macrophage mannose receptor (MR), which is a transmembrane C-type lectin expressed on the surface of many non-MZ macrophage subsets, endothelial cells, and DCs (Chao and MacPherson, 1990; Linehan et al., 1999). However, the classical MR was recently shown to be present in serum in a soluble form, generated and released from macrophages into the circulation by its proteolytic cleavage from the cell surface. This soluble MR binds to *Candida albicans*, and probably other microorganisms and carbohydrate structures (Martínez-Pomares et al., 1998). Marginal metallophilic macrophages bear receptors for this soluble form of the classical MR, so that the soluble MR effectively acts as a partially site-specific opsonin, targeting mannose-bearing antigens to macrophages in the MZ (Martínez-Pomares et al., 1996; Martínez-Pomares et al., 1998). The binding of the soluble truncated mannose receptor to mannosylated antigens in vivo may thereby serve to increase the thymic-independent immune response by delivering them to cells in the splenic MZ (Linehan et al., 1999). Thus, there are several mechanisms by which polysaccharide antigens are targeted to MZ macrophages and B-cells.

During the humoral immune response to a soluble thymus-dependent antigen (TD, one that requires T-cell help), antigen becomes localized in a finely dispersed pattern in primary follicles, after which germinal centers begin forming. This tissue distribution reflects the presence of antigen on FDCs, and was originally thought to be the major source of antigen for initiating the B-cell response. FDCs take up antigen only in the form of Ig- and complement-containing immune complexes (MacLennan, 1994). These immune complexes bind primarily through complement receptors CR1 (CD35) and CR2 (CD21) on FDC (Reynes et al., 1985), although some binding can also occur directly to Fc receptors (Yoshida et al., 1993). FDCs do not phagocytose or otherwise degrade antigen, but retain it on the cell surface in a stable state for long periods of time, at least many months, and probably years. FDCs in lymphoid follicles may be the only site in the host in which native, unprocessed protein antigen can be retained for long periods of time. Because of the requirement for pre-existing antibody, follicular localization of most antigens must be preceded by a B-cell response and antigen-specific Ig secretion elsewhere, as described below. Once lodged on the surface of the FDC, in the presence of T-cell help, this antigen is presented to the resting B-cell expressing a corresponding antigen-specific B-cell receptor, resulting in B-cell activation, proliferation, and differentiation. A possible exception to the requirement for pre-existing antibody is that some carbohydrate-containing antigens may be bound via receptors for the soluble MR. This is the same receptor just described that is expressed by cells in the MZ, and mannose-containing antigens may therefore be bound to FDCs in the same manner (Martínez-Pomares et al., 1996; Martínez-Pomares et al., 1998; Linehan et al., 1999).

Since blood does not pass directly through the splenic B-cell areas, antigen:antibody complexes must somehow be transported into the follicles after they are first localized in the MZ. MZ macrophages have been observed migrating into the white pulp, some of which enter germinal centers (Kotani et al., 1985; Matsuno et al., 1985), which suggested that antigen taken up by these macrophages could be carried into lymphoid follicles and deposited onto FDCs. MZ B-cells have also been observed to migrate into primary B-cell follicles in the spleen (Gray et al., 1984). Because immune complexes bearing C3 fragments bind to MZ B-cells, it is likely that such cells could migrate to follicles and then transfer antigen to the complement receptor-bearing FDC. The regeneration of the capacity to trap antigen in the follicles of irradiated rats corresponded temporally to the reconstitution of MZ B-cells on d 5 after irradiation, consistent with a dependence of antigen localization upon an intact MZ B-cell compartment (Kroese et al., 1986). In contrasting experiments, follicular trapping of antigen was demonstrated after the chemical depletion of MZ macrophages and marginal metallophilic macrophages. These authors favored the view that immune complexes passively diffuse through the MZ and into the follicles (Laman et al., 1990). A parallel role for MZ B-cells in antigen transport, however, was not ruled out in this study. Transfer of carbohydrate-containing antigens may also occur through binding of the soluble mannose receptor described above. Thus, glycoconjugates bound to soluble MR would be delivered to cells in the MZ bearing ligands for the MR, followed by migration of these cells into nascent germinal centers. Putative transport cells with a dendritic morphology, and expressing a surface ligand for the soluble MR, have been observed to migrate to follicles during the immune response to ovalbumin (Martínez-Pomares et al., 1996).

Directly demonstrating the presence of intact thymus-dependent (TD) protein antigen in the T-cell-rich zone of the spleen is generally difficult (Van den Eertwegh et al., 1992). However, the relevant form of antigen for the stimulation of T-cells is not the intact protein, but proteolytic fragments associated with MHC on the surface of the APC. Therefore, antigen can be demonstrated

functionally, even in the absence of visible histochemical evidence of antigen. After the iv injection of soluble protein antigen, Crowley et al. (1990) tested various cell populations from the spleen for their ability to stimulate antigen-specific T-cells in vitro. DCs from the PALS of these primed mice were capable of activating T-cells, showing that they contained immunogenic peptide in vivo. Protein antigen could access the periarteriolar T-cell zone in two ways. Circulating antigen can be taken up by DCs in the MZ, followed by cell migration into the PALS, processing of the antigen, with differentiation into IDCs, the mature tissue form of DC. The IDCs in the PALS would then present the transported and processed antigen to the surrounding T-cells. For antigens present in peripheral tissues, antigen can be taken up by local DCs. These cells can then migrate through lymphatics to draining lymph nodes, or through the bloodstream to the spleen (Kupiec-Weglinski et al., 1988). DCs derived from a vascularized cardiac allograft were shown to migrate to the PALS, in which they associated with CD4 T-cells, thus stimulating an immune response to the allogeneic tissue (Larsen et al., 1990). In a separate study, within 24 h of the iv injection of purified DCs, they were localized in the T-cell area of the white pulp, again demonstrating a mechanism by which these cells could transport and present peripheral antigen to splenic T-cells (Austyn et al., 1988).

Mature DCs and IDCs are the most potent APCs for priming naïve T-lymphocytes (Banchereau and Steinman, 1998), but, like B-cells, they do not have the intracellular machinery to break down complex particulate antigens. Such antigens must be phagocytosed, broken down, and the proteins processed by macrophages before presentation to T-cells (Dal Monte and Szoka, 1989; van Rooijen, 1990). For example, in a study of the presentation of *Listeria monocytogenes* antigens, macrophage processing was required for the activation of T-cells by intact organisms or synthetically aggregated antigen, but not for presentation of soluble Listerial antigens (Ziegler, Orlin and Cluff, 1987). Although macrophages can present antigen to T-cells, they are much less efficient in doing so than DCs or B-cells (Francotte and Urbain, 1985). Particulate antigens have been demonstrated to be phagocytosed by macrophages, degraded, then transferred to secondary APCs (Roska and Lipsky, 1985; Kapsenberg et al., 1986; Wright et al., 1987). Particulate antigens can be degraded by macrophages in the MZ, then transferred to B-cells or DCs, which would then transport antigen into the white pulp. Such particulates could also be broken down by phagocytes in the periphery and transferred to DCs, followed by traffic to the spleen. Thus, as suggested by van Rooijen (1990), the sequential processing of some antigens by different cell types may play a critical role in the induction of T-cell immune responses.

4.5. PROTOTYPIC IMMUNE RESPONSES IN THE SPLEEN

4.5.1. T-INDEPENDENT B-CELL RESPONSES
The immune response to most protein antigens requires the participation of antigen-specific CD4 helper T-cells. Humans and experimental animals with a selective deficiency of the T-cell system, however, can nonetheless make good antibody responses to many bacteria. Thymus-independent (TI) antigens can directly activate B-lymphocytes to proliferate, secrete Ig, and differentiate into plasma cells, without the need for T-lymphocytes. As previously discussed, bacterial capsular polysaccharides, with repetitively arranged antigenic structures (epitopes), can crosslink receptors for antigen

on the B-cell surface, and are classical TI-2 antigens. However, other antigens, which are more commonly considered as being thymic-dependent, such as some viruses, can have a TI component to their response, if they display a high density of repeating epitopes (Ochsenbein et al., 2000). Although not requiring T-cells, TI-2 responses are enhanced by cytokines that can be provided by accessory cells, such as natural killer cells, DCs, and macrophages (Mond et al., 1995; Snapper et al., 1995; Chelvarajan et al., 1998). TI type 1 (TI-1) antigens also elicit responses in the absence of T-cells, but the response results from inherent mitogenic activity that polyclonally activates most B-cells, independent of the binding specificity of their surface Ig. At low concentrations, which probably are attained in vivo, these TI-1 antigens activate only B-cell clones that also have specificity for the antigen, because the surface B-cell receptor binds epitopes on the molecule and effectively concentrates the antigen, which then can deliver a mitogenic signal. Bacterial lipopolysaccharide is a potent TI-1 antigen. Monomeric soluble proteins are rarely TI, because they lack the polyvalent epitopes necessary for crosslinking B-cell receptors.

The spleen is a major site of production of immune responses to TI-2 antigens; it is more difficult to elicit such responses from lymph nodes (Goud et al., 1988; Ochsenbein et al., 2000). Splenectomized mice and humans are deficient in their antibody response to the model TI-2 antigens DNP-Ficoll and DNP-hydroxyethyl starch (Amlot et al., 1985; Amlot and Hayes, 1985). The response to model TI antigens injected subcutaneously is greater in the spleen than lymph nodes, even though antigen drains directly into the latter before reaching the spleen through the circulation (Delemarre et al., 1989). B-cells in the spleen are therefore particularly specialized for TI responses to carbohydrate, independent of the mode of antigen injection. As might be inferred by the selective localization of TI-2 antigens in the MZ (see Subheading 4.3.2.), considerable data have indicated that this compartment has particular importance in such responses (Claassen et al., 1986). In experiments in which clodronate-containing liposomes were used to eliminate spleen macrophages chemically, the ability to mount a TI response to a particulate bacterial antigen did not return as the red pulp was repopulated with macrophages. In contrast, when macrophages in the MZ were reconstituted, TI responsiveness returned (Buiting et al., 1996), which emphasizes the importance of the MZ in maintaining responsiveness to particulate TI antigens. However, disruption of MZ macrophages or B-cells does not decrease the B-cell response to all TI-2 antigens, and the exact role of the MZ in the TI response is not yet fully defined. Some of these differences may result from the nature of the antigen. For example, the response to neutral polysaccharides, which localize more selectively in the MZ than do acidic polysaccharides (Humphrey and Grennan, 1981), may have different dependence on the splenic MZ (Cohn and Schiffman, 1987). Experiments in the rat have demonstrated that all pneumococcal carbohydrates examined, when opsonized by complement, could localize to the MZ by binding to complement receptor-positive B-cells (Harms et al., 1996; Peset Llopis et al., 1996). This suggests that antigens that can directly activate complement, or are recognized by receptors for mannans (Chao and MacPherson, 1990), would localize appropriately for a MZ B-cell response.

Antibody responses are important for the resolution of many viral infections; others are cleared primarily by CD8 T-lymphocytes. Even though the immune response to most proteins requires CD4 helper T-cells, recent studies have demonstrated a role for TI Ig responses to several viruses (Bachmann et al., 1995; Szomolanyi-Tsuda and Welsh, 1998). Infection of T-cell-deficient mice with polyomavirus elicited a protective neutralizing IgG response; animals with combined B- and T-cell deficiency succumbed to infection (Szomolanyi-Tsuda and Welsh, 1996). Immunization with noninfectious virus-like particles induced a strong IgM response, 10-fold higher than soluble capsid antigens, demonstrating that viral antigens with structured repeating epitopes are necessary for inducing the optimal TI antibody response (Szomolanyi-Tsuda et al., 1998). However, only infection by live virus was capable of causing a switch to the IgG antibody class in these mice. TI neutralizing antibody responses to other viruses have also been described (Szomolanyi-Tsuda and Welsh, 1998). Of particular interest is the finding that a mucosal IgA response against rotavirus, a major pediatric pathogen, can take place in mice in the absence of T-cell help (Borrow et al., 1996). Although isotype switch from IgM to other Ig classes is enhanced by help from CD4 T-cells, experiments have shown that cytokines, such as interferon-γ from natural killer cells, which are activated during virus infection, may also induce class switching.

In an interesting series of experiments, Ochsenbein et al. (1999b) examined the humoral immune response to a murine neurotropic virus, the vesicular stomatitis virus (VSV). An early neutralizing antibody response is required to block virus spread to the central nervous system and to prevent lethal encephalitis in infected mice. The early IgM response to this virus is TI, and depends on activation of the classical pathway of complement, in such a manner that the response is markedly decreased in both C3 and C4 knockout mice. VSV antigen was found to localize heavily in macrophages in the splenic MZs within 1 d of injection into normal mice. However, no such localization was seen in the absence of complement component C3, thus showing a correlation between complement-mediated antigen trapping in the MZ and a protective TI antibody response. Even though these viruses can stimulate a TI response, in the presence of T-cell help, even stronger responses are subsequently formed, and effective long-term memory is generated.

In additional experiments, the requirements for TD and TI responses were compared, using VSV, lymphocytic choriomeningitis virus (LCMV), and poliovirus (Ochsenbein et al., 2000). Iv infection with high doses of all of these agents resulted in strong TI antibody responses; low doses resulted in a primarily TD responses. These TI responses were associated with the localization of viral antigen in the MZ, and by 48 h the formation of foci of proliferating B-cells in the MZ. A similar dependence of the type of response on dose was found for purified VSV antigen. Virus infection through the subcutaneous route resulted in only TD responses, as did iv infection in splenectomized mice, showing that the TI antibody response depends on the presence of the spleen. The TI response to inactivated virion particles, which exhibit epitopes in a rigid, repetitive form, is 1000-fold higher than that to an equivalent dose of soluble recombinant VSV protein. Together, these experiments showed that the induction of early TI responses depends not only on the presence of an antigenic structure with repeating epitopes, but also requires that a sufficient dose of antigen be trapped in the MZ of the spleen. The MZ, therefore, is specialized for trapping viral antigen, particularly when bound to activated complement components. After localization in the MZ, the high antigen density on macrophages can crosslink the antigen receptors of MZ B-cells and lead to a rapid neutralizing antibody response.

4.5.2. THYMUS-DEPENDENT IMMUNE RESPONSES Antibody responses to most soluble protein antigens require interaction between B-cells and antigen-specific T-cells. Although TD responses take longer to develop than TI, they generally give rise to higher titers of Ig, and antibody of a higher binding affinity. In addition, these responses are characterized by effective long-term memory, with memory B- and T-lymphocytes persisting in the host and providing long-term protection against secondary exposure to a pathogen. Since T-lymphocytes respond almost exclusively to processed peptide epitopes, T-cells generally cannot recognize polysaccharide antigens. They can, however, provide specific help to increase the antibody response to carbohydrate or other moieties present as haptenic groups on carrier proteins. Unlike TI responses, for which the splenic architecture is particularly well-suited, TD responses are induced equally well in lymph nodes, as well as other lymphoid tissues, the origin of the response depending on the site of introduction of antigen.

TD responses in the spleen involve three distinct steps: trapping of antigen followed by binding of antigen to complementary receptors on B-cells, thus providing the first signal for B-cell activation; the processing of antigen by APCs and presentation to T-lymphocytes; and interaction between antigen-specific B-cells and activated T-cells, and the exchange of signals resulting in further B-cell stimulation. These steps occur sequentially in specialized microenvironments within the spleen (Kelsoe, 1996; Camacho et al., 1998; MacLennan, 1998). B-cells may bind antigen first, as they recirculate through the PALS, or in the MZ, followed by their migration into the PALS. Regardless of the initial site of encounter, these B-cells first become activated and begin proliferating in the T-cell-rich zone (Gray, 1988; Liu et al., 1991; Jacob and Kelsoe, 1992). Antigen binding to the B-cell receptor provides the initial activating signal, and if complement component C3d is fixed to the antigen, permitting additional signaling through CD21, then the threshold for cell activation is markedly lowered (Fischer et al., 1996; Carroll, 2000). Concomitant with this, APCs that contain antigen process it into immunogenic oligopeptides, which they then transport to the cell surface associated with MHC-II molecules. For the primary immune response, activation of helper T-cells is dependent on interaction with antigen-bearing IDCs in the PALS. Naïve antigen-specific T-lymphocytes migrate toward IDCs that secrete chemotactic chemokines, such as SLC (Willimann et al., 1998). The IDC then present the processed antigen and deliver co-stimulatory signals, resulting in activation of the T-cells. B-lymphocytes that have taken up the same antigen also present immunogenic peptides with MHC-II. When one of these B-cells encounters an activated T-cell of the same specificity, membrane-mediated interactions take place, and soluble factors are released, which provide the second signal required for full B-cell activation. Some of these B-cells begin to secrete antibody, and go on to form antibody-secreting plasma cells in the red pulp and bone marrow (Eikelenboom et al., 1982). This early antibody generally has a low affinity of binding to antigen. Other activated B-cells migrate to the boundary between the B- and T-cell zones, begin secreting chemokines that attract activated T-cells (Cyster, 1999; Krzysiek et al., 1999), and later move into the adjacent primary follicles in response to FDC-derived chemotactic cytokines (Forster et al., 1996; Gunn et al., 1998; Ansel et al., 2000).

Once localized in the B-cell follicle, the activated B-cells interact with antigen that has been trapped by FDC, and are stimulated further, giving rise to germinal centers by d 6 postimmunization.

Each germinal center is oligoclonal, being derived from 1–3 antigen-specific precursor B-cells (Liu et al., 1991; Kelsoe, 1996). As described previously, antigen binds to the FDC only in the form of immune complexes. Thus, in the absence of pre-existing specific Ig, whether natural antibody (Ehrenstein et al., 1998; Ochsenbein et al., 1999) or from a previous immune response, the trapping of antigens on FDC requires the early antibody response first initiated in the nearby T-cell zone (van Rooijen and Kors, 1985; Yoshida et al., 1993). The antigen-specific helper T-cells activated in the PALS downregulate the chemokine receptor CCR7, lose their responsiveness to the T-cell zone chemokine SLC, and migrate away from the IDC in the PALS (Randolph et al., 1999). These T-cells then migrate to the outer rim of the follicles, together with the stimulated B-cells, in response to B-cell-secreted chemokines (Cyster, 1999). A small number of antigen-specific T-cells then migrate into the germinal centers where they are further stimulated by antigen on dendritic cells, and then deliver additional help to proliferating B-cells (Grouard et al., 1996; Zheng et al., 1996).

The overall result of this helper T-cell–B-cell interaction is to increase the proliferation and clonal expansion of antigen-specific B-cells. In addition, cytokines secreted by the T-cells, such as interleukin-4 and -5, induce class switching in B-cells, resulting in an increase in IgE, IgA, and some IgG subclasses. Within the germinal center, B-cell Ig genes undergo hypermutation, and antigen, CD4 T-cells, and FDCs select for B-cells that express Ig with progressively increasing affinity for antigen (Kelsoe, 1996; Tew et al., 1997; Takahashi et al., 1998). A subset of these high-affinity cells subsequently differentiates into memory B-cells. Thus, germinal centers function both to increase the efficacy of the primary immune response and also to prime the host for an enhanced rapid response to subsequent challenge by antigen at a later time.

The secondary immune response differs somewhat from the primary response described above. Pre-existing antibody causes more rapid antigen localization in follicles. In addition, memory B-cells located in the MZ migrate in large numbers into the PALS, become stimulated by activated memory T-cells, and these blasts then migrate to follicles and initiate the germinal center response (Liu et al., 1991). In addition, in the secondary response, there are many more B-cells that can trap antigen through their antigen-specific surface B-cell receptor. Because B-lymphocytes can process soluble protein antigen, these B-cells are major antigen-presenting cells for T-cells in the secondary response. The subsequent bidirectional T–B-cell signaling thereby results in both T- and B-cell stimulation and proliferation. Thus, the previously primed and expanded population of memory T- and B-cells gives rise to rapid high-titer antibody responses.

Naïve T-lymphocytes that encounter antigen in the spleen can also differentiate into effector T-cells that have little or no role in helping B-cells. The Th1 subset of CD4 T-cells secrete proinflammatory cytokines, such as interferon-γ, and mediate a variety of inflammatory reactions. Naïve T-cells, activated by DCs in the central PALS, can differentiate into Th1 cells, then migrate to sites of antigen deposition in the periphery (Randolph et al., 1999). Similarly, CD8 T-cells recirculate through the PALS and, if they come into contact with cognate antigen on APCs, they undergo activation, clonal expansion, and differentiation into cytotoxic T-cells (Willfuhr et al., 1990). Localization of CD8 T-cells in the central PALS, in which they contact antigen, and their egress after activation and differentiation, is controlled by the regulated expression of chemokine receptors and responsiveness to PALS-associated chemokines (Potsch et al., 1999), as described for CD4 T-cells. The resulting CD8 effector T-cells are important in a variety of host responses, including allograft rejection and protection against many viral infections.

4.6. THE IMMUNE RESPONSE IN AUTOIMMUNE THROMBOCYTOPENIAS

A number of syndromes are associated with potentially life-threatening thrombocytopenia of immune origin. Thus, platelet destruction may be mediated by circulating antibodies to normal platelet plasma membrane antigens or to drug-induced neo-antigens. The clearest example of an antibody-mediated disease is idiopathic thrombocytopenic purpura (ITP). In this disease, antibodies that are produced principally in the spleen, and are predominantly of the IgG class, bind to platelet surface antigens. The most common of these autoantigens are the integrin glycoprotein IIb/IIIa and the gpIb/IX complex (Tomiyama et al., 1987). Autoantibodies to gpIIb/IIIa or the Ib-IX complex, both of which mediate platelet adhesion, can result in platelet dysfunction. In ITP, sensitization of the platelet with IgG results in a decrease in platelet survival, usually in the absence of complement fixation. Since approx one-third of circulating platelets are in the spleen at any time, in the presence of locally produced antibody, they are recognized and phagocytosed by Fc receptor-bearing macrophages in the red pulp. A more complete discussion of thrombocytopenia is presented in Chapter 12.

The human IgG Fc receptors FcγRI, FcγRA, and FcγRIIIA, are independently able to bind and take up opsonized antigens, and it is likely that all three receptors are simultaneously engaged by Ig, and can remove platelets in vivo (McKenzie and Schreiber, 1998). A rare exception might be for platelets opsonized exclusively by IgG$_2$, which binds well only to FcγRIIA. In addition to binding the Fc regions of Ig on the platelet surface, these receptors transduce an activating signal that further increases phagocytic activity. Macrophages also express Fc receptors (FcγRIIB) that transduce inhibitory signals, potentially downregulating some macrophage responses. However, there is no evidence that ligation of these receptors on phagocytes downregulates the opsonization response, unlike the FcγRIIB-mediated inhibition observed in B-lymphocyte responses to antigen (Heyman, 2000).

The roles of antibodies and Fc receptors have been examined in murine models of ITP. In (NZW x BXSB)F1 mice, natural antiplatelet antibody induces thrombocytopenia, which is chiefly corrected by splenectomy (Mizutani et al., 1990; Mizutani et al., 1992). Mice injected with a rat monoclonal antibody specific for a platelet surface antigen become moderately thrombocytopenic, but less so than with polyclonal antibody (Burstein et al., 1992). Platelet depletion in response to antibody injection is unchanged in animals deficient in complement components C3 and C4, which is consistent with clinical observations that platelet clearance does not depend on complement activation (Sylvestre et al., 1996) (a possible role for complement in some cases of ITP in humans is discussed in Chapter 12, Subheading 3.2.). However, in animals with genetic deficiency in Fcγ receptors, the response to cytotoxic antibodies was markedly diminished, thus substantiating the role of Fcγ receptors in removing opsonized platelets. In order to study the role of human FcR in platelet clearance, a transgene for human FcγRIIA was expressed in FcR γ-chain knockout mice. In these animals, the only phagocytosis-competent receptor is therefore of human origin. When these mice were injected with the above-

described monoclonal rat anti-mouse platelet antibody, platelets were rapidly cleared from the circulation, resulting in severe thrombocytopenia, considerably more pronounced than in normal FcR$^+$ mice (McKenzie et al., 1999). These experiments suggest that human FcγRIIA, a single-chain receptor that does not have a counterpart in the mouse, is especially active in removing antibody-sensitized platelets from the circulation. This is despite the lower affinity of binding of this receptor to IgG (approx 50-fold less than FcγRI), because the avidity of multipoint binding to coated platelets would still be high. In addition, since mice deficient in the FcR γ chain still express the inhibitory FcγRIIIB, these results suggest that the inhibitory receptor does not downmodulate phagocytosis mediated by the activating receptor, FcγRIIA.

4.6.1. IMMUNOLOGIC TREATMENT OF ITP   The commonly used therapies for ITP have in common the goals of reducing the autoimmune antibody response to platelet self-antigens, and also of blocking the effector phase of the response (i.e., Fc receptor-mediated phagocytic clearance, which causes platelet destruction.) Glucocorticoid treatment decreases autoantibody production, but platelet counts frequently increase before antibody levels fall. The early increase in platelet survival therefore may be related to the ability of corticosteroids to cause downregulation of macrophage FcR expression (Fries et al., 1983). Splenectomy removes both the major source of autoantibody production and the principal site of platelet destruction, and usually results in a rapid increase in platelet counts. In patients in whom splenectomy has little therapeutic benefit, antibody production has mostly shifted to the bone marrow, with platelet destruction then occurring primarily in the marrow and liver.

One treatment of a variety of immune disorders, including ITP, is the administration of high doses of Ig pooled from many donors. This intravenous immunoglobulin (IVIg) therapy is effective in inducing substantial increases in circulating platelet levels in many patients with chronic ITP. Despite considerable ongoing basic research, the mechanisms of action of IVIg remain unclear. This is not because of a lack of meaningful information, but, rather, there are many plausible mechanisms, several of which probably do play independent roles in modulating the host response to platelets (Mouthon et al., 1996; Rhoades et al., 2000). In an early study in patients with ITP, IVIg was found to increase platelet survival. At the same time, the clearance of antibody-sensitized autologous erythrocytes was markedly prolonged (Fehr et al., 1982). This supported the hypothesis that the decreased destruction of opsonized platelets and RBC induced by IVIg results from nonantigen-specific blockade of the reticuloendothelial system, because of competitive inhibition between normal and pathogenic Ig for binding to Fc receptors. Given the high levels of donor Ig reached, and the fact that some of this is in dimeric and multimeric form, thereby increasing its avidity of binding to FcR, this would seem a reasonable explanation for temporary clinical improvement in platelet counts. However, the successful induction of long-term remissions in some patients, persisting long after donor Ig would have been cleared, indicates that IVIg must modify the ongoing immune response in some more fundamental way than simply producing a transient inhibition of the effector phase of platelet destruction. Considerable interest has therefore been expressed in defining the immunomodulatory activities of IVIg.

Normal serum and commercial, pooled IVIg preparations have been shown to contain natural antibodies to many normal self-antigens, including cell surface proteins that have major roles in the induction and regulation of immune responses (Guilbert et al., 1982; Mouthon et al., 1996). Many of these antibodies have shown biological activity in modifying immune reactions, e.g., antibody in IVIg that binds to human CD4 on T-cells inhibits proliferative responses in mixed lymphocyte reactions and the infection of CD4 T-cells by HIV (Hurez et al., 1994). Ig with specificities to MHC antigens (Kaveri et al., 1996), β_2 microglobulin (Vincent and Revillard, 1983), CD5 (Vassilev et al., 1993) and B- and T-cell receptors (Marchalonis et al., 1994) have also been found. In addition to inhibiting spontaneous and cytokine-dependent lymphocyte proliferation at therapeutic levels in vitro (van Schaik et al., 1992; Amran et al., 1994), IVIg also inhibits the secretion of several T-cell and macrophage cytokines (Abe et al., 1994; Andersson et al., 1994; Nachbaur et al., 1997). Blocking the action of such cytokines would be expected to have widespread regulatory effects in the immune system in vivo. The natural anti-Arg-Gly-Asp peptide antibody present in IVIg binds to the Arg-Gly-Asp (RGD) peptide sequence, which is the recognition site on many integrin ligands. This antibody activity completely inhibits adenosine-diphosphate-induced gpIIb/IIIa integrin-mediated platelet aggregation, the adhesion of unstimulated platelets to fibrinogen, and of thrombin-stimulated platelets to von Willebrand factor, potentially resulting in decreased platelet activity that could be beneficial in patients with thrombotic diseases (Vassilev et al., 1999).

The normal repertoire of Igs includes antibodies against exogenous antigens, as well as nonpathogenic antibodies against some autoantigens. In addition, there exists a special set of natural antibodies specific for epitopes in the antigen combining sites in the variable regions of other serum antibodies. Such anti-idiotypic antibodies can suppress specific antibody responses (Kohler et al., 1977), and, when directed against the V regions of T-cell receptors, can inhibit specific T-cell-mediated immune reactions (McKearn, 1974; Stuart et al., 1982; Marchalonis et al., 1992). Rowley et al. (1980) have proposed that a major immune regulatory mechanism involves homeostatic interactions between idiotypic and anti-idiotypic antibodies, with each new immune response generating a new wave of idiotypic interactions exerting positive and negative feedback. An autoimmune response represents in part an abnormal skewing of this equilibrium, resulting in an increase in pathogenic autoantibodies or clones of self-reactive T-cells.

IVIg has been shown to contain anti-idiotypic antibodies that bind to autoantibodies of several specificities (Rossi and Kazatchkine, 1989; Kaveri et al., 1997), including some that bind to anti-platelet IgG (Berchtold et al., 1989). One conceptually straightforward mechanism by which autoantibody titers can be reduced is by binding to neutralizing anti-idiotypic IgG in the infused IVIg, the resulting complexes subsequently being removed by phagocytes of the reticuloendothelial system (Rhoades et al., 2000). Anti-idiotypic antibody in IVIg can thus block binding of antibody to the platelet autoantigen. Other mechanisms, however, must be invoked to explain the more long-lasting therapeutic effects of IVIg persisting beyond the lifetime of the donor Ig. One possible activity of the heterologous Ig in IVIg could be to bind to platelet-specific B-cell antigen receptors, and perhaps to receptors on helper T-cells, and cause perturbations in the host regulatory idiotype network, resulting in suppression of the humoral response to platelet autoantigens (Lacroix-Desmazes et al., 1996). The pooled normal Ig in commercial IVIg contains antibody that binds to both T- and B-cell receptors, with a clonally restricted idiotypic specificity that could serve such an immunomodulatory function

(Marchalonis et al., 1992; Marchalonis et al., 1994). In order to examine these anti-idiotypic Igs in detail, Fischer et al. (1999) used a phage-display system to determine the specificities of a large number of Ig clones from three patients with ITP, whose antibodies reacted with IVIg. Many of the patients' antibodies that bound to Ig in the IVIg also bound strongly to the surface of platelets, and many of the clones shared sequence homology in the complementarity-determining region of their variable regions, as well as to previously sequenced antiplatelet autoantibodies. IVIg-reactive antibody from controls did not bind to platelets, but they nonetheless preferentially used the same set of germline variable region genes (Hoffmann et al., 2000). This suggests that Ig in normal serum and IVIg preferentially interacts with and regulates a subset of B-cells expressing a favored subset of self-reactive B-cell receptors, including B-cells with specificity for platelet membrane antigens.

The administration of IVIg has been shown to have a direct effect on autoimmune diseases in several animal models. Injection of myelin basic protein into rats induces the T-cell-mediated demyelinating syndrome experimental allergic encephalomyelitis. Injection of IVIg blocks induction of the disease, and induces antigen-specific unresponsiveness in CD4 T-cells, so that they cannot transfer the disease to normal recipients (Pashov et al., 1998). Immunodeficient (SCID) mice, reconstituted with T-cells from a patient with myasthenia gravis and boosted 1 d later with acetylcholine receptor (AchR), develop autoantibodies that cause experimental myasthenia gravis. Injection of normal human Ig suppresses the anti-AchR antibody, and inhibits the loss of motor end plate AchR (Vassilev et al., 1999). Because IVIg has been shown to contain anti-idiotypic Igs that bind to pathogenic anti-AchR antibodies (Liblau et al., 1991), it is probable that the immune regulation seen in these SCID mice results from modulation of the idiotype network and selection against autoreactive B-cells. Pooled normal human serum contains anti-idiotypic antibodies of the IgM class that neutralize autoimmune IgG in vitro. When injected into rats immunized with a retinal antigen, this normal IgM protected against the induction of autoimmune uveitis, probably by anti-idiotypic blocking of rat lymphocytes bearing Ig idiotypes crossreactive with those in humans (Hurez et al., 1997).

Clearly, from the above observations, IVIg contains natural antibodies with a broad array of specificities against lymphocyte surface regulatory molecules and idiotypic specificities against antibodies expressed in both normal subjects and patients with autoimmune thrombocytopenia. Such antibodies would probably act in the short term by neutralizing platelet autoantibodies. Although it is difficult to prove that IVIg deviates the immune repertoire by modulating the idiotypic network, considerable experimental evidence provides precedents for such an effect, and it remains a prime candidate for the mechanism of long-term suppression of autoreactive antibodies and clinical improvement in patients with ITP.

4.7. IMMUNE CONSEQUENCES OF THE HYPOSPLENIC STATE

The most important sequela of the loss of spleen function is an increase in the risk of overwhelming bacterial sepsis, particularly from encapsulated pneumococcus, *Hemophilus influenzae*, and meningococcus (Bisno and Freeman, 1970), as well as from some rarer organisms (Garnham, 1980; *see also* Chapter 11). Even in asplenic, infected patients who receive prompt therapy, the case fatality rate for fulminant pneumococcal sepsis remains at 50–80% (Nuorti et al., 1997). The risk of postsplenectomy infection is higher for infants and young children (King and Schumaker, 1952; Eraklis and Filler, 1972). There is also a correlation between the relative risk of infection and the underlying disease state responsible for the splenic disorder. Thus, patients splenectomized as a result of hematologic malignancy or patients with hemoglobinopathies (Chilcote et al., 1976) are at much greater risk than are otherwise healthy persons. However, even patients who have been previously splenectomized for trauma retain a small, but significantly elevated, lifelong risk of bacteremia (Gopal and Bisno, 1977). Part of the reason for the lower rate of infection in adults splenectomized for trauma is the frequent regrowth of functional splenic tissue in the abdomen (splenosis) after splenic rupture (Pearson et al., 1978). Although splenectomy is the most common cause of loss of spleen function, other processes can result in functional asplenia, including congenital splenic hypoplasia and sickle cell anemia (see Chapters 10 and 15). Both splenic hypofunction and atrophy, with increased risk of sepsis, occur in patients with systemic lupus erythematosus (Dillon et al., 1982; Hamburger et al., 1982) and inflammatory bowel disease (Ryan et al., 1981; Foster et al., 1982). Severe splenic fibrosis and atrophy also occur in patients who have received splenic irradiation, and the resulting hyposplenism can result in fulminant pneumococcal sepsis and disseminated intravascular coagulation (Dailey et al., 1980; Dailey et al., 1981).

Considerable experimental evidence confirms the importance of the spleen in host resistance to bacteremia. In splenectomized mice, clearance of injected pneumococcus is slowed, resulting in fatal sepsis (Loggie et al., 1985). Similarly, asplenic rats do not clear iv pneumococcus rapidly and succumb to infection (Leung et al., 1972). Other organs in the reticuloendothelial system, such as the liver and bone marrow, filter blood and are capable of removing microorganisms. What then is special about the spleen that makes it so important in defense of the host against serious bacteremia? As previously discussed, the spleen is the only organ that serves both as a phagocytic filter that removes particulate antigens from the bloodstream, and also as a lymphoid organ that can mount an adaptive immune response against these organisms. The most important first line of defense is the filtration of bacteria and their destruction by red pulp or MZ macrophages, and this process must be rapid in order to overcome the speed at which bacteria can replicate. A key property of splenic phagocytosis is that, unlike the liver, it is effective in removing poorly opsonized particles from the bloodstream, an antigen-nonspecific process mediated in part by receptors of the innate immune system (van der Laan et al., 1999; see also Subheading 4.3.2.). The uptake process is markedly enhanced in the presence of antibody and the activation of complement, the resulting immune complexes then being taken up avidly by macrophage Fc and complement receptors (Brown et al., 1983). Thus, preimmunization of animals with pneumococcal antigen induces secretion of opsonizing antibody and increases bacterial clearance and decreases mortality (Leung et al., 1972; Hosea et al., 1980). Kupffer cells in the liver are much less able to take up antigen in the absence of antibody or complement (Schulkind et al., 1967). After iv injection of ^{125}I-labeled pneumococcus into normal rabbits, most of the organisms localized in the spleen (Brown et al., 1981). In contrast, in immune animals, most of the label was taken up by the liver. The clearance of *Escherichia coli* by the liver is similarly dependent on opsonizing antibody (Benacerraf et al., 1959). Studies of the clearance of labeled erythrocytes in humans confirmed that the spleen is the major site of red blood cell destruction in the absence of antibody, and that the relative amount of

removal in the liver is enhanced as the amount of antibody increases (Jandl and Kaplan, 1960; Oliver et al., 1999). Thus, in the nonimmune host, the distinctive phagocytic capacity of the spleen is essential for the effective clearance of encapsulated bacteria. Furthermore, the spleen plays an increasingly important role in the clearance of more virulent organisms, which resist phagocytosis, and for which the liver is unable to compensate in the absence of specific antibody.

The major antibody class secreted in responses to bacterial polysaccharides in humans is IgG_2, which is particularly important in resistance to infection by encapsulated bacteria (Scott et al., 1988; Sanders et al., 1995). IgG_2, bound to the bacterial surface, increases binding to phagocyte FcR in the spleen, as well as liver, thus stimulating increased uptake. One additional factor to be considered is that allelic polymorphisms in human Fc receptors affect their binding of Ig and immune complexes. There are two major alleles of the FcγRIIA gene, which are co-dominantly expressed on all phagocytes. FcγRIIA is the only type that binds well to the IgG_2 subclass, and it has been shown that the allele with arginine at position 131 (FcγRIIA-R^{131}) binds IgG_2 much less well than the isoform containing histidine (FcγRIIA-H^{131}) at the same position (Warmerdam et al., 1990; Warmerdam et al., 1991). Consistent with this poor IgG_2 binding, the FcγRIIA-R^{131} allelic form is markedly deficient in its ability to mediate the phagocytic uptake of IgG_2-coated erythrocytes (Salmon et al., 1992). More importantly, the uptake of IgG_2-opsonized pneumococcus, *Staphylococcus aureus*, and *H. influenzae*, by neutrophils and monocytes isolated from persons expressing the FcγRIIA-R^{131} allele, is much lower than in individuals homozygous for the H^{131} allele (Bredius et al., 1993; Sanders et al., 1995). Because the major isotype responding to polysaccharides is IgG_2, and IgG_2 is particularly important in resistance to bacterial infection (Scott et al., 1988; Sanders et al., 1995), Fc receptor polymorphism might be expected to influence the host responses in vivo. Several studies have shown that FcγRIIA polymorphism does indeed have substantial clinical importance. Expression of the low-IgG_2-binding allele is associated with an increased prevalence of chronic bacterial infections in children and invasive pneumococcal infections in patients with systemic lupus erythematesus (Sanders et al., 1994; Yee et al., 1997). FcγRIIA-R^{131} is also strongly associated with increased risk of bacteremia in patients with pneumococcal pneumonia, and with a higher mortality rate in patients who become bacteremic (Yee et al., 2000). The R^{131} allotype also confers a higher risk of meningococcal sepsis (Bredius et al., 1994). These observations emphasize the critical role of antibody- and Fc receptor-mediated phagocytosis in the optimal clearance of encapsulated bacteria.

The ability of iv antigens to elicit a specific immune response is deficient in asplenic patients. Patients with functional or anatomic asplenia, injected with the nonreplicating virus ΦX174, a particulate antigen, responded with lower antibody titers than normal controls (Jandl and Kaplan, 1960; Oliver et al., 1999). Iv heterologous erythrocytes also induced markedly diminished responses in asplenic children (Kevy et al., 1968). There are conflicting data regarding to the ability of healthy asplenic subjects to respond to immunization with polysaccharides. Hosea et al. (1981) showed decreased IgG and IgM responses to direct challenge with 8/9 pneumococcal polysaccharides (Hosea et al., 1981), which is similar to the poor responses to pneumococcal antigens seen in splenectomized mice (Cohn and Schiffman, 1987; Aaberge and Lovik, 1996; Leemans et al., 1999), although the responses to some polysaccharides were better than others. The deficient response to some capsular polysaccharides could result from their different chemical structures and different compartmental localization in the spleen, as described in Subheading 5.1. The response of splenectomized humans injected with the synthetic TI-2 carbohydrate antigen, DNP-Ficoll, was reduced by 90%, compared to eusplenic controls (Amlot and Hayes, 1985). However, in patients primed with the antigen before splenectomy, the antibody response to subsequent rechallenge was normal. Thus, the initial response to certain TI antigens is localized to the spleen, but subsequent responses to subcutaneous antigen can arise from spleen-derived precursor B-cells that have recirculated to other lymphoid organs (van Rees et al., 1987). In spite of the lower response to some carbohydrate antigens, most asplenic patients over the age of 2 yr who are immunized subcutaneously with current commercial pneumococcal vaccines respond with antibody titers comparable to those obtained in healthy persons of the same age, and they experience significantly fewer episodes of bacteremia (reviewed in Nuorti et al., 1997). This responsiveness to nonintravascular pneumococcal polysaccharides may be caused in part by prior exposure to pneumococcal or crossreactive environmental antigens, with subsequent peripheralization of antigen-reactive B-cells, before splenectomy.

During an infection localized in peripheral tissues, the innate immune system can usually mediate control for a sufficient amount of time for the immune system to generate antibody, which then effects bacterial clearance. In immune subjects, circulating antibody can promote the rapid removal of bacteria replicating in the bloodstream, which is almost always sufficient to prevent severe bacteremia and sepsis. However, an important unresolved question is whether, in the naïve host, with no pre-existing circulating antibody, activation of an immune response is important for the clearance of bacteria that rapidly gain entry to the bloodstream. As previously discussed, the MZ in the spleen is particularly efficient for trapping antigen and rapidly activating B-cell responses in the absence of T-cell help, which takes several days to develop. With their high expression of the co-activating receptor, CD21, MZ B-cells are poised for rapid activation by complement-opsonized antigens, implicating them in the earliest humoral response to antigen (Timens et al., 1989; Dempsey et al., 1996; Oliver et al., 1999). Recent experiments have shown that MZ B cells and B-1 B cells act together to generate early responses to intravascular T-independent antigens (Martin et al., 2001). The spleen dependency of immune responses to iv antigens was shown in studies by Rowley (1950a,b), who demonstrated that, when a low dose of antigen is presented intravenously, as would occur in the initial stage of bacteremia, both splenectomized rats and humans are incapable of mounting a significant antibody response, in contrast to the normal responses in eusplenic controls.

Any adaptive B-cell response would have to be rapid in onset to mediate effective resistance to a rapidly progressing bloodstream infection, in which death frequently occurs within 24 h of the onset of symptoms. Unfortunately, there are few data on early immune responses, and most experimental studies begin measuring antibody responses no earlier than 48–72 h postinjection. In a study of the response to several viruses, for example, T-independent neutralizing antibodies were easily detectable at titers up to 2^6 at 48 h after infection, suggesting that significant levels may have been present considerably earlier (Ochsenbein et al., 2000). Antibodies to SRBCs can be detected 24 h after iv injection (Liacopoulos et al., 1971). A few studies have examined the early response to pneumococcus in animal models. Ellis and Smith (1966) showed that rabbits immunized with 5×10^3 killed pneumococci developed type-

specific resistance to subsequent challenge with a lethal dose of viable organisms, as shown by their rapid clearance from the bloodstream and protection from death. This resistance was seen as early as 8 h after immunization, but the same priming regimen did not protect previously splenectomized animals. A similar spleen-dependent development of resistance to type 25 pneumococcus was also observed in rats, although the earliest time-point examined was 3 d (Leung et al., 1972). An agglutinin response to pneumococcus was observed within 5 h of an intraperitoneal injection (Nunes, 1950), a route by which antigen gains rapid access to the circulation. Taken together, these data suggest that at least some T-independent antibody can be secreted very early in response to bacteria or other particulate antigens that are delivered directly through the circulation into the spleen. These antibodies would opsonize the bacteria and target them for phagocytosis. Possibly, very low levels of antibody could opsonize only particles present locally in the spleen. Antibody secreted by B-cells in follicles can cause antigen trapping by adjacent Fc receptor-bearing cells (van Rooijen and Kors, 1985). Thus, low concentrations of anti-bacterial antibody could be secreted by MZ B-cells, bind to organisms as they are filtered through the spleen, and cause their phagocytosis by macrophages in the MZ or red pulp. According to this hypothesis, such splenic clearance could begin within hours of the onset of bacteremia, long before there is a sufficient systemic level of antibody to effect phagocytosis by Kupffer cells in the liver.

The immature immune system in children less than 2 yr old responds poorly to TI polysaccharide antigens, both in natural infections and with pneumococcal vaccine (Nuorti et al., 1997). In addition, young children have low levels of circulating natural antibody against pneumococcus and *H. influenzae*, presumably because of their lack of prior exposure. Children are therefore at higher risk for fulminant infection by encapsulated organisms, and, since serum opsonins are critical for the hepatic clearance of virulent bacteria, they are at particularly high risk in the absence of a functioning spleen. Neonatal B-cells express lower levels of surface CD21, which explains in part their poor response to TI antigens (Rijkers et al., 1998). Furthermore, the MZ is the last splenic compartment to organize, and it does not become mature until 18–24 mo of age, the time at which children become responsive to polysaccharide antigens (Timens et al., 1989). Because antigen localization in MZ macrophages and B-cells is involved in inducing the response to carbohydrate antigens, their responses to encapsulated bacteria are poor (Peset Llopis et al., 1996). The high risk of sepsis in young asplenic children therefore results from their low levels of pre-existing circulating antibody, an inability to mount a sufficiently rapid antibody response to intravascular antigens, and lack of the major organ that is capable of phagocytosing unopsonized bacteria. Infection by Gram-negative organisms is less common, because of the earlier appearance of natural antibody to enteric organisms, and hence more effective clearance by the liver.

4.8. CONCLUSION

The spleen is the largest secondary lymphoid organ, and, because of its direct connection to the bloodstream and the architecture of the splenic cords and sinuses, it has a special role in the clearance of circulating bacteria, even under conditions in which other phagocytic organs are ineffective. In addition, the spleen has a major role in generating antigen-specific immune responses to polysaccharide antigens. In the otherwise healthy adult, lack of a functioning spleen results in only a small predisposition to fulminant infection.

In the very young and in those with other serious underlying diseases, however, the ability of the spleen to phagocytose and kill organisms is critically important in host resistance to overwhelming bacterial sepsis. In addition to its filtration function, a key to this protection against bloodborne infection may lie in the ability of the spleen to trap antigen and activate B-cells rapidly enough to provide the opsonizing antibody that is necessary for optimal bacterial clearance. No other organ in the body has this unique dual capacity to trap and concentrate intravascular antigen and mount rapid humoral immune responses.

REFERENCES

Aaberge, I. S. and Lovik, M. (1996) The antibody response after immunization with pneumococcal polysaccharide vaccine in splenectomized mice: the effect of re-immunization with pneumococcal antigens. *APMIS* **104**, 307–317.

Abe, Y., Horiuchi, A., Miyake, M., and Kimura, S. (1994) Anti-cytokine nature of natural human immunoglobulin: one possible mechanism of the clinical effect of intravenous immunoglobulin therapy. *Immunol. Rev.* **139**, 5–19.

Allman, D. M., Ferguson, S. E., and Cancro, M. P. (1992) Peripheral B cell maturation. I. Immature peripheral B cells in adults are heat-stable antigen^{hi} and exhibit unique signaling characteristics. *J. Immunol.* **149**, 2533–2540.

Amlot, P. L., Grennan, D., and Humphrey, J. H. (1985) Splenic dependence of the antibody response to thymus-independent (TI-2) antigens. *Eur. J. Immunol.* **15**, 508–512.

Amlot, P. L. and Hayes, A. E. (1985) Impaired human antibody response to the thymus-independent antigen, DNP-Ficoll, after splenectomy. Implications for post-splenectomy infections. *Lancet* **1**, 1008–1011.

Amran, D., Renz, H., Lack, G., Bradley, K., and Gelfand, E. W. (1994) Suppression of cytokine-dependent human T-cell proliferation by intravenous immunoglobulin. *Clin. Immunol. Immunopathol.* **73**, 180–186.

Andersson, U., Bjork, L., Skansen-Saphir, U., and Andersson, J. (1994) Pooled human IgG modulates cytokine production in lymphocytes and monocytes. *Immunol. Rev.* **139**, 21–42.

Ansel, K. M., McHeyzer-Williams, L. J., Ngo, V. N., McHeyzer-Williams, M. G., and Cyster, J. G. (1999) In vivo-activated CD4 T cells upregulate CXC chemokine receptor 5 and reprogram their response to lymphoid chemokines. *J. Exp. Med.* **190**, 1123–1134.

Ansel, K. M., Ngo, V. N., Hyman, P. L., Luther, S. A., Forster, R., Sedgwick, J. D., et al. (2000) A chemokine-driven positive feedback loop organizes lymphoid follicles. *Nature* **406**, 309–314.

Austyn, J. M., Kupiec-Weglinski, J. W., Hankins, D. F., and Morris, P. J. (1988) Migration patterns of dendritic cells in the mouse. Homing to T cell-dependent areas of spleen, and binding within marginal zone. *J. Exp. Med.* **167**, 646–651.

Bachmann, M. F., Hengartner, H., and Zinkernagel, R. M. (1995) T helper cell-independent neutralizing B cell response against vesicular stomatitis virus: role of antigen patterns in B cell induction? *Eur. J. Immunol.* **25**, 3445–3451.

Banchereau, J. and Steinman, R. M. (1998) Dendritic cells and the control of immunity. *Nature* **392**, 245–252.

Benacerraf, B., Sebestyen, M., and Schlossman, S. (1959) A quantitative study of the kinetics of blood clearance of P^{32}-labelled *Eschirichia coli* and *Staphylococci* by the reticuloendothelial system. *J. Exp. Med.* **110**, 27–48.

Berchtold, P., Dale, G. L., Tani, P., and McMillan, R. (1989) Inhibition of autoantibody binding to platelet glycoprotein IIb/IIIa by antiidiotypic antibodies in intravenous gammaglobulin. *Blood* **74**, 2414–2417.

Bisno, A. L. and Freeman, J. C. (1970) The syndrome of asplenia, pneumococcal sepsis, and disseminated intravascular coagulation. *Ann. Int. Med.* **72**, 389–393.

Boes, M., Prodeus, A. P., Schmidt, T., Carroll, M. C., and Chen, J. Z. (1998) A critical role of natural immunoglobulin M in immediate defense against systemic bacterial infection. *J. Exp. Med.* **188**, 2381–2386.

Bofill, M., Janossy, G., Janossa, M., Burford, G. D., Seymour, G. J., Wernet, P., and Kelemen, E. (1985) Human B cell development. II. Subpopulations in the human fetus. *J. Immunol.* **134**, 1531–1538.

Borrow, P., Tishon, A., Lee, S., Xu, J. C., Grewal, I. S., Oldstone, M. B. A., and Flavell, R. A. (1996) CD40L-deficient mice show deficits in antiviral immunity and have an impaired memory CD8$^+$ CTL response. *J. Exp. Med.* **183**, 2129–2142.

Bredius, R. G., de Vries, C. E., Troelstra, A., van Alphen, L., Weening, R. S., van de Winkel, J. G., and Out, T. A. (1993) Phagocytosis of *Staphylococcus aureus* and *Haemophilus influenzae* type B opsonized with polyclonal human IgG1 and IgG2 antibodies. Functional hFcγ RIIa polymorphism to IgG2. *J. Immunol.* **151**, 1463–1472.

Bredius, R. G., Derkx, B. H., Fijen, C. A., de Wit, T. P., de Haas, M., Weening, R. S., van de Winkel, J. G., and Out, T. A. (1994) Fc-γ receptor IIa (CD32) polymorphism in fulminant meningococcal septic shock in children. *J. Infec. Dis.* **170**, 848–853.

Briles, D. E., Nahm, M., Schroer, K., Davie, J., Baker, P., Kearney, J., and Barletta, R. (1981) Antiphosphocholine antibodies found in normal mouse serum are protective against intravenous infection with type 3 streptococcus pneumoniae. *J. Exp. Med.* **153**, 694–705.

Brown, E. J., Hosea, S. W., and Frank, M. M. (1981) The role of the spleen in experimental pneumococcal bacteremia. *J. Clin. Invest.* **67**, 975–982.

Brown, E. J., Hosea, S. W., and Frank, M. M. (1983) The role of antibody and complement in the reticuloendothelial clearance of pneumococci from the bloodstream. *Rev. Infec. Dis.* **5(Suppl 4)**, S797–S805.

Buiting, A. M., De Rover, Z., Kraal, G., and Van Rooijen, N. (1996) Humoral immune responses against particulate bacterial antigens are dependent on marginal metallophilic macrophages in the spleen. *Scand. J. Immunol.* **43**, 398–405.

Burke, J. S. and Simon, G. T. (1970) Electron microscopy of the spleen. II. Phagocytosis of colloidal carbon. *Am. J. Pathol.* **58**, 157–181.

Burstein, S. A., Friese, P., Downs, T., and Mei, R. L. (1992) Characteristics of a novel rat anti-mouse platelet monoclonal antibody: application to studies of megakaryocytes. *Exp. Hematol.* **20**, 1170–1177.

Camacho, S. A., Kosco-Vilbois, M. H., and Berek, C. (1998) The dynamic structure of the germinal center. *Immunol. Today* **19**, 511–514.

Carroll, M. C. (2000) The role of complement in B cell activation and tolerance. *Adv. Immunol.* **74**, 61–88.

Chadburn, A. (2000) The spleen: anatomy and anatomical function. *Semin. Hematol.* **37**, 13–21.

Chan, E. Y. and MacLennan, I. C. (1993) Only a small proportion of splenic B cells in adults are short-lived virgin cells. *Eur. J. Immunol.* **23**, 357–363.

Chao, D. and MacPherson, G. G. (1990) Analysis of thymus-independent type 2 antigen uptake by marginal zone macrophages in thin slices of viable lymphoid tissue in vitro. *Eur. J. Immunol.* **20**, 1451–1455.

Chaplin, D. D. and Fu, Y. (1998) Cytokine regulation of secondary lymphoid organ development. *Curr. Opin. Immunol.* **10**, 289–297.

Chelvarajan, R. L., Gilbert, N. L., and Bondada, S. (1998) Neonatal murine B lymphocytes respond to polysaccharide antigens in the presence of IL-1 and IL-6. *J. Immunol.* **161**, 3315–3324.

Chilcote, R. R., Baehner, R. L., and Hammond, D. (1976) Septicemia and meningitis in children splenectomized for Hodgkin's disease. *N. Engl. J. Med.* **295**, 798–800.

Christensen, B. E., et al. (1978) Traffic of T and B-lymphocytes in the normal spleen. *Scand. J. Haematol.* **20**, 246–257.

Ciavarra, R. P., Buhrer, K., Van Rooijen, N., and Tedeschi, B. (1997) T cell priming against vesicular stomatitis virus analyzed *in situ*: red pulp macrophages, but neither marginal metallophilic nor marginal zone macrophages, are required for priming CD4+ and CD8+ T cells. *J. Immunol.* **158**, 1749–1755.

Claassen, E., Kors, N., and Van Rooijen, N. (1986) Influence of carriers on the development and localization of anti-2,4,6-trinitrophenyl (TNP) antibody-forming cells in the murine spleen. II. Suppressed antibody response to TNP-Ficoll after elimination of marginal zone cells. *Eur. J. Immunol.* **16**, 492–497.

Cohn, D. A. and Schiffman, G. (1987) Immunoregulatory role of the spleen in antibody responses to pneumococcal polysaccharide antigens. *Infect. Immun.* **55**, 1375–1380.

Cook, M. C., Korner, H., Riminton, D. S., Lemckert, F. A., Hasbold, J., Amesbury, M., et al. (1998) Generation of splenic follicular structure and B cell movement in tumor necrosis factor-deficient mice. *J. Exp. Med.* **188,** 1503–1510.

Coon, J. and Hunter, R. (1973) Selective induction of delayed hypersensitivity by a lipid conjugated protein antigen which is localized in thymus dependent lymphoid tissue. *J. Immunol.* **110,** 183–190.

Crowley, M., Inaba, K., and Steinman, R. M. (1990) Dendritic cells are the principal cells in mouse spleen bearing immunogenic fragments of foreign proteins. *J. Exp. Med.* **172,** 383–386.

Cyster, J. G. (1999) Chemokines and cell migration in secondary lymphoid organs. *Science* **286,** 2098–2102.

Dailey, M. O., Coleman, C. N., and Fajardo, L. F. (1981) Splenic injury caused by therapeutic irradiation. *Am. J. Surg. Pathol.* **5,** 325–331.

Dailey, M. O., Coleman, C. N., and Kaplan, H. S. (1980) Radiation-induced splenic atrophy in patients with Hodgkin's disease and non-Hodgkin's lymphomas. *N. Engl. J. Med.* **302,** 215–217.

Dailey, M. O., Post, W., and Hunter, R. L. (1977) Induction of cell-mediated immunity to chemically modified antigens in guinea pigs. II. The interaction between lipid-conjugated antigens, macrophages, and T lymphocytes. *J. Immunol.* **118,** 963–970.

Dal Monte, P. and Szoka, F. C. Jr. (1989) Effect of liposome encapsulation on antigen presentation in vitro. Comparison of presentation by peritoneal macrophages and B cell tumors. *J. Immunol.* **142,** 1437–1443.

De Bruyn, P. P. H. and Farr, A. G. (1980) Lymphocyte-RES interactions and their fine-structural correlates. In: *The Reticuloendothelial System,* vol. I (Carr, I. and Daems, W. T., eds.), Plenum, New York, pp. 499–523.

Delemarre, F. G., Claassen, E., and Van Rooijen, N. (1989) Primary *in situ* immune response in popliteal lymph nodes and spleen of mice after subcutaneous immunization with thymus-dependent or thymus-independent (type 1 and 2) antigens. *Anat. Rec.* **223,** 152–157.

Dempsey, P. W., Allison, M. E., Akkaraju, S., Goodnow, C. C., and Fearon, D. T. (1996) C3d of complement as a molecular adjuvant: bridging innate and acquired immunity. *Science* **271,** 348–350.

Dijkstra, C. D. (1982) Characterization of nonlymphoid cells in rat spleen, with special reference to strongly Ia-positive branched cells in T-cell areas. *J. Reticuloendothel. Soc.* **32,** 167–178.

Dillon, A. M., Stein, H. B., and English, R. A. (1982) Splenic atrophy in systemic lupus erythematosus. *Ann. Int. Med.* **96,** 40–43.

Dunn-Walters, D. K., Isaacson, P. G., and Spencer, J. (1995) Analysis of mutations in immunoglobulin heavy chain variable region genes of microdissected marginal zone (MGZ) B cells suggests that the MGZ of human spleen is a reservoir of memory B cells. *J. Exp. Med.* **182,** 559–566.

Ehlenberger, A. G. and Nussenzweig, V. (1977) The role of membrane receptors for C3b and C3d in phagocytosis. *J. Exp. Med.* **145,** 357–371.

Ehrenstein, M. R., O'Keefe, T. L., Davies, S. L., and Neuberger, M. S. (1998) Targeted gene disruption reveals a role for natural secretory IgM in the maturation of the primary immune response. *Proc. Natl. Acad. Sci. USA* **95,** 10,089–10,093.

Eikelenboom, P., Boorsma, D. M., and van Rooijen, N. (1982) The development of IgM- and IgG-containing plasmablasts in the white pulp of the spleen after stimulation with a thymus-independent antigen (LPS) and a thymus-dependent antigen (SRBC). *Cell Tissue Res.* **226,** 83–95.

Ellis, E. F. and Smith, R. T. (1966) The role of the spleen in immunity. With special reference to the post-splenectomy problem in infants. *Pediatrics* **37,** 111–119.

Eraklis, A. J. and Filler, R. M. (1972) Splenectomy in childhood: a review of 1413 cases. *J. Pediatr. Surg.* **7,** 382–388.

Fehr, J., Hofmann, V., and Kappeler, U. (1982) Transient reversal of thrombocytopenia in idiopathic thrombocytopenic purpura by high-dose intravenous gamma globulin. *N. Engl. J. Med.* **306,** 1254–1258.

Fischer, M. B., Ma, M., Goerg, S., Zhou, X., Xia, J., Finco, O., et al. (1996) Regulation of the B cell response to T-dependent antigens by classical pathway complement. *J. Immunol.* **157,** 549–556.

Fischer, P., Jendreyko, N., Hoffmann, M., Lerch, H., Uttenreuther-Fischer, M. M., Chen, P. P., and Gaedicke, G. (1999) Platelet-reactive IgG antibodies cloned by phage display and panning with IVIG from three patients with autoimmune thrombocytopenia. *Br. J. Haemotol.* **105,** 626–640.

Forster, R., Mattis, A. E., Kremmer, E., Wolf, E., Brem, G., and Lipp, M. (1996) A putative chemokine receptor, BLR1, directs B cell migration to defined lymphoid organs and specific anatomic compartments of the spleen. *Cell* **87,** 1037–1047.

Forster, R., Schubel, A., Breitfeld, D., Kremmer, E., Renner-Muller, I., Wolf, E., and Lipp, M. (1999) CCR7 coordinates the primary immune response by establishing functional microenvironments in secondary lymphoid organs. *Cell* **99,** 23–33.

Foster, K. J., Devitt, N., Gallagher, P. J., and Abbott, R. M. (1982) Overwhelming pneumococcal septicaemia in a patient with ulcerative colitis and splenic atrophy. *Gut* **23,** 630–632.

Francotte, M. and Urbain, J. (1985) Enhancement of antibody response by mouse dendritic cells pulsed with tobacco mosaic virus or with rabbit antiidiotypic antibodies raised against a private rabbit idiotype. *Proc. Natl. Acad. Sci. USA* **82,** 8149–8152.

Fraser, I. P., Koziel, H., and Ezekowitz, R. A. (1998) The serum mannose-binding protein and the macrophage mannose receptor are pattern recognition molecules that link innate and adaptive immunity. *Semin. Immunol.* **10,** 363–372.

Fries, L. F., Brickman, C. M., and Frank, M. M. (1983) Monocyte receptors for the Fc portion of IgG increase in number in autoimmune hemolytic anemia and other hemolytic states and are decreased by glucocorticoid therapy. *J. Immunol.* **131,** 1240–1245.

Fu, Y. X., Huang, G., Wang, Y., and Chaplin, D. D. (1998) B lymphocytes induce the formation of follicular dendritic cell clusters in a lymphotoxin α-dependent fashion. *J. Exp. Med.* **187,** 1009–1018.

Fu, Y. X., Molina, H., Matsumoto, M., Huang, G., Min, J., and Chaplin, D. D. (1997) Lymphotoxin-α (LTα) supports development of splenic follicular structure that is required for IgG responses. *J. Exp. Med.* **185,** 2111–2120.

Futterer, A., Mink, K., Luz, A., Kosco-Vilbois, M. H., and Pfeffer, K. (1998) The lymphotoxin beta receptor controls organogenesis and affinity maturation in peripheral lymphoid tissues. *Immunity* **9,** 59–70.

Garnham, P. C. C. (1980) Human babesiosis: European aspects. *Trans. R. Soc. Trop. Med. Hyg.* **74,** 153–155.

Gopal, V. and Bisno, A. L. (1977) Fulminant pneumococcal infections in 'normal' asplenic hosts. *Arch. Int. Med.* **137,** 1526–1530.

Goud, S. N., Muthusamy, N., and Subbarao, B. (1988) Differential responses of B cells from the spleen and lymph node to TNP-Ficoll. *J. Immunol.* **140,** 2925–2930.

Gray, D. (1988) Recruitment of virgin B cells into an immune response is restricted to activation outside lymphoid follicles. *Immunology* **65,** 73–79.

Gray, D., Kumararatne, D. S., Lortan, J., Khan, M., and MacLennan, I. C. (1984) Relation of intra-splenic migration of marginal zone B cells to antigen localization on follicular dendritic cells. *Immunology* **52,** 659–669.

Gray, D., MacLennan, I. C., Bazin, H., and Khan, M. (1982) Migrant $\mu^+\delta^+$ and static $\mu^+\delta^-$ B lymphocyte subsets. *Eur. J. Immunol.* **12,** 564–569.

Grouard, G., Durand, I., Filgueira, L., Banchereau, J., and Liu, Y. J. (1996) Dendritic cells capable of stimulating T cells in germinal centres. *Nature* **384,** 364–367.

Guilbert, B., Dighiero, G., and Avrameas, S. (1982) Naturally occurring antibodies against nine common antigens in human sera. I. Detection, isolation and characterization. *J. Immunol.* **128,** 2779–2787.

Gunn, M. D., Ngo, V. N., Ansel, K. M., Ekland, E. H., Cyster, J. G., and Williams, L. T. (1998) B-cell-homing chemokine made in lymphoid follicles activates Burkitt's lymphoma receptor-1. *Nature* **391,** 799–803.

Hamburger, M. I., Lawley, T. J., Kimberly, R. P., Plotz, P. H., and Frank, M. M. (1982) A serial study of splenic reticuloendothelial system Fc receptor functional activity in systemic lupus erythematosus. *Arthritis Rheum.* **25,** 48–54.

Harms, G., Hardonk, M. J., and Timens, W. (1996) In vitro complement-dependent binding and in vivo kinetics of pneumococcal polysaccharide TI-2 antigens in the rat spleen marginal zone and follicle. *Infect. Immun.* **64**, 4220–4225.

Hayakawa, K. and Hardy, R. R. (1988) Normal, autoimmune, and malignant CD5+ B cells: the Ly-1 B lineage? *Ann. Rev. Immunol.* **6**, 197–218.

Hayakawa, K. and Hardy, R. R. (2000) Development and function of B-1 cells. *Curr. Opin. Immunol.* **12**, 346–353.

Hayward, A. R. and Ezer, G. (1974) Development of lymphocyte populations in the human foetal thymus and spleen. *Clin. Exp. Immunol.* **17**, 169–178.

Heyman, B. (2000) Regulation of antibody responses via antibodies, complement, and Fc receptors. *Ann. Rev. Immunol.* **18**, 709–737.

Hoffmann, M., Uttenreuther-Fischer, M. M., Lerch, H., Gaedicke, G., and Fischer, P. (2000) IVIG-bound IgG and IgM cloned by phage display from a healthy individual reveal the same restricted germ-line gene origin as in autoimmune thrombocytopenia. *Clin. Exp. Immunol.* **121**, 37–46.

Hosea, S. W., Brown, E. J., and Frank, M. M. (1980) The critical role of complement in experimental pneumococcal sepsis. *J. Infect. Dis.* **142**, 903–909.

Hosea, S. W., Burch, C. G., Brown, E. J., Berg, R. A., and Frank, M. M. (1981) Impaired immune response of splenectomised patients to polyvalent pneumococcal vaccine. *Lancet* **1**, 804–807.

Hsu, S. M., Cossman, J., and Jaffe, E. S. (1983) Lymphocyte subsets in normal human lymphoid tissues. *Am. J. Clin. Pathol.* **80**, 21–30.

Humphrey, J. H. and Grennan, D. (1981) Different macrophage populations distinguished by means of fluorescent polysaccharides. Recognition and properties of marginal-zone macrophages. *Eur. J. Immunol.* **11**, 221–228.

Hurez, V., Kaveri, S. V., Mouhoub, A., Dietrich, G., Mani, J. C., Klatzmann, D., and Kazatchkine, M. D. (1994) Anti-CD4 activity of normal human immunoglobulin G for therapeutic use. (Intravenous immunoglobulin, IVIg). *Ther. Immunol.* **1**, 269–277.

Hurez, V., Kazatchkine, M. D., Vassilev, T., Ramanathan, S., Pashov, A., Basuyaux, B., et al. (1997) Pooled normal human polyspecific IgM contains neutralizing anti-idiotypes to IgG autoantibodies of autoimmune patients and protects from experimental autoimmune disease. *Blood* **90**, 4004–4013.

Jacob, J. and Kelsoe, G. (1992) *In situ* studies of the primary immune response to (4-hydroxy-3-nitrophenyl)acetyl. II. A common clonal origin for periarteriolar lymphoid sheath-associated foci and germinal centers. *J. Exp. Med.* **176**, 679–687.

Jandl, J. H. and Kaplan, M. E. (1960) The destruction of red cells by antibodies in man, III. Quantitative factors influencing the patterns of hemolysis *in vivo. J. Clin. Invest.* **39**, 1145–1156.

Jones, J. F. (1983) Development of the spleen. *Lymphology* **16**, 83–89.

Kamps, W. A. and Cooper, M. D. (1982) Microenvironmental studies of pre-B and B cell development in human and mouse fetuses. *J. Immunol.* **129**, 526–531.

Kapsenberg, M. L., Teunissen, M. B., Stiekema, F. E., and Keizer, H. G. (1986) Antigen-presenting cell function of dendritic cells and macrophages in proliferative T cell responses to soluble and particulate antigens. *Eur. J. Immunol.* **16**, 345–350.

Kaveri, S., Prasad, N., Vassilev, T., Hurez, V., Pashov, A., Lacroix-Desmazes, S., and Kazatchkine, M. (1997) Modulation of autoimmune responses by intravenous immunoglobulin (IVIg). *Multiple Sclerosis* **3**, 121–128.

Kaveri, S., Vassilev, T., Hurez, V., Lengagne, R., Lefranc, C., Cot, S., et al. (1996) Antibodies to a conserved region of HLA class I molecules, capable of modulating CD8 T cell-mediated function, are present in pooled normal immunoglobulin for therapeutic use. *J. Clin. Invest.* **97**, 865–869.

Kelsoe, G. (1996) Life and death in germinal centers (redux). *Immunity* **4**, 107–111.

Kevy, S. V., Tefft, M., Vawier, G. F., and Rosen, F. S. (1968) Hereditary splenic hypoplasia. *Pediatrics* **42**, 752–757.

King, H. and Schumaker, H. B. (1952) Splenic studies; I. Susceptibility to infection after splenectomy performed in infancy. *Ann. Surg.* **136**, 239–242.

Kohler, H., Rowley, D. A., DuClos, T., and Richardson, B. (1977) Complementary idiotypy in the regulation of the immune response. *Fed. Proc.* **36**, 221–224.

Koni, P. A., Sacca, R., Lawton, P., Browning, J. L., Ruddle, N. H., and Flavell, R. A. (1997) Distinct roles in lymphoid organogenesis for lymphotoxins a and b revealed in lymphotoxin beta-deficient mice. *Immunity* **6**, 491–500.

Kotani, M., Matsuno, K., and Ezaki, T. (1986) Marginal zone bridging channels as a pathway for migrating macrophages from the red towards the white pulp in the rat spleen. *Acta Anat.* **126**, 193–198.

Kotani, M., Matsuno, K., Miyakawa, K., Ezaki, T., Hayama, T., and Ekino, S. (1985) Migration of macrophages from the marginal zone to germinal centers in the spleen of mice. *Anat. Rec.* **212**, 172–178.

Kraal, G. (1992) Cells in the marginal zone of the spleen. *Int. Rev. Cytol.* **132**, 31–74.

Kraal, G., Rodrigues, H., Hoeben, K., and Van Rooijen, N. (1989) Lymphocyte migration in the spleen: the effect of macrophage elimination. *Immunology* **68**, 227–232.

Kraal, G., Schornagel, K., Streeter, P. R., Holzmann, B., and Butcher, E. C. (1995) Expression of the mucosal vascular addressin, MAdCAM-1 on sinus-lining cells in the spleen. *Am. J. Pathol.* **147**, 763–771.

Kraal, G., Ter Hart, H., Meelhuizen, C., Venneker, G., and Claassen, E. (1989b) Marginal zone macrophages and their role in the immune response against T-independent type 2 antigens: modulation of the cells with specific antibody. *Eur. J. Immunol.* **19**, 675–680.

Kraal, G., Weissman, I. L., and Butcher, E. C. (1982) Germinal centre B cells: antigen specificity and changes in heavy chain class expression. *Nature* **298**, 377.

Kroese, F. G., Wubbena, A. S., and Nieuwenhuis, P. (1986) Germinal centre formation and follicular antigen trapping in the spleen of lethally X-irradiated and reconstituted rats. *Immunology* **57**, 99–104.

Krzysiek, R., Lefevre, E. A., Zou, W., Foussat, A., Bernard, J., Portier, A., Galanaud, P., and Richard, Y. (1999) Antigen receptor engagement selectively induces macrophage inflammatory protein-1 alpha (MIP-1a) and MIP-1b chemokine production in human B cells. *J. Immunol.* **162**, 4455–4463.

Kumararatne, D. S., Bazin, H., and MacLennan, I. C. (1981) Marginal zones: the major B cell compartment of rat spleens. *Eur. J. Immunol.* **11**, 858–864.

Kupiec-Weglinski, J. W., Austyn, J. M., and Morris, P. J. (1988) Migration patterns of dendritic cells in the mouse. Traffic from the blood, and T cell-dependent and -independent entry to lymphoid tissues. *J. Exp. Med.* **167**, 632–645.

Lacroix-Desmazes, S., Mouthon, L., Spalter, S. H., Kaveri, S., and Kazatchkine, M. D. (1996) Immunoglobulins and the regulation of autoimmunity through the immune network. *Clin. Exp. Rheumatol.* **14(Suppl 15)**, S9–S15.

Laman, J. D., Kors, N., Van Rooijen, N., and Claassen, E. (1990) Mechanism of follicular trapping: localization of immune complexes and cell remnants after elimination and repopulation of different spleen cell populations. *Immunology* **71**, 57–62.

Langman, J. (1969). *Medical Embryology. Human Development: Normal and Abnormal*, Williams and Wilkins, Baltimore, pp. 283–284.

Larsen, C. P., Morris, P. J., and Austyn, J. M. (1990) Migration of dendritic leukocytes from cardiac allografts into host spleens. A novel pathway for initiation of rejection. *J. Exp. Med.* **171**, 307–314.

Leemans, R., Harms, G., Rijkers, G. T., and Timens, W. (1999) Spleen autotransplantation provides restoration of functional splenic lymphoid compartments and improves the humoral immune response to pneumococcal polysaccharide vaccine [see comments]. *Clin. Exp. Immunol.* **117**, 596–604.

Leung, L. S., Szal, G. J., and Drachman, R. H. (1972) Increased susceptibility of splenectomized rats to infection with Diplococcus pneumoniae. *J. Infect. Dis.* **126**, 507–513.

Levine, M. H., Haberman, A. M., Sant'Angelo, D. B., Hannum, L. G., Cancro, M. P., Janeway, C. A., Jr., and Shlomchik, M. J. (2000) A B-cell receptor-specific selection step governs immature to mature B cell differentiation. *Proc. Natl. Acad. Sci. USA* **97**, 2743–2748.

Liacopoulos, P., Amstutz, H., and Gille, F. (1971) Early antibody-forming cells of double specificity. *Immunology* **20,** 57–66.

Liblau, R., Gajdos, P., Bustarret, F. A., el Habib, R., Bach, J. F., and Morel, E. (1991) Intravenous gamma-globulin in myasthenia gravis: interaction with anti-acetylcholine receptor autoantibodies. *J. Clin. Immunol.* **11,** 128–131.

Linehan, S. A., Martínez-Pomares, L., Stahl, P. D., and Gordon, S. (1999) Mannose receptor and its putative ligands in normal murine lymphoid and nonlymphoid organs: In situ expression of mannose receptor by selected macrophages, endothelial cells, perivascular microglia, and mesangial cells, but not dendritic cells. *J. Exp. Med.* **189,** 1961–1972.

Liu, Y. J., Oldfield, S., and MacLennan, I. C. (1988) Memory B cells in T cell-dependent antibody responses colonize the splenic marginal zones. *Eur. J. Immunol.* **18,** 355–362.

Liu, Y. J., Zhang, J., Lane, P. J., Chan, E. Y., and MacLennan, I. C. (1991) Sites of specific B cell activation in primary and secondary responses to T cell-dependent and T cell-independent antigens. *Eur. J. Immunol.* **21,** 2951–2962.

Loder, F., Mutschler, B., Ray, R. J., Paige, C. J., Sideras, P., Torres, R., Lamers, M. C., and Carsetti, R. (1999) B cell development in the spleen takes place in discrete steps and is determined by the quality of B cell receptor-derived signals. *J. Exp. Med.* **190,** 75–89.

Loggie, B. W., Hauer-Pollack, G., and Hinchey, E. J. (1985) Influence of splenectomy on lethal effects of pneumococcal infection. *Can. J. Surg.* **28,** 213–215.

Lyons, A. B. and Parish, C. R. (1995) Are murine marginal-zone macrophages the splenic white pulp analog of high endothelial venules? *Eur. J. Immunol.* **25,** 3165–3172.

Mackay, F., Majeau, G. R., Lawton, P., Hochman, P. S., and Browning, J. L. (1997) Lymphotoxin but not tumor necrosis factor functions to maintain splenic architecture and humoral responsiveness in adult mice. *Eur. J. Immunol.* **27,** 2033–2042.

MacLennan, I. C. (1994) Germinal centers. *Ann. Rev. Immunol.* **12,** 117–139.

MacLennan, I. C. (1998) B-cell receptor regulation of peripheral B cells. *Curr. Opin. Immunol.* **10,** 220–225.

Marchalonis, J. J., Kaymaz, H., Dedeoglu, F., Schluter, S. F., Yocum, D. E., and Edmundson, A. B. (1992) Human autoantibodies reactive with synthetic autoantigens from T-cell receptor b chain. *Proc. Natl. Acad. Sci. USA* **89,** 3325–3329.

Marchalonis, J. J., Kaymaz, H., Schluter, S. F., and Yocum, D. E. (1994) Naturally occurring human autoantibodies to defined T-cell receptor and light chain peptides. *Adv. Exp. Med. Biol.* **347,** 135–145.

Martínez-Pomares, L., Kosco-Vilbois, M., Darley, E., Tree, P., Herren, S., Bonnefoy, J. Y., and Gordon, S. (1996) Fc chimeric protein containing the cysteine-rich domain of the murine mannose receptor binds to macrophages from splenic marginal zone and lymph node subcapsular sinus and to germinal centers. *J. Exp. Med.* **184,** 1927–1937.

Martin, F., Oliver, A. M., and Kearney, J. F. (2001) Marginal zone and B1 B cells unite in the early response against T-independent blood-borne particulate antigens. *Immunity* **14,** 617–629.

Martínez-Pomares, L., Mahoney, J. A., Kaposzta, R., Linehan, S. A., Stahl, P. D., and Gordon, S. (1998) Functional soluble form of the murine mannose receptor is produced by macrophages in vitro and is present in mouse serum. *J. Biol. Chem.* **273,** 23,376–23,380.

Matsumoto, M., Fu, Y. X., Molina, H., Huang, G., Kim, J., Thomas, D. A., Nahm, M. H., and Chaplin, D. D. (1997) Distinct roles of lymphotoxin a and the type I tumor necrosis factor (TNF) receptor in the establishment of follicular dendritic cells from non-bone marrow-derived cells. *J. Exp. Med.* **186,** 1997–2004.

Matsumoto, M., Mariathasan, S., Nahm, M. H., Baranyay, F., Peschon, J. J., and Chaplin, D. D. (1996) Role of lymphotoxin and the type I TNF receptor in the formation of germinal centers. *Science* **271,** 1289–1291.

Matsuno, K., Miyakawa, K., and Kotani, M. (1985) Macrophages migrate from the marginal zone into the germinal centre of the rodent spleen. *Adv. Exp. Med. Biol.* **186,** 421–426.

McKearn, T. J. (1974) Antireceptor antiserum causes specific inhibition of reactivity to rat histocompatibility antigens. *Science* **183,** 94–96.

McKenzie, S. E. and Schreiber, A. D. (1998) Fc? receptors in phagocytes. *Curr. Opin. Hematol.* **5,** 16–21.

McKenzie, S. E., Taylor, S. M., Malladi, P., Yuhan, H., Cassel, D. L., Chien, P., et al. (1999) The role of the human Fc receptor FcγRIIA in the immune clearance of platelets: a transgenic mouse model. *J. Immunol.* **162,** 4311–4318.

Mitchell, J. and Abbot, A. (1971) Antigens in immunity. XVI. A light and electron microscope study of antigen localization in the rat spleen. *Immunology* **21,** 207–224.

Mizutani, H., Furubayashi, T., Kashiwagi, H., Honda, S., Take, H., Kurata, Y., et al. (1992) Effects of splenectomy on immune thrombocytopenic purpura in (NZW x BXSB) F1 mice: analyses of platelet kinetics and anti-platelet antibody production. *Thromb. Haemost.* **67,** 563–566.

Mizutani, H., Furubayashi, T., Kuriu, A., Take, H., Tomiyama, Y., Yoshida, H., et al. (1990) Analyses of thrombocytopenia in idiopathic thrombocytopenic purpura-prone mice by platelet transfer experiments between (NZW x BXSB)F1 and normal mice. *Blood* **75,** 1809–1812.

Mond, J. J., Vos, Q., Lees, A., and Snapper, C. M. (1995) T cell independent antigens. *Curr. Opin. Immunol.* **7,** 349–354.

Mouthon, L., Kaveri, S. V., Spalter, S. H., Lacroix-Desmazes, S., Lefranc, C., Desai, R., and Kazatchkine, M. D. (1996) Mechanisms of action of intravenous immune globulin in immune-mediated diseases. *Clin. Exp. Immunol.* **104(Suppl 1),** 3–9.

Murphy, M., Walter, B. N., Pike-Nobile, L., Fanger, N. A., Guyre, P. M., Browning, J. L., Ware, C. F., and Epstein, L. B. (1998) Expression of the lymphotoxin b receptor on follicular stromal cells in human lymphoid tissues. *Cell Death Differ.* **5,** 497–505.

Nachbaur, D., Herold, M., Eibl, B., Glassl, H., Schwaighofer, H., Huber, C., et al. (1997) A comparative study of the in vitro immunomodulatory activity of human intact immunoglobulin (7S IVIG), F(ab')2 fragments (5S IVIG) and Fc fragments. Evidence for post-transcriptional IL-2 modulation. *Immunology* **90,** 212–218.

Namikawa, R., Mizuno, T., Matsuoka, H., Fukami, H., Ueda, R., Itoh, G., Matsuyama, M., and Takahashi, T. (1986) Ontogenic development of T and B cells and non-lymphoid cells in the white pulp of human spleen. *Immunology* **57,** 61–69.

Ngo, V. N., Korner, H., Gunn, M. D., Schmidt, K. N., Riminton, D. S., Cooper, M. D., et al. (1999) Lymphotoxin a/b and tumor necrosis factor are required for stromal cell expression of homing chemokines in B and T cell areas of the spleen. *J. Exp. Med.* **189,** 403–412.

Nieuwenhuis, P. and Ford, W. L. (1976) Comparative migration of B- and T-Lymphocytes in the rat spleen and lymph nodes. *Cell. Immunol.* **23,** 254–267.

Nossal, G. J., Austin, C. M., Pye, J., and Mitchell, J. (1966) Antigens in immunity. XII. Antigen trapping in the spleen. *Int. Arch. Allergy Appl. Immunol.* **29,** 368–383.

Nunes, D. S. (1950) Demonstration of agglutinins 5 hours after intraperitoneal injection of pneumococcus type 1 in guinea pigs. *Can. J. Res.* **28,** 298–306.

Nuorti, P. J., Butler, J. C., and Breiman, R. F. (1997) Prevention of pneumococcal disease: recommendations of the Advisory Committee on Immunization Practices (ACIP). *MMWP* **46,** 1–25.

Ochsenbein, A. F., Fehr, T., Lutz, C., Suter, M., Brombacher, F., Hengartner, H., and Zinkernagel, R. M. (1999a) Control of early viral and bacterial distribution and disease by natural antibodies. *Science* **286,** 2156–2159.

Ochsenbein, A. F., Pinschewer, D. D., Odermatt, B., Carroll, M. C., Hengartner, H., and Zinkernagel, R. M. (1999b) Protective T cell-independent antiviral antibody responses are dependent on complement. *J. Exp. Med.* **190,** 1165–1174.

Ochsenbein, A. F., Pinschewer, D. D., Odermatt, B., Ciurea, A., Hengartner, H., and Zinkernagel, R. M. (2000) Correlation of T cell independence of antibody responses with antigen dose reaching secondary lymphoid organs: implications for splenectomized patients and vaccine design. *J. Immunol.* **164,** 6296–6302.

Oliver, A. M., Martin, F., and Kearney, J. F. (1999) IgM^high CD21^high lymphocytes enriched in the splenic marginal zone generate effector cells more rapidly than the bulk of follicular B cells. *J. Immunol.* **162,** 7198–7207.

Pashov, A., Dubey, C., Kaveri, S. V., Lectard, B., Huang, Y. M., Kazatchkine, M. D., and Bellon, B. (1998) Normal immunoglobulin G protects against experimental allergic encephalomyelitis by inducing transferable T cell unresponsiveness to myelin basic protein. *Eur. J. Immunol.* **28,** 1823–1831.

Pasparakis, M., Kousteni, S., Peschon, J., and Kollias, G. (2000) Tumor necrosis factor and the p55TNF receptor are required for optimal development of the marginal sinus and for migration of follicular dendritic cell precursors into splenic follicles. *Cell. Immunol.* **201,** 33–41.

Pearson, H. A., Johnston, D., Smith, K. A., and Touloukian, R. J. (1978) The born-again spleen. Return of splenic function after splenectomy for trauma. *N. Engl. J. Med.* **298,** 1389–1392.

Peset Llopis, M. J., Harms, G., Hardonk, M. J., and Timens, W. (1996) Human immune response to pneumococcal polysaccharides: complement-mediated localization preferentially on CD21-positive splenic marginal zone B cells and follicular dendritic cells. *J. Allergy Clin. Immunol.* **97,** 1015–1024.

Potsch, C., Vöhringer, D., and Pircher, H. (1999) Distinct migration patterns of naive and effector CD8 T cells in the spleen: correlation with CCR7 receptor expression and chemokine reactivity. *Eur. J. Immunol.* **29,** 3562–3570.

Qian, Q., Jutila, M. A., Van Rooijen, N., and Cutler, J. E. (1994) Elimination of mouse splenic macrophages correlates with increased susceptibility to experimental disseminated candidiasis. *J. Immunol.* **152,** 5000–5008.

Randolph, D. A., Huang, G. M., Carruthers, C. J. L., Bromley, L. E., and Chaplin, D. D. (1999) The role of CCR7 in TH₁ and TH₂ cell localization and delivery of B cell help in vivo. *Science* **286,** 2159–2162.

Reynes, M., Aubert, J. P., Cohen, J. H., Audouin, J., Tricottet, V., Diebold, J., and Kazatchkine, M. D. (1985) Human follicular dendritic cells express CR1, CR2, and CR3 complement receptor antigens. *J. Immunol.* **135,** 2687–2694.

Rhoades, C. J., Williams, M. A., Kelsey, S. M., and Newland, A. C. (2000) Monocyte-macrophage system as targets for immunomodulation by intravenous immunoglobulin. *Blood Rev.* **14,** 14–30.

Rijkers, G. T., Sanders, E. A., Breukels, M. A., and Zegers, B. J. (1998) Infant B cell responses to polysaccharide determinants. *Vaccine* **16,** 1396–1400.

Rose, M. L., Birbeck, M. S. C., Wallis, V. J., Forrester, J. A., and Davies, A. J. S. (1980) Peanut lectin binding properties of germinal centres of mouse lymphoid tissue. *Nature* **284,** 364–366.

Roska, A. K. and Lipsky, P. E. (1985) Dissection of the functions of antigen-presenting cells in the induction of T cell activation. *J. Immunol.* **135,** 2953–2961.

Rossi, F. and Kazatchkine, M. D. (1989) Antiidiotypes against autoantibodies in pooled normal human polyspecific Ig. *J. Immunol.* **143,** 4104–4109.

Rouse, R. V., Ledbetter, J. A., and Weissman, I. L. (1982) Mouse lymph node germinal centers contain a selected subset of T cells: the helper phenotype. *J. Immunol.* **128,** 2243–2246.

Rowley, D. A. (1950a) The effect of splenectomy on the formation of circulating antibody in the adult male albino rat. *J. Immunol.* **64,** 289–295.

Rowley, D. A. (1950b) The formation of circulating antibody in the splenectomized human being following injection of heterologous erythrocytes. *J. Immunol.* **65,** 515–521.

Rowley, D. A., Kohler, H., and Cowan, J. D. (1980) An immunologic network. *Contemp. Top. Immunobiol.* **9,** 205–230.

Ryan, F. P., Jones, J. V., Wright, J. K., and Holdsworth, C. D. (1981) Impaired immunity in patients with inflammatory bowel disease and hyposplenism: the response to intravenous phi X174. *Gut* **22,** 187–189.

Salmon, J. E., Edberg, J. C., Brogle, N. L., and Kimberly, R. P. (1992) Allelic polymorphisms of human Fc γ receptor IIA and Fc γ receptor IIIB. Independent mechanisms for differences in human phagocyte function. *J. Clin. Invest.* **89,** 1274–1281.

Sanders, L. A., Feldman, R. G., Voorhorst-Ogink, M. M., de Haas, M., Rijkers, G. T., Capel, P. J., Zegers, B. J., and van de Winkel, J. G. (1995a) Human immunoglobulin G (IgG) Fc receptor IIA (CD32) polymorphism and IgG2-mediated bacterial phagocytosis by neutrophils. *Infect. Immun.* **63,** 73–81.

Sanders, L. A., Rijkers, G. T., Tenbergen-Meekes, A. M., Voorhorst-Ogink, M. M., and Zegers, B. J. (1995b) Immunoglobulin isotype-specific antibody responses to pneumococcal polysaccharide vaccine in patients with recurrent bacterial respiratory tract infections. *Pediatr. Res.* **37,** 812–819.

Sanders, L. A., van de Winkel, J. G., Rijkers, G. T., Voorhorst-Ogink, M. M., de Haas, M., Capel, P. J., and Zegers, B. J. (1994) Fcg receptor IIa (CD32) heterogeneity in patients with recurrent bacterial respiratory tract infections. *J. Infec. Dis.* **170,** 854–861.

Schulkind, M. L., Ellis, E. F., and Smith, R. T. (1967) Effect of antibody upon clearance of I-125-labelled pneumococci by the spleen and liver. *Pediatr. Res.* **1,** 178–184.

Scott, M. G., Shackelford, P. G., Briles, D. E., and Nahm, M. H. (1988) Human IgG subclasses and their relation to carbohydrate antigen immunocompetence. *Diag. Clin. Immunol.* **5,** 241–248.

Snapper, C. M., Moorman, M. A., Rosas, F. R., Kehry, M. R., Maliszewski, C. R., and Mond, J. J. (1995) IL-3 and granulocyte-macrophage colony-stimulating factor strongly induce Ig secretion by sort-purified murine B cell activated through the membrane Ig, but not the CD40, signaling pathway. *J. Immunol.* **154,** 5842–5850.

Sprent, J. (1973) Circulating T and B lymphocytes of the mouse. I. Migratory properties. *Cell. Immunol.* **7,** 10–39.

Stein, H., Bonk, A., Tolksdorf, G., Lennert, K., Rodt, H., and Gerdes, J. (1980) Immunohistologic analysis of the organization of normal lymphoid tissue and non-Hodgkin's lymphomas. *J. Histochem. Cytochem.* **28,** 746–760.

Steiniger, B., Barth, P., Herbst, B., Hartnell, A., and Crocker, P. R. (1997) The species-specific structure of microanatomical compartments in the human spleen: strongly sialoadhesin-positive macrophages occur in the perifollicular zone, but not in the marginal zone. *Immunology* **92,** 307–316.

Stuart, F. P., Fitch, F. W., and McKearn, T. J. (1982) Enhancement of rat renal allografts with idiotypic and antiidiotypic monoclonal alloantibodies. *Transplant. Proc.* **14,** 313–315.

Su, D. and Van Rooijen, N. (1989) The role of macrophages in the immunoadjuvant action of liposomes: effects of elimination of splenic macrophages on the immune response against intravenously injected liposome-associated albumin antigen. *Immunology* **66,** 466–470.

Sylvestre, D., Clynes, R., Ma, M., Warren, H., Carroll, M. C., and Ravetch, J. V. (1996) Immunoglobulin G-mediated inflammatory re-sponses develop normally in complement-deficient mice. *J. Exp. Med.* **184,** 2385–2392.

Szomolanyi-Tsuda, E., Le, Q. P., Garcea, R. L., and Welsh, R. M. (1998) T-cell-independent immunoglobulin G responses in vivo are elicited by live-virus infection but not by immunization with viral proteins or virus-like particles. *J. Virol.* **72,** 6665–6670.

Szomolanyi-Tsuda, E. and Welsh, R. M. (1996) T cell-independent antibody-mediated clearance of polyoma virus in T cell-deficient mice. *J. Exp. Med.* **183,** 403–411.

Szomolanyi-Tsuda, E. and Welsh, R. M. (1998) T-cell-independent antiviral antibody responses. *Curr. Opin. Immunol.* **10,** 431–435.

Takahashi, Y., Dutta, P. R., Cerasoli, D. M., and Kelsoe, G. (1998) *In situ* studies of the primary immune response to (4-hydroxy-3-nitrophenyl)acetyl. V. Affinity maturation develops in two stages of clonal selection. *J. Exp. Med.* **187,** 885–895.

Tew, J. G., Wu, J., Qin, D., Helm, S., Burton, G. F., and Szakal, A. K. (1997) Follicular dendritic cells and presentation of antigen and costimulatory signals to B cells. *Immunol. Rev.* **156,** 39–52.

Timens, W., Boes, A., and Poppema, S. (1989) Human marginal zone B cells are not an activated B cell subset: strong expression of CD21 as a putative mediator for rapid B cell activation. *Eur. J. Immunol.* **19,** 2163–2166.

Timens, W., Boes, A., Rozeboom-Uiterwijk, T., and Poppema, S. (1989) Immaturity of the human splenic marginal zone in infancy. Possible contribution to the deficient infant immune response. *J. Immunol.* **143,** 3200–3206.

Timens, W. and Poppema, S. (1985) Lymphocyte compartments in human spleen. An immunohistologic study in normal spleens and uninvolved spleens in Hodgkin's disease. *Am. J. Pathol.* **120,** 443–454.

Tomiyama, Y., Kurata, Y., Mizutani, H., Kanakura, Y., Tsubakio, T., Yonezawa, T., and Tarui, S. (1987) Platelet glycoprotein IIb as a target antigen in two patients with chronic idiopathic thrombocytopenic purpura. *Br. J. Haematol.* **66,** 535–538.

Van den Berg, T. K., Dopp, E. A., Daha, M. R., Kraal, G., and Dijkstra, C. D. (1992) Selective inhibition of immune complex trapping by follicular dendritic cells with monoclonal antibodies against rat C3. *Eur. J. Immunol.* **22,** 957–962.

Van den Eertwegh, A. J. M., Boersma, W. J. A., and Claassen, E. (1992) Immunological functions and *in vivo* cell-cell interactions of T cells in the spleen. *Crit. Rev. Immunol.* **11,** 337–380.

van der Laan, L. J., Dopp, E. A., Haworth, R., Pikkarainen, T., Kangas, M., Elomaa, O., et al. (1999) Regulation and functional involvement of macrophage scavenger receptor MARCO in clearance of bacteria in vivo. *J. Immunol.* **162,** 939–947.

van Ewijk, W., Rozing, J., Brons, N. H., and Klepper, D. (1977) Cellular events during the primary immune response in the spleen. A fluorescence- light- and electronmicroscopic study in germfree mice. *Cell Tissue Res.* **183,** 471–489.

van Furth, R. and Diesselhoff-den Dulk, M. M. (1984) Dual origin of mouse spleen macrophages. *J. Exp. Med.* **160,** 1273–1283.

van Rees, E. P., Dijkstra, C. D., and van Rooijen, N. (1987) The early postnatal development of the primary immune response in rat popliteal lymph node, stimulated with thymus-independent type-1 and type-2 antigens. *Cell Tissue Res.* **250,** 695–699.

van Rooijen, N. (1977) Immune complexes in the spleen: three concentric follicular areas of immune complex trapping, their interrelationships and possible function. *J. Reticuloendothel. Soc.* **21,** 143–151.

van Rooijen, N. (1990) Antigen processing and presentation in vivo: the microenvironment as a crucial factor. *Immunol. Today* **11,** 436–439.

van Rooijen, N. and Kors, N. (1985) Mechanism of follicular trapping: double immunocytochemical evidence for a contribution of locally produced antibodies in follicular trapping of immune complexes. *Immunology* **55,** 31–34.

van Schaik, I. N., Lundkvist, I., Vermeulen, M., and Brand, A. (1992) Polyvalent immunoglobulin for intravenous use interferes with cell proliferation in vitro. *J. Clin. Immunol.* **12,** 325–334.

Vassilev, T., Gelin, C., Kaveri, S. V., Zilber, M. T., Boumsell, L., and Kazatchkine, M. D. (1993) Antibodies to the CD5 molecule in normal human immunoglobulins for therapeutic use (intravenous immunoglobulins, IVIg). *Clin. Exp. Immunol.* **92,** 369–372.

Vassilev, T., Yamamoto, M., Aissaoui, A., Bonnin, E., Berrih-Aknin, S., Kazatchkine, M. D., and Kaveri, S. V. (1999) Normal human immunoglobulin suppresses experimental myasthenia gravis in SCID mice. *Eur. J. Immunol.* **29,** 2436–2442.

Vassilev, T. L., Kazatchkine, M. D., Van Huyen, J. P., Mekrache, M., Bonnin, E., Mani, J. C., et al. (1999) Inhibition of cell adhesion by antibodies to Arg-Gly-Asp (RGD) in normal immunoglobulin for therapeutic use (intravenous immunoglobulin, IVIg). *Blood* **93,** 3624–3631.

Veerman, A. J. and van Rooijen, N. (1975) Lymphocyte capping and lymphocyte migration as associated events in the in vivo antigen trapping process. An electron-microscopic autoradiographic study in the spleen of mice. *Cell Tissue Res.* **161,** 211–217.

Vincent, C. and Revillard, J. P. (1983) Auto-antibodies specific for β2 microglobulin in normal human serum. *Mol. Immunol.* **20,** 877–884.

von Andrian, U. H. and Mackay, C. R. (2000) Advances in immunology: T-cell function and migration: two sides of the same coin. *N. Engl. J. Med.* **343,** 1020–1033.

Warmerdam, P. A., van de Winkel, J. G., Gosselin, E. J., and Capel, P. J. (1990) Molecular basis for a polymorphism of human Fc γ receptor II (CD32). *J. Exp. Med.* **172,** 19–25.

Warmerdam, P. A., van de Winkel, J. G., Vlug, A., Westerdaal, N. A., and Capel, P. J. (1991) Single amino acid in the second Ig-like domain of the human Fc γ receptor II is critical for human IgG2 binding. *J. Immunol.* **147,** 1338–1343.

Willfuhr, K. U., Westermann, J., and Pabst, R. (1990) Absolute numbers of lymphocytes subsets migrating through the compartments of the normal and transplanted rat spleen. *Eur. J. Immunol.* **20,** 903–911.

Willimann, K., Legler, D. F., Loetscher, M., Roos, R. S., Delgado, M. B., Clark-Lewis, I., Baggiolini, M., and Moser, B. (1998) The chemokine SLC is expressed in T cell areas of lymph nodes and mucosal lymphoid tissues and attracts activated T cells via CCR7. *Eur. J. Immunol.* **28,** 2025–2034.

Wright, M. D., Wood, P. R., Coia, G., and Cheers, C. (1987) Particulate antigens may be reprocessed after initial phagocytosis for presentation to T cells in vivo. *Immunol. Cell Biol.* **65,** 505–510.

Yee, A. M., Ng, S. C., Sobel, R. E., and Salmon, J. E. (1997) FcgRIIA polymorphism as a risk factor for invasive pneumococcal infections in systemic lupus erythematosus. *Arthritis Rheum.* **40,** 1180–1182.

Yee, A. M., Phan, H. M., Zuniga, R., Salmon, J. E., and Musher, D. M. (2000) Association between FcgRIIa-R131 allotype and bacteremic pneumococcal pneumonia. *Clin. Infec. Dis.* **30,** 25–28.

Yoshida, K., van den Berg, T. K., and Dijkstra, C. D. (1993) Two functionally different follicular dendritic cells in secondary lymphoid follicles of mouse spleen, as revealed by CR1/2 and FcRgII-mediated immune-complex trapping. *Immunology* **80,** 34–39.

Zhang, J., Liu, Y. J., MacLennan, I. C., Gray, D., and Lane, P. J. (1988) B cell memory to thymus-independent antigens type 1 and type 2: the role of lipopolysaccharide in B memory induction. *Eur. J. Immunol.* **18,** 1417–1424.

Zheng, B., Han, S., and Kelsoe, G. (1996) T helper cells in murine germinal centers are antigen-specific emigrants that downregulate Thy-1. *J. Exp. Med.* **184,** 1083–1091.

Ziegler, H. K., Orlin, C. A., and Cluff, C. W. (1987) Differential requirements for the processing and presentation of soluble and particulate bacterial antigens by macrophages. *Eur. J. Immunol.* **17,** 1287–1296.

5 The Role of the Spleen in Hemostasis

W. JEAN DODDS, DVM

5.1. INTRODUCTION

The reticuloendothelial system, particularly in the liver and spleen, was first implicated in storage, synthesis, and regulation of hemostatic components over 40 years ago (Graham et al., 1951; Penick et al., 1951; Pool and Spaet, 1954; Webster et al., 1975). An intensive period of research followed, and focused on the sites of synthesis of plasma antihemophilic factor (factor VIII) and Christmas factor (factor IX) (Dodds, 1973; Dodds and Hoyer, 1974a; Webster et al., 1975; Bloom, 1979), and the splenic storage of platelets (Penny et al., 1966). This effort was temporarily abandoned in the late 1970s, to await development of the more advanced biotechnology, biochemistry, and molecular genetics that have since generated definitive answers (Losier and High, 1990; Jamison and Degen, 1991; Nakanishi et al., 1991; Hoeben et al., 1992; Yu and Slayter, 1994; Oh et al., 1995; Yasuda et al., 1995; Tefferi et al., 1997). Today, the structural genes coding for factors VIII and IX and von Willebrand factor have been isolated and cloned by recombinant techniques (Davie, 1995; Walter and High, 1997). The respective proteins have been sequenced, and cDNA probes have been used to locate and identify the missing or mutant amino acids or sequences in a variety of mutants of hemophilias A and B and von Willebrand disease (Davie, 1987, 1995; Lozier and High, 1990; Walter and High, 1997). This chapter summarizes data, collected during this four-decade period, on the relationship of the spleen to hemostasis and thrombosis.

5.2. COAGULATION FACTORS

5.2.1. FACTOR VIII (Antihemophilic Factor)
The search for the exact cell site(s) of factor VIII synthesis began in earnest in the early 1950s (Penick et al., 1970; Dodds and Hoyer, 1974a; Bloom, 1979), and remains controversial today (Dodds, 1997). Investigators at the University of North Carolina utilized normal dogs exposed to total body irradiation, chloroform, and carbon tetrachloride (Graham et al., 1951; Penick et al., 1951), and hemophilic dogs (Graham et al., 1951), to show that factor VIII levels were not significantly affected by marrow failure and hepatotoxins. By contrast, platelet counts were severely depressed and prothrombin utilization was impaired. Parallel studies by Pool and Spaet (1954) showed that rats treated with ethionine, but not pancreatectomy, had decreased factor VIII levels, thereby suggesting the reticu-

loendothelial system as a possible source of factor VIII. When the chloroform toxicity studies were repeated with an improved method of measuring factor VIII levels, decreased levels were observed. However, blockade of reticuloendothelial phagocytic function with methyl palmitate failed to alter factor VIII levels (Penick et al., 1970).

These conflicting data spawned the hypothesis that the spleen was the organ controlling circulating factor VIII levels (Webster et al., 1975; Bloom, 1979). In the early 1960s, hematologists in Great Britain and France observed elevated factor VIII levels, following exercise or adrenaline injection (Goudemand et al., 1964; Libre et al., 1968; Rizza and Eipe, 1971), and these effects appeared to be abolished by splenectomy in some (Goudemand et al., 1964; Libre et al., 1968), but not all, (Webster et al., 1975; Rizza and Eipe, 1971) studies. When splenectomized normal dogs were cross-circulated with hemophilic dogs (Weaver et al., 1964), the factor VIII levels of the normal dogs dropped to about 50%. Similarly, factor VIII levels in the counterpart intact hemophilic parabiosis rose to about 60%. Splenectomized hemophilic heterozygotes (carrier female dogs) had a transient change in their factor VIII levels, from ~50% prior to surgery to as low as 5% afterwards. The normal control dogs, treated in a similar fashion, showed essentially no change in activity. Thus, the spleen was somehow involved in regulating or maintaining factor VIII levels, although it was not the sole source of factor VIII, because splenectomy of normal humans or animals did not produce a hemophilic state (Weaver et al., 1964; Webster et al., 1975).

Pool (1966) provided direct evidence of the prominent role of the spleen in controlling factor VIII levels. In her studies, extracts of splenic (but not other) tissue slices generated factor VIII activity. The following year, two other groups independently corroborated her findings, using isolated organ perfusion techniques (Norman et al., 1967; Webster et al., 1967b). This technology was adopted by our own laboratory, and by others, from the late 1960s to the mid-1970s (Dodds, 1969a,b; Kelly et al., 1970; Dodds and Hoyer, 1974a,b; Webster et al., 1975). The studies by Webster et al., at the University of North Carolina, showed that the amount of factor VIII activity produced by perfusion of normal dog spleens with hemophilic dog blood was ~5× greater than that observed for hepatic perfusion (Webster et al., 1967b, 1975). Little activity was generated by perfusion of the hind limb, and none was obtained from normal perfused lungs or kidneys, or from hemophilic dog spleens. Norman et al. (1967), in Boston, perfused normal pig spleens with hemophilic human blood, and generated about 18% of normal activity after 4 h; activity was also produced from perfused

From: *The Complete Spleen: A Handbook of Structure, Function, and Clinical Disorders* Edited by: A. J. Bowdler © Humana Press Inc., Totowa, NJ

livers. In 1968, the North Carolina group showed that peptidase extracts of dog kidneys contained factor VIII activity, and suggested that a monomeric form of the protein was synthesized by this organ (Webster et al., 1975).

Our lab, meanwhile, had developed the isolated, perfused rabbit organ model (Dodds, 1969a), and demonstrated production of both factors VIII and IX activity by the liver, spleen, and kidney. The appearance of these activities was greatest in the spleen, and was prevented by addition of inhibitors of protein synthesis (puromycin, cycloheximide, actinomycin D) to the perfusate. The production of clotting factor activity by the liver and spleen was regulated by negative feedback (Dodds, 1973; Dodds and Hoyer, 1974a,b), and hepatic perfusates contained independent stimulators of the factors VIII and IX produced by perfused spleens (Dodds, 1969b, 1973). These findings indicated that the liver produced specific precursor proteins that enhanced splenic synthesis and/or release of factors VIII and IX. The factor VIII stimulator had a mol wt between 115,000 and 300,000 Daltons; the factor IX stimulator was smaller, ~30,000–100,000 Daltons (Dodds et al., 1972). These data are compatible with what is known today about the sizes of the structural subunits of each of these coagulation proteins (Davie, 1987, 1995).

Kelly et al. (1970) reported that perfused pig spleens generated puromycin-sensitive factor VIII activity, with a half-life of about 10 h. This was followed by the work of Ponn et al. (1971), demonstrating that cultured rabbit splenic macrophages produced factor VIII activity for up to 9 d. Similar culture studies with leukocytes and fibroblasts recovered a factor VIII-like activity, but it was not decreased by incubation with antifactor VIII antibody (Dodds, 1973). This procoagulant activity was later shown to be the tissue factor that shortened the end point in clotting assays (Webster et al., 1975).

The discovery that procoagulant activity, generated by tissue culture systems or perfused organs, could reflect production of nonspecific thromboplastic material, or activation in the test system or assay, confirmed long-standing concerns plaguing this area of research. Thus, the question of whether the coagulation activity, produced by in vitro systems, represented *de novo* biosynthesis or storage and release of preformed activity, remained unresolved.

More definitive studies of the site(s) of factor VIII (and factor IX) synthesis involved organ transplantation (Webster et al., 1973; Webster et al., 1975). Orthotopic and heterotopic transplantation of liver, spleen, kidney, and bone marrow were performed. These studies showed that the liver was the primary organ site of factors VIII and IX production, and that extrahepatic production of factor VIII, but not factor IX, also occurred (Walter and High, 1997; Dodds, 1997). This conclusion was firmly established when transplantation of livers from dogs with either hemophilia A (factor VIII deficiency) or B (factor IX deficiency), into normal dogs, produced a reduction in circulating factor VIII levels to ~20% of normal, but not lower. In contrast, factor IX levels became <1% after the counterpart hemophilia B transplant. Furthermore, neither the kidney nor bone marrow transplants were able to correct the defect in hemophilic dogs.

With respect to the spleen, transplants were performed between normal and hemophilic dogs and normal and hemophilic human patients. The first of these landmark experiments was undertaken by Webster et al. (1967a), in which normal dog spleens were transplanted into two hemophilic dogs that survived for only 52 and 72 h, respectively. During this time, factor VIII activity increased from <1%, prior to transplantation, to 5–10% in one animal and 3–7% in the other. Because of the short duration of these preliminary studies, a distinction between release of stored factor VIII and new biosynthesis could not be made. However, Norman et al. (1968) successfully transplanted normal spleens into three dogs with a milder form of hemophilia, and one survived for 6 mo. The authors reported sustained factor VIII activity, based on assays using human, rather than canine, plasma controls, and concluded that the spleen synthesized factor VIII. This was followed rapidly by seven more studies in dogs (Marchioro et al., 1969; McKee et al., 1970; Penick et al., 1970; Sise et al., 1970; Webster et al., 1971; Hampton et al., 1973; Groth et al., 1974), and one in humans (Hathaway et al., 1969) which failed to demonstrate anything beyond a transient rise in factor VIII activity. Thus, splenic transplants in hemophilic recipients released sufficient stored factor VIII to maintain hemostasis during the postoperative period, but levels never exceeded 20%, and were not sustained. It was concluded that the spleen serves as a storage site of factor VIII, which is released at times of stress or hemostatic demand (Webster et al., 1975).

Following this work, other lymphatic tissues (vascularized lymph node grafts) were transplanted into hemophilic dogs, with short-term graft viability and transient factor VIII production (Groth et al., 1974). Similarly, human splenic cell suspensions or homogenates failed to sustain factor VIII production when administered to hemophiliacs (Hathaway et al., 1969). Overall, the disappointing results of these complicated and expensive experiments caused this approach to be abandoned in the mid-1970s.

Interest in identifying the cell site(s) of synthesis of factor VIII has continued. Bloom et al., in Wales, localized production of factor VIII to several human tissues by antibody neutralization (Bloom and Giddings, 1972; Bloom, 1979), and Kelly et al. (1984) and Hoyer and Dodds (1985) detected factor VIII immunologically in tissue extracts and perfused organs from the liver, spleen, lung, and kidney of guinea pigs. Additional evidence that factor VIII is synthesized by several different tissues comes from work of Van der Kwast et al. (1983) and Wion et al. (1985), who used specific immunohistochemical staining techniques and mRNA to localize factor VIII in human hepatic sinusoidal endothelial cells, and mononuclear, nonlymphoid cells of the spleen, lung, and lymph nodes. Retrovirus-mediated transfer of a human factor VIII gene, into murine hematopoietic progenitor cells, showed that most of the infected spleen colonies contained the factor VIII vector (Hoeben et al., 1992). However, although the vector sequences were immediately expressed, transcription was repressed. Recent studies on the induction of factor VIII protein synthesis in mice, regulated by a metalloprotein promoter-driven eukaryotic expression vector, showed increased expression of factor VIII in liver, spleen, and lung (Oh et al., 1995).

The exact cell(s) source of plasma factor VIII is still not established (Dodds, 1997). Several cell types and organs, including the spleen, remain likely candidates. Synthesis of von Willebrand factor, the companion protein of the circulating plasma factor VIII complex, is known to take place in endothelial cells and megakaryocytes (Davie, 1987, 1995; Lozier and High, 1990; Walter and High, 1997). Recent studies of neoplastic lymphocytes in the blood and spleen of a human patient showed that they strongly expressed von Willebrand factor and platelet glycoprotein Ib (Tefferi et al., 1997).

5.2.2. FACTOR IX (Christmas Factor)   Interest in the site of factor IX synthesis developed in parallel to that of factor VIII, but was not as actively pursued, because the mutation of hemophilia B is much less common than that of hemophilia A, in humans and other species (Webster et al., 1975; Dodds, 1997). Early observations, in the late 1950s, from studies of coumarin-induced deficiency states and hepatic disease, implicated the liver as the major site of factor IX production. Factor IX was produced by rat liver slices in vitro, and by isolated perfused rat and rabbit livers (Dodds, 1969a; Webster et al., 1975) and rabbit kidneys and spleens (Dodds, 1969a). The latter studies, performed in our lab, suggested that organs other than the liver could be involved in synthesis, release, and regulation of factor IX, as was shown to pertain to factor VIII, and as discussed previously. A similar negative feedback control of factor IX production in perfused organs was found, and an independent hepatic stimulator of factor IX production from perfused spleens was identified (Dodds, 1969b; Dodds et al., 1972; Dodds and Hoyer, 1974a,b).

The evidence for extrahepatic production of factor IX has come solely from isolated organ perfusion and tissue extraction studies. Failure to confirm these findings, by subsequent organ transplantation studies between normal and hemophilia B dogs (Webster et al., 1975), indicated that the coagulation activity produced in these in vitro systems resulted from release of preformed activity in tissue stores.

Webster et al. (1975) showed that two normal canine recipients of livers from hemophilia B dogs could not maintain their circulating factor IX levels after transplantation. Levels fell to less than 1% of normal, and remained undetectable for the length of the experiment (up to 53 d). Thus, the liver was identified as the sole source of factor IX, and the cell site of synthesis was likely to be the hepatocyte. Since these earlier studies, cloning of human and canine factor IX genes has localized the hepatocyte as the cell site for factor IX biosynthesis (Furie and Furie, 1995; Walter and High, 1997).

5.2.3. OTHER COAGULATION FACTORS

Most of the other plasma coagulation factors are synthesized solely in the liver, with the exception of factors V and XIII (fibrin stabilizing factor), and possibly factor II (prothrombin) (Jamison and Degen, 1991; Dodds, 1997). At one time, factor V was believed to be produced by the liver, but to be influenced by the spleen, because the low circulating factor V levels of cirrhotics rebounded, if the patients were splenectomized for associated hypersplenism (Vergoz et al., 1967). Current information has identified the sites of factor V production as endothelial cells, megakaryocytes, and hepatocytes (Davie, 1987, 1995). Factor XIII is synthesized by hepatocytes, peripheral blood monocytes, and monocytes and macrophages from other tissues (Weisberg et al., 1987; Dodds, 1997). Clonal and sequence analysis of cDNA clones from bovine aortic endothelial cell transglutaminase (factor XIII) showed hybridization to a single mRNA species in liver, lung, spleen, and heart, but not brain (Nakanishi et al., 1991). Prenatal and postnatal expression of mRNA coding for rat prothrombin was studied by Jamison and Degen (1991). These authors found prothrombin mRNA in many tissues, including the liver and spleen, during fetal development.

5.3. PLATELETS

The spleen has been assigned many roles in the control of platelet kinetics in health and disease (Penny et al., 1966; Shulman and Jordan, 1987; Tefferi et al., 1997). In hypersplenism, thrombocytopenia has been attributed to excessive platelet sequestration, inhibition of thrombopoiesis, and pooling within the enlarged organ

(Aster, 1965; Penny et al., 1966). In the latter study, three decades ago, the increase in platelet pool size in splenomegaly was the sole reason for thrombocytopenia in most of their patients. In myeloproliferative disorders, on the other hand, the spleen may be the site of platelet production. A recent investigation of a patient with splenic lymphoma found that her neoplastic lymphocytes strongly expressed platelet glycoprotein Ib, as well as von Willebrand factor (Tefferi et al., 1997).

Plateletpheresis in normal and asplenic humans and animals has been performed for therapeutic reasons, and to evaluate platelet reserve. The exchangeable platelet pool in the spleen has been calculated to be about one-third of the total number of circulating platelets, by this and other techniques using radiolabeled platelets (Shulman and Jordan, 1987). Platelet production is normal, or even slightly enhanced, in asplenic subjects after plateletpheresis. However, temporary platelet pooling, after platelet depletion, may delay entrance of newly formed platelets into the circulation. In rabbits and dogs, the larger younger platelets are preferentially retained by the spleen; after splenectomy, the number of large platelets circulating is increased (Shulman and Jordan, 1987).

Platelets leaving the circulation permanently, during physiological turnover, are taken up equally by the liver and spleen. However, the relative number of platelets sequestered by each organ in pathologic situations varies with the degree of platelet injury (Shulman and Jordan, 1987).

Platelet survival is usually normal or only slightly reduced in the thrombocytopenia of hypersplenism. The nearly normal total platelet mass, in the presence of low peripheral platelet counts, suggests that total mass, rather than concentration, is the factor controlling feedback regulation of thrombopoiesis (Shulman and Jordan, 1987).

Studies of platelet kinetics suggest that splenic pooling is probably caused by delay during the transit of platelets through the spleen. Splenic transit time of platelets is about 10 min, and appears to be independent of splenic size or blood flow (Peters et al., 1980).

The thrombocytopenia of hypersplenism may or may not be of sufficient severity to cause spontaneous bruising or bleeding. Conversely, the thrombocytosis of myeloproliferative disorders can produce either bleeding or thrombotic tendencies, the mechanism of which remains poorly understood (Shulman and Jordan, 1987).

5.4. FIBRINOLYTIC COMPONENTS

The major precursor zymogen of the fibrinolytic system is plasminogen (Verstraete, 1995). Despite years of intensive studies in animals (Highsmith, 1980), identification of the specific cell sites of plasminogen synthesis in humans was a recent event (Robbins, 1987). Both the liver and kidney are sites of plasminogen synthesis in humans and other species, although considerable species variation exists, and multiple sites have been implicated in plasminogen storage and regulation (Highsmith, 1980).

Eosinophils, especially of the bone marrow, and other types of granulocytes were reported in early studies to produce and release plasma and tissue plasminogen and its activators (Shulman and Jordan, 1987). These findings have not been substantiated by more recent experiments using sophisticated molecular techniques (Kimata et al., 1991; Verstraete, 1995).

Highsmith (1980) reported the kidney to be the primary source of plasminogen following acute depletion studies in cats. As in the earlier work with granulocytes, the spleen was not among other tissues implicated in the metabolic regulation or fate of plasminogen. Tissue plasminogen activator, on the other hand, has been shown to localize on experimental microthrombi in various organs (kidneys, liver, lung, and spleen) of rats, with disseminated intravascular coagulation (Kimata et al., 1991).

5.5. ANTICOAGULANTS (COAGULATION AND FIBRINOLYSIS INHIBITORS)

Of the six major protease inhibitors of blood, four have inhibitory action against one or more clotting factors. These are antithrombin III, Cl activator, α_2-macroglobulin, and α_1-antitrypsin; each is synthesized in the liver. Although the spleen was previously not known to play a role in the synthesis, regulation, or metabolic fate of the inhibitors, recent molecular studies showed splenic tissue localization and mRNA expression of several inhibitors. Endogenous rat antithrombin III activity was localized in a variety of tissues, including the spleen (Xu and Slayter, 1994). Activated protein C and its co-factor, protein S, serve as regulators of blood coagulation. Expression of rat protein S mRNA was studied by RNA blot analysis, and found to occur not only in rat liver, but also in lung, spleen, testis, and uterus (Yasuda et al., 1995).

In some patients with systemic lupus erythematosus, the spleen has been implicated in the production of the thromboplastic globulin known as the "lupus anticoagulant" (Walsh and Schmaier, 1987).

5.6. CLINICAL MANIFESTATIONS

5.6.1. BLEEDING   Because the spleen is not a primary organ for production of coagulation proteins, depletion of clotting activity and bleeding are not usually associated with splenic disease or removal. The significant role of the spleen as a source of platelet reserve, however, places patients at risk of bleeding when thrombocytopenia becomes moderate to severe in the absence of a spleen or normal splenic function (Shulman and Jordan, 1987). Similarly, the thrombocytopenia associated with hypersplenism may be clinically expressed as a bleeding tendency, if some other factor or condition compromising hemostasis is also present (such as von Willebrand disease, coumadin therapy, or the hyperfibrinolysis of cryptogenic splenomegaly).

In immune thrombocytopenic states, the spleen is often the focal organ of platelet destruction, and splenectomy may be advisable. This may well induce remission of the immunologic disorder, but removal of the spleen has also removed the splenic platelet pool as a future reserve to protect the patient in the event of recurrence (Penny et al., 1966).

5.6.2. THROMBOSIS   Thrombosis is a more common manifestation than bleeding, during the course of splenic disease. Myeloproliferative disorders, hypersplenism, and other neoplasms, especially of hematological or vascular origin (lymphoma–leukemia complex, hemangiosarcomas), which involve the spleen, are often associated with a thrombotic tendency (Colman et al., 1987).

REFERENCES

Aster, R. H. (1965) Splenic platelet pooling as a cause of 'hypersplenic' thrombocytopenia. *Trans. Assoc. Am. Physicians* **78**, 362–373.

Bloom, A. L. (1979) The biosynthesis of factor VIII. *Clin. Haematol.* **8**, 53–77.

Bloom, A. L. and Giddings, J. C. (1972) Factor VIII (antihaemophilic factor) in tissues detected by antibody neutralization. *Br. J. Haematol.* **23**, 157–165.

Colman, R. W., Hirsh, J., Marder, V. J., and Salzman, E. W., eds. (1987) Section A. Pathogenesis of thrombosis. In: *Hemostasis and Thrombosis*, 2nd ed., Lippincott, Philadelphia, pp. 1063–1184.

Davie, E. W. (1987) The blood coagulation factors: their cDNA's, genes, and expression. In: *Hemostasis and Thrombosis*, 2nd ed. (Colman, R. W., Hirsh, J., Marder, V. J., and Salzman, E. W., eds.), Lippincott, Philadelphia, pp. 242–267.

Davie, E. W. (1995) Biochemical and molecular aspects of the coagulation cascade. *Thromb. Haemost.* **74**, 1–6.

Dodds, W. J. (1969a) Storage, release and synthesis of coagulation factors in isolated perfused organs. *Am. J. Physiol.* **217**, 879–883.

Dodds, W. J. (1969b) Hepatic influence of splenic synthesis of coagulation factors in isolated perfused organs. *Science* **166**, 882,883.

Dodds, W. J. (1973) Organ perfusion studies in hemophilia. In: *Haemophilia* (Ala, F. and Denson, K. W. E., eds.), Excerpta Medica, Amsterdam, pp. 39–49.

Dodds, W. J. and Hoyer, L. W. (1974a) Factors regulating the production of coagulation activities in perfused organs. In: *Proceedings, National Conference on Research Animals in Medicine,* National Institutes of Health, Washington, DC, pp. 463–472.

Dodds, W. J. and Hoyer, L. W. (1974b) Coagulation activities in perfused organs: regulation by addition of animal plasmas. *Br. J. Haematol.* **26**, 497–509.

Dodds, W. J., Raymond, S. L., Moynihan, A. C., and Fenton, J. W. II. (1972) Independent stimulators regulating the production of coagulation factors VIII and IX in perfused spleens. *J. Lab. Clin. Med.* **79**, 770–777.

Dodds, W. J. (1997) Hemostasis. In: *Clinical Biochemistry of Domestic Animals*, 5th ed. (Kaneko, J. J., Harvey, J. W., and Bruss, M. L., eds.), Academic, San Diego, pp. 241–283.

Furie, B. C. and Furie, B. (1995) Biosynthesis of factor IX: implications for gene therapy. *Thromb. Haemost.* **74**, 274–277.

Goudemand, M., Foucaut, M., Habay, D., et al. (1964) Les variations du taux de factor VIII au cours de l'exercise musculaire. *Nouv. Rev. Fr. Hematol.* **4**, 315–319.

Graham, J. B., Collins, P. L. Jr., Godwin, J. D., and Brinkhous, K. M. (1951) Assay of plasma antihemophilic activity in normal and heterozygous (hemophilic) and prothrombinopenic dogs. *Proc. Soc. Exp. Biol. Med.* **77**, 294–296.

Groth, C. G., Hathaway, W. E., Gustafsson, A., et al. (1974) Correction of coagulation in the hemophilic dog by transplantation of lymphatic tissue. *Surgery* **75**, 725–733.

Hampton, J. W., Buckner, R. G., Gunn, C. G., Miller, L. K., and Mayes, J. W. (1973) Canine hemophilia in beagles: genetics, site of factor VIII synthesis, and attempts at experimental therapy. In: *Haemophilia* (Ala, F. and Denson, K. W. E., eds.), Excerpta Medica, Amsterdam, pp. 26–32.

Hathaway, W. E., Mull, M. M., Githens, J. H., Groth, C. G., Marchioro, T. L., and Starzl, T. E. (1969) Attempted spleen transplant in classical hemophilia. *Transplantation* **7**, 73–75.

Highsmith, R. F. (1980) Origin of plasminogen and metabolic fate. In: *Fibrinolysis* (Kline, D. L. and Reddy, K. N. H., eds.), CRC, Boca Raton, FL, pp. 151–164.

Hoeben, R. C., Einerhand, M. P., Briet, E., et al. (1992) Toward gene therapy in haemophilia A: retrovirus-mediated transfer of a factor VIII gene into murine haematopoietic progenitor cells. *Thromb. Haemost.* **67**, 341–345.

Hoyer, L. W. and Dodds, W. J. (1985) Unpublished observations.

Jamison, C. S. and Degen, S. J. F. (1991) Prenatal and postnatal expression of messenger RNA coding for rat prothrombin. *Biochim. Biophys. Acta* **1088**, 208–216.

Kelly, D. A., Summerfield, J. A., and Tuddenham, E. G. D. (1984) Localization of factor VIIIC: antigen in guinea pig tissues and isolated liver cell fractions. *Br. J. Haematol.* **56**, 535–543.

Kelly, G., Pechet, L., and Eiseman, B. (1970) Synthesis of antihemophilic globulin by the isolated perfused spleen. *Surg. Gyn. Obst.* **131**, 473–485.

Kimata, H., Koide, T., Nakajima, K., and Kondo, S. (1991) Localization of tissue plasminogen activator on experimental microthrombi in rats. Micro-autoradiographic observations. *J. Pharmacobiodyn.* **14**, 25–33.

Libre, E. P., Cowan, D. H., Watkins, S. P. Jr., and Shulman, N. R. (1968) Relationships between spleen, platelets, and factor VIII levels. *Blood* **31**, 358–368.

Lozier, J. N. and High, K. A. (1990) Molecular basis of hemophilia. *Hematol. Pathol.* **4**, 1–26.

Marchioro, T. L., Hougie, C., Ragde, H., Epstein, R. B., and Thomas, E. D. (1969) Hemophilia: role of organ homografts. *Science* **163**, 188–190.

McKee, P. A., Coussons, R. T., Buckner, R. G., et al. (1970) Effect of the spleen on canine factor VIII levels. *J. Lab. Clin. Med.* **75**, 391–402.

Nakanishi, K., Nara, K., Hagiwara, H., et al. (1991) Cloning and sequence analysis of cDNA clones for bovine aortic- endothelial- cell transglutaminase. *Eur. J. Biochem.* **202**, 15–21.

Norman, J. C., Covelli, V. H., and Sise, H. S. (1968) Transplantation of the spleen: experimental cure of hemophilia. *Surgery* **64**, 1–14.

Norman, J. C., Lambilliotte, J. P., Kojima, Y., and Sise, H. S. (1967) Antihemophilic factor release by perfused liver and spleen: relationship to hemophilia. *Science* **158**, 1060–1061.

Oh, S., Kim, S., Min, Y., et al. (1995) Construction of metallothionein-I promoter inserted human blood coagulation factor VIII expression vector and the induction of factor VIII protein synthesis in mouse. *Kor. J. Biochem.* **27**, 199–208.

Penick, G. D., Cronkite, E. P., Godwin, I. D., and Brinkhous, K. M. (1951) Plasma antihemophilic activity following total body irradiation. *Proc. Soc. Exp. Biol. Med.* **78**, 732–734.

Penick, G. D., Webster, W. P., Peacock, E. E., Hutchin, P., and Zukoski, C. F. (1970) Organ transplantation in animal hemophilia. In *Hemophilia and New Hemorrhagic States* (Brinkhous, K. M., ed.), University of North Carolina Press, Chapel Hill, pp. 97–105.

Penny, R., Rozenberg, M. C., and Firkin, B. G. (1966) The splenic platelet pool. *Blood* **27**, 1–16.

Peters, A. M., Klonizakis, I., Lavender, J. P., and Lewis, S. M. (1980) Use of [111] indium-labelled platelets to measure spleen function. *Br. J. Haematol.* **46**, 587–593.

Ponn, R. B., Kellogg, E. A., Korff, J. M., et al. (1971) The role of the splenic macrophage in antihemophilic factor (factor VIII) synthesis. *Arch. Surg.* **103**, 398–401.

Pool, J. G. (1966) Antihemophilic globulin (AHG, factor VIII) activity in spleen. *Fed. Proc.* **25**, 317.

Pool, J. G. and Spaet, T. H. (1954) Ethionine-induced depression of plasma antihemophilic globulin in the rat. *Proc. Soc. Exp. Biol. Med.* **87**, 54–57.

Rizza, C. R. and Eipe, J. (1971) Exercise, factor VIII and the spleen. *Br. J. Haematol.* **20**, 629–635.

Robbins, K. C. (1987) The plasminogen-plasmin enzyme system. In: *Hemostasis and Thrombosis*, 2nd ed. (Colman, R. W. Hirsh, J., Marder, V. J., and Salzman, E. W., eds.), Lippincott, Philadelphia, pp. 162–181.

Shulman, N. R. and Jordan, J. V. Jr. (1987) Platelet kinetics. In: *Hemostasis and Thrombosis*, 2nd ed. (Colman, R. W., Hirsh, J., Marder. V. J., and Salzman, E. W., eds.), Lippincott, Philadelphia, pp. 431–451.

Sise, H. S. Joison, J. Pegg, C. A. S., and Norman, J. C. (1970) Potential of the transplanted spleen in canine hemophilia. In: *Hemophilia and New Hemorrhagic States* (Brinkhous, K. M., ed.), University of North Carolina Press, Chapel Hill, pp. 106–115.

Tefferi, A., Hanson, C. A., Kurtin, P. J., et al. (1997) Acquired von Willebrand's disease due to aberrant expression of platelet glycoprotein Ib by marginal zone lymphoma cells. *Br. J. Haematol.* **96**, 850–853.

Van der Kwast, T. H., Stel, H. V., and Veerman, E. C. L. (1983) Localization of VIII:C Ag using different monoclonal antibodies against VIII: C. *Thromb. Haemost.* **50**, 17.

Vergoz, D., Levy, V. G., Najman, A., and Caroli, J. (1967) Variations du facteur V au cours des splenectomies dans les cirrhoses.[Changes in factor V during splenectomies for cirrhosis]. *Rev. Fr. d'Etudes Clin. Biol.* **12**, 725–731 (French).

Verstraete, M. (1995) The fibrinolytic system: from Petri dishes to genetic engineering. *Thromb. Haemost.* **74**, 25–35.

Walsh, P. N. and Schmaier, A. H. (1987) Platelet coagulant protein interactions. In *Hemostasis and Thrombosis*, 2nd ed. (Colman, R. W., Hirsh, J., Marder, V. J., and Salzman, E. W., eds.), Lippincott, Philadelphia, pp. 689–709.

Walter, J. and High, K. A. (1997) Gene therapy for the hemophilias. *Adv. Vet. Med.* **40**, 119–134.

Webster, W. P., Penick, G. D., and Mandel, S. R. (1973) Orthotopic and heterotopic organ transplantation in hemophilia A. In: *Haemophilia* (Ala, F. and Denson, K. W. E., eds.), Excerpta Medica, Amsterdam, pp. 33–38.

Weaver, R. A., Price, R. E., and Langdell, R. D. (1964) Antihemophilic factor in cross-circulated normal and hemophilic dogs. *Am. J. Physiol.* **206**, 335–337.

Webster, W. P., Penick, G. V., Peacock, E. E., and Brinkhous, K. M. (1967a) Allotransplantation of spleen in hemophilia. *NC Med. J.* **28**, 505–507.

Webster, W. P., Reddick, R. L., Roberts, H. R., and Penick, G. D. (1967b) Release of factor VIII (antihaemophilic factor) from perfused organs and tissues. *Nature* **213**, 1146,1147.

Webster, W. P., Zukoski, C. F., Hutchin, P., et al. (1971) Plasma factor VIII synthesis and control as revealed by canine organ transplantation. *Am. J. Physiol.* **220**, 1147–1154.

Webster, W. P., Dodds, W. J., Mandel, S. K., and Penick, G. D. (1975) Biosynthesis of factors VIII and IX: organ transplantation and perfusion studies. In: *Handbook of Hemophilia*, Part I (Brinkhous, K. M. and Hemker, H. C., eds.), Excerpta Medica, Amsterdam, pp. 149–163.

Weisberg, L. J., Shiu, D. T., Conkling, P. R., and Shuman, M. A. (1987) Identification of normal peripheral blood monocytes and liver as sites of synthesis of coagulation factor XIII a-chain. *Blood* **70**, 579–582.

Wion, K. L., Kelly, D., and Summerfield, J. A. (1985) Distribution of factor VIII mRNA and antigen in human liver and other tissues. *Nature* **317**, 725–728.

Xu, T. and Slayter, H. S. (1994) Immunocytochemical localization of endogenous anti-thrombin III in the vasculature of rat tissues reveals locations of anticoagulantly active heparan sulfate proteoglycans. *J. Histochem. Cytochem.* **42**, 1365–1376.

Yasuda, F., Hayashi, T., Tanitame, K., Nishioka, J., and Suzuki, K. (1995) Molecular cloning and functional characterization of rat plasma protein S. *J. Biochem. (Tokyo)* **117**, 374–383.

CHARACTERISTICS OF THE DISORDERED SPLEEN

II

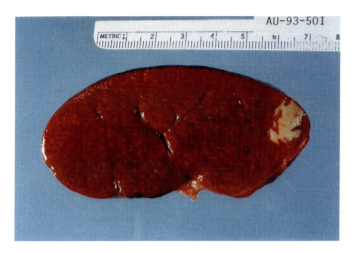

Color Plate 1. Organizing splenic infarct in a patient who died of bacterial endocarditis with septic emboli.

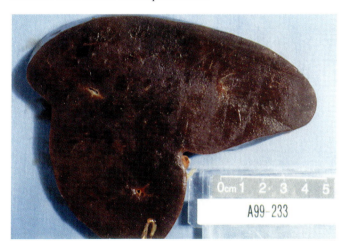

Color Plate 2. Spleen with extensive amyloid deposits from a patient with longstanding history of primary amyloidosis. Notice the waxy appearance of the splenic cut surface. (Courtesy of Dr. Michelle Barry, University of Iowa).

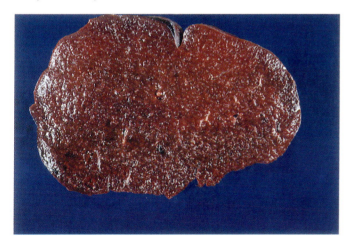

Color Plate 3. Splenic congestion. The cut surface is meaty, firm, and red with indistinct white pulp.

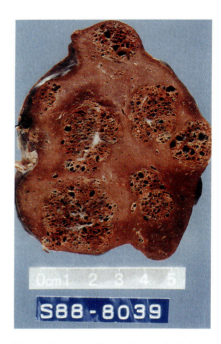

Color Plate 4. Splenic hemangioma. Most splenic hemangiomas are single but they can be multiple as in this case. Notice the red spongy appearance of the cut surface.

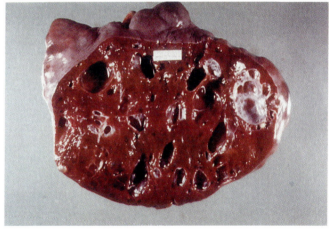

Color Plate 5. Lymphangioma. Cystic areas with a "Swiss cheese" appearance of the cut surface are typical of this vascular proliferation.

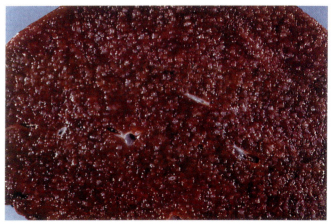

Color Plate 6. Splenic involvement by follicular lymphoma. The uniformly distributed small nodules are seen throughout. This so-called miliary pattern is also typically seen in other small lymphoid cell lymphomas involving the spleen (*see* color plates 7 and 8).

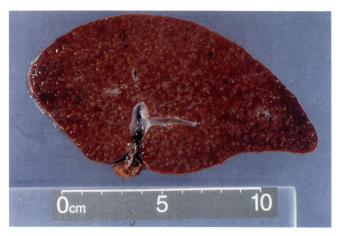

Color Plate 7. Chronic lymphocytic leukemia involving the spleen. This leukemia, in contrast to other types of leukemias, exhibits a miliary pattern of involvement reminiscent of other small lymphoid cell lymphomas.

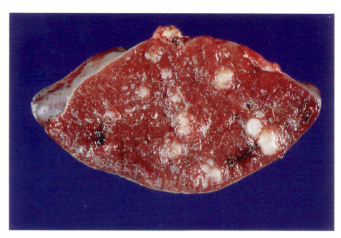

Color Plate 10. Hodgkin's lymphoma involving the spleen. Similar to large cell non-Hodgkin's lymphomas, isolated or confluent nodules are the characteristic pattern of splenic involvement in this lymphoma.

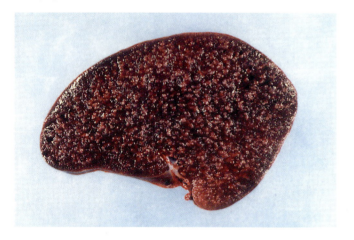

Color Plate 8. Splenic marginal zone lymphoma. Similarly to other small lymphoid cell lymphomas, a predominantly white pulp involvement with a miliary pattern is seen.

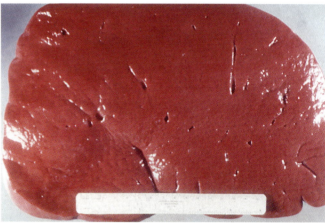

Color Plate 11. Chronic myeloid leukemia. Red homogeneous firm cut surface with obliteration of white pulp are typical of the cut surface in this type of leukemia.

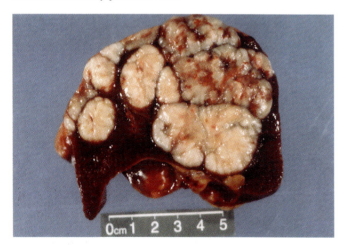

Color Plate 9. Diffuse large B-cell lymphoma involving the spleen. In contrast to small lymphoid cell processes large nodular masses are typically present in large cell lymphomas in the spleen.

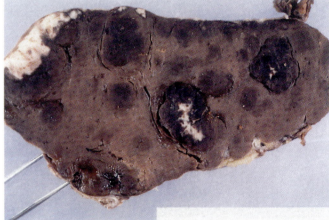

Color Plate 12. Primary splenic angiosarcoma. Partially necrotic, red, nodular masses are seen in this example.

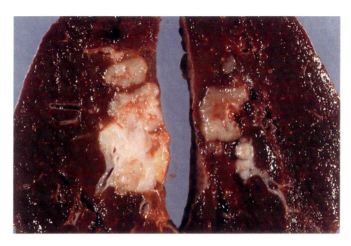

Color Plate 13. Involvement of spleen by metastatic carcinoma originating from a papillary serous carcinoma of the ovary.

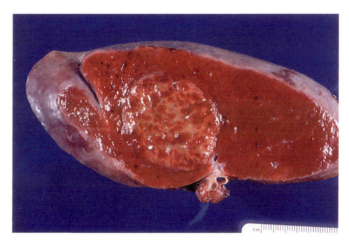

Color Plate 14. Spleen with myeloid metaplasia. The cut surface is red and firm with indistinct white pulp. The circumscribed bulging nodule in the center showed microscopic features of a hamartoma, also with myeloid metaplasia.

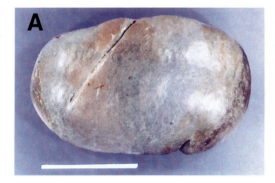
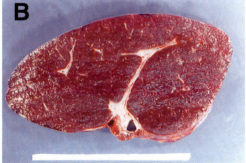

Color Plate 15. Spleen in idiopathic myelofibrosis. The patient had a longstanding history of myelofibrosis. The spleen weighed 5.5 kilogram and had a very firm cut surface. **(A)** External surface showing subcapsular hemorrahages; **(B)** Gross appearance of splenic cut surface.

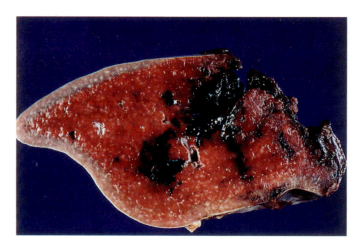

Color Plate 16. Splenic rupture, traumatic. The cut surface illustrates inadequate fixation because the specimen was left in formalin overnight without prior slicing.

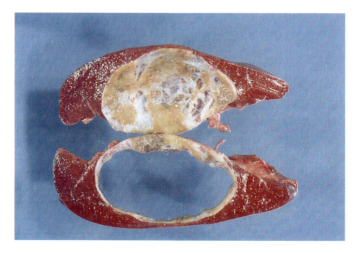

Color Plate 17. Epidermoid cyst. This primary splenic cyst was unilocular and lined by a stratified squamous epithelium.

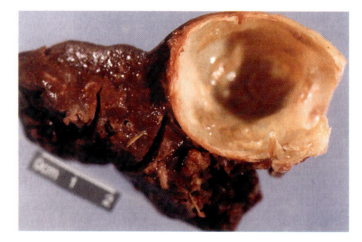

Color Plate 18. Splenic pseudocyst. This type of cyst does not have any gross or microscopically identifiable lining. In this example, the wall of the cyst was entirely calcified.

6 The Pathology of the Spleen*

MOHAMMAD A. VASEF, MD AND CHARLES E. PLATZ, MD

6.1. INTRODUCTION

The pathology of the spleen, as defined by morbid anatomy, is dependent on the examination of the surgically removed spleen or the spleen examined at autopsy. Although this process certainly does not provide the only information relevant to defining the pathology of the spleen, it is the purpose of this chapter to review the knowledge about the spleen gained by such examinations.

The spleen has long been regarded as a mysterious organ that was mostly examined postmortem, and only rarely during life. Two centuries ago, in his text on morbid pathology, Mathew Baillie (1793) described pathologic alterations involving the spleen, including the appearance of the surface and changes in texture and size. Although Dr. Baillie's text was limited to only a few pages, it provided accurate descriptions of entities including acute splenitis and splenic congestion. He accurately pointed out that a hard spleen was secondary to congestion and not scarring. He also described rare conditions involving the spleen, such as splenic cysts, stony concretions, and "wasting" of the organ. Thus, it appears that, by 1793, many splenic abnormalities described in today's textbooks had already been recognized. The chapters on the spleen in more recent surgical pathology textbooks remain relatively brief. The gross anatomy of the organ, as well as splenic functions, have been well-described (see, e.g., Chapters 1, 2, and 12). However, there has been a significant lag in our understanding of some histomorphologic processes in many conditions, because of lack of opportunity for the study of surgical and autopsy specimens, particularly in rare conditions. During the last four decades, several authors have attempted to bring together the pathology of the spleen in specific monographs or textbooks (Blaustein, 1963; Macpherson et al., 1973; Wolf and Neiman, 1988; Neiman and Orazi, 1999), as well as in chapters in general or surgical pathology texts.

Traditionally, discussions of splenic pathology have been organized according to the anatomic distribution of pathologic findings into two major categories: pathologic states involving the white pulp and those involving the red pulp. This chapter attempts to classify pathologic processes on the basis of the gross changes in

size and weight, as well as alterations in splenic function, and to correlate the pathologic processes with these alterations and deviations from normal. In so doing, we intend to relate pathology more closely to clinical evaluation, in which spleen size has long been an important indicator of splenic disorder, and in which pathophysiology has been a major concern. In some conditions, spleen size may be small, normal, or large, so some degree of overlap occurs in this format, which is noted when relevant. Because several pathologic changes in the spleen have been covered in other chapters, we will not attempt comprehensive coverage in this chapter, but make additional complementary discussion to individual topics presented elsewhere in this book.

6.2. EXAMINATION OF THE SPLEEN

6.2.1. PROCESSING AND HANDLING OF THE SPLENECTOMY SPECIMEN
Because the spleen contains a significant amount of blood, and is rich in histiocytes, special attention needs to be taken in handling and processing of this organ, in order to obtain optimal morphology, and to avoid autolysis. The spleen should be transferred to the pathology laboratory as soon as it is removed from the patient, and processed immediately. Before measuring and weighing the organ, the hilar fat should be removed and searched for lymph nodes. Identification and processing of the hilar lymph nodes may prove useful for a precise evaluation, particularly in cases suspected of involvement by malignant lymphoma. After weighing and measuring, the spleen should be sliced at 3–5 mm intervals, and fixed in an ample amount (10–20× its volume) of formalin overnight. Adequate fixation is crucial, in order to assess fine nuclear detail, particularly when evaluating hematolymphoid processes. Any suspicious nodule or lesion should be removed and fixed in a separate container overnight. A representative piece of any suspicious lesion should be snap-frozen and kept at −70°C, for possible additional studies, such as frozen section immunohistochemistry and/or molecular genetic studies. Also, portions of suspicious areas can be transferred into appropriate media for conventional cytogenetics, as well as for electron microscopy, if indicated.

Fine-needle aspiration biopsy of the spleen is a common procedure in many parts of the world, and is claimed to be relatively safe in clinically relevant patients (Lampert, 1983). This procedure, however, is neither popular nor widely performed in the United States, except for rare cases in which there is suspicion of solid tumor, including metastatic carcinoma.

6.2.2. SPLENIC SIZE
Enlargement of the spleen (splenomegaly) remains the most important finding that may indicate abnormality.

*A revision and extension of the chapter in the 1st edition entitled "Chapter 7: The Pathology of the Spleen" by Stebbins B. Candor, MD, formerly Chairman of Pathology, Marshall University School of Medicine, Huntington, WV.

From: *The Complete Spleen: A Handbook of Structure, Function, and Clinical Disorders* Edited by: A. J. Bowdler © Humana Press Inc., Totowa, NJ

79

Table 6.1
The Weight of the Histologically Normal Spleen

Spleen Weight (g): Sex and Age Variables*

Age	Males	Females
3rd decade	96–364	65–300
8th decade	66–234	70–195

Ethnic and Sex Variables in Spleen Weight (g)†

	Mean age (yrs)	Median weight (g)	Mean weight (g)	Range weight (g)
Males, white	54	140	145	75–245
Males, black	38	100	105	40–200
Females, white	54	115	115	55–190
Females, black	39	90	95	35–190

*From Boyd (1933). The range of weights given as normal is between the 2.5 and 97.5 percentiles in grams.

†From Myers and Segal (1974). The range of weights given as normal is between the 5th and 95th percentiles in grams.

Using palpation or percussion, splenomegaly is detected by the examining physician when the organ extends beyond defined anatomical limits (*see* Chapter 9, Subheading 4.1.). More accurate estimates of splenic volume can be made by two-dimensional sonography or radiography, particularly by computed tomography (CT) imaging. A recent study has shown that three-dimensional ultrasonography can provide improved accuracy over the traditional two-dimensional sonographic techniques (De Odorico et al., 1999). Using CT images, a significant correlation has been shown between splenic volume and body weight. Also, there appears to be good correlation between splenic volume and age. The ratio of splenic volume to body weight decreases with age (Watanabe et al., 1997).

The size of the spleen is important to the pathologist as well, because it may serve as an indicator of splenic disease. However, the weight of the normal spleen has a relatively wide range (Kayser, 1987; Myers and Segal, 1974; Boyd, 1933; DeLand, 1970; McCormick and Kashgarian, 1965), which may create difficulty in establishing the presence or absence of enlargement. For example, a spleen with a weight at the lower end of the normal range may enlarge 2–3× in size, and still fall within the normal range. For adults, a normal mean weight between 120 and 200 gm is often quoted (McCormick and Kashgarian, 1965; Whitley et al., 1966; Blendis et al., 1969; Miale, 1971). In general, spleen weight is higher in the young and in males, and whites tend to have larger spleens than blacks (Table 1).

6.2.3. NORMAL MICROSCOPIC ANATOMY OF THE SPLEEN

At the light microscopic level, the pathologist may find no specific morphologic changes in a spleen that is larger or smaller than normal, or that shows functional disorder. Although the spleen is divided into two structurally and functionally distinct components, designated "red pulp" and "white pulp," these two components are closely related to the splenic vasculature as a whole (*see* Chapter 1). After entering the spleen, the splenic artery divides into trabecular arteries, which further divide into central arteries, and enter the marginal zones and white pulp. The arterioles then terminate either in a sinus of the red pulp (direct or closed connections) or in the splenic cords (indirect or open connections). The cells released to the splenic cords eventually pass into the sinuses, and from there into the venous circulation. Relatively slow circulation through the cords permits the removal of senescent or structurally altered red blood cells by macrophages. The macrophages within the splenic cords phagocytose abnormal red blood cells, such as sickle cells and spherocytes, by a process of culling (Molnar and Rappaport, 1972; Crosby, 1957), and remove inclusions, such as Heinz bodies and malarial parasites, by a process of so-called "pitting" (Schnitzer et al., 1972; Rifkind, 1965). In addition, these macrophages induce red blood cell fragmentation in such conditions as autoimmune hemolytic anemia (Bowdler, 1976), thalassemia (Sen Gupta et al., 1960), and hemoglobin H disease (Wennberg and Weiss, 1968). The close relationship between splenic cords, splenic sinuses, and macrophages can best be illustrated by scanning electron microscopy (*see* Chapter 2), and is thought to be central to an understanding of splenic pathology. Normal red blood cells while traveling from cord to sinus, undergo considerable deformation, demonstrable by scanning and transmission electron microscopy (Bishop and Lansing, 1982). In contrast to normal red blood cells, cells with decreased cell membrane elasticity or altered cellular configuration will not be able to travel as easily from cord to sinus, and therefore will expand the cords, which is histologically described as cordal sequestration. This process is particularly apparent in sickle cell disease, spherocytosis, and elliptocytosis, and may also be observed in autoimmune hemolytic anemias (*see also* Chapter 7).

The white pulp is composed of lymphoid aggregates, which are, as noted above, intimately associated with the splenic arterial circulation. Surrounding the central arteries is a mixture of B- and T-lymphocytes, the periarterial lymphoid sheath (PALS). The size and structure of the lymphoid aggregates are variable, depending on the age of the subject and the status of antigenic stimulation. In the immunologically stimulated state, an active germinal center is present, surrounded by a darkly staining cuff of mantle zone cells and an outer rim of pale staining lymphoid cells, designated the "marginal zone." The lymphoid aggregates of the white pulp in infancy and in unstimulated adult spleens, are, in general, hypoplastic and lack germinal centers (*see also* Chapter 4).

The immunoarchitecture of the spleen has been extensively studied and characterized (Christensen et al., 1978; Weissman, 1976; Grogan et al., 1984; Hsu, 1983; Timens and Poppema, 1985; Van Ewijk and Nieuwenhuis, 1985). The majority of B-cells are found in the germinal centers and mantle zone, and, to a lesser extent, in the marginal zone. The B-cells in mantle and marginal zones express surface immunoglobulin (Ig) M or D. The red pulp contains abundant monocyte-derived cells, including macrophages.

6.3. ANATOMIC VARIATIONS

The normal spleen may show fetal lobulation, which may be confused with infarction. However, in contrast to infarction, fetal lobulation is not associated with thickening of the capsule. Complete absence of spleen is discussed in Subheading 4.1.1.1.

6.3.1. ACCESSORY SPLEEN Accessory spleen refers to one or more small foci of splenic tissue in the presence of an otherwise normal-sized spleen. Accessory splenic tissue can be found in approx 10–15% of the population. Accessory spleens are more commonly found in younger individuals, probably because they later become less prominent with the involutional effect of aging. Accessory spleens have histologic features similar to the primary spleen, and are functional (Fig. 1). Therefore, therapeutic splenectomy may be unsuccessful, if the accessory splenic tissue is not

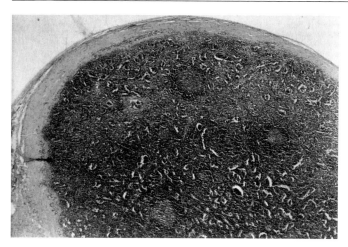

Fig. 6.1. Accessory spleen. A well-formed capsule distinguishes this from splenosis.

identified and removed at the time of surgery. In 90% of cases, accessory spleens are single, but they may also be multiple. Splenic hilum, lienorenal and gastrosplenic ligaments, jejunal wall, the tail of the pancreas, mesentery, and omentum are the most common sites for accessory splenic tissue.

6.3.2. POLYSPLENIA Polysplenia is a condition in which multiple spleens are present. As with the accessory spleen, these splenunculi are functional. A strong association with congenital cardiac anomalies and gastrointestinal malformations has been documented. From 146 autopsied cases of polysplenia studied by Peoples et al. (1983), at least half revealed congenital cardiovascular anomalies. The abnormalities included bilateral superior vena cava, interruption of inferior vena cava with azygos continuation, ventricular septal defect, ostium primum defect, and left ventricular outflow obstruction. However, in many cases, the cardiac abnormalities are not complex, and not all patients with polysplenia have cardiac anomalies. Abdominal heterotaxia is reported to be associated with 55% of cases (Peoples et al., 1983). Other noncardiac abnormalities associated with polysplenia syndrome include duodenal atresia (Raff and Schwartz, 1983); biliary atresia (Varela-Fascinetto et al., 1998; Maggard et al., 1999); and congenital short pancreas (Wainwright and Nelson, 1993).

A case of an (11) (q13.5;q25) inversion has been recently reported in a 9-mo-old male infant with polysplenia, complex cyanotic heart defects, altered lung lobation, and symmetric liver (Iida et al., 2000). As yet, however, no consistent chromosomal abnormalities, known to be specific for polysplenia and associated malformations, have been described.

6.3.3. SPLENOSIS A second form of ectopic splenic tissue results from the regeneration of splenic fragments implanted at suitably supportive sites for growth, usually following traumatic rupture of the organ, but also, less commonly, following splenic surgery. This appears to be a form of autotransplantation, and its extent is broadly related to the extent of the trauma to the organ (Stovall and Ling, 1988). By far the most common site of regrowth is the peritoneal cavity, but other sites, some widely distributed, may also be involved. Vento et al. (1999) reported a case of splenosis in a 45-year-old man, involving thorax, abdomen, pelvis, and hepatic parenchyma. This patient had a history of splenectomy 25 years earlier.

Occurrence of splenosis in unusual sites can create diagnostic problems by mimicking primary or metastatic tumors. Foroudi et al. (1999) reported a case of splenosis in the liver, mimicking metastatic nodules. Because of a prior history of breast cancer, this patient was extensively investigated for presumed liver metastases, before the diagnosis of splenosis was made. The patient had a history of traumatic rupture of the spleen some years before the development of her breast cancer. Turk et al. (1988) describe a case of splenosis presenting as a renal mass, and review the further complications of this condition. A unique case of cerebral splenosis, with a presumptive diagnosis of meningioma, and subsequently surgically excised, has also been described (Rickert et al., 1998). In addition, pelvic splenosis, with low abdominal pain mimicking endometriosis, has been reported (Zitzer et al., 1998). We have seen, in consultation, a case of splenosis that occurred in the axillary region.

Unlike the accessory spleen, these ectopic nodules are usually multiple, and may be numerous. Generally, there is no hilum, and the capsule and fibrous trabeculae lack muscle and elastic tissue, so that the individual nodule is less well defined than an accessory spleen. The red pulp is histologically similar to that of the normal spleen, but the white pulp is generally poorly defined and decreased in amount.

There is some residual functional capacity in the nodules of splenosis, and their capacity to take up radionuclide during liver–spleen scanning indicates that they have phagocytic function. However, their capacity to compensate effectively for the loss of the filtration function, following splenectomy, is in some doubt. Their deficiency in filtration function probably results from abnormality of the vascular structures that evolve during regeneration.

Pedunculated forms of splenic remnants may undergo torsion with infarction (Fleming et al., 1976). Also, clearly, that the nodules of splenosis may be involved in disease processes comparable to those affecting the structurally normal spleen. This is usually seen in relation to the hematological sequelae of hereditary spherocytosis, hypersplenism, and immune thrombocytopenia, but has also been observed in other disorders, such as malaria.

6.4. PATHOLOGICAL PROCESSES AFFECTING THE SPLEEN

The range of disorders recognized as affecting the spleen is now so wide that it is necessary to select relatively few to illustrate how pathological processes affect the organ. Two principal changes occur: in structure, which usually results in enlargement of the organ (splenomegaly), or, less commonly, in a decrease in size; and in the activity of the organ, which may be expressed either as a decrease (hyposplenism) or an apparent increase (hypersplenism) in activity (*see also* Chapters 9 and 10). A number of conditions affecting the spleen are shown in Table 2, which outlines those that result in enlargement of the organ.

A decrease in spleen size is usually accompanied by a reduction in the expression of splenic function. This may result in diminished efficiency of the filtration of abnormal particles (such as red blood cells made abnormal by heat treatment, sulfhydryl-blocking agents, or warm antibodies), ineffective pitting of intracellular inclusions, such as Howell-Jolly bodies; decreased phagocytosis (as shown by the intensity of radionuclide uptake in liver–spleen scanning), and by an increased susceptibility to bacterial infection, especially with polysaccharide-encapsulated bacteria (*see* Chapter 10).

Table 6.2
The Causes of Splenomegaly

A. INFECTION
  1. Acute.
    Infectious mononucleosis; viral hepatitis; cytomegalovirus infection; septicemia (including tuberculous); salmonelloses; relapsing fever; tularemia; splenic abscess; toxoplasmosis.
  2. Subacute and chronic
    Chronic septicemias; tuberculous splenomegaly, leprosy; Yersinia; subacute bacterial endocarditis; brucellosis; syphilis; malaria; leishmaniasis; schistosomiasis; systemic fungal disease; inflammatory pseudotumor.

B. IMMUNE PROLIFERATIONS AND NONINFECTIOUS GRANULOMATOUS DISORDERS
Angioimmunoblastic lymphadenopathy; angiofollicular hyperplasia; systemic lupus erythematosus; rheumatoid arthritis; Still's disease; rheumatic fever; Behcet's syndrome; serum sickness; sarcoidosis; berylliosis; necrotizing splenic granulomas.

C. VASCULITIDES
Polyarteritis nodosa; leukocytoclastic angiitis; peliosis.

D. CONGESTIVE SPLENOMEGALY
  1. Intrahepatic.
    Portal cirrhosis; postnecrotic scarring; biliary cirrhosis; Wilson's disease; hemochromatosis; veno-occlusive disease; congenital fibrosis; bilharziasis.
  2. Portal vein obstruction
    Thrombosis, stenosis, atresia; cavernous malformation; arteriovenous aneurysm; obstructive lesions at porta hepatis.
  3. Splenic vein obstruction.
    Thrombosis, stenosis, atresia; angiomatous malformation; obstruction by pancreatic disease, splenic arterial aneurysm and retroperitoneal fibrosis.
  4. Hepatic vein occlusion.
    Budd-Chiari syndrome.
  5. Cardiac.
    Acute, chronic or recurrent congestive cardiac failure; constrictive pericarditis (Banti's syndrome).

E. HEMATOLOGICAL DISORDERS
  1. Hemolytic disorders.
    Hereditary red blood cell membrane disorders; thalassemia; sickle–thalassemia; sickle cell disease (early stages); hemoglobin-SC disease.
  2. Myeloproliferative disorders.
    Primary (agnogenic myeloid metaplasia); polycythemia vera (variable); essential thrombocythemia (variable).
  3. Miscellaneous.
    Primary splenic hyperplasia; megaloblastic anemias; iron deficiency.

F. NEOPLASM
  1. Hematolymphoid.
    Acute leukemias; chronic leukemias; prolymphocytic leukemia; hairy cell leukemia; malignant lymphoma; dendritic cell tumors; systemic mastocytosis; plasma cell myeloma.
  2. Metastatic.
    Carcinoma, especially lung and breast; melanoma; neuroblastoma; malignant teratoma; choriocarcinoma.
  3. Benign.
    Hamartoma (single, multiple); hemangioma (capillary, cavernous); lymphangioma; lipoma

G. MISCELLANEOUS
  1. Storage diseases.
    Gaucher's disease; Neimann-Pick disease; ceroid histiocytosis; Tangier disease; Hurler's syndrome; Hunter's syndrome.
  2. Cysts.
    Pseudocyst; epidermoid (epithelial) cyst; echinococcal (hydatid) cyst.
  3. Others.
    Amyloidosis; Albers-Schönberg disease; hereditary hemorrhagic telangiectasia; hyperthyroidism.

Adapted with permission from Bowdler (1983).

An increase in spleen size may result in one or more forms of cytopenia in the peripheral blood. If it does, and there is accompanying evidence of adequate production of the relevant cells by the bone marrow, then it may be appropriate to identify a state of hypersplenism as present, which can be confirmed if splenectomy is shown to correct the deficit. Clearly, "hypersplenism" is essentially a descriptive term, and does not imply a single specific mechanism: pooling of blood cells with maldistribution, increased blood volume, and shortened cell life-span may all contribute in varying degrees to the syndrome. Examples of concurrent changes in the size of the spleen and its functional activity are given in the following subheadings.

6.4.1. DIMINISHED SPLEEN FUNCTION WITH SMALL-TO-NORMAL SPLEEN SIZE
Conditions with diminished splenic activity are described further in Chapter 10. They include both congenital and acquired conditions, and also disorders in which the spleen is involved as part of a more generalized immune deficiency.

6.4.1.1. Congenital Disorders with Hyposplenism

6.4.1.1.1. Congenital Absence of the Spleen (Asplenia) This rare condition may be seen as an isolated defect or, more often, as part of a syndrome that includes congenital anomalies, such as heart defects and heterotaxy (Applegate et al., 1999; Razzouk et al., 1995). Sporadic, isolated congenital asplenia is usually diagnosed after death caused by pneumococcal infection (Ferlicot et al., 1997; Kanthan 1999). Previously healthy children, who clinically deteriorate rapidly, should have a blood smear done as part of their work up. The peripheral blood smear may demonstrate Howell-Jolly bodies, an indicator of asplenia. The suspected asplenia then can be confirmed by abdominal image analysis. More commonly, asplenia is part of a syndrome that may include partial or complete situs inversus viscerum, severe cardiovascular anomalies, including total anomalous pulmonary venous connection (Yasukochi et al., 1997), interrupted inferior vena cava (Ruscazio et al., 1998), and pulmonary malformations, including accessory lobes. Rare cases of asplenia co-existing with a horseshoe adrenal gland have been reported (Shafaie et al., 1997; Herman, 1999). Putschar and Manion (1956) discussed the various combinations reported in the literature, and eight cases not previously reported. It is more commonly seen in males, and presents clinical problems in and of itself, because of increased susceptibility to infection.

The *Hox11* gene, involved in T-cell leukemia, has also been documented to play an essential role in normal development and functions of the spleen (Dear et al., 1995). Although *Hox11* gene is not required for initiation of splenic development, it is essential for survival of splenic precursors during organogenesis. Newborn *Hox11*⁻/⁻ mice exhibit asplenia. A consistent molecular genetic abnormality underlying asplenia syndrome has not been detected in humans; however, isolated cases of asplenia syndrome with molecular abnormalities, such as t(11;20) translocation (Freeman et al., 1996) and deleted ring chromosome 4 (Hou and Wang, 1996), have been reported.

6.4.1.1.2. Splenic Hypoplasia   Less uncommon, this disorder may be associated with other signs of a lack of normal development of mesenchymal organs, and with Fanconi's anemia. Kevy et al. (1968) reported three such cases, and described one with a small spleen weighing 1 gm, with the white pulp seen only at one pole. Other lymphoid structures were considered normal.

6.4.1.2. Immunodeficiency Disorders   The immunodeficiency disorders are systemic diseases of the immune system, which are expressed in the spleen principally as disorders of the white pulp. The red pulp appears to remain unaffected. Although most current knowledge is concentrated on the function of the spleen in these disorders, structural changes have also been identified and described. The histopathology of the spleen in immunodeficiency disorders varies, depending on the nature of the disorder. The PALS is usually empty in cases of T-cell deficiency, such as DiGeorge syndrome. In severe combined immunodeficiency disease (SCID), the spleen is generally small, and without discernible malpighian corpuscles or white pulp grossly and microscopically. However, in some patients with SCID, the PALS may contain lymphocytes of B-cell origin, immunoblasts, plasma cells, and plasmacytoid cells, but no T-cells. In this situation, T-cells in the PALS area are thought to be replaced by B-lymphocytes (van Houte et al., 1990). Follicles with germinal centers are typically absent. Lack of follicles with germinal centers is also seen in X-linked agammaglobulinemia, although, in late-onset agammaglobulinemia, the spleen may exhibit follicles, but no plasma cells (Huber, 1992). de Vries et al. (1968) describe splenic histology in two brothers with Swiss-type agammaglobulinemia, and illustrate a spectrum of white pulp changes. In the older sibling, there was severe depletion of the white pulp with only a few cells showing nuclear pyknosis and karyorrhexis; in the younger, there was a normal number of follicles, some of which were enlarged, with germinal centers cuffed by lymphocytes. The illustrations show differences, but do not clearly illustrate germinal center formation. In common variable immunodeficiency about one-third of the patients may present with splenomegaly. The white pulp may reveal large lymphoid aggregates with active and prominent germinal centers. The red pulp macrophages may show decreased lysozyme and sarcoid-like granulomas (Neiman, 1977; Edelstein et al., 1978). In several other immunodeficiency states, clusters of epithelioid histiocytes may be present. In chronic granulomatous disease, the spleen shows extensive granulomatous infiltrate. Sarcoid-like granulomas can also be seen in selective IgA deficiency (Edelstein et al., 1978; Urmacher and Nielsen, 1985).

In some of the less common immunologic deficiencies, a mixed splenic pathology has been described. In the initial case of the syndrome that carries his name, Nezelof described the spleen of a 14-mo-old male dying with thymic dysplasia (Nezelof et al., 1964; Nezelof, 1968). The spleen was slightly reduced in size, and grossly consisted of red pulp. The malpighian bodies were visible microscopically, but consisted essentially of large reticular cells, without germinal center formation. Scattered plasma cells were present in the red pulp.

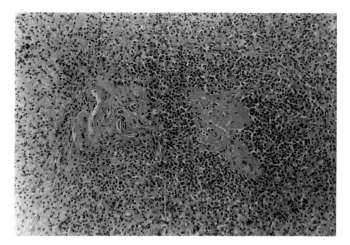

Fig. 6.2.   Follicular involution in the spleen of a patient dying with AIDS. Lymphoid follicles are atrophic and contain mostly hyalinized material and a few small lymphocytes and plasma cells.

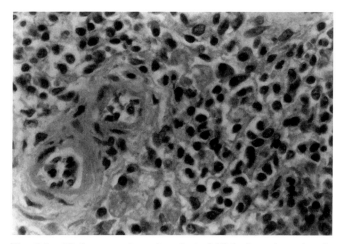

Fig. 6.3.   High-power view of a splenic follicle from the patient in Fig. 2. Lymphocytes and plasma cells are seen, but no transformed/activated cells are present.

Snover et al. (1981) described the histologic findings in the Wiskott-Aldrich syndrome, another uncommon immunodeficiency. As others have noted in other deficiencies, "the findings in the spleen tended to parallel those in the lymph nodes." The only consistent finding was the lymphoid depletion about the arterioles. A reticulum stain demonstrated the collapse of the supporting structure about the vessels secondary to cell loss. The next most common finding was extramedullary hematopoiesis, and a few cases showed hemophagocytosis and sequestration of red blood cells. There was no consistent relationship between these two findings. Eosinophilia was seen in more than one-half the cases, and was prominent in most of these. Occasionally, plasmacytosis with atypia was seen. As noted in other deficiencies, the germinal centers of lymphoid follicles reveal a spectrum of changes, ranging from hyperplasia with mitoses and active macrophages, to depletion and predominance of epithelioid cells and PAS-positive extracellular material. The terminal stage of the acquired immunodeficiency syndrome (AIDS) shows similar histology, and this end stage is illustrated in Figs. 2 and 3.

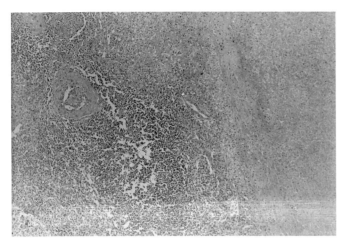

Fig. 6.4. Vasculitis with infarction. The vessel on the left is partially occluded by an organized thrombus, but occlusion of another vessel has produced the infarct on the right side of the photomicrograph.

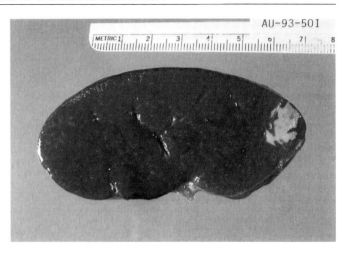

Color plate 1. Organizing splenic infarct in a patient who died of bacterial endocarditis with septic emboli.

One type of immunodeficiency may in fact represent a specific defect in splenic function (Ambrosino et al., 1987). A 30-year-old male showed decreased immune responsiveness to polysaccharides, resulting in repeated infections with *Haomophilus influenzae*. Upon challenge with polysaccharide antigens, there was essentially no response, although other immune responses appeared to be intact. Timens and Poppema (1987) have emphasized that the marginal zone of the splenic white pulp may be a unique structure that is important to the host's ability to respond to this type of antigen. This concept is based on their earlier work (Timens and Poppema, 1985), in which normal spleens were examined by immunohistochemistry. Splenic lymphoid tissue proved to be similar in lymphocyte phenotyping to other lymphoid organs, except for the marginal zone, which zone differs in containing circulating and noncirculating B-cells and helper T-cells, and most are medium-sized lymphocytes. Perhaps failure to form this zone normally may be responsible for increased susceptibility to certain organisms in neonates, and in congenital immunologic deficiencies.

6.4.1.3. Acquired Splenic Atrophy and Infarction Atrophy and infarction are the principal causes of a small spleen. Atrophy occurs in many disorders, and is sometimes found in idiopathic form in elderly individuals. The configuration of the spleen is normal, but the capsule is diffusely wrinkled, and the cut surface is depressed in relation to the capsule.

Old infarction results in an irregularly shaped and distorted spleen, with focal thickening of the capsule; the loss of tissue can be related in most instances to occlusion of vessels. In sickle cell disease, the small blood vessels are obstructed by the sickled cells (*see* Chapter 15). In essential thrombocythemia, the occluding material consists of platelets; in malaria, it is the parasites or thrombi. Infarcts may be seen in leukemic and myeloproliferative disorders, but here it is thought that vessels are compressed, rather than occluded. In rare instances, a localized or systemic arteritis may produce thrombosis and subsequent infarction (Fig. 4); this generally does not produce a significant loss of spleen size or diminished function. Infarcts vary in number and size, but are similar in gross appearance, being wedge-shaped, with the base at the capsule, and occupying the area corresponding to the distribution of the affected vessel (Color plate 1). They are well-delineated,

firm, and dark red, and, in the early stages, bulge from the cut surface. The capsule may show loss of its usual glistening character, and present a dull, shaggy appearance. Later the infarct develops central pallor and softening, with the formation of a distinct red border. Resolution comes in the form of a scar, with white, firm retracted tissue being visible on the external and cut surface. Microscopically, there is early diffusion of red blood cells and subsequent necrosis and repair. If an infection is superimposed, as may occur with an infected embolus, the area will be grossly less red, and softer from the outset. If small branches of the arterial system are involved, as with *in situ* infectious thrombosis, the areas will appear more like small spots, an appearance termed a "Fleckmilz spleen."

Atrophy occurs as a complication of several disorders, including idiopathic steatorrhea, dermatitis herpetiformis, and autoimmune disorders (*see* Chapter 10). It may also follow radiation therapy and cytotoxic chemotherapy.

6.4.2. DIMINISHED SPLEEN FUNCTION WITH SPLENIC ENLARGEMENT This is a commonly found situation, although few disorders contribute to it. The basic pathophysiologic mechanism is infiltration of the spleen, either by cells or noncellular substances, which can both interfere with its function and cause enlargement of the organ (Steinberg et al., 1983).

6.4.2.1. Neoplasms Hematolymphoid neoplasms have the capacity to diminish the functional activity of the spleen, because of their potential for diffuse replacement of the organ. This may occur in leukemias, lymphomas, and, less commonly, in splenic involvement by plasma cell myeloma. The spleen involved by leukemia exhibits an irregularly thickened capsule and a bulging gray-red cut surface. Microscopically, there is a diffuse infiltration of both cords and sinuses by leukemic cells, with effacement of normal splenic architecture. A similar picture may be seen in aggressive forms of plasma cell myeloma, although splenomegaly occurs in only 5–10% of cases. In malignant lymphoma, there may be multiple small tumor nodules or a large single mass, as discussed later in this chapter.

6.4.2.2. Sarcoidosis A definite histologic diagnosis of sarcoidosis is not possible, because of the lack of specific histologic features for the sarcoid granuloma. The diagnosis is established by exclusion of other causes of noncaseating granulomas, and by clinico-pathological correlation. Extensive involvement of the spleen by sarcoidosis may lead to splenomegaly and decreased function (Guyton and Zumwalt, 1975). Sarcoid spleens have weighed up to 800 gm. The cut surface is often dark red, with large gray nodules. These epithelioid granulomas tend to be localized to the white pulp.

6.4.2.3. Germinal Center Hypoplasia
This disorder of genetic origin is characterized by paucity of the germinal centers in splenic white pulp (Weisdorf and Krivit, 1982). It was present in three generations of a family in which most members had splenomegaly. The spleens were often massive, with poorly developed or absent lymphoid follicles. Recurrent bacterial sepsis and autoimmune disorders were also part of the clinical picture.

McKinley et al. (1987) describe a similar disorder in a family with splenomegaly and germinal center hypoplasia, apparently inherited as an autosomal dominant trait. In one case, the spleen weighed 1750 g. Microscopically, there was an expanded white pulp, but no germinal centers. Plasma cells were present. Immunoperoxidase stains revealed B- and T-cells in their usual location, as well as dendritic cells. The initial pancytopenia resolved after splenectomy; there appeared to be an overall defect in the helper T-cell population.

6.4.2.4. Follicular Involution in AIDS
The acquired counterpart to the inherited hypoplasia of germinal centers is the late stage AIDS. The spleen is often enlarged, but the lymphocyte population declines significantly during the course of the disease (Klatt and Meyer, 1987). In two reviews, the mean spleen weight was 315 gm (Reichert et al., 1983; Niedt and Schinella, 1985). In the early stage of the disease, there is follicular hyperplasia, but later the gross appearance of the cut surface is red and meaty, without discernible malpighian corpuscles, reflecting loss of the lymphoid tissue. Initially, the lymphoid follicles show active germinal centers with active cell turnover and numerous tingible body macrophages. The lymphoid follicles then become less cellular and exhibit deposits of eosinophilic amorphous material. There is gradual loss of the cells in the periarteriolar sheaths, with replacement by fibrous tissue (Figs. 2 and 3). Erythrophagocytosis and foci of hematopoiesis may be evident. In the red pulp there is congestion and an increase in cells, predominantly plasma cells, immunoblasts, and histiocytes. Hemosiderin may be present, both intra- and extracellularly. The red pulp also shows an increase in vascularity, which is possibly one factor increasing the potential for spontaneous rupture of spleen (noted later).

Patients testing positively for human immunodeficiency virus (HIV) may present with idiopathic thrombocytopenic purpura (ITP) in the prodromal phase of AIDS. Histologically, the white pulp shows nonspecific lymphoid follicular hyperplasia. However, using immunohistochemistry, an increase in cytotoxic/suppressor lymphocytes, with a decreased CD4:CD8 ratio, is noted in the germinal centers (Rousselet et al., 1988). In addition, retroviral-like particles have been detected within the germinal centers, by electron microscopic examination. Except for an increase in the CD8 population, a decrease in CD4:CD8 ratio, and the finding of virus particles ultrastructurally, most of the morphologic changes in the spleen in the early stages of AIDS are not distinguishable from those of control HIV-negative patients with ITP.

In addition to AIDS-associated morphologic changes, the spleen may demonstrate a variety of neoplastic and nonneoplastic lesions in the AIDS population. The nonneoplastic lesions are largely composed of infectious processes, which include those of

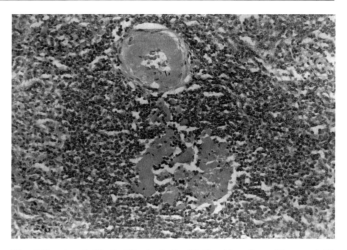

Fig. 6.5. Amyloidosis. The typical subintimal location of the amyloid is shown. In later stages, and in severe forms, extensive amyloid deposits can be identified throughout the spleen (*see* Color plate 2).

Mycobacterium avium intracellulare (MAI), splenic abscesses caused by *Salmonella* group D, and cytomegalovirus (Mathew et al., 1989), splenic abscess caused by *Mycobacterium tuberculosis* (Wolff et al., 1991), and cat scratch disease or bacillary (epithelioid) angiomatosis (Schwartzman et al., 1990). Some infectious processes in the AIDS population may exhibit a tumor-like presentation, including mycobacterial infection presenting as a spindle-cell pseudotumor of the spleen (Suster et al., 1994), and bacillary angiomatosis mimicking Kaposi's sarcoma (Steeper et al., 1992). The distinction between bacillary angiomatosis and other vascular proliferations is important, because the former lesions will respond to antibiotic therapy. A case of simultaneous bacillary angiomatosis and Kaposi's sarcoma of the skin, and hepatosplenic bacillary angiomatosis, in an AIDS patient, has also been reported (Steeper et al., 1992).

Kaposi's sarcoma, the most common neoplasm found in AIDS patients, may also involve the spleen (Gonzalez-Lopez et al., 1996). Other neoplastic processes in the AIDS population, which may involve the spleen, include high-grade lymphomas, and, less commonly, smooth muscle tumors (Barbashina et al., 2000). Epstein-Barr virus (EBV), which has been commonly detected in these neoplastic processes in the setting of AIDS, is thought to play a role in the development of these tumors.

6.4.2.5. Amyloidosis
Amyloidosis occasionally infiltrates the spleen to a degree sufficient to cause hyposplenism; it is probably the commonest substance to produce a large hypofunctioning spleen (Gertz et al., 1983). The minimal lesion occurs as a subintimal deposit of the pulp arteries (Fig. 5). The macroscopic pattern of infiltration ranges from grossly visible small nodular deposits, referred to as a "sago spleen," to a hard, yellow, waxy organ produced by diffuse deposits of amyloid throughout the red pulp (Color plate 2). The extensive involvement of the red pulp results in hyposplenism. Rarely, amyloid forms a distinct tumor mass, leaving the remaining splenic tissue normal (Chen et al., 1987). The diagnosis is suggested clinically by frequent infections associated with firm splenomegaly. Microscopically, the diagnostic feature is the dichroism with polarized light examination of a Congo red stain. Electron microscopic examination reveals the distinct β

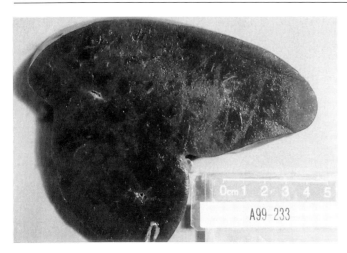

Color plate 2.   Spleen with extensive amyloid deposits from a patient with long-standing history of primary amyloidosis. Notice the waxy appearance of the splenic cut surface. (Courtesy of Dr. Michelle Barry, University of Iowa).

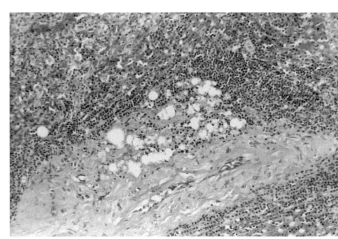

Fig. 6.6.   Lipogranuloma. Variably sized fat droplets are seen in typical periarteriolar location.

pleating of the fibrillary pattern. Immunohistochemical analysis can also be used to document the presence of light chains or A substance.

6.4.3. NORMAL SPLENIC FUNCTION WITH DECREASED OR NORMAL SIZE   These conditions of the spleen usually produce little change in the functional activity of the organ, and, rarely, enlargement, so that they are unlikely to present clinically. Some, however, are accessible to radiological diagnosis, and are described further in Chapter 17.

6.4.3.1. Lipogranuloma   Lipogranuloma, also known as "mineral oil lipidosis," is a common condition characterized by the presence of clusters of vacuolated cells in or about the white pulp (Fig. 6). Cruickshank (1984) and Cruickshank and Thomas (1984) reviewed the literature, and discussed the epidemiologic and histologic aspects. The entity is an acquired condition, which is rare before the age of 20 yr, and apparently unrelated to ethnic factors. The incidence of lipogranuloma ranges from 50%, in North America, Australia, and New Zealand, to nil, in Africa and Central and South America. It is more common in males than females. At one time, the condition was thought to be principally the result of disordered lipid metabolism, but at least some cases appear to be result from ingested mineral oil (Liber and Rose, 1967). There is an increased incidence of lipogranuloma in patients with peptic ulcer, and a decreased incidence in association with malignant lymphoma. Wanless and Geddie (1985) drew attention to a wide variability in the incidence of the lesion in autopsy studies, and also to an association between the presence of splenic lesions and similar lesions in the portal areas of the liver.

Histologically, the lesions consist of clusters of lipid droplets of variable size within macrophages, lymphocytes, and plasma cells. There is little epithelioid cell or fibroblastic reaction. Some observers have emphasized the occurrence of a sarcoid-like granulomatous lesion, but more recent reports are consistent in finding intracellular lipid droplets only within mononuclear cells. The lesion should be distinguished from other lipid lesions, such as the reaction to injected radio-opaque substances and Whipple's disease. In rare instances, granulomas related to an infectious agent may contain lipid, but these can be distinguished by the different pattern of cellular infiltrate.

Haber et al. (1988) reported the splenic histology of the fat overload syndrome. In this condition, intravenous fat emulsion therapy leads to several complications, including splenomegaly. The spleen is a homogeneous salmon-pink color, with small foci of necrosis noted on the cut surface. Microscopically, the red pulp shows distended acellular cords filled with Sudan black-positive material. Focally fat thrombi occlude small blood vessels, which may explain the focal necrosis of the white pulp.

6.4.3.2. Hamartoma   Hamartoma is defined as an abnormal or disorganized mixture of the mature tissues normally found in the affected organ. As such, splenic hamartomas consist of abnormally formed sinuses and cordal tissues. Splenic hamartomas are most commonly found in the elderly. The incidence is low: Lee et al. (1987) report ~100 cases in their literature review. On gross examination, the usually solitary hamartoma is round and appears well-circumscribed, compressing the surrounding tissue. The size can be one-to-several centimeters in diameter and involved spleens can weigh as much as 2 kg (Ross, 1971). Microscopically, they consist of slit-like vascular spaces (sinuses) intermixed with cord-like structures. The endothelial lining cells have ovoid nuclei and indistinct cytoplasm, and immunohistologic features of sinus lining cells, with CD8, factor VIII, and CD31 positivity, and CD68 negativity (Arber, 1997; Falk, 1989; Zukerberg, 1991). There is no capsule, and trabeculae are not evident. Silverman and LiVolsi (1978) point out that there may be fibrosis, lymphocytes, and eosinophils associated with these tumors, potentially causing confusion with Hodgkin's disease. Red blood cells are usually found in the vascular spaces, and hemosiderin deposits are seen in the periphery of some hamartomas. The surrounding parenchyma is normal, except for compression and occasional foci of extramedullary hematopoiesis. As noted previously, some hamartomas become symptomatic, and can cause detectable splenomegaly. Splenomegaly may occur because of the relatively uncommon feature of multiple hamartomas, as well as growth of one tumor (Morgenstern et al., 1984). Rarely, the spleen may rupture, resulting in an acute abdomen. Because most hamartomas consist of red pulp components, increase in function of the red pulp component can produce clinical problems related to sequestration (hypersplenism), as reported by Iozzo et al. (1980).

The histologic distinction of splenic hamartoma from hemangioma may be problematic. The presence of sinuses and splenic cord elements is characteristic of hamartoma, and the immunophenotypes of the lining cells appear to be different, because hemangiomas are CD8- and CD68-negative (Arber et al., 1997; Zukerberg, 1991).

6.4.3.3. Peliosis Peliosis is often found incidentally: Like lipidosis, it may be associated with liver changes, and, like the hamartoma, it is vascular in nature. This condition may cause enlargement of the spleen, although this is generally slight. Peliosis usually does not produce physical signs or symptoms. The process is visible on the cut surface of the organ, as multiple, small, round-to-oval, dark-red cystic spaces. The lesions may be localized or spread diffusely throughout the red pulp or, conversely, may be so small that they are not seen grossly (Tada et al., 1983).

Microscopically, the cystic spaces are more common in the parafollicular areas, often in the marginal zone, but they can be found throughout the red pulp. The spaces initially are round, and appear to be dilated sinuses lined by sinus lining cells and ring fibers. The lumina are filled with erythrocytes, and contain leukocytes and histiocytes. As the spaces enlarge, the lining cells may disappear, and some organization of the contents may occur. The cavities may exist either separately or in clusters, with no more than a thin layer of reticulum separating them. Occasionally, a communication is seen between a space and a venous channel, although this probably has no pathogenetic significance. If the process is extensive, there may be a decrease in the extent of the white pulp.

The condition must be distinguished from simple dilatation of the red pulp sinuses, which is commonly seen in various forms of splenic congestion. However, the parafollicular location of peliosis is distinctive. Usually there are similar lesions in the liver, which help to distinguish peliosis from other vascular lesions, but cases confined to the spleen have been described (Warfel and Ellis, 1982). Peliosis, Greek for "livid spot," or "black and blue," has been associated with several diseases and therapeutic modalities. Naeim et al. (1973) proposed anabolic steroids as a possible etiologic agent. Peliosis has also been found in patients with malignancy, tuberculosis, and cirrhosis (Bleiweiss et al., 1986). Toxic factors and congenital defects have also been suggested as etiologic factors. In some cases, peliosis can be clinically significant. Because of its vascularity, it can lead to splenic rupture with intraabdominal bleeding, requiring emergency medical attention (Garcia et al., 1982; Chen and Felix, 1986; Rege et al., 1998). Javier Penalver et al. (1998) report a case of splenic peliosis, with spontaneous rupture, in a patient with immune thrombocytopenia, who had been treated with danazol. These authors suggest a cause–effect relationship between danazol therapy and splenic peliosis. An isolated case of splenic peliosis has recently been reported in a patient who had undergone liver transplantation (Raghavan et al., 1999). The peliosis in this patient was diagnosed only after traumatic rupture of the spleen. Rarely, peliosis can produce hypersplenism, leading to a decrease in blood components, including platelets (Taxy, 1978; Lacson et al., 1979). An isolated case of extensive splenic peliosis, with massive splenomegaly, has also been reported recently (Supe et al., 2000).

6.4.4. NORMAL SPLENIC FUNCTION (WITH NORMAL OR INCREASED SPLENIC SIZE)

6.4.4.1. Congestion The various causes for splenic enlargement resulting from congestion are listed in Table 2. Regardless of the cause of the congestion, the principal change is enlargement of

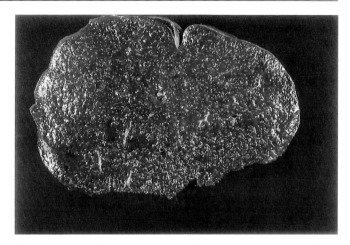

Color plate 3. Splenic congestion. The cut surface is meaty, firm, and red, with indistinct white pulp.

the red pulp by predominantly sinusoidal red blood cells without these being inherently abnormal, perhaps because of increased pressure in the venous system as a whole, as in congestive heart failure, in the portal system, or in the venous outflow at the level of the splenic vein. The organ is moderately enlarged, generally firm, and the capsule is thickened. The cut surface is meaty, firm, and dark gray-red, and the white pulp is indistinct (Color plate 3). In long-standing congestion, small, firm, brown-gray nodular deposits, Gamna-Gandy bodies, may be noted in the red pulp. Microscopically, the venous walls are thickened and cellular, with a proliferation of lining cells and fibroblasts. The cords are compressed and the sinuses dilated with red blood cells. The trabeculae are thickened by collagen or fibrous tissue. In areas where congestion has led to hemorrhage, red blood cells and hemosiderin deposits are present at an early stage, but, with the process of organization, there is an increase in fibrous tissue, with encrustation with iron and calcium salts on the elastic fibers and connective tissue, forming the Gamna-Gandy bodies. In later stages, collagen may be deposited in the cords, and extramedullary hematopoiesis may be seen.

6.4.4.2. Neoplasms Because the spleen consists principally of vascular channels and lymphoid tissue, the majority of primary neoplasms arise from one of these tissues. Benign and malignant vascular tumors make up the majority of primary splenic neoplasms. Primary splenic lymphoma is rare; however, both Hodgkin's lymphoma and non-Hodgkin's lymphomas often involve the spleen as part of the systemic manifestation of the diseases. Malignant nonlymphoid neoplasms may also be primary or secondary.

6.4.4.2.1. Benign Vascular Neoplasms

6.4.4.2.1.1. HEMANGIOMA The most common benign neoplasm of the spleen is the hemangioma (Rappaport, 1966), which generally occurs in young-to-middle-aged adults, and in males, without racial preference. Like the hamartoma, these tumors commonly do not produce clinical signs or symptoms, and a high percentage are seen as incidental findings at autopsy (Garvin and King, 1981). They are generally single, and only a few centimeters in diameter. They appear red, spongy, and well circumscribed (Color plate 4), unless infarction, thrombosis, or fibrosis has occurred. The microscopic pattern can be either capillary or cavernous, or a combination of both (Fig. 7). The vascular spaces are lined by flattened

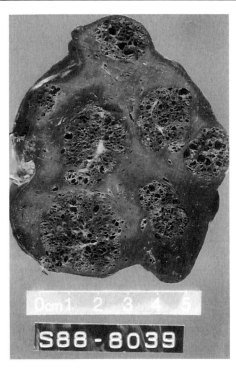

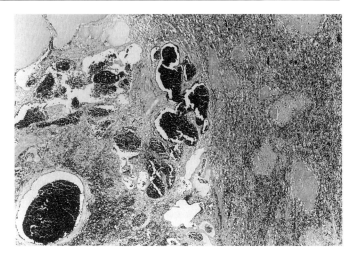

Fig. 6.7. Splenic hemangioma. Variably sized blood-filled vascular spaces are lined by flattened endothelial cells. Adjacent normal appearing splenic tissue is shown on the right side of the photomicrograph.

Color plate 4. Splenic hemangioma. Most splenic hemangiomas are single, but they can be multiple, as in this case. Notice the red, spongy appearance of the cut surface.

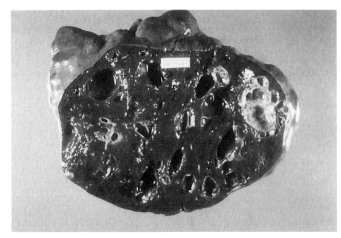

Color plate 5. Lymphangioma. Cystic areas, with a "Swiss cheese" appearance of the cut surface, is typical of this vascular proliferation.

endothelial cells, possibly of pulp cord, capillary or venous endothelial origin. These cells are generally CD31-, CD34-, and factor VIII-positive, and CD8- and CD68-negative (Zukerberg, 1991; Arber et al., 1997). They are filled with erythrocytes and proteinaceous material. Splenic cords are generally not found within the lesion, although lymphoid nodules may occasionally be seen. Splenic hemangiomas, which are very large or multiple, may produce the picture of hypersplenism with anemia or thrombocytopenia (Harris, 1985). Multiple splenic hemangiomas may be part of a systemic process in which other organs, such as the liver and skin, are also involved (Kagalwala et al., 1987). Rarely, the whole spleen may be replaced by a diffuse hemangiomatosis (Ruck et al., 1994).

6.4.4.2.1.2. LITTORAL CELL ANGIOMA   Littoral cell angioma is a rare but distinctive benign vascular tumor of the spleen (Falk et al., 1991). Most patients present with splenomegaly with or without hypersplenism. The littoral cell angioma consists of single or multiple blood-filled nodules, on gross examination. Histologically, it is composed of anastomosing vascular channels with focal pseudo-papillary patterns, and, often, anastomoses, with the normal splenic sinuses at the periphery (Warnke et al., 1995). Using paraffin immunohistochemistry, the lining cells are reported to be positive for CD21, CD31, factor VIII, and CD68, and negative for CD34 and CD8, which are characteristic of sinus lining cells (Arber et al., 1997; Falk et al., 1991). The lesion may have tall endothelial cells, but absence of cellular atypia and mitoses. The presence of architectural features of splenic sinuses is helpful in distinguishing this benign vascular proliferation from angiosarcoma.

6.4.4.2.1.3. LYMPHANGIOMA   Lymphangioma is an uncommon benign vascular proliferation. The neoplastic nature of this tumor is uncertain, and it is possible that it is, in fact, a hamartoma. Lymphangioma has a "Swiss cheese" pattern on radiologic examination (Ellison, 1980). Grossly, the lesion is spongy, cystic (Color plate 5),

or occasionally solid, and the spaces are filled with serous fluid. A subcapsular location is more common than with hemangioma (Hamoudi et al., 1975). The channels are lined by flattened endothelial cells, and the lumina contain proteinaceous material, but very few cells. Like hemangiomas, they may be capillary, cavernous, or cystic, depending on the size of the channels. The lymphangioma may be multiple (Pistoia and Markowitz, 1988), and concurrent involvement of other organs is common (Marymount and Knight, 1987).

6.4.4.2.2. Benign Nonvascular and Tumor-Like Lesions

6.4.4.2.2.1. LOCALIZED REACTIVE LYMPHOID HYPERPLASIA   Burke and Osborne (1983) described seven cases of localized florid reactive lymphoid hyperplasia, in which a single nodule was found in a normal-sized spleen. The nodules ranged from 0.1 to 1 cm in diameter, and were described as fleshy and white to gray-white. Microscopically, they exhibited varying degrees of lymphoid hyperplasia, characterized by multiple, reactive germinal centers or by a mixed infiltrate composed of sheets of small and large lymphocytes and plasma cells. Most follicles showed a mantle of small lymphocytes. In six cases, splenectomy had been performed as part of staging laparotomy for malignant lymphoma, and, in one case, because of autoimmune hemolytic anemia. In contrast, the usual reactive lymphoid hyperplasia is composed of generalized expansion of the white pulp, with multiple, relatively uniform nodules throughout the spleen. Lymphoid hyperplasia, presenting as a solitary nodule, may mimic malignant lymphoma, a potential problem, particularly in spleens removed as part of staging in patients known to have malignant lymphoma.

6.4.4.2.2.2. INFLAMMATORY PSEUDOTUMORS Inflammatory pseudotumors were first described in other organs, such as lung and gastrointestinal tract, but have subsequently been identified in the spleen, as well (Sheahan et al., 1988; McMahon, 1988). This process is usually associated with splenomegaly, and, on gross examination, single or multiple 0.5–1.5 cm nodules are present in or near malpighian corpuscles. The microscopic appearance varies, from a very heterogeneous cellular proliferation to one showing active fibrosis. Plasma cells are usually prominent, and some of them may exhibit atypia. Necrosis and granulomas with giant cells may also be present. There is no capsule formation, but the lesion compresses the surrounding parenchyma. Cultures and special stains are typically negative. The benign nature is further confirmed by the polyclonal pattern of staining of the B-cell population (McMahon, 1988).

6.4.4.2.2.3. OTHER RARE BENIGN TUMORS Other elements of the spleen are rarely the source of a benign tumor. These include lipoma (Easler and Dowlin, 1969) and fibroma (Rappaport, 1966).

6.4.4.2.3. Malignant Neoplasms

6.4.4.2.3.1. PRIMARY SPLENIC LYMPHOMAS Primary lymphomas of the spleen are relatively uncommon, and comprise about 1% of all lymphomas. Most are non-Hodgkin's lymphomas (Spier et al., 1985). Primary Hodgkin's lymphoma is rare (Zellers et al., 1990; Niv et al., 1986). The distinction between primary splenic lymphoma and primary nodal lymphoma with secondary splenic involvement is not always easy. There are no universally accepted criteria for definition of primary lymphomas of the spleen, and some published cases may represent disseminated lymphomas with secondary involvement. Using the strict criteria described by Brox et al. (1991) and Das Gupta et al. (1965), primary splenic lymphomas are limited to those with only spleen or spleen and splenic hilar lymph node involvement, without demonstrable lymphoma in other sites. Although we favor using these criteria in establishing a diagnosis of primary splenic lymphoma, possibly, occasional primary splenic lymphomas, with secondary involvement of sites other than splenic hilar lymph nodes may thus be excluded.

Using strict diagnostic criteria (i.e., lymphoma involvement limited to spleen and splenic hilar lymph nodes), Warnke et al. (1995), analyzed 47 reported cases of primary splenic non-Hodgkin's lymphomas. All the patients were adults (mean age 57 years), with slight male predominance. The patients presented with splenomegaly, and often with systemic symptoms, such as fever and weight loss. Two patients were HIV-positive. 30/47 cases (64%) were large-cell type (including anaplastic large-cell lymphoma); 15 cases (32%) were small-cell-type, including small lymphocytic, lymphoplasmacytoid, and mantle cell lymphoma; the remaining cases included 1 case of mixed-cell type, and 1 case of small-noncleaved cell type.

The spleen is usually enlarged, and may weigh up to several kilograms. In small-cell lymphomas, the cut surface may show no evident expansion of white pulp, or numerous small white nodules (miliary pattern) distributed uniformly throughout (Color plates

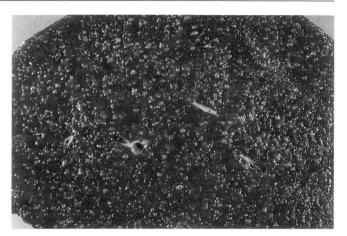

Color Plate 6. Splenic involvement by follicular lymphoma. The uniformly distributed small nodules are seen throughout. This so-called "miliary pattern" is also typically seen in other small lymphoid cell lymphomas involving the spleen (*see* Color plates 7 and 8).

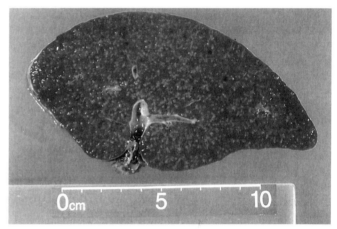

Color plate 7. CLL involving the spleen. This leukemia, in contrast to other types of leukemias, exhibits a miliary pattern of involvement reminiscent of other small lymphoid cell lymphomas.

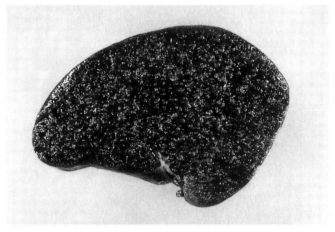

Color plate 8. Splenic marginal zone lymphoma. As with other small lymphoid cell lymphomas, a predominantly white pulp involvement with a miliary pattern is seen.

6–8), in large cell lymphomas, solitary or multiple large nodular masses are evident (Color plate 9). Audouin et al. (1988) discuss three gross appearances of primary lymphoma, including the

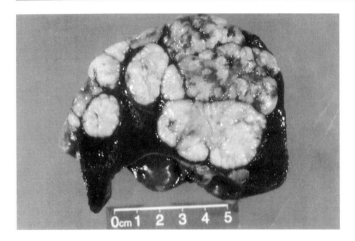

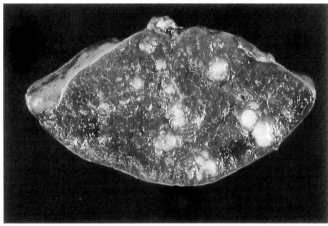

Color plate 9. Diffuse large B-cell lymphoma involving the spleen. In contrast to small lymphoid cell processes, large-cell lymphomas in the spleen typically presents with large nodular masses.

Color plate 10. Hodgkin's lymphoma involving the spleen. Similar to large cell non-Hodgkin's lymphomas, isolated or confluent nodules are the characteristic pattern of splenic involvement in this lymphoma.

diffuse, faintly nodular, the micronodular diffuse, and the micronodular focal. Some cases present as one large tumor mass, more typical of primary Hodgkin's disease of the spleen (Niv et al., 1986). The hilar and surrounding lymph nodes may be involved, and, on rare occasions, there may be direct extension into adjacent tissues. Microscopically, the small-cell proliferations primarily involve and expand the white pulp, but there may also be variable extension into the red pulp, occasionally sufficiently extensive to obscure the separation of red and white pulp on gross and microscopic examination. In small lymphocytic lymphoma, the neoplastic cells contain small, round, regular nuclei, with coarse chromatin and indistinct nucleoli. Occasional prolymphocytes and paraimmunoblasts may be identified. In mantle cell lymphoma, the neoplastic cells are uniform in size and shape, and large lymphoid cells are typically absent. The nuclei are irregular, and the chromatin is dense. The large-cell lymphomas are heterogeneous and in general show a more prominent diffuse growth pattern, with distortion of splenic architecture, and smaller numbers of large nodules, which may be confluent.

Most primary splenic lymphomas are reported to be of B-cell lineage. In one study, 14/17 splenic lymphomas were of B-lineage, and the remaining 3 of T-lineage (Falk and Stutte, 1990). Although rare, all subtypes of Hodgkin's lymphoma have been described with primary splenic involvement (Zellers et al., 1990; Niv et al., 1986).

6.4.4.2.3.2. SECONDARY SPLENIC LYMPHOMAS

6.4.4.2.3.2.1. Hodgkin's Lymphoma   Splenic involvement can be detected in more than a quarter of patients with Hodgkin's lymphoma. Isolated or confluent nodules are commonly found on gross examination (Color plate 10). All subtypes of Hodgkin's lymphoma commonly involve the spleen, except for the nodular lymphocyte predominance subtype. The white pulp is the usual site of involvement. Reed-Sternberg and Hodgkin cells, in an appropriate background composed of small lymphocytes, eosinophils, and plasma cells, are detected microscopically at the sites of involvement. However, diagnostic Reed-Sternberg cells are not an absolute requirement for establishment of splenic involvement in patients known to have Hodgkin's disease. In these cases, the presence of Reed-Sternberg cell variant/Hodgkin cells, in appropriate background, is considered adequate for the diagnosis (Lukes,

1971). Replacement of radiotherapy by systemic chemotherapy has resulted in a significant reduction in the rate of splenectomy in patients with Hodgkin's disease (Rosenberg, 1988).

6.4.4.2.3.2.2. Non-Hodgkin's Lymphoma   The frequency of splenic involvement by different types of lymphomas varies in different studies; however, in most studies, small lymphocytic lymphoma, follicular lymphoma, mantle cell lymphoma, and large-cell lymphoma are listed as lymphomas frequently involving the spleen (Kim and Dorfman, 1974; Warnke et al., 1995; Arber et al., 1997). Non-Hodgkin's lymphomas typically involve the white pulp, although red pulp involvement may also be seen to a lesser degree. Because of the normal nodular architecture of the white pulp, most lymphomas involving the spleen will exhibit a nodular pattern. Therefore, a nodular pattern alone should not be used for the classification of the lymphoma.

In small lymphocytic lymphoma, a predominantly white pulp distribution is seen, although the red pulp may also be extensively infiltrated by neoplastic cells, and, on occasion, residual white pulp nodules may be difficult to discern. The neoplastic cells contain small, round, regular nuclei with coarse chromatin. Occasional prolymphocytes and paraimmunoblasts are seen in most cases, but proliferation centers are not usually evident. Follicular lymphomas show a predominantly, and usually exquisitely, white pulp distribution with expansion of the malpighian corpuscles. Smaller nodules of neoplastic cells may also be present in the red pulp. The neoplastic cells have markedly irregular and cleaved nuclei. In the mixed-cell type, in addition to small cleaved cells, scattered larger lymphoid cells with open chromatin are seen. Mantle cell lymphoma expands the white pulp and often infiltrates splenic cords, leaving occasional residual germinal centers. The neoplastic cells contain irregular nuclei with a more open chromatin, compared to the dense chromatin seen in cells of small lymphocytic lymphoma. Prolymphocytes and paraimmunoblasts are typically absent, as are large lymphoid cells. Because of its more aggressive clinical course, mantle cell lymphoma needs to be distinguished from other low-grade B-cell neoplasms. At times, this distinction cannot be made reliably on purely morphologic grounds, particularly when neoplastic mantle cells infiltrate the pre-existing follicles and create a follicular lymphoma-like picture. For problematic cases,

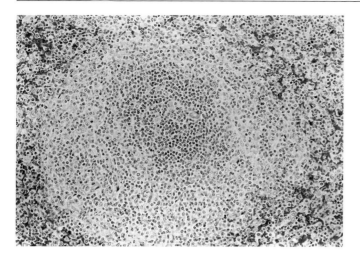

Fig. 6.8. Splenic lymphoma with circulating villous lymphocytes. The pattern of splenic involvement is predominantly white pulp although, as is illustrated here, the red pulp may also be variably involved.

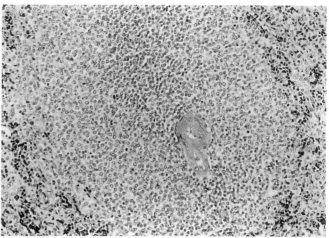

Fig. 6.9. Splenic marginal zone B-cell lymphoma. Although a marginal zone pattern may be evident, the neoplastic cells also infiltrate the mantle zone, and may replace the germinal centers, as illustrated here.

immunohistochemical staining for cyclin D1 protein can be very useful. Recent studies have shown that this protein is expressed in the majority of cases of mantle cell lymphoma, and is typically absent in other low-grade B-cell neoplasms (Vasef et al., 1997; Zukerberg et al., 1995). Some cases of lymphoplasmacytoid lymphoma may show prominent splenic involvement. Histologically, the white pulp is extensively involved by a mixed population of plasma cells, plasmacytoid cells, and transformed immunoblastic cells.

Splenic involvement by large cell lymphoma is characterized by solitary or multiple, often confluent, nodular masses with splenic architectural distortion (Color plate 9). Tumor nodules are surrounded by uninvolved white and red pulp and are typically separate from uninvolved splenic tissue. Large-cell lymphoma may show other patterns of involvement, including diffuse white pulp infiltration and variable red pulp involvement. Infrequently, a diffuse red pulp distribution is seen (Arber et al., 1997).

Although any histologic subtype of non-Hodgkin's lymphoma may present with splenomegaly, several distinct histologic subtypes are associated with significant splenomegaly. These include splenic B-cell lymphoma with circulating villous lymphocytes, marginal zone lymphoma, lymphoplasmacytoid lymphoma, and hepatosplenic T-cell lymphoma.

Splenic B-cell lymphoma with circulating villous lymphocytes (SLVL) was described by Melo et al., in 1987. A similar entity had been described by Nieman et al., in 1979, as "malignant lymphoma simulating leukemic reticuloendotheliosis." The disease is characterized by splenomegaly, circulating lymphoma cells, and minimal-to-no lymphadenopathy. The circulating lymphoma cells are slightly larger than small-lymphocytic lymphoma cells, and contain round-to-oval hyperchromatic nuclei and basophilic cytoplasm, with short villi concentrated in one pole of the cells. Some cells show plasmacytoid features. Bone marrow involvement is common, and a serum monoclonal protein is detectable in most cases. The pattern of splenic involvement is predominantly white pulp but red pulp is also variably involved (Fig. 8). This pattern is different from hairy cell leukemia, which has a predominantly red pulp pattern. Most patients with this lymphoma are elderly men, and the disease has an indolent course, with a 5-year survival

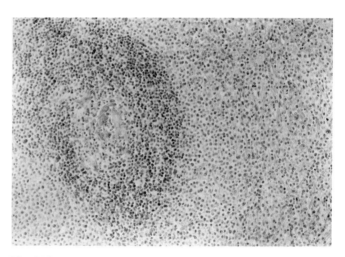

Fig. 6.10. Nodal monocytoid B-cell lymphoma involving the spleen. A distinct marginal zone distribution, with partial periarterial lymphocyte cuff preservation, is seen.

greater than 75% (Mulligan et al., 1991). In a minority of the cases, t(11;14)(q13;q32) translocation, with expression of *bcl-1* gene, has been detected (Jadayel et al., 1994).

Splenic marginal zone lymphoma is rare (Schmid et al., 1992). Patients with this type of lymphoma present with splenomegaly, anemia, and bone marrow involvement, and therefore, despite the designation, it is difficult to prove as being primary, using strict criteria. Histologically, the neoplastic cells in the spleen exhibit a marginal zone pattern, but may infiltrate the mantle zone and replace the germinal centers (Fig. 9). Cytologically, the neoplastic cells are similar to monocytoid B-cell lymphoma and low-grade B-cell lymphoma of mucosa-associated lymphoid tissue. Nodal monocytoid B-cell lymphoma may rarely involve the spleen (Vasef and Katzin, 1993; Traweek and Sheibani, 1992). The pattern of involvement has a distinct marginal zone distribution, with partial periarterial lymphocyte cuff preservation (Fig. 10). Cytologically, monocytoid B-cell lymphoma cells contain oval vesicular nuclei, indistinct nucleoli, and abundant clear cytoplasm. The cytologic

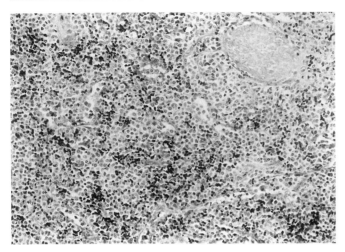

Fig. 6.11. Hairy cell leukemia. The neoplastic cells exhibit a predominantly splenic cord and sinus pattern. This pattern is distinctly different from lymphomas, which characteristically involve the white pulp.

features of monocytoid B-cell lymphoma are similar to the neoplastic cells of hairy cell leukemia; however, the pattern of splenic involvement in hairy cell leukemia is distinctly different, involving predominantly splenic cords and sinuses (Fig. 11); monocytoid B-cell lymphoma principally involves white pulp, often expanding or effacing the marginal zone.

Hepatosplenic T-cell lymphoma is a distinct entity that typically occurs in young adults, and has a poor prognosis (Wong et al., 1995). Clinical presentation includes hepatosplenomegaly, weight loss, fever, and cytopenia. This neoplasm is similar to another subtype of T-cell lymphoma, designated "erythrophagocytic T-γ lymphoma" (Kadin et al., 1981). However, the erythrophagocytic activity seen in erythrophagocytic T-γ lymphoma is not a feature of hepatosplenic T-cell lymphoma. The neoplastic cells infiltrate the red pulp and sinuses with a diffuse pattern. The pattern of bone marrow and liver involvement in this lymphoma is intrasinusoidal, and is similar to that seen in the spleen. The individual cells contain medium-sized, oval-to-folded nuclei, and moderate amounts of pale cytoplasm. The neoplastic cells express T-cell-associated antigens, including CD3, and they are often CD56-positive. They also express γ/δ T-cell receptors. Molecular analysis of T-cell receptor genes shows clonal rearrangements of γ or δ chain T-cell receptor gene. The β chain T-cell receptor gene is either in germline or rearranged configuration (Farcet et al., 1990). Hepatosplenic lymphoma of B-lineage has also been reported to arise in patients with hepatitis C virus infection. A possible association between hepatitis C virus and hepatosplenic B-cell lymphoma has been suggested (Murakami et al., 1988; Naschitz et al., 1994; Izumi et al., 1996; Izumi et al., 1997).

6.4.4.2.3.3. LEUKEMIAS   The spleen is commonly involved in leukemias; however, the degree of splenic involvement depends on the duration of the disease, as well as on the type of leukemia. In chronic leukemias, significant involvement of spleen is usually clinically evident; in acute leukemias, significant splenomegaly is not usually seen. Some types of leukemias, such as hairy cell leukemia, are associated with significant hypersplenism, but this rarely occurs in acute lymphoid leukemias. In some cases of severe cytopenia secondary to hypersplenism, therapeutic splenectomy may become necessary. Decreased splenic function can also be

seen in leukemias. Simoes et al. (1995) analyzed alteration in splenic function in patients with leukemia, and showed that, in greater than 50% of patients with acute leukemias, hyposplenism was present.

Grossly, the spleen involved by leukemia demonstrates enlargement that tends to be diffuse. The cut surface is homogeneous, except for areas of hemorrhage or infarction. The white pulp nodules are either totally absent or inconspicuous. The spleen can rupture as a result of extensive leukemic infiltrate or splenic infarction (Flood and Carpenter, 1961; Serur and Terjanian, 1992). Microscopically, leukemic involvement is predominantly red pulp, but a peritrabecular pattern may also be seen. Commonly, the leukemic cells infiltrate the splenic cords extensively, and sinuses may also be involved.

In general, the myeloid leukemias produce more splenic enlargement and infarction than the lymphoid leukemias.

All French-American-British (FAB) subtypes of acute myelogenous leukemias (AML) can involve the spleen. AML in the spleen can present as *de novo* disease, as a blast crisis in a chronic myeloproliferative disorder, or evolve from a myelodysplastic syndrome. The criteria for the FAB classification of AML are based on morphologic examination and cytochemical studies of bone marrow and peripheral blood (Bennett et al., 1985). Distinguishing between the various FAB subtypes of AML in the spleen, on morphologic grounds alone, is usually not possible. Paraffin immunohistochemical stains using antimyeloperoxidase and antilyzosyme antibodies, may be useful to confirm the granulocytic/monocytic nature of the neoplastic cells. For the FAB subtypes, M6 (erythroleukemia) and M7 (megakaryocytic leukemia), antibodies against hemoglobin for erythroleukemia (Neiman, 1980) and factor VIII for megakaryocytic leukemias may prove useful.

Marked granulocytic hyperplasia, with increased immature myeloid precursors in the spleen, can be induced by granulocyte colony-stimulating factor (G-CSF) (Figs. 12A,B). The histologic features may simulate a myeloid leukemic infiltrate (Vasef et al., 1998).

The spleen in chronic myeloid leukemia (CML) generally shows a red, homogenous, firm cut surface with obliterated white pulp (Color plate 11), although, occasionally, residual white pulp may be noted. Histologically, a spectrum of granulocytic cells at different stages of maturation is seen. Immature myeloid precursors can be detected using antimyeloperoxidase antibody. Most patients with CML eventually enter an aggressive phase known as "accelerated phase" or "blast crisis." The blasts in the majority of the cases are myeloblasts; however, in approx 30%, the blasts are lymphoblasts and express terminal deoxynucleotidyl transferase (TdT) (Muehleck et al., 1984).

Splenomegaly is present in approx 10% of acute lymphoid leukemia (ALL) cases, and is most frequent in T-lineage subtype (Neiman and Orazi, 1999). Histologically, the leukemic cells typically involve the red pulp with a patchy distribution. Immunophenotypically, the L1 and L2 FAB subtypes are TdT-positive, regardless of lineage. The mature B-cell ALL (L3) is usually TdT-negative.

Chronic lymphocytic leukemia (CLL) is the only leukemia with a predominantly white pulp pattern of splenic involvement. The mature-appearing small lymphoid cells in CLL expand and obliterate the white pulp nodules. Patients with CLL may develop cytopenia as a result of autoimmune hemolytic anemia/thrombocytopenia (Kaden et al., 1979), or, less frequently, cytopenia may develop

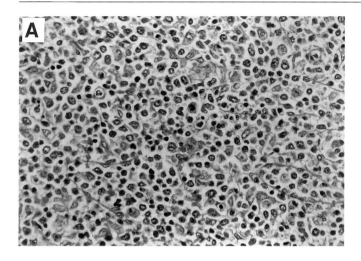

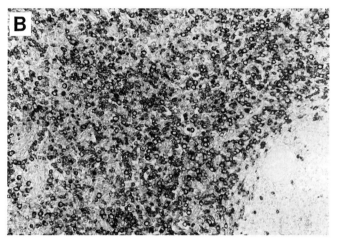

Fig. 6.12. Marked myeloid hyperplasia, with sheets of immature myeloid cells in the spleen induced by G-CSF administration, mimicking a myeloid leukemic infiltrate (**A**). The immature cells are myeloperoxidase-positive (**B**) (immunoperoxidase and hematoxylin counterstain).

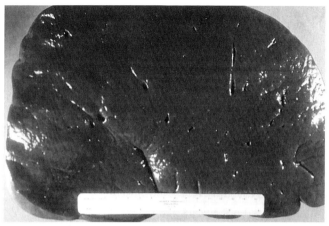

Color plate 11. Chronic myeloid leukemia. Red, homogeneous, firm cut surface, with obliteration of white pulp is typical of the cut surface in this type of leukemia.

secondary to splenomegaly and hypersplenism (Christensen, 1971). Massive splenic enlargement associated with severe anemia or thrombocytopenia has poor prognostic implications in CLL patients (Binet et al., 1977).

In prolymphocytic leukemia, the spleen may be very large, and the cut surface is deep red with a diffuse small nodular pattern (Bearman et al., 1978). Microscopically, cells that mark as B-lymphocytes are seen in the grossly defined nodules, in both the white and red pulp. A T-cell variant of prolymphocytic leukemia has also been recognized (Catovsky et al., 1973). On occasion, other leukemias may produce distinct nodules, as well as diffuse enlargement (Hogan et al., 1989). In four cases of myelocytic leukemia, small but distinct nodules were noted, varying from dark red, to pink, to brown.

Hairy cell leukemia characteristically presents with massive splenomegaly. The spleen usually weighs ~2000 g, and the capsule is tense, but not thickened. The cut surface is meaty, dark red, and without distinct malpighian corpuscles, and may have areas of apparent infarction (Burke et al., 1974). The prominent microscopic feature is a diffuse infiltrate of round-to-oval cells obscuring the white pulp and filling the red pulp sinusoids and cords (Fig. 11).

The cell population is fairly uniform, with abundant cytoplasm, and without significant mitotic activity. Ribosomal–lamellar complexes are present in the cytoplasm of hairy cells on electron microscopic examination (Burke et al., 1974). However, these complexes are not specific for hairy cells, and have been described in other lymphoid neoplasms (Brunning and Parkin, 1975). A distinctive feature is the formation of pseudosinuses, which range in size from that of slightly dilated sinuses to poorly delineated large masses of red blood cells, which are grossly visible. Nanba et al. (1977) demonstrated that these lesions are lined to varying degrees by neoplastic cells, without demonstrable splenic sinus or venous endothelium; consequently, they are termed "pseudosinuses." Hairy cell leukemia must be differentiated from mast cell disease, which has a similar cytologic appearance and pattern of splenic involvement. Hairy cell leukemic cells stain with B-cell-associated antigens, including CD20. Mast cells are KP-1 (CD68)-positive and CD20-negative. Marginal zone B-cell lymphoma/monocytoid B-cell lymphoma cells share cytologic appearance similar to hairy cells; however, the pattern of splenic involvement in these lymphomas is white pulp predominant, in contrast to the mostly red pulp involvement of hairy cell leukemia.

Another leukemic process, large granular lymphocytic (LGL) leukemia, with prominent involvement of the spleen, was described by McKenna et al. (1977) as a subtype of CLL. These cases showed marked neutropenia and splenomegaly, in addition to lymphocytosis. This entity has been characterized as a neoplastic proliferation of LGLs or T8 hyperlymphocytosis, with evidence that the neoplastic cells are probably responsible for the neutropenia (Grillot-Courvalin et al., 1987). The spleen may weigh up to 2000 g, and grossly have an intact, but thinned, capsule, and a firm, smooth, red cut surface. Microscopically there is diffuse infiltration or focal aggregates of the LGLs in the red pulp. The lymphoid follicles are present, usually in normal numbers, but they may lack germinal centers. The periarteriolar sheath may show depletion of lymphocytes (Loughran et al., 1985). Two subtypes of LGL leukemia have been described, based on distinct immunophenotypes of the neoplastic cells: T-LGL leukemias are CD3-, CD8-, CD16-, and CD57-positive, but CD56-negative. Natural killer (NK) LGL leukemias are CD3-, CD4-, CD8-, and CD57-negative, but CD16- and CD56-positive (Semenzato et al., 1997; Chan et al., 1986). Most patients with T-LGL exhibit an indolent course (Dhodapkar et al., 1994), but an aggressive variant has also been reported (Gentile et al., 1994). Patients with NK-LGL type usually present with massive hepatosplenomegaly, and have a poor prognosis. The majority of the patients with NK-LGL phenotype die of progressive disease within 1 year after diagnosis (Semenzato et al., 1987).

Adult T-cell leukemia/lymphoma commonly presents with hepatosplenomegaly, lymphadenopathy, and skin involvement. The disease was originally described in Japan (Uchiyama et al., 1977), but is also reported in West Africa and the West Indies, although less commonly (Catovsky et al., 1982). Patients with this disease usually present with a chronic course, but have a rapid course terminally. Extremely abnormal, hyperlobated circulating lymphocytes are characteristically found in the peripheral blood. In about 50% of the patients, the spleen is enlarged and infiltrated by leukemic cells (Kinoshita et al., 1982). Immunophenotypically, the neoplastic cells are of T-lineage (CD2-, CD3-, and CD5-positive). In the majority of the patients, the neoplastic cells express CD4 antigen, but in a minority a CD8 phenotype is seen. The neoplastic cells are TdT-negative. Sporadic cases of adult T-cell lymphoma/leukemia have been described in the United States.

In systemic mast cell disease, the spleen is often involved, and demonstrates numerous changes (Travis and Li, 1988). The spleens weigh up to 1140 g, and capsular thickening is usually seen. The cut surface shows small nodules in a diffuse pattern. Fibrosis, involving capsule and parenchyma, can be extensive, and calcification may be present. Pale-staining mast cells are most often seen about the trabeculae and follicles, and some degree of fibrosis and eosinophilia is generally present. Mast cell disease must be differentiated from other cytologically pale-staining hematolymphoid neoplasms, such as hairy cell leukemia, T-cell lymphomas, and marginal zone and monocytoid B-cell lymphomas.

6.4.4.2.3.4. NONHEMATOPOIETIC MALIGNANT NEOPLASMS

6.4.4.2.3.4.1. Primary Malignant Neoplasms   Primary sarcomas are rare in the spleen. Those reported include angiosarcoma (Smith et al., 1985), and rare examples of malignant fibrous histiocytoma (Govoni et al., 1980). Over 100 cases of primary splenic angiosarcoma have been reported, some under different designations, such as hemangiosarcoma and malignant hemangioendothelioma (Falk et al., 1993). The tumor is either confined to the spleen, or the organ contains the largest tumor mass, if multiple organs are involved. Metastatic disease is present in more than three-fourths of cases. Usually the spleen is enlarged, and this may have occurred as a sudden clinical event. These sarcomas appear as definable, firm, red nodular masses (Color plate 12), or as a generalized enlargement of the spleen. Microscopically, the appearances are quite variable; vascular spaces may be evident (Fig. 13), or the stromal sarcomatous element may predominate (Rappaport, 1966). Hemosiderin is generally present, often in significant amounts. Occasionally, extramedullary hematopoiesis may be seen in the tumor, and, clinically, some patients have a microangiopathic hemolytic anemia (Sordillo et al., 1981). Angiosarcoma cells exhibit endothelial immunohistologic features. They are usually factor VIII-, Ulex-, CD31-, and CD34-positive, and CD8- and CD68-negative (Arber et al., 1997; Falk et al., 1993). The prognosis is poor, with <1 yr survival from the time of diagnosis (Garvin and King, 1981).

Kaposi's sarcoma may also occur in the spleen, but this is rare, even in patients with AIDS (Ziegler and Dorfman, 1988). When present, the tumor follows the major blood vessels into the red pulp in a diffuse manner, rather than forming distinct tumor nodules.

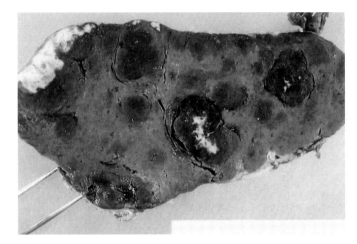

Color plate 12.   Primary splenic angiosarcoma. Partially necrotic, red, nodular masses are seen in this example.

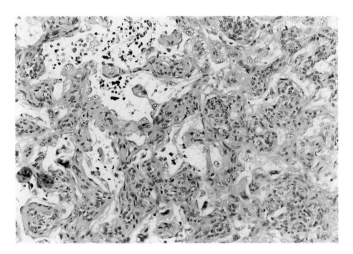

Fig. 6.13.   Splenic angiosarcoma. An anastomosing network of vascular channels, which communicate with each other, is shown.

Primary malignant epithelial tumors of the spleen are extremely rare, with only isolated cases reported. They include two cases of squamous cell carcinoma apparently arising from an epithelial cyst (Elit and Aylward, 1989, Masci et al., 1985), and a case of adenocarcinoma arising in heterotopic pancreatic tissue (Shuman and Bouterie, 1976).

6.4.4.2.3.4.2. Metastatic Malignant Neoplasms   The spleen is a uncommon site for nonhematopoietic metastatic disease. The exact cause of this resistance is still uncertain; however, a widely accepted theory, explaining the low incidence of metastases in the spleen, cites the absence of afferent lymphatic vessels (Warren and Davis, 1934). Therefore, it is thought that metastatic tumors in the spleen occur only hematogenously. The splenic capsule may be involved in abdominal carcinomatosis, and direct extension can occur from adjacent organs, but a distinct intrasplenic mass is rare. In most cases, it is an asymptomatic finding associated with diffuse and widespread carcinomatosis, most commonly originating from carcinoma of the breast, lung, or ovary (Color plate 13).

Secondary melanoma also occurs. Rare cases of neuroblastoma and teratoma involving the spleen have been reported (Marymount and Gross, 1963), as have metastatic seminoma (Willey et al., 1982), and choriocarcinoma (Carr et al., 1987). We have seen a case of

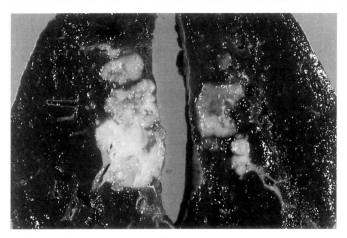

Color plate 13. Involvement of spleen by metastatic carcinoma originating from a papillary serous carcinoma of the ovary.

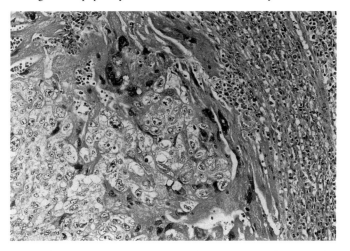

Fig. 6.14. Choriocarcinoma metastatic to spleen. A mixed population of neoplastic cells composed of syncytiotrophoblast, cytotrophoblast, and intermediate trophoblast is seen.

unexpected metastatic choriocarcinoma in a spleen removed from a patient who presented with intracranial bleeding thought to be caused by vasculitis, and treated with steroids, with subsequent thrombocytopenia (Fig. 14).

The overall autopsy frequency of splenic metastasis in cases of carcinoma is ~4%, but the actual percentage may be higher. The presence of metastatic disease during life may become better documented with newer radiologic techniques: Up to 50% of melanoma patients have abnormal liver and spleen scans (Klein et al., 1987). Most cases are asymptomatic, but painful splenomegaly and cytopenias may occur. Splenomegaly secondary to metastatic carcinoma may be the first indication of recurrent tumor, particularly in gynecologic neoplasms (Klein et al., 1987. Gilks et al., 1989; Jorgensen and Chrintz, 1988). Although not widely utilized in splenic disease, fine-needle aspiration has proved to be a useful method for confirmation of metastatic tumors (Zeppa et al., 1994).

6.4.4.3. Storage Diseases The spleen is a common site of involvement in most lysosomal storage diseases, including lipidoses and mucopolysaccharidoses. These infiltrative processes comprise a small portion of cases with splenomegaly, but are an important category, because they almost always represent a sign of systemic disease. The spleen is enlarged because of the accumulation of intra- or extracellular substances.

6.4.4.3.1. Lipidosis

6.4.4.3.1.1. GAUCHER'S DISEASE (GLUCOSYL CERAMIDE LIPIDOSIS) Like most lipid storage disorders, Gaucher's disease is inherited as an autosomal-recessive trait. Etiologically, a deficiency in the enzyme, glucocerebrosidase A, is present, which leads to intracellular accumulation of the glucocerebroside. The underlying genetic abnormality includes mutations at the enzyme locus on chromosome 1q21 (Mistry et al., 1992). In contrast to the rapidly fatal infantile type (type 2) (Glew et al., 1985), the adult type (type 1) exhibits a chronic course, and is compatible with long life. Another type of the disease (type 3) characteristically affects young adults, and has intermediate severity. The spleen is enlarged in all types of the disease; however, in type 1, it is usually a dominant presenting feature. In contrast to type 1, neurologic symptoms are the most prominent features in types 2 and 3. In Gaucher's disease, the spleen may be large, with a dry, firm, and pale-grey cut surface, with loss of defined pulp compartments. Histiocytes containing glucocerebroside fill the red pulp cords (Lee et al., 1977). The cells have round uniform nuclei, which are occasionally multiple, and abundant cytoplasm, which appears fibrillar. The cytoplasm in Gaucher cells is intensely PAS-positive, and the PAS positivity is diastase resistant (Lee et al., 1977).

6.4.4.3.1.2. NIEMANN-PICK DISEASE This includes a heterogeneous group of autosomal recessive disorders (Elleder, 1989; Weisz et al., 1994). Of the five described subtypes (A–E), two (A and B subtypes) result from sphingomyelinase deficiency (Schuchman and Desnick, 1995). In Nieman-Pick disease, sphengomyelin or cholesterol are accumulated, particularly in the spleen and neural tissue. Type A accounts for the majority of the cases, and usually will be evident by the age of 6 mo. Prominent splenomegaly, hepatomegaly, lymphadenopathy, central nervous system involvement associated with mental retardation, and cutaneous xanthomas are typical findings (Schuchman and Desnick, 1995). In type B, neural involvement is absent. In adults with type B disease, massive splenomegaly is typically found. Patients with type C Nieman-Pick disease are usually older and present with splenomegaly, hepatomegaly, and neural involvement (Pentchev et al., 1995). In a manner similar to Gaucher's disease, the affected spleen is pale. Histologically, the cells infiltrate the red pulp and have pale, vacuolated cytoplasm. The cells are paler than Gaucher cells on routine H&E stained sections, and are only weakly PAS-positive. Sudan black B, and oil red O stains are positive. Electron microscopy may demonstrate lamellated structures (Dumontel et al., 1993) and parallel structures designated as "zebra bodies." The intracellular lipid deposits demonstrate a yellow-green autofluorescence.

6.4.4.3.1.3. CEROID HISTIOCYTOSIS Ceroid deposits may accumulate in liver and spleen in the sea-blue histiocyte syndrome (Silverstein et al., 1970). This syndrome is characterized by prominent splenomegaly, and may present with an autosomal recessive inheritance pattern (Sawitsky et al., 1972). Rarely, central nervous system, pulmonary involvement, and skin pigmentation may be noted (Silverstein et al., 1970; Silverstein and Ellefson, 1972). Thrombocytopenia may also occur secondary to cordal widening and platelet sequestration. Ceroid-containing histiocytes accumulate in both the splenic cords and sinuses. In H&E-stained sections, the histiocytes contain cytoplasmic yellow-to-brown granules; in Romanovsky stained smears, they appear blue-green. The ceroid granules are PAS-positive and diastase resistant.

Ceroid histiocytosis can also occur as part of the familial Hermansky-Pudlak syndrome (Schinella et al., 1985), as well as in several other disorders, including CLL (Dosik et al., 1972), chronic granulomatous disease of childhood (Bartman et al. 1967), ITP (Chandra et al., 1973), and some subtypes of hyperlipidemia (Parker et al., 1976).

6.4.4.3.2. Gangliosidoses

6.4.4.3.2.1. TAY-SACHS DISEASE The most common of the gangliosidoses is Tay-Sachs disease, which is characterized by accumulation of a sphingolipid, GM2 ganglioside. The underlying cause is deficiency of the enzyme, hexosaminidase A, because of a mutation in the α subunit locus located on chromosome 15 (Sandhoff et al., 1989). The dominant sites of involvement include the peripheral and central nervous system, and other organs, such as the heart, may also be involved. Splenomegaly may also be present. The cells contain fine cytoplasmic vacuoles, and stain positively with Sudan black B.

6.4.4.3.2.2. FABRY DISEASE Fabry disease is unique among the sphingolipidoses, in being transmitted by an X-linked structural gene, evidently responsible for the gene product, α-galactosidase A. Deficiency leads to the accumulation of the sphingolipid, ceramide trihexoside, particularly in the heart and kidney, and, to a lesser extent, in lymphoid organs (Desnick and Bishop, 1989). Prominent splenomegaly is not usually a feature of this disease. The involved organs contain foamy histiocytes.

6.4.4.3.2.3. WOLMAN'S DISEASE In Wolman's disease, foamy histiocytes involve several organs, including the spleen. Triglyceride and cholesterol esters accumulate in the cells, because of deficiency of the enzyme acid, esterase (Lough et al., 1970). Foamy cells can also accumulate in the spleens of patients with "von Gierke disease" (Chen and Burchell, 1995), and in tuberous sclerosis (Bender and Yunis, 1982).

6.4.5. INCREASED SPLENIC FUNCTION WITH NORMAL OR DECREASED SIZE

6.4.5.1. Idiopathic Thrombocytopenic Purpura ITP almost invariably presents with a spleen that is not enlarged, or at most only minimally so, but there is increased activity of the spleen in platelet destruction and antibody formation (McMillan et al., 1974). In a review of 12 patients undergoing splenectomy, Tavassoli and McMillan (1975) found that the spleens ranged in weight from 80 to 424 g. The two weighing over 250 g were enlarged for reasons other than ITP. Gross examination is usually unremarkable. Microscopically, the prominent feature is reactive hyperplasia of the white pulp with prominence of the germinal centers, which typically have a starry sky appearance (Fig. 15). Intrafollicular PAS-positive material may be present. The marginal zone is expanded, and transformed lymphocytes and plasma cells constitute part of this expansion. Red pulp sinuses and cords contain scattered foamy macrophages, attributed to the phagocytosis of platelets (Tavassoli and McMillan, 1975). The junction of the marginal zone and red pulp is the site of most such activity, since this is the first site of antigen–antibody encounter. Plasmacytosis is also seen in the red pulp. If steroid therapy has been given, there may be lymphoid depletion and more histiocytes than normal. Periarterial fibrosis is reported to occur in some cases (Berendt et al., 1986).

6.4.6. INCREASED SPLENIC FUNCTION WITH NORMAL OR INCREASED SIZE

6.4.6.1. Hypersplenism The term "hypersplenism" has been widely used to refer to the excess destruction of circulating blood cells by the spleen. It does not indicate a specific mechanism for the disorder, but represents a syndrome that may have any number of causes. Historically, some cases were thought to be congenital

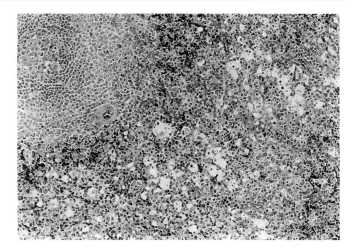

Fig. 6.15. ITP. Reactive lymphoid hyperplasia of white pulp with expanded marginal zone is present. The adjacent red pulp contains scattered macrophages.

or idiopathic (Doan and Wright, 1945; Dacie et al., 1978). However, few, if any, of these are now recognized if primary splenic pathology, and autoimmune or other abnormalities of the circulating cells are excluded (Bowdler, 1983).

Dameshek (1955) proposed four criteria for the diagnosis of hypersplenism: peripheral blood cytopenia, bone marrow hyperplasia, splenomegaly, and reversal of cytopenia following splenectomy. Some types of hypersplenism do not meet all four criteria, but are included under the term (Jacob, 1974; Amorosi, 1965). Splenic sequestration and destruction of red blood cells has been considered the main mechanism of the cytopenias (Crosby, 1962; Christensen, 1973). Abnormal red blood cells account for the majority of disorders in which abnormal cells are entrapped in normal splenic cords. It may be argued that such cases should not be considered hypersplenism. Alternatively, abnormality in the spleen itself may result in increased destruction of normal cells. The spleen in either case shows splenic cords expanded by the cells that are being destroyed, and increased numbers of cordal macrophages. In immune hemolytic anemia, the antibody-coated red blood cells are sequestered and destroyed within splenic cords (Sokol et al., 1992). A similar mechanism is responsible for hypersplenism related to immune thrombocytopenia, as well as for some cases of immune-related neutropenia (Laszlo et al., 1978). Any process that diffusely or extensively involves the spleen, resulting in expansion or abnormality of the cords, may result in increased destruction, including connective tissue (fibrocongestive splenomegaly), macrophages (Gaucher's or other storage diseases), neoplastic infiltrative processes (leukemia, lymphomas), or primary splenic lesions, such as hemangioma, hematoma, and angiosarcoma (Rappaport, 1970; see also Chapters 8, 9, and 12 for discussion).

6.4.6.2. Congenital Hemolytic Disorders In hereditary spherocytosis, the spleen is enlarged, with a thin, tense capsule and few adhesions. The cut surface is dark-red and firm. The malpighian corpuscles are not prominent, but may still be visible as small white specks. Microscopically, the white pulp is intact, but dispersed by the widened red pulp. There is marked congestion of Billroth's cords (cordal sequestration), with an increase in reticulum fibers. The red pulp sinuses are patent, and appear empty. Overt phagocytosis of red blood cells is usually not a prominent

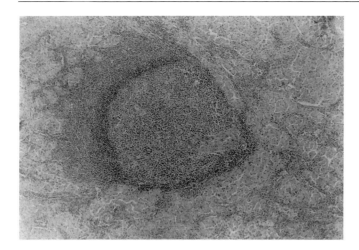

Fig. 6.16. Advanced activated immune response. Note the polarized germinal center characteristic of a reactive germinal center. The spleen is from a patient with Gaucher's disease.

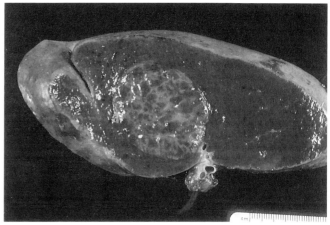

Color plate 14. Spleen with myeloid metaplasia. The cut surface is red and firm, with indistinct white pulp. The circumscribed bulging nodule in the center showed microscopic features of a hamartoma, also with myeloid metaplasia.

feature, but hemosiderin deposits are present (Chapter 7). Spherocytes can be easily identified on H&E-stained sections. In a related condition, hereditary elliptocyosis, the splenic changes are similar. This pattern also holds true for the hemoglobinopathies, although, in thalassemia, evidence of perisplenitis may be found. In early sickle cell disease with splenomegaly, the spleen is noted to be more spherical, and the cut surface is dark red and dry; the malpighian corpuscles are not prominent. Blaustein (1963) also comments that sickle-cell-trait spleens from severely hypoxic patients may undergo massive necrosis and hemorrhage, so that they may resemble, grossly, a "bag of blood."

6.4.6.3. Immune Hyperfunction In immune hyperfunction, splenic enlargement is generally uncommon, and the prominence of the white pulp is more evident microscopically than grossly. The white pulp tends to go through stages of morphologic change during prolonged stimulation. Unstimulated white pulp is composed of small lymphoid aggregates around the arterioles. Early in the course of stimulation, the lymphocytes undergo transformation, and immunoblasts are seen. In the second stage, active germinal center formation, with mantle zones, and intermixed plasma cells, become evident. The lymphoid follicles with active germinal centers gradually enlarge and show the same changes as in lymph nodes with reactive follicular hyperplasia, often demonstrating a "starry sky" pattern secondary to tingible body macrophages scattered among the transforming lymphoid cells (Fig. 16). The immune system reaches a height of activity, then starts to decline; at this time, there is lymphoid depletion, with an increase in epithelioid histiocytes and acellular hyaline deposits.

6.4.6.4. Extramedullary Hematopoiesis (Myeloid Metaplasia) With the exception of the proliferation of lymphocytes in the stimulated spleen, the adult human spleen does not normally play an active role in hematopoiesis. However, it is an appropriate environment for extramedullary hematopoiesis in pathologic conditions. This is particularly evident in so-called "agnogenic (primary) myeloid metaplasia," which is discussed in detail in Chapter 14. In this condition, extreme splenomegaly can occur. The capsular surface is smooth and shiny, except for those areas that overlie infarcts. The cut surface is generally dark red-brown and firm (Color plate 14), unless the organ is heavily infiltrated with leukocytes, in which

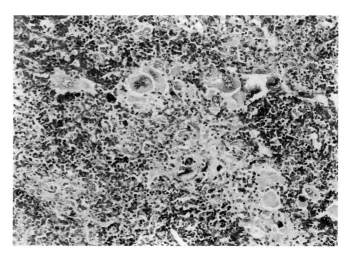

Fig. 6.17. Extramedullary hematopoiesis (myeloid metaplasia). Notice the large numbers of megakaryocytic precursors.

case it is pale red. The malpighian corpuscles are indistinct and dispersed. Microscopically, the hematopoietic precursors are evident, initially, predominantly in the sinuses, but later in the cords of Billroth. The erythroid precursors are easily detected, because of their darkly staining round nuclei, and some observers have proposed that these cells predominate in the sinuses and that myeloid precursors locate to the cords. Scattered megakaryocytic precursors are also present, often in prominent numbers (Fig. 17). Various splenic cells show reactive changes, and macrophages are usually prominent and contain cellular debris. These cells are particularly prominent with special stains or by electron microscopy (Tavassoli and Weiss, 1973). The reticular structure of the spleen remains intact. Prior therapy may alter the splenic pathology.

Extramedullary hematopoiesis (myeloid metaplasia) in the spleen occurs in a variety of other pathologic states, including idiopathic myelofibrosis (Wolf and Neiman, 1985; Color plate 15A,B), metastatic carcinoma (O'Keane et al., 1989), and following administration of cytokines, such as G-CSF (Vasef et al., 1998).

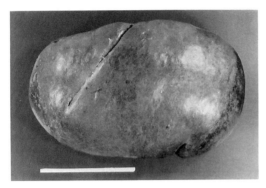
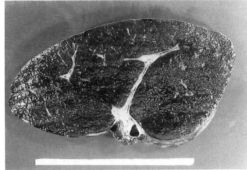

Color plate 15. Spleen in idiopathic myelofibrosis. The patient had a long-standing history of myelofibrosis. The spleen weighed 5.5 kg, and had a very firm cut surface. (**A**) External surface showing subcapsular hemorrhages; (**B**) gross appearance of splenic cut surface.

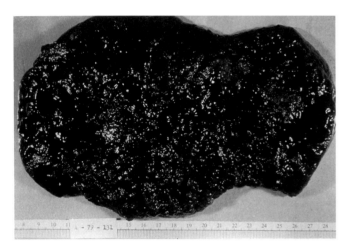

Fig. 6.18. Acute splenitis. The soft splenic parenchyma spills over the edge of the capsule.

Because there is no documentation of a splenic role in normal hematopoiesis in the adult human, it is thought that the hematopoietic precursor cells found in a variety of pathologic states originate from the bone marrow (Neiman and Orazi, 1999). The circulating precursor cells are presumably released into the peripheral blood, then are filtered by the spleen. Splenic extramedullary hematopoiesis is a common finding in patients with bone marrow transplantation who have received CD34-positive stem cells by intravenous infusion (Arnold et al., 1985). Similarly, stimulation of the bone marrow by cytokines, and subsequent release of stem cells into peripheral blood, appears to be the underlying mechanism of splenic extramedullary hematopoiesis following administration of these agents (Siena et al., 1989).

6.4.6.5. Infectious Processes The enlarged spleen of acute splenitis has been familiar to physicians for centuries. Acute splenitis presents as a large, soft, diffluent spleen with a thinly stretched capsule (Fig. 18). The cut surface is grey-pink, and may bulge above the capsule. The pulp scrapes away easily, leaving the trabeculae visible, or it may ooze from the cut surface. The white pulp is not discernible, grossly, but, microscopically, it shows varying degrees of hyperplasia. The macrophages of the red pulp show active phagocytosis. Neutrophils and eosinophils may be seen in the sinuses; with prolonged infections, plasma cells are also found.

The spectrum of these nonspecific changes in children is described by Gadaleanu (1981) in 221 spleens from children with bronchopulmonary inflammatory diseases. A generalized hyperplasia of lymphoid follicles and periarteriolar lymphocytes, and increased numbers of plasma cells in the red pulp were noted in about one-third of the cases. The germinal centers were composed of a mixture of transformed lymphoid cells (immunoblasts) and tingible body macrophages cuffed by smaller lymphocytes. In most cases, the hyperplasia was focal and moderate. In about 20% of the cases, lymphoid depletion was found, usually relating to a more severe or longer clinical course.

Some infectious agents produce more distinctive changes, as observed by Blaustein (1963). Streptococcal infections may produce a grey coloration and a soft spleen. *Clostridium welchii* produces proliferation of the reticuloendothelial (RE) cells in the cords, so that the sinuses appear empty and the malpighian corpuscles spread apart. In brucellosis, the RE cells become enlarged and form a sarcoid-like reaction in the red pulp. In spirochetal diseases, there is a spectrum of changes. Congenital syphilis produces a large, red, hyperemic spleen, with fibrosis and infiltration of macrophages and plasma cells. Plasma cells are also prominent in secondary syphilis, together with hyperplasia of the white pulp. Gummas can be seen in tertiary syphilis. In louse-borne relapsing fever, the large, firm spleen shows multiple grey foci on the cut surface, which represent microabscesses in the white pulp (Judge et al., 1974). In Lyme disease, red pulp hyperplasia and spirochetes are seen (Cimmino et al., 1988). Viral diseases, such as infectious mononucleosis, can also produce areas of necrosis, as well as marked hyperplasia of the white pulp. The immunoblastic reaction can involve the red pulp as well, and can produce cells similar to Reed-Sternberg cells. Such changes may be marked enough to raise the question of lymphoma, particularly Hodgkin's lymphoma. These features may also be seen in brucellosis.

Tuberculosis is often less active in producing a reaction with enlargement, compared with the diseases already discussed, but granulomas are evident as yellow-to-white, irregular, nodular areas on the cut surface. Granulomas are found in other infectious diseases, and are also associated with neoplastic conditions, such as Hodgkin's disease. Kuo and Rosai (1974), however, were able to demonstrate tuberculosis or a fungal disease in only 3/20 cases with granulomatous inflammation.

In drug addicts, a variety of splenic changes have been described (Kringsholm and Christoffersen, 1984). Spleen weight increases with the duration of drug addiction. A distinctive microscopic feature is the presence of refractile or birefringent material found in the histiocytes near the central arterioles, the frequency of which increases with the chronicity of drug use. As in other reactive conditions, germinal centers are prominent.

6.4.6.6. Idiopathic Tropical Splenomegaly Idiopathic tropical splenomegaly syndrome (TSS) is characterized by significant splenomegaly, hepatomegaly, elevated erythrocyte sedimentation rate, elevation of serum IgM, and often the presence of antibodies to malarial parasites. Patients with TSS are in areas endemic for malaria, but clearly, there are several etiologies, often related to the geographical area, and not all cases of TSS have malaria. The spleen often weighs 4000 g or more, and the capsule is thin and smooth (Geary et al., 1980). The cut surface is firm and red, although malaria, when present, may produce a dark-brown color in the acute stage, because of malarial pigment. In TSS, the sinuses are dilated and filled with histiocytes, which show phagocytic activity. In various endemic forms in different countries, there may be different or additional findings. Lowenthal et al. (1980) report that TSS in northern Zambia showed marked red blood cell sequestration, and plasma cells or plasmacytoid lymphocytes in the intersinusoidal tissue of the spleen.

In chronic malaria, the spleen has a thick, grey-white capsule, and the cut surface is firm and grey-black. Microscopically, fibrosis and pigment deposition replace the reactive lymphoid hyperplasia seen in the early stages. Also, in early disease, the parasites may be visibly occluding arterioles. Recent studies have shown that the γ/δ T-cell subset plays a significant role in cell-mediated immunity against malaria (Nakazawa et al., 1994).

6.4.6.7. Autoimmune Disorders In autoimmune hemolytic anemia of warm antibody type, the spleen is generally enlarged, with a smooth capsule showing focal thickening. The cut surface is smooth and red, and the malpighian corpuscles are dispersed. Microscopically, the white pulp shows reactive lymphoid hyperplasia and, often, prominent marginal zones. The splenic cords are congested with red blood cells, and scattered lymphocytes, and hemosiderin-laden macrophages are present. Erythrophagocytosis is often seen, and occasionally extramedullary hematopoiesis is found.

In rheumatoid arthritis (RA) complicated by neutropenia (Felty syndrome), the enlarged hyperactive spleen may play a role in inducing neutropenia; however, several other mechanisms have also been claimed to be involved, such as decreased neutrophil production (Gupta et al., 1975). The spleen may be enlarged in uncomplicated RA, because of increased lymphoid tissue with prominent follicular hyperplasia. The arterioles within the follicles may show hyaline thickening of their walls, with swelling of the endothelial cells. Amyloidosis, particularly in the vessel walls, may occur. The systemic vasculitis found in severe active rheumatoid disease can involve the spleen, as well.

Vasculitis involving the spleen can also be found in patients with periarteritis nodosum (PAN) and systemic lupus erythematosus (SLE). In PAN, the larger vessels tend to be involved; in SLE, chiefly the arterioles are affected. The characteristic "onion-skin" lesion of SLE may be the healed stage of a vasculitis involving the smaller arterial vessels. This change may be very prominent, and may lead to obliteration of the follicular structures.

6.4.7. MISCELLANEOUS LESIONS
6.4.7.1. Rupture of the Spleen Rupture of the spleen can occur regardless of the size or functional status of the organ. Although the most frequent cause of rupture is trauma (Color plate 16), rupture may also occur spontaneously (nontraumatic rupture) in many diseases. Massad et al. (1988) have summarized the various causes

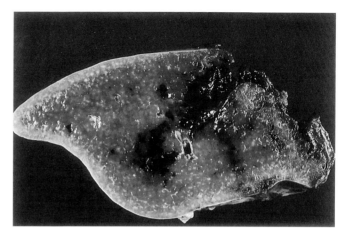

Color plate 16. Splenic rupture, traumatic. The cut surface illustrates inadequate fixation, because the specimen was left in formalin overnight, without prior slicing.

Table 6.3
Disorders Associated
With Spontaneous Rupture of the Spleen

Hematological disorders
    Hemoglobin C disease, Hodgkin's disease, polycythemia vera, hemolytic anemias, hereditary ovalocytosis
Malignant tumors
    Leukemias, hemangiosarcoma, metastatic hepatoma
Infections
    Infectious mononucleosis, malaria, infective endocarditis, chickenpox mumps, hepatitis A, influenza, aspergillosis
Inflammatory disorders
    Crohn's disease, chronic pancreatitis
Connective tissue disorders
    Systemic lupus erythematosus, rheumatoid disease
Miscellaneous
    Sarcoidosis, portal hypertension, amyloidosis, pregnancy, acquired immunodeficiency syndrome

Adapted with permission from Massad et al. (1988).

of splenic rupture, which include hematologic disorders, malignant tumors, inflammatory diseases, infections, and connective tissue diseases (Table 3). Infectious diseases are among the more common causes. In a spleen infected by Epstein-Barr virus (infectious mononucleosis), the inflammatory process involves and compromises the integrity of the capsule, making the acutely enlarged spleen prone to rupture. The same process probably underlies the fragility of the spleen in many other disorders, including AIDS (Mirchandani et al., 1985). Splenic rupture has also been reported following mumps infection. A recent review reports 10 cases of rupture in splenic amyloidosis (Kozicky et al., 1987). A rare cause of rupture of an unenlarged spleen is thrombolytic agents. Wiener and Ong (1989) described a ruptured spleen weighing only 76 g, which led to hemoperitoneum and death, in a patient treated with streptokinase for myocardial infarction.

Although patients with splenic rupture usually present with an acute abdomen and/or shock, in some cases, significant delays have been reported before medical attention is obtained (Prager et al., 1971). These patients may present with a palpable mass. A

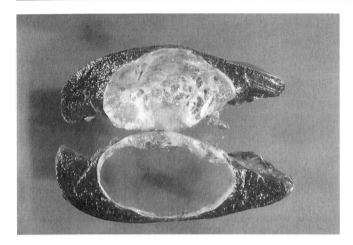

Color plate 17. Epidermoid cyst. This primary splenic cyst was unilocular and lined by a stratified squamous epithelium.

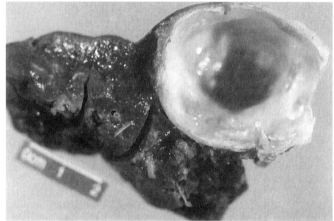

Color plate 18. Splenic pseudocyst. This type of cyst does not have any gross or microscopically identifiable lining. In this example, the wall of the cyst was entirely calcified.

subcapsular hematoma or free hemorrhage in the peritoneal cavity may be found. The hematoma may have developed a reactive capsule. Therefore, this lesion should be considered in the differential diagnosis of a hemorrhagic mass.

6.4.7.2. Abscess   Like other lymphoid organs, the spleen is an uncommon site for abscess formation. Chulay and Lankerani (1976) found only 10 cases of splenic abscess in 10 years in a busy hospital. Pain, fever, and left-upper-quadrant tenderness are among the presenting symptoms. With newer radiologic techniques, the diagnosis can be made antemortem more frequently than a decade ago (Lawhorne and Zuidema, 1976). Three basic pathophysiologic conditions for abscess formation have been proposed: The protective capacity of the spleen may be overwhelmed; internal damage may have occurred; or there may have been extension from adjacent sites of infection. In the first category are cases secondary to infective endocarditis, sepsis, or a depressed immune system. Internal damage may be either trauma, hematoma formation, or infarction (Epstein and Omar, 1983). Least common is the third, in which external infection penetrates into the spleen. Not all cases are caused by infection, because vasculitides and sterile inflammatory reactive conditions can lead to abscess formation.

6.4.7.3. Cysts   Splenic cysts are rare, and are divided into primary and secondary types (Dawes and Malangoni, 1986). The primary forms include those with epithelial (or mesothelial) lining (Color plate 17) and those associated with parasites (parasitic cysts), e. g., Echinococcus. The secondary form is the pseudocyst (Color plate 18), also called "traumatic cyst," which presumably results from the resolution of hematoma following trauma (Garvin and King, 1981). The wall of the pseudocyst has no distinct lining on gross or microscopic examination, and the inner surface is usually shaggy, with attached fibrin. The surrounding fibrous wall contains hemosiderin or calcium deposits. Pseudocysts tend to occur in younger individuals. There is a male predominance, with the mean age at diagnosis in the range of 28 to 33 yr. 75% of patients complain of either an abdominal mass or pain. Cysts may become infected, with an inflammatory response in the surrounding pulp or capsule (Didlake and Miller, 1986).

6.4.7.4. Capsular Changes   As described by Baillie (1793), the splenic capsule occasionally shows fibrosis in the form of a diffuse thickening or a fibrous plaque formation. Adhesions may be seen

if an inflammatory process has been present. Wanless and Bernier (1983) have reviewed the changes in the capsule. The thickening of the capsule is more evident with advancing age. Increase in splenic vein pressure, as the result of congestive heart failure or intrahepatic fibrosis, may be a contributory factor. Histologically, the thickening is usually dense hyaline acellular fibrous tissue superficial to the elastica of the capsule. In some cases, bands of collagen extended internally. Hemosiderin deposits are often present, as well as small blood vessels, particularly in early lesions.

REFERENCES

Ambrosino, D. M., Siber, G. R., Chilmonczyk, B. A., Jernberg, J. B., and Finberg, R. W. (1987) An immunodeficiency characterized by impaired antibody responses to polysaccharides. *N. Engl. J. Med.* **316**, 790–793.

Amorosi, E. L. (1965) Hypersplenism. *Semin. Hematol.* **2**, 249–285.

Applegate, K. E., Goske, M. J., Pierce, G., and Murphy, D. (1999) Situs revisited: imaging of the heterotaxy syndrome. *Radiographics* **19**, 837–852.

Arber, D. A., Rappaport, H., and Weiss, L. M. (1997) Non-Hodgkin's lymphoproliferative disorders involving the spleen. *Mod. Pathol.* **10**, 18–32.

Arber, D. A., Strickler, J. G., Chen, Y. Y., and Weiss, L. M. (1997) Splenic vascular tumors: a histologic, immunophenotypic, and virologic study. *Am. J. Surg. Pathol.* **21**, 827–835.

Arnold, R., Calvo, W., Heymer, B., Schmeiser, T., Heimpel, H., and Kubanek, B. (1985) Extramedullary haemopoiesis after bone marrow transplantation. *Scand. J. Haematol.* **34**, 9–12.

Audouin, J., Diebold, J., Schwartz, H., Le Tourneau, A., Bernadou, A., and Zittoun, R. (1988) Malignant lymphoplasmacytic lymphoma with prominent splenomegaly (primary lymphoma of the spleen). *J. Pathol.* **155**, 17–33.

Baillie, M. (1793) *The Morbid Anatomy of Some of the Most Important Parts of the Human Body* (Johnson, J. and Nicol, G., eds.). London.

Barbashina, V., Heller, D. S., Hameed, M., et al. (2000) Splenic smooth-muscle tumors in children with acquired immunodeficiency syndrome: report of two cases of this unusual location with evidence of an association with Epstein-Barr virus. *Virchows Arch.* **436**, 138–139.

Bartman, J., van de Velde, R. L., and Friedman, F. (1967) Pigmented lipid histiocytosis and susceptibility to infection: ultrastructure of splenic histiocytes. *Pediatrics* **40**, 1000–1002.

Bearman, R. M., Pangales, G. A., and Rappaport, H. (1978) Prolymphocytic leukemia. Clinical, histopathological, and cytochemical observations. *Cancer* **42**, 2360–2372.

Bender, B. L. and Yunis, E. J. (1982) The pathology of tuberous sclerosis. *Pathol. Ann.* **17,** 339–382.

Bennett, J. M., Catovsky, D., Daniel, M. T., Flandrin, G., Galton, D. A., Gralnick, H. R., and Sultan, C. (1985) Proposed revised criteria for the classification of acute myeloid leukemia. A report of the French-American-British Cooperative Group. *Ann. Intern. Med.* **103,** 620–625.

Berendt, H. L., Mant, M. J., and Jewell, L. D. (1986) Periarterial fibrosis in the spleen in idiopathic thrombocytopenic purpura. *Arch. Pathol. Lab. Med.* **110,** 1152–1154.

Binet, J. L., Lepoprier, M., Dighiero, G., Charron, D., D'Athis, P., Vaugier, G., et al. (1977) Clinical staging system for chronic lymphocytic leukemia: prognostic significance. *Cancer* **40,** 855–864.

Bishop, M. B. and Lansing, L. S. (1982) The spleen: a correlative overview of normal and pathologic anatomy. *Hum. Pathol.* **13,** 334–342.

Blaustein, A. (1963) *The Spleen.* McGraw-Hill, New York.

Bleiweiss, I. J., Thung, S. N., and Goodman, J. D. (1986) Peliosis of the spleen in a patient with cirrhosis of the liver. *Arch. Pathol. Lab. Med.* **110,** 669–671.

Blendis, L. M., Williams, R., and Kreel, L. (1969) Radiological determination of spleen size. *Gut* **10,** 433–435.

Bowdler, A. J. (1976) Role of the spleen and splenectomy in autoimmune hemolytic disease. *Sem. Hematol.* **13,** 335–348.

Bowdler, A. J. (1983) Splenomegaly and hypersplenism. *Clin. Haematol.* **12,** 467–488.

Boyd, E. (1933) Normal variability in weight of the adult liver and spleen. *Arch. Pathol.* **16,** 350–372.

Brox, A., Bishinsky, J. I., and Berry, G. (1991) Primary non-Hodgkin lymphoma of the spleen. *Am. J. Hematol.* **38,** 95–100.

Brunning, R. D. and Parkin, J. (1975) Ribosome-lamella complexes in neoplastic hematopoietic cells. *Am. J. Pathol.* **79,** 565–578.

Burke, J. S., Byrne, G. E. Jr., and Rappaport, H. (1974) Hairy cell leukemia (leukemic reticuloendotheliosis). I. A clinical pathologic study of 21 patients. *Cancer* **33,** 1399–1410.

Burke, J. S. and Osborne, B. M. (1983) Localized reactive lymphoid hyperplasia of the spleen simulating malignant lymphoma. A report of seven cases. *Am. J. Surg. Pathol.* **4,** 373–380.

Carr, A. J., Jacob, G., Glanfield, P. A., and Rogers, K. (1987) Male chorio-carcinoma of the spleen: a case report. *Eur. J. Surg. Oncol.* **13,** 75–76.

Catovsky, D., Galetto, J., Okos, A., Galton, D. A., Wiltshaw, E., and Stathopoulos, G. (1973) Prolymphocytic leukaemia of B and T cell type. *Lancet* **2,** 232–234.

Catovsky, D., Greaves, M. F., Rose, M., Galton, D. A., Goolden, A. W., McCluskey, D. R., et al. (1982) Adult T-cell lymphoma-leukaemia in Blacks from the West Indies. *Lancet* **1,** 639–643.

Chan, W. C., Link, S., Mawle, A., Check, I., Brynes, R. K., and Winton, E. F. (1986) Heterogeneity of large granular lymphocyte proliferations: delineation of two major subtypes. *Blood* **68,** 1142–1153.

Chandra, P., Rosner, F., and Sawitsky, A. (1973) Sea-blue histiocytes in thrombocytopenic purpura. *Ann. Intern. Med.* **79,** 901–902.

Chen, K. T. and Felix, E. L. (1986) Splenic peliosis. *Arch. Pathol. Lab. Med.* **110,** 1122.

Chen, K. T., Flam, M. S., and Workman, R. D. (1987) Amyloid tumor of the spleen. *Am. J. Surg. Pathol.* **11,** 723–725.

Chen Y.-T. and Burchell, A. (1995) Glycogen storage diseases. In: *The Metabolic and Molecular Bases of Inherited Disease,* 7th ed., vol. 1 (Scriver, C. R., Beaudet, A. L., Sly, W. S., and Valle, D., eds.), McGraw-Hill, New York, pp. 935–965.

Christensen, B. E. (1971) Effects of an enlarged splenic erythrocyte pool in chronic lymphocytic leukemia: mechanisms of erythrocyte sequestration in the spleen and liver. *Scand. J. Haematol.* **8,** 92–103.

Christensen, B. E. (1973) Pathophysiology of the "hypersplenism syndrome." Remarks about definition and estimation of the splenic erythrocyte pool. *Scand. J. Haematol.* **11,** 5–7.

Christensen, B. E., Jonsson, V., and Matre, R. (1978) Traffic of T and B lymphocytes in the normal spleen. *Scand. J. Haematol.* **20,** 246–257.

Chulay, J. D. and Lankerani, M. R. (1976) Splenic abscess. Report of 10 cases and review of the literature. *Am. J. Med.* **61,** 513–522.

Cimmino, M. A., Azzolini, A., Tobia, F., and Pesce, C. M. (1989) Spirochetes in the spleen of a patient with chronic Lyme disease. *Am. J. Clin. Pathol.* **91,** 95–97.

Crosby W. H. (1962) Hypersplenism. *Ann. Rev. Med.* **13,** 127–146.

Crosby, W. H. (1957) Siderocytes and the spleen. *Blood* **12,** 165–170.

Cruickshank, B. (1984) Follicular (mineral oil) lipidosis: I. Epidemiologic studies of involvement of the spleen. *Hum. Pathol.* **15,** 724–730.

Cruickshank, B. and Thomas, M. J. (1984) Mineral oil (follicular) lipidosis: II. Histologic studies of spleen, liver, lymph nodes, and bone marrow. *Hum. Pathol.* **15,** 731–737.

Dacie, J. V., Galton, D. A. G., Gordon-Smith, E. C., and Harrison, C. V. (1978) Non-tropical "idiopathic splenomegaly": a follow-up study of ten patients described in 1969. *Br. J. Haematol.* **38,** 185–193.

Dameshek, W. (1955) Hypersplenism. *Bull. NY Acad. Med.* **31,** 113.

Das Gupta, T., Coombes, B., and Brasfeld, R. D. (1965) Primary malignant neoplasms of the spleen. *Surg. Gynecol. Obstet.* **120,** 947–960.

Dawes, L. G. and Malangoni, M. A. (1986) Cystic masses of the spleen. *Am. Surg.* **52,** 333–336.

Dear, T. N., Colledge, W. H., Carlton, M. B., Lavenir, I., Larson, T., Smith, A. J., et al. (1995) Hox11 gene is essential for cell survival during spleen development. *Development* **121,** 2909–2915.

DeLand, F. H. (1970) Normal spleen size. *Radiology* **97,** 589–592.

De Odorico, I., Spaulding, K. A., Pretorius, D. H., Lev-Toaff, A. S., Bailey, T. B., and Nelson, T. R. (1999) Normal splenic volumes estimated using three-dimensional ultrasonography. *J. Ultrasound Med.* **18,** 231–236.

Desnick, R. J. and Bishop, D. F. (1989) Fabry disease: α-galactosidase deficiency; Schindler disease: α-N-acetylgalactosaminidase deficiency. In: *The Metabolic Basis of Inherited Disease,* 6th ed. (Scriver, C. R., Beaudet, A. L., Sly, W. S., and Valle, D., eds.), McGraw-Hill, New York, pp. 1751–1796.

de Vries, M. J., Dooren, L. J., and Cleton, F. J. (1968) Graft-versus-host or autoimmune lesions in the Swiss type of agammaglobulinemia: their relation to a deficient development of the thymic epithelium. In: *Immunologic Deficiency Diseases in Man* (Bergsma, D., ed.), The National Foundation, New York, pp. 173–187.

Dhodapkar, M. V., Li, C. Y., Lust, J. A., Tefferi, A., and Phyliky, R. L. (1994) Clinical spectrum of clonal proliferations of T-large granular lymphocytes: a T-cell clonopathy of undetermined significance? *Blood* **84,** 1620–1627.

Didlake, R. H. and Miller, R. C. (1986) Epidermoid cyst of the spleen manifested as an abdominal abscess. *South. Med. J.* **79,** 635–637.

Doan, C. A. and Wright, C. S. (1946) Primary congenital and secondary acquired splenic panhematopenia. *Blood* **1,** 10–26.

Dosik, H., Rosner, F., and Sawitsky, A. (1972) Acquired lipidosis: Gaucher-like cells and "blue cells" in chronic granulocytic leukemia. *Semin. Hematol.* **9,** 309–316.

Dumontel, C., Girod, C., Dijoud, F., Dumez, Y., and Vanier, M. T. (1993) Fetal Niemann-Pick disease type C: ultrastructural and lipid findings in liver and spleen. *Virchows Arch. A Pathol. Anat. Histopathol.* **422,** 253–259.

Easler, R. E. and Dowlin, W. M. (1969) Primary lipoma of the spleen: a case report. *Arch. Pathol.* **88,** 557–559.

Edelstein, A. D., Miller, A., Zimelman, A. P., Rocklin, R. E., and Neiman, R. S. (1978) Adult severe combined immunodeficiency and sarcoidlike granulomas with hypersplenism. *Am. J. Hematol.* **5,** 55–62.

Elit, L. and Aylward, B. (1989) Splenic cyst carcinoma presenting in pregnancy. *Am. J. Hematol.* **32,** 57–60.

Elleder, M. (1989) Niemann-Pick disease. *Pathol. Res. Pract.* **185,** 293–328.

Ellison, R. B. (1980) Radiologic Seminar CCI. Cystic lymphangioma: a consideration in asymptomatic, massive, cystic splenomegaly. *J. Miss. State Med. Assoc.* **21,** 67–68.

Epstein, B. M. and Omar, G. M. (1983) Infective complications of splenic trauma. *Clin. Radiol.* **34,** 91–94.

Falk, S., Krishnan, J., and Meis, J. M. (1993) Primary angiosarcoma of the spleen: a clinicopathologic study of 40 cases. *Am. J. Surg. Pathol.* **17,** 959–970.

Falk, S. and Stutte, H. J. (1990) Primary malignant lymphomas of the spleen, a morphological and immunohistochemical analysis of 17 cases. *Cancer* **66,** 2612–2619.

Falk, S., Stutte, H. J., and Frizzera, G. (1991) Littoral cell angioma, a novel splenic lesion demonstrating histiocytic differentiation. *Am. J. Surg. Pathol.* **15,** 1023–1033.

Farcet, J.-P., Gaulard, P., Marolleau, J.-P., Le Couedic, J.-P., Henni, T., Gourdin, M.-F., et al. (1990) Hepatosplenic T-cell lymphoma: sinusal/sinusoidal localization of malignant cells expressing the T-cell receptor γ/δ. *Blood* **75**, 2213–2219.

Ferlicot, S., Emile, J. F., Le Bris, J. L., Cheron, G., and Brousse, N. (1997) Congenital asplenia. A childhood immune deficit often detected too late. *Ann. Pathol.* **17**, 44–46.

Fleming, C. R., Dickson, E. R., and Harrison, E. G. (1976) Splenosis: autotransplantation of splenic tissue. *Am. J. Med.* **61**, 414–419.

Flood, M. J. and Carpenter, R. A. (1961) Spontaneous rupture of the spleen in acute myeloid leukemia. *Br. Med. J.* **1**, 35–36.

Foroudi, F., Ahern, V., and Peduto, A. (1999) Splenosis mimicking metastases from breast carcinoma. *Clin. Oncol. (R. Coll. Radiol.)* **11**, 190–192.

Freeman, S. B., Muralidharan, K., Pettay, D., Blackston, R. D., and May, K. M. (1996) Asplenia syndrome in a child with balanced reciprocal translocation of chromosomes 11 and 20 [46,XX,t(11;20)(q13.1;q13.13)]. *Am. J. Med. Genet.* **61**, 340–344.

Gadaleanu, G. (1981) Spleen immunomorphologic behavior in primary and secondary acute bronchopulmonary inflammations of children. Comparative analysis of the lung and hilar tracheobronchial lymph node reactions. *Morphol. Embryol.* **27**, 219–225.

Garcia, R. L., Khan, M. K., and Berlin, R. B. (1982) Peliosis of the spleen with rupture. *Hum. Pathol.* **13**, 177–179.

Garvin, D. F. and King, F. M. (1981) Cysts and nonlymphomatous tumors of the spleen. *Pathol. Ann.* **16**, 61–80.

Geary, C. G., Clough, V., and MacIver, J. E. (1980) Tropical splenomegaly. *Br. J. Hosp. Med.* **24**, 419–421.

Gentile, T, C., Uner, A. H., Hutchison, R. E., et al. (1994) CD3+, CD56+ aggressive variant of large granular lymphocyte leukemia. *Blood* **84**, 2315–2321.

Gertz, M. A., Kyle, R. A., and Greipp, P. R. (1983) Hyposplenism in primary systemic amyloidosis. *Ann. Intern. Med.* **98**, 475–477.

Gilks, G. B., Acker, B. D., and Clement, P. B. (1989) Recurrent endometrial adenocarcinoma: presentation as a splenic mass mimicking malignant lymphoma. *Gynecol. Oncol.* **33**, 209–211.

Glew, R. H., Basu, A., Prence, E. M., and Remaley, A. T. (1985) Lysosomal storage diseases. *Lab. Invest.* **53**, 250–269.

Gonzalez-Lopez, A., Fernandez-Martin, J. I., Gordillo, I., and Dronda, F. (1996) Disseminated Kaposi's sarcoma with hepatosplenic involvement in AIDS. *Med. Clin. (Barc)* **106**, 622–623.

Govoni, E., Bazzochi, F., Pileri, S., and Martinelli, G. (1980) Primary malignant fibrous histiocytoma of the spleen: an ultra-structural study. *Histopathology* **6**, 351–361.

Grillot-Courvalin, C., Vinci, G., Tsapis, A., Dokhelar, M. C., Vainchenker, W., and Brouet, J. C. (1987) The syndrome of T8 hyperlymphocytosis: Variation in phenotype and cytotoxic activities of granular cells and evaluation of their role in associated neutropenia. *Blood* **69**, 1204–1210.

Grogan, T. M., Rangel, C. S., Richter, L. C., Wirt, D. P., and Villar, H. V. (1984) Further delineation of the immunoarchitecture of the human spleen. *Lymphology* **17**, 61–68.

Gupta, R., Robinson, W. A., and Albrecht, D. (1975) Granulopoietic activity in Felty's syndrome. *Ann. Rheum. Dis.* **34**, 156–161.

Guyton, J. R. and Zumwalt, R. E. (1975) Pneumococcemia with sarcoid-infiltrated spleen. *Ann. Intern. Med.* **82**, 847–848.

Haber, L. M., Hawkins, E. P., Seilheimer, D. K., and Saleem, A. (1988) Fat overload syndrome. An autopsy study with evaluation of the coagulopathy. *Am. J. Clin. Pathol.* **90**, 223–237.

Harris, N. (1985) Case Records of the Massachusetts General Hospital. Weekly clinicopathological exercises. Case 48-1985. A 69-year-old man with peripheral vascular disease and hypersplenism. *N. Engl. J. Med.* **313**, 1405–1412.

Hamoudi, A. B., Vassay, L. E., and Morse, T. S. (1975) Multiple lymphangioendotheliomata of the spleen in a 13-year-old girl. *Arch. Pathol.* **99**, 605–606.

Herman, T. E. (1999) Special imaging casebook. Neonate with osteogenesis imperfecta and asplenia syndrome with horseshoe adrenal. *J. Perinatol.* **19**, 543–545.

Hogan, S. F., Osborne, B. M., and Butler, J. J. (1989) Unexpected splenic nodules in leukemic patients. *Hum. Pathol.* **20**, 62–68.

Hou, J. W. and Wang, T. R. (1996) Amelia, dextrocardia, asplenia, and congenital short bowel in deleted ring chromosome 4. *J. Med. Genet.* **33**, 879–881.

Hsu, S. M., Cossman, J., and Jaffe, E. S. (1983) Lymphocyte subsets in normal human lymphoid tissues. *Am. J. Clin. Pathol.* **80**, 21–30.

Huber, J., Zegers, B. J., and Schuurman, H. J. (1992) Pathology of congenital immunodeficiencies. *Semin. Diagn. Pathol.* **9**, 31–62.

Iida, A., Emi, M., Matsuoka, R., Hiratsuka, E., Okui, K., Ohashi, H., et al. (2000) Identification of a gene disrupted by inv(11)(q13.5;q25) in a patient with left-right axis malformation. *Hum. Genet.* **106**, 277–287.

Iozzo, R. V., Haas, J. E., and Chard, R. L. (1980) Symptomatic splenic hamartoma: a report of two cases and review of the literature. *Pediatrics* **66**, 261–265.

Izumi, T., Sasaki, R., Miura, Y., and Okamoto, H. (1996) Primary hepatosplenic lymphoma: association with hepatitis C virus infection. *Blood* **87**, 5380–5381.

Izumi, T., Sasaki, R., Tsunoda, S., Akutsu, M., Okamoto, H., and Miura, Y. (1997) B cell malignancy and hepatitis C virus infection. *Leukemia* **3(Suppl)** 516–518.

Jacob, H. S. (1974) Hypersplenism: Mechanisms and management. *Br. J. Haematol.* **27**, 1–5.

Jadayel, D., Matutes, E., Dyer, M. J., Brito-Babapulle, V., Khohkar, M. T., Oscier, D., and Catovsky, D. (1994) Splenic lymphoma with villous lymphocytes: analysis of BCL-1 rearrangements and expression of the cyclin D1 gene. *Blood* **83**, 3664–3671.

Javier Penalver, F., Somolinos, N., Villanueva, C., Sanchez, J., Monteagudo, D., and Gallego, R. (1998) Splenic peliosis with spontaneous splenic rupture in a patient with immune thrombocytopenia treated with danazol. *Haematologica* **83**, 666–667.

Jorgensen, L. N. and Chrintz, H. (1988) Solitary metastatic endometrial carcinoma of the spleen. *Acta. Obstet. Gynecol. Scand.* **67**, 91–92.

Judge, D. M., Samuel, I., Perine, P. L., Vukotic, D., and Ababa, A. (1974) Louse-borne relapsing fever in man. *Arch. Pathol.* **97**, 136–140.

Kaden, B. R., Rosse, W. F., and Hauch, T. W. (1979) Immune thrombocytopenia in lymphoproliferative diseases. *Blood* **53**, 545–551.

Kadin, M. E., Kamoun, M., and Lamberg, J. (1981) Erythrophagocytic T-gamma lymphoma: a clinicopathologic entity resembling malignant histiocytosis. *N. Engl. J. Med.* **304**, 648–653.

Kagalwala, T. Y., Vaidya, V. U., Bharucha, B. A., Pandya, A. L., and Kumta, N. B. (1987) Cavernous hemangiomas of the liver and spleen. *Indian Pediatr.* **24**, 427–430.

Kanthan, R., Moyana, T., and Nyssen, J. (1999) Asplenia as a cause of sudden unexpected death in childhood. *Am. J. Forensic Med. Pathol.* **20**, 57–59.

Kayser, K. *Height and weight in human beings: autopsy report.* (1987) Verlag fuer angewante Wissenschaften, Munich.

Kevy, S. V., Tefft, M., Vawier, G. F., and Rosen, F. S. (1968) Hereditary splenic hypoplasia. *Pediatrics* **42**, 752–757.

Kim, H. and Dorfman, R. F. (1974) Morphological studies of 84 untreated patients subjected to laparatomy for the staging of non-Hodgkin's lymphomas. *Cancer* **33**, 657–674.

Kinoshita, K., Kamihira, S., Ikeda, S., Yamada, Y., Muta, T., Kitamura, T., Ichimaru, M., and Matsuo, T. (1982) Clinical, hematologic and pathologic features of leukemic T-cell lymphoma. *Cancer* **50**, 1554–1562.

Klatt, E. C. and Meyer, P. R. (1987) Pathology of the spleen in the acquired immunodeficiency syndrome. *Arch. Pathol. Lab. Med.* **111**, 1050–1053.

Klein, B., Stein, M., Kuten, A., Steiner, M., Barshalom, D., Robinson, E., and Gal, D. (1987) Splenomegaly and solitary spleen metastasis in solid tumors. *Cancer* **60**, 100–102.

Kozicky, O. J., Brandt, L. J., Lederman, M., and Milcu, M. (1987) Splenic amyloidosis: a case report of spontaneous splenic rupture with a review of the pertinent literature. *Am. J. Gastroenterol.* **82**, 582–587.

Kringsholm, B. and Christoffersen, P. (1984) Spleen and portal lymph node pathology in fatal drug addiction. *Forensic Sci. Int.* **25**, 233–244.

Kuo, T. and Rosai, J. (1974) Granulomatous inflammation in splenectomy specimens. *Arch. Pathol.* **98**, 261–268.

Lacson, A., Berman, L. D., and Neiman, R. S. (1979) Peliosis of the spleen. *Am. J. Clin. Pathol.* **71**, 586–590.

Lampert, I. A. (1983) Splenectomy as a diagnostic technique. *Clin. Haematol.* **12**, 535–563.

Laszlo, J., Jones, R., and Silberman, H. R. (1978) Splenectomy for Felty's syndrome: clinicopathologic study of 27 patients. *Arch. Intern. Med.* **138**, 597–602.

Lawhorne, T. W. Jr. and Zuidema, G. D. (1976) Splenic abscess. *Surgery* **79**, 686–689.

Lee, J. K., Tai, D. I., Chen, W. J., Sheen-Chen, S. M., Lee, T. Y., and Wan, Y. L. (1987) Splenic hamartoma; report of a case and review of the literature. *Taiwan I Hsueh Hui Tsa Chih [J. Formosan Med. Assoc.]* **86**, 1125–1128.

Lee, R. E., Peters, S. P., and Glew, R. H. (1977) Gaucher's disease: clinical, morphologic and pathogenic considerations. *Pathol. Ann.* **2**, 309–324.

Liber, A. F. and Rose, H. G. (1967) Saturated hydrocarbons in follicular lipidosis of the spleen. *Arch. Pathol.* **83**, 116–122.

Lough, J., Fawcett, L., and Weigensberg, B. (1970) Wolman's disease. *Arch. Pathol.* **89**, 103–110.

Loughran, T. P. Jr., Kadin, M. E., Starkebaum, G., Abkowitz, J. L., Clark, E. A., Disteche, C., Lum, L. G., and Slichter, S. J. (1985) Leukemia of large granular lymphocytes: association with clonal chromosomal abnormalities and autoimmune neutropenia, thrombocytopenia, and hemolytic anemia. *Ann. Intern. Med.* **102**, 169–175.

Lowenthal, M. N., Hutt, M. S., Jones, I. G., Mohelsky, V., and O'Riordan, E. C. (1980) Massive splenomegaly in northern Zambia. I. Analysis of 344 cases. *Trans. R. Soc. Trop. Med. Hyg.* **74**, 91–98.

Lukes, R. J. (1971) Criteria for involvement of lymph node, bone marrow, spleen, and liver in Hodgkin's disease. *Cancer Res.* **31**, 1755–1767.

Macpherson, A. I. S., Richmond, J., and Stuart, A. E. (1973) *The Spleen.* American Lecture Series, No. 893. Charles C Thomas, Springfield, IL.

Maggard, M. A., Goss, J. A., Swenson, K. L., McDiarmid, S. V., and Busuttil, R. W. (1999) Liver transplantation in polysplenia syndrome: use of a living-related donor. *Transplantation* **68**, 1206–1209.

Marymount, J. H. Jr. and Gross, S. (1963) Patterns of metastatic cancer in the spleen. *Am. J. Clin. Pathol.* **40**, 58–66.

Masci, P., Ciardi, A., Pozza, D., Alessi, A., and Nanni, E. (1985) Acute abdomen caused by rupture of the spleen due to an apparently primary squamous carcinomas [Italian]. *Ann. Ital. Chir.* **57**, 137–142.

Marymount, J. V. and Knight, P. J. (1987) Splenic lymphangiomatosis: a rare cause of splenomegaly. *J. Pediatr. Surg.* **5**, 461–462.

Massad, M., Murr, M., Razzouk, B., Nassourah, Z., Sankari, M., and Najjar, F. (1988) Spontaneous splenic rupture in an adult with mumps: a case report. *Surgery* **103**, 381–382.

Mathew, A., Raviglione, M. C., Niranjan, U., Sabatini, M. T., and Distenfeld, A. (1989) Splenectomy in patients with AIDS. *Am. J. Hematol.* **32**, 184–189.

McCormick, W. F. and Kashgarian, M. (1965) The weight of adult human spleen. *Am. J. Clin. Pathol.* **43**, 332–333.

McKenna, R. W., Parkin, J., Kersey, J. H., Gajl-Peczalska, K. J., Peterson, L., and Brunning, R. D. (1977) Chronic lymphoproliferative disorder with unusual clinical, morphologic, ultrastructural and membrane surface marker characteristics. *Am. J. Med.* **62**, 588–596.

McKinley, R. A., Kwan, Y. L., and Lam-Po-Tang, P. R. L. (1987) Familial splenomegaly syndrome with reduced circulating T helper cells and splenic germinal center hypoplasia. *Br. J. Haematol.* **67**, 393–396.

McMahon, R. F. T. (1988) Inflammatory pseudotumor of spleen. *J. Clin. Pathol.* **41**, 734–736.

McMillan, R., Longmire, R. L., Yelenosky, R., Donnell, R. L., and Armstrong, S. (1974) Quantitation of platelet binding IgG produced in vitro by spleens from patients with idiopathic thrombocytopenic purpura. *N. Engl. J. Med.* **291**, 812–817.

Melo, J. V., Hegde, U., Parreira, A., Thompson, I., Lampert, I. A., and Catovsky, D. (1987) Splenic B-cell lymphoma with circulating villous lymphocytes: differential diagnosis of B-cell leukaemias with large spleens. *J. Clin. Pathol.* **40**, 642–651.

Miale, J. B. (1971) Hemopoietic system: reticuloendothelium, spleen, lymph nodes, and bone marrow. In: *Pathology*, 6th ed. (Anderson, W. A. D., ed.), C.V. Mosby, St. Louis, pp. 1483–1574.

Mirchandani, H. G., Mirchandani, I. H., and Pak, M. S. Y. (1985) Spontaneous rupture of the spleen due to acquired immunodeficiency syndrome in an intravenous drug abuser. *Arch. Pathol. Lab. Med.* **109**, 1114–1116.

Mistry, P. K., Smith, S. J., Ali, M., Hatton, C. S., McIntyre, N., and Cox, T. M. (1992) Genetic diagnosis of Gaucher's disease. *Lancet* **339**, 889–892.

Molnar, Z. and Rappaport, H. (1972) Fine structure of the red pulp of the spleen in hereditary spherocytosis. *Blood* **39**, 81–98.

Morgenstern, L., McCafferty, L., Rosenberg, J., and Michel, S. L. (1984) Hamartomas of the spleen. *Arch. Surg.* **119**, 1291–1293.

Muehleck, S. D., McKenna, R. W., Arthur, D. C., Parkin, J. L., and Brunning, R. D. (1984) Transformation of chronic myelogenous leukemia: clinical, morphologic, and cytogenetic features. *Am. J. Clin. Pathol.* **82**, 1–14.

Mulligan, S. P., Matutes, E., Dearden, C., and Catovsky, D. (1991) Splenic lymphoma with villous lymphocytes: natural history and response to therapy in 50 cases. *Br. J. Haematol.* **78**, 206–209.

Murakami, Y., Hotei, H., Tsumura, H., et al. (1988) A case of primary splenic malignant lymphoma and a review of 98 cases reported in Japan. *J. Jpn. Soc. Clin. Surg.* **49**, 716–722.

Myers, J. and Segal, R. J. (1974) Weight of the spleen. I. Range of normal in a non-hospital population. *Arch. Pathol.* **98**, 33–35.

Naeim, F., Copper, P. H., and Semion, A. A. (1973) Peliosis hepatis. Possible etiologic role of anabolic steroids. *Arch. Pathol.* **95**, 284–285.

Nakazawa, S., Brown, A. E., Maeno, Y., Smith, C. D., and Aikawa, M. (1994) Malaria-induced increase of splenic gamma delta T cells in humans, monkeys, and mice. *Exp. Parasitol.* **79**, 391–398.

Nanba, K., Soban, E. J., Bowling, M. C., and Berard, C. W. (1977) Splenic pseudosinuses and hepatic angiomatous lesions. Distinctive features of hairy cell leukemia. *Am. J. Clin. Pathol.* **67**, 415–426.

Naschitz, J. E., Zuckerman, E., Elias, N., and Yeshurun, D. (1994) Primary hepatosplenic lymphoma of the B-cell variety in a patient with hepatitis C liver cirrhosis. *Am. J. Gastroenterol.* **89**, 1915–1916.

Neiman, R. S. (1980) Erythroblastic transformation in myeloproliferative disorders: confirmation by an immunohistologic technique. *Cancer* **46**, 1636–1640.

Neiman, R. S. and Orazi, A. (1999) Leukemias. In: *Disorders of the Spleen*, 2nd ed. Saunders, Philadelphia, pp. 192–214.

Neiman, R. S. (1977) Incidence and importance of splenic sarcoid-like granulomas. *Arch. Pathol. Lab. Med.* **101**, 518–521.

Neiman, R. S., Sullivan, A. L., and Jaffe, R. (1979) Malignant lymphoma simulating leukemic reticuloendotheliosis: a clinicopathologic study of ten cases. *Cancer* **43**, 329–342.

Nezelof, C., Jammet M.-L., Lortholary, P., Labrune, B., and Lamy, M. (1964) L'hypoplasie hereditaire du thymus: sa place et sa responsibilite dans une observation d' aplasie lymphocytaire normoplasmocytaire et normoglobulinemique du nourrisson. *Arch. Fr. Pediatr.* **21**, 897–920.

Nezelof, C. (1968) Thymic dysplasia with normal immunoglobulins and immunologic deficiency: *pure alymphocytosis*. In: *Immunologic Deficiency Diseases in Man* (Bergsma, D., ed.), Birth Defects Original Article Series, IV, No.1, The National Foundation, New York, pp. 104–115.

Niedt, G. W. and Schinella, R. (1985) Acquired immunodeficiency syndrome. *Arch. Pathol. Lab. Med.* **109**, 727–734.

Niv, Y., Abu-Avid, S., and Oren, M. (1986) Primary Hodgkin's disease of the spleen. *Am. J. Med.* **81**, 1120–1121.

O'Keane, J. C., Wolf, B. C., and Neiman, R. S. (1989) The pathogenesis of splenic extramedullary hematopoiesis in metastatic carcinoma. *Cancer* **63**, 1539–1543.

Parker, A. C., Bain, A. D., Brydon, W. G., Harkness, R. A., Smith, A. F., Smith, I. I., and Boyd, D. H. A. (1976) Sea-blue histiocytosis associated with hyperlipidemia. *J. Clin. Pathol.* **29**, 634–638.

Pentchev, P. G., Vanier, M. T., Suzuki, K., and Patterson, M. C. (1995) Niemann-Pick disease type C: A cellular cholesterol lipidosis. In:

The Metabolic Basis of Inherited Disease (Scriver, C. R., Beaudet, A. L., Sly, W. S., and Valle, D, eds.), McGraw-Hill, New York, pp. 2625–2639.

Peoples, W. M., Moller, J. H., and Edwards, J. E. (1983) Polysplenia: a review of 146 cases. *Pediatr. Cardiol.* **4,** 129–137.

Pistoia, F. and Markowitz, S. K. (1988) Splenic lymphangiomatosis: CT diagnosis. *Am. J. Roentgenol.* **150,** 121–122.

Prager, D., Morel, D., and Dex, W. (1971) The syndrome of chronic occult rupture of the spleen. *JAMA* **218,** 1824,1825.

Putschar, W. G. T. and Manion, W. C. (1956) Congenital absence of the spleen and associated anomalies. *Am. J. Clin. Pathol.* **26,** 429–470.

Raff, L. J. and Schwartz, S. T. (1983) Polysplenia complex and duodenal atresia. *Arch. Pathol. Lab. Med.* **107,** 202–203.

Raghavan, R., Alley, S., Tawfik, O., Webb, P., Forster, J., and Uhl, M. (1999) Splenic peleosis: a rare complication following liver transplantation. *Dig. Dis. Sci.* **44,** 1128–1131.

Rappaport, H. (1966) Tumors of the hematopoietic system. In: *Atlas of Tumor Pathology*, Armed Forces Institute of Pathology, Section III, Fascicle 8, pp. 357–388.

Rappaport, H. (1970) Pathologic anatomy of the splenic red pulp. In: *Die Milz* (Lennert, K. and Harms, D., eds.), Springer-Verlag, Berlin, pp. 24–43.

Razzouk, A. J., Gundry, S. R., Chinnock, R. E., Larsen, R. L., Ruiz, C., Zuppan, C. W., and Bailey, L. L. (1995) Orthotopic transplantation for total anomalous pulmonary venous connection associated with complex congenital heart disease. *J. Heart Lung Transplant.* **14,** 713–717.

Rege, J. D., Kavishwar, V. S., and Mopkar, P. S. (1998) Peliosis of spleen presenting as splenic rupture with haemoperitoneum: a case report. *Indian J. Pathol. Microbiol.* **41,** 465–467.

Reichert, C. M., O'Leary, T. J., Levens, D. L., Simrell, C. R., and Macher, A. M. (1983) Autopsy pathology in the acquired immune deficiency syndrome. *Am. J. Pathol.* **112,** 357–382.

Rickert, C. H., Maasjosthusmann, U., Probst-Cousin, S., August, C., and Gullotta, F. (1998) A unique case of cerebral spleen. *Am. J. Surg. Pathol.* **22,** 894–896.

Rifkind, R. A. (1965) Heinz body anemia: an ultrastructural study. II. Red cell sequestration and destruction. *Blood* **26,** 433–448.

Rosenberg, S. A. (1988) Exploratory laparatomy and splenectomy for Hodgkin's disease: a commentary. *J. Clin. Oncol.* **6,** 574–575.

Rousselet, M. C., Audouin, J., Le Tourneau, A., Bouchard, I., Espinoza, P., Kazatchkine, M., and Diebold, J. (1988) Idiopathic thrombocytopenic purpura in patients at risk for acquired immunodeficiency syndrome. Histopathologic study, immunohistochemistry, and ultrastructural study on six spleens. *Arch. Pathol. Lab. Med.* **112,** 1242–1250.

Ruck, P., Horny, H. P., Xiao, J. C., Baijinski, R., and Kaiserling, E. (1994) Diffuse sinusoidal hemangiomatosis of the spleen. A case report with enzyme-histochemical, immunohistochemical, and electron-microscopic findings. *Pathol. Res. Pract.* **190,** 708–714.

Ruscazio, M., Van Praagh, S., Marrass, A. R., et al. (1998) Interrupted inferior vena cava in asplenia syndrome and a review of the hereditary patterns of visceral situs abnormalities. *Am. J. Cardiol.* **81,** 111–116.

Sandhoff, K., Conzelmann, E., Neufeld, E. F., Kaback, M. M., and Suzuki, K. (1989) The GM2 gangliosidoses. In: *The Metabolic Basis of Inherited Disease*, 6th ed., vol. II (Scriver, C. R., Beaudet, A. L., Sly, W. S., and Valle, D., eds.), McGraw-Hill, New York, pp. 1824–1839.

Sawitsky, A., Rosner, F., and Chodsky, S. (1970) The sea-blue histiocyte syndrome. *N. Engl. J. Med.* **282,** 1100–1101.

Schinella, R. A., Greco, M. A., Garay, S. M., Lackner, H., Wolman, S. R., and Fazzini, E. P. (1985) Hermansky-Pudlak syndrome: a clinicopathologic study. *Hum. Pathol.* **16,** 366–376.

Schmid, C., Kirkham, N., Diss, T., and Isaacson, P. G. (1992) Splenic marginal zone cell lymphoma. *Am. J. Surg. Pathol.* **16,** 455–466.

Schnitzer, B., Sodeman, T., Mead, M. L., and Contacos, P. G. (1972) Pitting function of the spleen in malaria: ultrastructural observations. *Science* **177,** 175–177.

Schuchman, E. H. and Desnick R. T. (1995) Niemann-Pick Disease Types A and B: acid sphingomyelinase deficiencies. In: *The Metabolic and*

Molecular Bases of Inherited Disease, 7th ed. vol. II (Scriver, C. R., Beaudet, A. L., Sly, W. S., and Valle, D., eds.), McGraw-Hill, New York, pp. 2601–2624.

Schwartzman, W. A., Marchevsky, A., and Meyer, R. D. (1990) Epithelioid angiomatosis or cat scratch disease with splenic and hepatic abnormalities in AIDS: case report and review of the literature. *Scand. J. Infect. Dis.* **22,** 121–133.

Semenzato, G., Pandolfi, F., Chisesi, T., De Rossi, G., Pizzolo, G., Zambello, R., et al. (1987) Lymphoproliferative disease of granular lymphocytes. A heterogeneous disorder ranging from indolent to aggressive conditions. *Cancer* **60,** 2971–2978.

Semenzato, G., Zambello, R., Starkebaum, G., Oshimi, K., and Loughran, T. P. Jr. (1997) The lymphoproliferative disease of granular lymphocytes: updated criteria for diagnosis. *Blood* **89,** 256–260.

Sen Gupta, P. C., Chatterjea, J. B., Mukherjee, A. M., and Chatterji, A. (1960) Observations on the foam cell in thalassemia. *Blood* **16,** 1039–1044.

Serur, D. and Terjanian, T. (1992) Spontaneous rupture of the spleen as the initial manifestation of acute myeloid leukemia. *NY State J. Med.* **92,** 160–161.

Shafaie, F. F., Katz, M. E., and Hannaway, C. D. (1997) A horseshoe adrenal gland in an infant with asplenia. *Pediatr. Radiol.* **27,** 591–593.

Sheahan, K., Wolf, B. C., and Neiman, R. (1988) Inflammatory pseudotumor of the spleen: a clinicopathologic study of three cases. *Hum. Pathol.* **19,** 1024–1031.

Shuman, R. L. and Bouterie, R. L. (1976) Cystadenocarcinoma of the pancreas presenting as a splenic cyst. *Surgery* **80,** 652–654.

Siena, S., Bregni, M., Brando, M., Ravagnani, F., Bonadonna, G., and Gianni, A. M. (1989) Circulation of CD34+ hematopoietic stem cells in the peripheral blood of high-dose cyclophosphamide-treated patients: enhancement by intravenous recombinant human granulocyte-macrophage colony-stimulating factor. *Blood* **74,** 1905–1914.

Silverman, M. L. and LiVolsi, V. A. (1978) Splenic hamartoma. *Am. J. Clin. Pathol.* **70,** 224–229.

Silverstein, M. N., Ellefson, R. D., and Ahern, E. J. (1970) The syndrome of the sea-blue histiocyte. *N. Engl. J. Med.* **282,** 1–4.

Silverstein, M. N. and Ellefson, R. D. (1972) The syndrome of the sea-blue histiocyte. *Semin. Hematol.* **9,** 299–307.

Simoes, B. P., Tone, L. G., Zago, M. A., and Figueiredo, M.S. (1995) Splenic function in acute leukemia. *Acta Haematol.* **94,** 123–127.

Smith, V. C., Eisenberg, B. L., and McDonald, E. C. (1985) Primary splenic angiosarcoma. Case report and literature review. *Cancer* **55,** 1625–1627.

Snover, D. C., Frizzera, G., Spector, B. D., Perry, G. S. III, and Kersey, J. H. (1981) Wiskott-Aldrich syndrome: histopathologic findings in the lymph nodes and spleens of 15 patients. *Hum. Pathol.* **12,** 821–831.

Sokol, R. J., Booker, D. J., and Stamps, R. (1992) The pathology of autoimmune hemolytic anemia. *J. Clin. Pathol.* **45,** 1047–1052.

Sordillo, E. M., Sordillo, P. P., and Hajdu, S. I. (1981) Primary hemangiosarcoma of the spleen: report of four cases. *Med. Pediatr. Oncol.* **9,** 319–324.

Spier, C. M., Kjeldsberg, C. R., Eyre, H. J., and Behm, F. G. (1985) Malignant lymphoma with primary presentation in the spleen. A study of 20 patients. *Arch. Pathol. Lab. Med.* **109,** 1076–1080.

Steeper, T. A., Rosenstein, H., Weiser, J., Inampudi, S., and Snover, D. C. (1992) Bacillary epithelioid angiomatosis involving the liver, spleen, and skin in an AIDS patient with concurrent Kaposi's sarcoma. *Am. J. Clin. Pathol.* **97,** 713–718.

Steinberg, M. H., Gatling, R. R., and Tavassoli, M. (1983) Evidence of hyposplenism in the presence of splenomegaly. *Scand. J. Haematol.* **5,** 437–439.

Stovall, T. G. and Ling, F. W. (1988) Splenosis: report of a case and review of the literature. *Obstet. Gynecol. Surg.* **43,** 69–72.

Supe, A., Desai, C., Rao, P. P., Madiwale, C., and Joshi, A. (2000) Isolated massive splenic peliosis. *Indian J. Gastroenterol.* **19,** 87–88.

Suster, S., Moran, C. A., and Blanco, M. (1994) Mycobacterial spindle-cell pseudotumor of the spleen. *Am. J. Clin. Pathol.* **101,** 539–542.

Tada, T., Wakkabayashi, T., and Kishimoto, H. (1983) Peliosis of the spleen. *Am. J. Clin. Pathol.* **79,** 708–713.

Tavassoli, M. and McMillan, R. (1975) Structure of the spleen in idiopathic thrombocytopenic purpura. *Am. J. Clin. Pathol.* **64**, 180–191.

Tavassoli, M. and Weiss, L. (1973) An electron microscopic study of the spleen in myelofibrosis with myeloid metaplasia. *Blood* **42**, 267–279.

Taxy, J. B. (1978) Peliosis: a morphologic curiosity becomes an iatrogenic problem. *Hum. Pathol.* **9**, 331–340.

Timens, W. and Poppema, S. (1985) Lymphocyte compartments in human spleen. An immunohistologic study in normal spleens and uninvolved spleens in Hodgkin's disease. *Am. J. Pathol.* **120**, 443–54.

Timens, W. and Poppema, S. (1987) Impaired immune response to polysaccharides. *N. Engl. J. Med.* **317**, 837–838.

Travis, W. D. and Li, C. Y. (1988) Pathology of the lymph node and spleen in systemic mast cell disease. *Mod. Pathol.* **1**, 4–14.

Traweek, S. T. and Sheibani, K. (1992) Monocytoid B-cell lymphoma: the biologic and clinical implications of peripheral blood involvement. *Am. J. Clin. Pathol.* **97**, 591–598.

Turk, C. O., Lipson, S. B., and Brandt, T. D. (1988) Splenosis mimicking a renal mass. *Urology* **24**, 248–250.

Uchiyama, T., Yodoi, J., Sagawa, K., Takatsuki, K., and Uchino, H. (1977) Adult T-cell leukemia: clinical and hematological features of 16 cases. *Blood* **50**, 481–492.

Urmacher, C. and Nielsen, S. (1985) The histopathology of the acquired immune deficiency syndrome. *Pathol. Annu.* **20**, 197–220.

Van Ewijk, W. and Nieuwenhuis, P. (1985) Compartments, domains, and migration pathways of lymphoid cells in the splenic pulp. *Experientia* **41**, 199–208.

Van Houte, A. J., Schuurman, H. J., Huber, J., van der Meer, J., van der Vegt, J. H., Kuis, W., Jambroes, G., and de Weger, R. A. (1990) The periarteriolar lymphocyte sheath in immunodeficiency. T- or B-lymphocyte area? *Am. J. Clin. Pathol.* **94**, 318–322.

Varela-Fascinetto, G., Castaldo, P., Fox, I. J., Sudan, D., Heffron, T. G., Shaw, B. W., and Langnas, A. N. (1998) Biliary atresia-polysplenia syndrome: surgical and clinical relevance in liver transplantation. *Ann. Surg.* **227**, 583–589.

Vasef, M. and Katzin, W. E. (1993) Monocytoid B-cell lymphoma with a distinctive clinical presentation. *Hum. Pathol.* **24**, 558–561.

Vasef, M. A., Medeiros, L. J., Koo, C., McCourty, A., and Brynes, R. K. (1997) Cyclin D1 immunohistochemical staining is useful in distinguishing mantle cell lymphoma from other low-grade B-cell neoplasms in bone marrow. *Am. J. Clin. Pathol.* **108**, 302–307.

Vasef, M. A., Neiman, R. S., Meletiou, S. D., and Platz, C. E. (1998) Marked granulocytic proliferation induced by granulocyte colony-stimulating factor in the spleen simulating a myeloid leukemic infiltrate. *Mod. Pathol.* **11**, 1138–1141.

Vento, J. A., Peng, F., Spencer, R. P., and Ramsey, W. H. (1999) Massive and widely distributed splenosis. *Clin. Nucl. Med.* **24**, 845–846.

Wainwright, H. and Nelson, M. (1993) Polysplenia syndrome and congenital short pancreas. *Am. J. Med. Genet.* **47**, 318–320.

Wanless, I. R. and Bernier, V. (1983) Fibrous thickening of the splenic capsule. *Arch. Pathol. Lab. Med.* **107**, 595–599.

Wanless, I. R. and Geddie, W. R. (1985) Mineral oil lipogranulomata in liver and spleen. *Arch. Pathol. Lab. Med.* **109**, 283–286.

Warfel, K. A. and Ellis, G. H. (1982) Peliosis of the spleen. *Arch. Pathol. Lab. Med.* **106**, 99–100.

Warnke, R. A., Weiss, L. M., Chan, J. K. C., et al. (1995) Lymphomas of the spleen. In: *Tumors of the lymph nodes and spleen. Atlas of Tumor Pathology,* third series, fascicle 14, Armed Forces Institute of Pathology, Washington, DC, 495-6. p. 411–406.

Warren, S. and Davis, H. (1934) Studies on tumor metastasis. V. The metastases of carcinoma to the spleen. *Am. J. Cancer* **21**, 517–533.

Watanabe, Y, Todani, T, Noda, T., and Yamamoto, S. (1997) Standard splenic volume in children and young adults measured from CT images. *Surg. Today* **27**, 726–728.

Weisdorf, S. A. and Krivit, R. (1982) Paucity of splenic germinal centers: a new and unique splenomegaly syndrome including dysfunctional immune system. *Clin. Immunol. Immunopathol.* **23**, 492–500.

Weissman, I. L. (1976) T cell maturation and the ontogeny of splenic lymphoid architecture. In: *Immune Aspects of the Spleen.* (Battisto, J. R. and Streilen, J. W., eds.), North Holland, Amsterdam, p. 77.

Weisz, B., Spirer, Z., and Reif, S. (1994) Niemann-Pick disease: newer classification based on genetic mutations of the disease. *Adv. Pediatr.* **41**, 415–426.

Wennberg, E. and Weiss, L. (1968) Splenic erythroclasia: an electron microscopic study of hemoglobin H disease. *Blood* **31**, 778–790.

Whitley, J. E., Maynard, C. D., and Rhyne, A. L. (1966) A computer approach to the prediction of spleen weight from routine films. *Radiology* **86**, 73–76.

Wiener, R. S. and Ong, L. S. (1989) Streptokinase and splenic rupture. *Am. J. Med.* **86**, 249.

Willey, R. F., Rodger, A., and Webb, J. N. (1982) Seminoma presenting as gross splenomegaly. *Scot. Med. J.* **27**, 254–255.

Wolf, B. C. and Neiman, R. S. (1989) *Disorders of the Spleen.* Saunders, Philadelphia.

Wolf, B. C. and Neiman, R. S. (1985) Myelofibrosis with myeloid metaplasia: pathophysiologic implication of the correlation between bone marrow changes and progression of splenomegaly. *Blood* **65**, 803–809.

Wolff, M. J., Bitran, J., Northland, R. G., and Levy, I. L. (1991) Splenic abscesses due to mycobacterium tuberculosis in patients with AIDS. *Rev. Infect. Dis.* **13**, 373–375.

Wong, K. F., Chan, J. K., Matutes, E., et al. (1995) Hepatosplenic gamma delta T-cell lymphoma. A distinctive aggressive lymphoma type. *Am. J. Surg. Pathol.* **6**, 718–726.

Yasukochi, S., Satomi, G., and Iwasaki, Y. (1997) Prenatal diagnosis of total anomalous pulmonary venous connection with asplenia. *Fetal. Diagn. Ther.* **12**, 266–269.

Zellers, R. A., Thibodeau, S. N., and Banks, P. M. (1990) Primary splenic lymphocyte- depletion Hodgkin's disease. *Am. J. Clin. Pathol.* **94**, 453–457.

Zeppa, P., Vetrani, A., Luciano, L., Fulciniti, F., Troncone, G., Rotoli, B., and Palombini, L. (1994) Fine needle aspiration biopsy of the spleen: a useful procedure in the diagnosis of splenomegaly. *Acta Cytol.* **38**, 299–309.

Ziegler, J. L. and Dorfman, R. F. (1988) *Kaposi's Sarcoma: Pathophysiology and Clinical Management.* Marcel Dekker, New York.

Zitzer, P., Pansky, M., Maymon, R., Langer, R., Bukovsky, I., and Golan, A. (1998) Pelvic splenosis mimicking endometriosis, causing low abdominal mass and pain. *Hum. Reprod.* **13**, 1683–1685.

Zukerberg, L. R., Yang, W., Arnold, A., and Harris, N. L. (1995) Cyclin D1 expression in non-Hodgkin's lymphoma: detection by immunohistochemistry. *Am. J. Clin. Pathol.* **103**, 756–760.

7 Splenic Pooling and Survival of Blood Cells*

ANTHONY J. BOWDLER, MD, PhD, FRCP, FRCPATH, FACP
AND FRANK GARY RENSHAW, DO

7.1. INTRODUCTION

The high frequency with which deficits in the principal cell lines occur in the blood counts of patients with splenomegaly has indicated a special relationship between the spleen and the composition of the circulating blood. To some, this has suggested a humoral controlling mechanism whereby the spleen could affect the rates of hemopoietic production and delivery of cells to the circulation (Dameshek and Estren, 1947; Dameshek, 1955), but until now, no convincing evidence has been presented that there is such an effect, at least to the extent that it would be of clinical significance (Bowdler, 1983).

To others, the relationship appeared to depend on an increased rate of cell destruction by the spleen (Doan, 1949); this was widely regarded as an exaggeration of the normal splenic function of destroying effete blood cells reaching the end of their normal lifespan. There was an implicit assumption that increased splenic mass would increase the rate of cell destruction, but this leaves to be explained why hemolysis of detectable degree is so variable among subjects with comparable degrees of splenic enlargement. Furthermore, it did not explain those conditions with active, or even aggressive, hemolysis, which may be associated with minor degrees of splenomegaly.

A more detailed insight into the relationship between the spleen and circulating blood cells evolved when effective blood-cell-labeling techniques became available in the 1950s. Of these, (^{51}Cr)-labeling has been the most productive (Gray and Sterling, 1950): In the measurement of red blood cell life-span, it has the disadvantage of providing only approximate estimates, because of the variable elution of radionuclide from cells, for which only approximate corrections can be made. However, the nuclide is detectable, with a suitably collimated γ counter, at the body surface, and this has made it possible to track cells during the various phases of their passage through, and their interaction with, the spleen and other organs, and, in conjunction with surface counting of plasma albumin labeled with iodine-131 (^{131}I), to determine the relative concentration of red blood cells and plasma in different regions of the body, expressed as the "regional hematocrit" (Bowdler 1969).

*This chapter is revised from the First Edition, Chapter 8, previously written by Anthony J. Bowdler and the late Professor Auge Videbaek.

From: *The Complete Spleen: A Handbook of Structure, Function, and Clinical Disorders* Edited by: A. J. Bowdler © Humana Press Inc., Totowa, NJ

These methods showed that the radionuclide labeling of red blood cells could, in various circumstances, reflect several phases of red blood cell interaction with the spleen. In normal circumstances, the first phase occurs during the first 2–3 min following the injection of labeled cells into the circulation, during the period in which these are mixing with, and being diluted by, the unlabeled cells of the general circulation. There is a rapid and immediate rise in the radioactivity detectable over the spleen, which characteristically has a half-life (T_{50}) of 1 min or slightly longer, and is accompanied by a simultaneous fall in the radioactivity of venous blood samples (Fig. 1). These changes terminate in plateaux of both the venous and the splenic radioactivity, when the mixing of injected red blood cells with the unlabeled red blood cells in the circulation is complete. In pathological circumstances, a second rising phase, following the initial rise in radioactivity over the spleen, is often detectable, especially when the spleen is enlarged (Harris et al., 1958; Motulsky et al., 1958; Toghill, 1964; Christensen, 1973). This secondary phase usually shows a slower rate of rise than the first, with a half-life between 5 min and 60 min or more (Figs. 1 and 2). This arises from the mixing of the labeled cells with a splenic pool of unlabeled red blood cells which slowly exchanges with the red blood cells of the general circulation. Comparable pooling has not been detected in other organs (Bowdler, 1962).

Following this, on a time-scale of days rather than minutes, there is often a slight but detectable net increase in radioactivity over the spleen, which may result from radionuclide adsorbed to the tissues from a fraction of the labeled red blood cells after their destruction *in situ*. In the presence of active hemolysis, with a large splenic red blood cell pool, there may also be demonstrated at this time rising activity in the region of the liver, indicating the destruction of red blood cells conditioned for hemolysis by the splenic pool, but released to complete the process elsewhere.

Platelets also show a pooling phenomenon, but in this case splenic pooling is present in the normal subject, and the size of the pool expands when the organ enlarges pathologically. There is also good evidence for the pooling of granulocytes in the normal spleen, the pool being in dynamic equilibrium with circulating granulocytes, and in large part constituting a component of the marginating granulocyte pool (Peters et al., 1985a). The mean transit times through the spleen for platelets and granulocytes are similar, at approx 6–12 min, which is considerably shorter than is found in most cases of pathologically pooled red blood cells (*see also* Chapter 12, Subheadings 3–5).

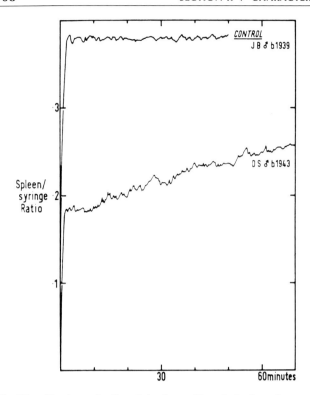

Fig. 7.1. Tracings of radioactivity detectable at the body surface over the spleen with a collimated scintillation counter following the intravenous injection of ^{51}Cr-labeled red blood cells. The control tracing (J.B.) is from a subject without detectable splenomegaly, and shows a rapid rise to an early plateau, which reflects the mixing of the nuclide-labeled cells with the red blood cells in the circulation. A single phase tracing of this type is typically found in normal subjects. The lower tracing (D.S.) is from a subject with warm-antibody autoimmune hemolytic anemia. The surface radioactivity rises in two phases: The first is a rapid rise comparable to that of the normal subject. The slower secondary rise reflects the exchange of red blood cells with the splenic red pool, and is abnormal. Ordinate: surface radioactivity in arbitrary units, related to the radioactivity of the syringe containing the labeled red blood cells, assayed with a standard geometrical relationship to the scintillation counter. Abscissa: time in minutes from injection. (Reproduced with permission from Bowdler, 1966.)

7.2. PATHOLOGICAL POOLING OF RED BLOOD CELLS

7.2.1. ANALYSIS OF RADIONUCLIDE UPTAKE BY SURFACE COUNTING

The slowly rising component in surface radio-activity over the spleen, after the injection of ^{51}Cr-labeled red blood cells can be reduced to a simple exponential expression. If A_t is the surface activity at any time, t, and A_e is the activity when equilibrium is attained, then $(A_e - A_t)/A_e$ expresses the shortfall in radioactivity from the equilibrium level, A_e, at any time, t, as a proportion of the final level of radioactivity (Fig. 2). The logarithm of the expression can be plotted graphically in sequence against time, most conveniently on a semilogarithmic plot, to give a curve that declines in two phases. The second phase reflects the slow secondary rise in splenic radioactivity, and, using numerical data from points beyond the primary rise in activity, it is possible to define the second phase as the calculated regression line of log $([A_e - A_t]/A_e)$. This can be extrapolated to the ordinate: the antilog of the point at which it meets the ordinate gives the fraction

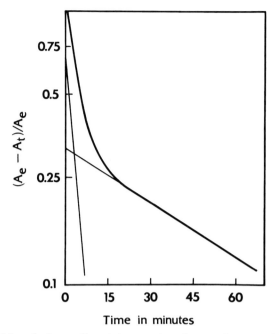

Fig. 7.2. Surface radioactivity over the spleen can be recognized as having two components in cases such as D.S. in Fig. 1. Plotting sequentially the radioactivity at time, t, as its difference from the final equilibrial activity, A_e, gives two phases. By semilogarithmic plotting, the second phase can be linearized, and its regression line characterized to give best estimates of the fraction of the radioactivity attributable to the pool and its half-life of development. Subtraction of the secondary (slow phase) curve from the total curve by conventional curve peeling gives the curve for the initial phase. Ordinate: surface radioactivity expressed as log $(A_e - A_t)/A_e$. Abscissa: time in minutes.

of the total radioactivity that can be ascribed to the slow phase. This line can be further characterized by the time taken for its value to fall to half the value at zero time (T_{50}). By a conventional "curve-peeling" process, the initial phase of the curve can be corrected by subtracting the values of the extrapolated slow-phase regression line from the total curve. The residual values can then be expressed as the "fast-phase" regression line, and characterized as the fraction of total activity so represented and its half-life for disappearance.

7.2.2. PATHOLOGICAL CONDITIONS PRODUCING SPLENIC RED BLOOD CELL POOLING

Red blood cell pooling, demonstrated by radionuclide studies, has been found predominantly in two circumstances: First, it tends to be well-developed in certain conditions characterized by active hemolysis associated with overt abnormalities of the red blood cells (type 1). Second, it occurs in disorders with marked splenic enlargement, which often show less overt evidence of accelerated red blood cell destruction (type 2). Included in type 1 are conditions such as hereditary spherocytosis, hemolytic cases of hereditary elliptocytosis, warm antibody autoimmune hemolytic disease, thalassemia major, and pernicious anemia. The inherent properties of the red blood cell, (shape, and so on) appear to determine the development of pooling, presumably because they impede flow of the affected cells through the pathways of the spleen. With respect to hereditary spherocytosis, and some cases of autoimmune hemolytic anemia, the spherocytic (or, more precisely, stomatocytic) shape may itself reduce deformability of the cell, and diminish the probability of a normal passage through sites such as the potential interendothelial spaces of the walls of the splenic sinuses. In addition, it is possible that poorly deformable cells are also impeded in passage elsewhere in the splenic circulation, e.g., in more proximal channels of the red pulp (*see* Chapters 2, Subheading 3.2.2.3, Fig. 6 and Chapter 3, Subheadings 3.4 and 3.12 for a more detailed discussion).

Although red blood cell shape appears to be the principal identifiable characteristic affecting flow through the spleen, other factors may include membrane rigidity (in hereditary spherocytosis), the adherence of cell surface-attached antibody to the Fc receptors of pulp macrophages (in autoimmune hemolysis), and intraerythrocytic viscosity (in sickle cell syndromes). In these conditions, normal red blood cells will not pool significantly on infusion into affected subjects, with the exception of a slow splenic uptake in immunohemolytic disorders, in which the infused cells may be modified in the circulation by antibody adhering to the cell surface. Conversely, infusion of the abnormal cells into the circulation of a normal subject produces prompt splenic pooling, showing that the pathophysiological infrastructure for pooling is present in the normal spleen.

Type 2 pooling appears to depend on a structural disorder in the affected spleen. Autologous cells have been found to pool in cases of myeloproliferative disorders (especially primary myeloid metaplasia, chronic myeloid leukemia, and cases of primary polycythemia showing more than slight splenic enlargement), lymphoproliferative disorders (although usually to a lesser degree than in the myeloproliferative disorders), congestive splenomegaly, primary hypersplenism (nontropical idiopathic splenomegaly), and tropical splenomegaly. Normal red blood cells infused into subjects with structural splenic pooling, will also demonstrate slow-phase accumulation in the spleen, although not necessarily to the same extent as is found with autologous cells.

In both types of pooling conditions, it seems most probable that the principal site of the red blood cell pool is the red pulp (Stutte, 1990; Pearson et al., 1969). The pathological changes in the spleen which interrupt the pathways of flow for blood cells, remain to be defined in many conditions. Possibly, the sinus reticular coat is abnormal and alters the dimensions of the interendothelial slits of the sinuses in conditions such as chronic myeloid leukemia (Björkman, 1947). In other cases, it appears that the arteriolar terminations, which are normally close to the external aspects of the sinus walls, have been distracted from their normal orientation, so that directed flow toward the sinuses is interrupted. Other areas of the pulp flow pathways may be diverted by cellular accumulations, and spleens may be found in which dense pathological cellular infiltrates (as in lymphomata and Gaucher's disease) so completely occupy the spaces of the red pulp that flow is impaired, to the extent that an exchangeable pool can no longer be demonstrated.

7.2.3. THE CONCEPT OF RED BLOOD CELL POOL: ITS QUANTITATION
Comparison of the rise in surface radioactivity over the spleen, with the corresponding simultaneous fall in the radioactivity in the blood, shows that the loss of red blood cells to the spleen may greatly exceed the numbers that could be sustainable by red blood cell production in a steady state. Clearly, therefore, the secondary rise in splenic radioactivity must reflect an exchange of viable cells rather than a unidirectional loss of cells to the spleen, which suggests the exchange of red blood cells between two pools, the one present in the general circulation and the other in a splenic pool of viable cells.

The volume of red blood cells in the exchanging red blood cell pool in the spleen can be estimated by three principal methods:

1. The volume of distribution of labeled red blood cells can be measured from blood samples taken by venipuncture at 3 min after injection of the labeled red blood cells, and again after surface counting over the spleen shows that the pool has equilibrated. The difference in the volumes of distribution approximates to the red blood cell volume in the pool. The error of the method is increased when the rate of equilibration is high and the T_{50} of the slow phase short, because significant pooling may have occurred before the first blood sample is taken. This method essentially measures the exchanging red blood cell pool, and does not include any intact red blood cells irreversibly trapped in the spleen, or those with very slow exchange rates.

2. The pool volume may be estimated by measurements of surface radioactivity, calibrated against a phantom (or model) of the spleen with known amounts of activity (Glass et al., 1968; Christensen, 1971). Scanning techniques may be used to provide a more accurate estimate of spleen volume (Rasmussen et al., 1973).

3. A third method of estimating the volume and turnover time is to analyze the fall in circulating red blood cell activity following the intravenous injection of labeled red blood cells. This is an elaboration of the first method, using a mathematical model that assumes first-order exchange kinetics between circulating red blood cells and the pooled cells, and applies the calculations of two-compartment exchange (Solomon, 1953; Bowdler, 1962).

The structural basis for red blood cell pooling has been discussed in detail in Chapter 3, Subheading 3.12; radionuclide studies have not provided a unique solution to the question of the required structure, although evidence of a high degree of red blood cell concentration in the pool suggested a parallel with the storage pool found in many mammals, such as dog, horse, and bovine. Harris et al. (1958) suggested that the fast phase of the surface equilibration curve reflected flow through the direct splenic vascular pathways between arterioles and venous sinuses, and that slow phase was the result of flow through the indirect (pulp) pathways. However, it has not been possible to define a mechanism by which cells would be differentially directed into the appropriate pathway, when their characteristics were abnormal, and it seems more probable that the spleen functions by passive filtration, rather than by an active sorting mechanism (Fig. 3). This concept holds that the majority of red blood cells are presented to the same pathway through the red pulp circulation, and that their flow rate is determined either by intrinsic characteristics of the cells, or by the proximity of the arteriolar capillaries to the sinus walls.

The volumes of red blood cells in the splenic pool are variable, and vary from 5% of the total red blood cell mass to more than 40%, so that, in some cases in which red blood cell production is impaired, the diversion of cells away from the active extrasplenic circulation may be a supplementary cause of anemia. Taking all causes of splenomegaly together, there is no close correlation between spleen size and the volume of the red blood cell pool. However, within fairly broad limits there is a tendency for the pool size to increase with spleen weight (Christensen, 1975).

7.2.4. THE CELL ENVIRONMENT IN THE POOLING SPLEEN
Measurements of the body hematocrit, expressed as the fraction of total blood volume consisting of red blood cells, show that it tends to be lower than the venous hematocrit, which is representative of

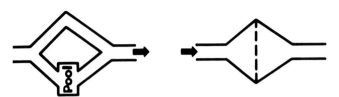

Fig. 7.3. Concepts of splenic pooling of red blood cells. The diagram on the left shows two potential routes of blood flow through the spleen, the one providing for unobstructed fast flow, and the second an anatomically separate, slowly flowing compartment. The diagram on the right suggests a functional barrier to flow, which may permit differential flow, either on the basis of the characteristics of the red blood cells, or the variable relationships of the afferent arterial capillaries to the efferent vessels (sinuses). (Adapted with permission from Bowdler, 1983.)

large vessel blood. The ratio of the body hematocrit to venous hematocrit is normally remarkably constant at about 0.91 ± 0.02 (Mollison et al., 1987). In the presence of marked splenomegaly, the body hematocrit rises in relation to the venous hematocrit, indicating the presence of a region containing blood with a high hematocrit. Surface counting studies, with labeled red blood cells and plasma, have shown this zone with a high proportion of red blood cells to be in the spleen (Bowdler, 1969), where the regional hematocrit is highest. This shows that the splenic red blood cell environment is one that is relatively poor in plasma, and through which the flow is exceptionally slow. Some have suggested that this creates an adverse environment for the red blood cells, with a tendency to low glucose levels and pH, creating metabolic stress and depletion of intracellular adenosine triphosphate (Jandl and Aster, 1967; Murphy, 1967; Wennberg and Weiss, 1969; *see also* Chapter 3, Subheading 3.6).

7.2.5. SPLENIC RED BLOOD CELL POOLING AND HEMOLYSIS The adverse physical characteristics of the environment of pooled red blood cells may have a direct influence on the viability of the pooled cells: This has been demonstrated for the red blood cells in hereditary spherocytosis, in which comparable conditions in vitro produce accelerated fragmentation of the red blood cell membrane, and increase sphering of the cells, with loss of membrane area in excess of the loss of volume (Weed and Bowdler, 1966). This appears to be the basis for the conditioning of the red blood cells to hemolysis in the spleen and elsewhere. However, the red blood cell membrane is especially vulnerable in this condition, and the extent to which this occurs in other disorders is uncertain.

In immunohemolytic conditions, the red blood cells in the splenic pool remain in close proximity to the macrophages of the spleen, in flow conditions that produce minimal disturbance to the process of adherence of red blood cells to the surface of the phagocytes. This appears to be capable of enhancing partial or complete phagocytosis of sensitized cells. The low volume of plasma in the pool, a result of skimming of plasma before blood reaches the cordal environment, may be an additional factor promoting phagocytosis, in that it reduces the inhibitory effect of ambient immunoglobulins.

However, in other conditions, and especially where pooling is caused by to structural disorders, the degree of red blood cell concentration is variable, and the proportion of the life-span of the red blood cell spent in the pool may be low. The critical period of retention in the spleen required to produce deleterious changes in the

normal red blood cell remains to be defined. In the majority of cases in which there is significant splenomegaly without a defined red blood cell defect, the red blood cell survival tends to be diminished (Ferrant, 1983), often to a life-span of 20–30 d. However, although this can frequently be corrected by splenectomy, this is not always the case (Bowdler, 1963), and the conditions required to produce the low-grade "splenopathic" anemia are clearly not present in all cases of splenic enlargement.

Christensen (1975) has shown that the volume of red blood cells in the splenic pool tends to correlate positively with the rates of destruction of red blood cells by the spleen for specific disorders. However, the relationship apparently shows marked differences between groups of disorders, e.g., the rate of cell destruction is much higher for a given size of red blood cell pool in myeloproliferative disorders than in lymphoproliferative disorders. This indicates that there are properties of the microenvironment of the pool that affect red blood cell survival, and which need more detailed definition than is currently available.

7.3. POOLING OF PLATELETS IN THE SPLEEN

Binet and Kaplan (1923) demonstrated that adrenaline injected intravenously in dogs causes an immediate but transient increase in the platelet count of the peripheral blood; this effect could be repeated 60–90 min after the first injection. Further, they showed that adrenaline had mobilized platelets from the spleen, since a rise in blood platelet count did not occur in splenectomized dogs, and therefore concluded that there existed a splenic pool of platelets exchangeable with platelets in the bloodstream.

The importance of the spleen to the adrenaline response was confirmed by demonstrating that the increase in platelet count, following adrenaline failed to appear in splenectomized human subjects (Wright et al., 1951; Aster, 1966; Kotilainen, 1969; Branehög et al., 1973). Aster (1965) showed that 25–50% of reinjected ^{51}Cr-labeled platelets are pooled in the human spleen, and that entry of platelets into the spleen is delayed by the administration of adrenaline prior to platelet infusion. This finding was confirmed by Freedman and Karpatkin (1975b). Conversely, ^{51}Cr-labeled platelets, once pooled in the spleen, can to some extent be mobilized by adrenaline (Fig. 4): This was shown by the increase in ^{51}Cr-platelet radioactivity that occurs in the blood following the administration of adrenaline (Aster, 1966; Branehög et al., 1973; Fredén et al., 1978a; Vilén et al., 1980), and the concomitant decrease in the platelet radioactivity detectable by surface counting over the spleen (Aster, 1966; Kotilainen, 1969).

When other agents with autonomic effects were investigated, some apparent paradoxes were discovered. The ability of adrenaline to release platelets from the spleen is shared by the β_1-receptor blocking agent, metoprolol (Kutti et al., 1977); whereas the β_1-receptor stimulator, isoprenaline, has the opposite effect, and leads to trapping of platelets in the spleen (Olsson et al., 1976; Fredén et al., 1978; Fredén et al., 1978). Peters and Lavender (1983) suggested that the apparently conflicting results could be explained by the effects of these agents on splenic blood flow, which decreases after adrenaline and increases after isoprenaline. However, adrenaline also diminishes spleen size (Doan and Wright, 1946), and, in 13 human subjects, Schaffner et al. (1985) showed a highly significant correlation between contraction of the spleen, as measured by ultrasound, and the mobilization of platelets ($r = 0.185, p < 0.002$).

Vilén et al. (1980) observed that a portion of the adrenaline-mobilizable platelet pool is located outside the spleen: After hav-

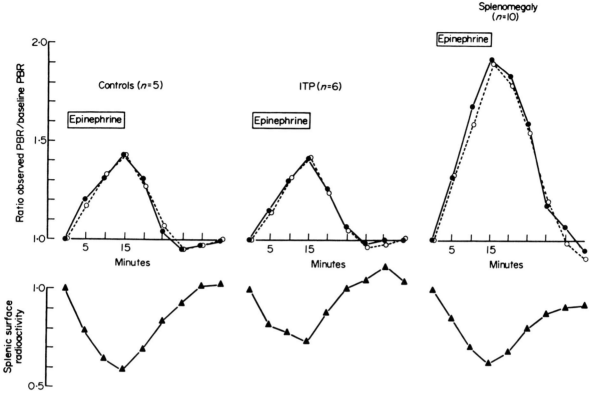

Fig. 7.4. Platelet pooling in the spleen: the response to epinephrine. Blood samples were drawn for the determination of venous platelet count and platelet bound radioactivity (upper figures), and surface radioactivity over the spleen, was recorded during the experiments. Baseline values are given as 1.0, and subsequent values are given in relation this. Relative platelet counts: O----O. Relative platelet bound radioactivity: ●----●. Relative splenic surface radioactivity: ▲----▲. (Reproduced with permission from Branehög, 1973.)

ing reinfused ^{51}Cr-labeled platelets into three normal and three splenectomized healthy men, adrenaline was given, and the blood platelet count and peripheral platelet radioactivity were measured. In the nonsplenectomized men, platelet counts increased by 40%; the asplenic men also showed an increase in platelet count and radioactivity, but this was limited to a mean value of only 8% (*see* Fig. 5).

Adrenaline and related substances are not the only agents able to mobilize a considerable fraction of the splenic platelet pool. Short-term, vigorous physical exercise can induce similar, and sometimes marked, changes, appearing immediately after the stress, and disappearing after 10–15 min rest (Sarajas et al., 1961). Dawson and Ogston (1969) investigated 12 intact and 6 splenectomized subjects, before and after exercise. Some of the asplenic subjects showed a well-marked transient thrombocytosis, indicating the existence of an extrasplenic exchangeable platelet pool. In humans undertaking physical exercise, Freedman et al. (1977) noted a transient platelet response. The total mobilizable pool of platelets was calculated to be at least 29% of the total platelet mass. However, splenectomized subjects still show a significant platelet response. On the day following reinjection of ^{111}In-oxine labeled platelets, Schmidt and Rasmussen (1984) investigated 15 healthy subjects who then carried out a defined pattern of vigorous physical work. Platelet radioactivity in the blood increased by about 15%, and that measured over the spleen showed an equivalent fall, which confirmed that the splenic platelet pool was mobilizable by exercise. Clearly, there is a substantial fraction of the total platelet popula-

tion that is held in platelet reservoirs located principally, but not exclusively, in the spleen, and which can be restored to the general circulation by certain definable and reproducible stimuli.

7.3.1. PLATELET RECOVERY When radionuclide-labeled platelets tagged with ^{51}Cr or ^{111}In are reinfused, they mix with the platelets present in the circulation. The initial mixing takes place within a matter of minutes (Aster, 1965; Kotilainen, 1969), but this is slower than the equilibration of ^{131}I-albumin with plasma. Because of the delay in complete mixing, the hypothetical zero time activity of labeled platelets must be measured indirectly. The disappearance curve of radioactivity can be extrapolated back to a zero time value. Alternatively, the blood radioactivity caused by platelets can be estimated after mixing is complete, and this value taken as 100% of initial activity (Fig. 5). Later estimations of platelet activity are then expressed in relation to the initial activity. Plotting the remaining blood radioactivity against time will then demonstrate the platelet disappearance curve. The immediate fall in radioactivity which occurs in the first 3 min, reflects initial mixing. Following this, the curve slowly reaches a minimum; in normal circumstances, this occurs within 10–20 min of the labeled platelets being infused. Surface activity recorded over the spleen will increase, and reach a plateau simultaneously with the blood activity curve reaching its minimum (Fig. 6). Following this, there is an equilibrium phase, which tends to be more or less constant for some hours, with the exception of circumstances such as acute idiopathic thrombocytopenia. The spleen and blood curves approach stable values, with almost identical monoexponential time-courses.

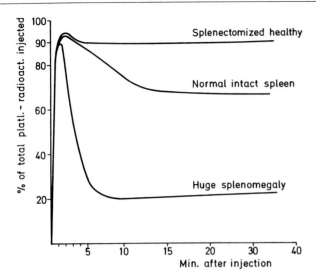

Fig. 7.5. [51]Cr platelet radioactivity in the peripheral blood during the first minutes following injection of labeled platelets into normal, splenomegalic, and splenectomized human subjects.

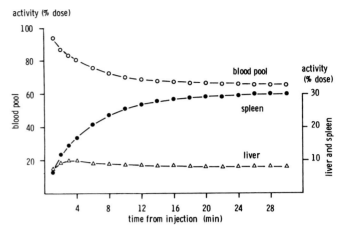

Fig. 7.6. Radioactivity curves recorded in relation to the cardiac blood pool, spleen, and liver following the injection of autologous ^{111}In-labeled platelets in a normal subject. Ordinate (left): blood pool as percentage of dose. Ordinate (right): liver and spleen activity as percentage of dose. Blood: O----O, Spleen: ●----● Liver: ▲----▲. (Reproduced with permission from Peters et al., 1984.)

Aster (1966) introduced the term "platelet recovery," defined as the percentage of infused radioactively-labeled platelets remaining in the peripheral circulation, when equilibrium with the splenic pool is complete. Platelet recovery is calculated from the formula:

Platelet recovery = Platelet activity
in the total blood volume × 100 / Platelet activity infused

In practice this can be calculated as:

Platelet activity/mL blood × blood volume (mL) × 100 /
Infused platelet suspension activity/mL × volume infused (mL)

Platelet recovery has been studied in healthy individuals, splenectomized subjects, and patients with splenomegaly from various causes and of differing degrees: An outline of the data is given in Table 1. In normal subjects, estimates of platelet recovery show a reliable consensus of ~60%, with only slight differences between studies using ^{51}Cr or ^{111}In as the label. However, variations between individuals can be considerable. The majority of unrecovered platelets is present in the spleen, with an average calculated value of 27% (Penny et al., 1966).

[111]In-oxine, and the later introduced ^{111}In-troponate, offer significant advantages over ^{51}Cr, including higher labeling efficiency, less dependence on available platelet numbers, and better external scintigraphic recording (McAfee and Thakur, 1976; Peters and Lavender, 1982; Danpure et al., 1982; Kiefel et al., 1985). Since 1979, ^{111}In has mostly replaced ^{51}Cr as the platelet label; however, few postsplenectomy platelet recovery studies have been undertaken using this nuclide (Heyns et al., 1980a; Hill-Zobel et al., 1986), and in these recovery values are marginally higher than those obtained by using ^{51}Cr platelets.

In splenectomized subjects (Fig. 5), the platelet disappearance curve shows no further fall after the initial mixing phase, following platelet infusion. This curve lacks the downslope seen when the spleen is present, and platelet recovery is close to 90% in these subjects (Heyns et al., 1980a; Hill-Zobel et al., 1986). These findings indicate that, in these circumstances, an average of 13% of

platelet radioactivity, with a range of 8 to 20%, is pooled outside the general circulation. Platelet recovery thus provides an indirect estimate of the splenic platelet pool, since the difference between the total platelet radioactivity infused and platelet recovery represents the sum of the platelet pool in the spleen and the 13% not recovered in asplenic individuals. Because the platelet pools are exchangeable (Aster, 1966; Kotilainen, 1969; Heyns et al., 1980b; Peters et al., 1980), it is apparent that platelets in healthy individuals spend between one-fourth and one-third of their life-span in the spleen.

The anatomical site of the splenic platelet pool was investigated by scanning electron microscopy (Weiss, 1974): Platelets appear to adhere to the surface of the endothelium of the sinuses and reticulum cells of the cords, marginal zone and white pulp.

A special affinity for the spleen is shown by the youngest platelets, which spend the first 1½–2 d, after release from the bone marrow, in the spleen (Shulman et al., 1965; Schulman et al., 1968). This constitutes a platelet pool distinct from the freely exchangeable pool. After splenectomy, no preferential retention of young platelets is found. Adrenaline injection in intact animals mobilizes young platelets (megathrombocytes) from the spleen (Freedman and Karpatkin, 1975b). Likewise, phenylhydrazine-induced hemolysis in dog and rabbit prevents the retention of megathrombocytes, by blockade of the macrophage system (Freedman and Karpatkin, 1975a), which produces a 1.68-fold increase in the total peripheral platelet count, and a 2.08-fold increase in the peripheral megathrombocytes. In splenectomized rabbits, macrophage blockade is followed by an equal increase (1.2-fold) in both platelet categories (Karpatkin, 1983). Wichmann and Gerhardts (1981) found that the preferential storage of young platelets fully explains the terminal tail (sagging) of the physiological platelet survival curve (Fig. 7). Watson and Ludlam (1986) confirmed the heterogeneity of circulating platelets: High density (young) platelets were shown to be preferentially retained in the spleen. Probably, young platelets in the spleen undergo a late maturation process analogous to the process of late development of the reticulocyte population in the spleen.

Table 7.1
Platelet Recovery Studies at Equilibrium in Healthy Splenomegalic and Splenectomized Subjects

Author(s)	Normal		Splenomegalic		Splenectomized		Normal Pooling	
							Platelet activity not accounted for* (% of total)	Splenic platelet pool+ (% of of total)
	n	Mean (%)	n	Mean(%)	n	Mean(%)		
^{51}Cr-labeling								
Aster (1965)	50	62	14	23	6	92	8	30
Kotilainen (1969)	10 (49–76)	58	15	25	8	85 (51–110)	15	27
Harker and Finch (1969)	15	65	4	12	4	88 (77–99)	12	23
Harker (1970)					10	91 (SD 7)		
Gehrmann and Elbers (1970)	10	58	8	17	5	83	17	25
Kummer and Bucher (1971)	22	62	23	37	4	91	9	29
Kutti and Weinfeld (1971a)	18	52 (SD 3)			9	80	20	28
Abrahamsen (1968b, 1972)	10	58 (45–68)	12	38 (20–63)	12	90	10	32
Gardner (1972)	14	68	8	31	12	88	12	20
Ries and Price (1974)	6	69	8	(8–29)				
Branehög et al. (1973)	18	60 (SD 2)						
Kutti and Safai-Kutti (1975)	10	60			6	90	10	30
Slichter and Harker (1976)	16	59 (SD 4)						
Heaton et al. (1979)	10	47 (SD 7)						
Totals (n)	209		85		76		66	66
Calculated means		60%		29%		87%	13%	27%
^{111}In-labeling								
Heaton et al. (1979)	10	71 (SD 4)						
Hawker et al. (1980)	4	69 (SD 3)						
Heyns et al. (1980a,b)	6	72 (SD 16)						
Robertson et al. (1981)	5	70 (SD 21)						
Scheffel et al (1982)	9	57 (SD 11)						
Bautista et al. (1984) 12 76								
Schmidt and Rasmussen (1985)	25	56 (42–49)						
Wessels et al. (1985)	28	61 (SD 12)						
Hill-Zobel et al. (1986)	12	59 (SD 9)	4	26 (SD 6)	4	98 (SD 9.8)	2	39
Totals	111		4		8		8	8
Calculated means		63%		26%		94%	7%	28%

*"Uncovered" platelets in splenectomized subjects (%).
+Total "unrecovered" platelets in normal subjects less "uncovered" platelets in splenectomized subjects (%).

7.3.2. PLATELET RECOVERY IN SPLENOMEGALY Splenomegaly is accompanied by an increase in the splenic platelet pool. This is shown by the following:

1. The early fall in peripheral ^{51}Cr platelet radioactivity following infusion of labeled platelets, is more rapid than in subjects with a spleen of normal size (Aster, 1965; Kotilainen, 1969).

2. In the presence of splenomegaly, the disappearance curve for blood platelet radioactivity finally stabilizes at a lower level than normal (Fig. 5).

3. In the presence of splenomegaly, the splenic surface radioactivity following infusion of radioactive platelets reaches equilibrium later, and at a higher level, than in normal subjects. The time for equilibrium to occur may be postponed for 1–2 h following infusion (Aster, 1965; Kotilainen, 1969; Abrahamsen, 1972).

4. The mobilization of platelets by adrenaline (Fig. 4) is greater in subjects with splenomegaly than when the spleen is of normal size (Aster, 1965; Kotilainen, 1969).

5. There is a negative relationship (Fig. 8) between spleen size and platelet recovery (Penny et al., 1966; Kutti et al., 1972; Abrahamsen, 1972).

6. Removal of an enlarged spleen results in a greatly increased platelet recovery to the level found in splenectomized, but otherwise healthy, subjects (Table 1).

Calculation of platelet recovery, based on the ^{51}Cr method in patients with splenomegaly, shows a mean value of 29%, compared to a calculated normal recovery of 60%. Evidently, recovery values of splenomegalic subjects vary principally because of differences in spleen size. In cases of marked splenomegaly, platelet recovery may be as low as 5% (Kotilainen et al., 1971). In other cases, Harker and Finch (1969) reported a platelet recovery of 12% before and 88% after splenectomy, and Abrahamsen (1972) 38% before and 90% after splenectomy (Fig. 9). A positive relationship between the size of the spleen and size of the platelet pool has also been shown, experimentally, by investigations of methyl cellulose-induced splenomegaly in rats (Aster, 1967; De Gabriele and Penington, 1967; Harker, 1969; Rolovic and Baldini, 1970).

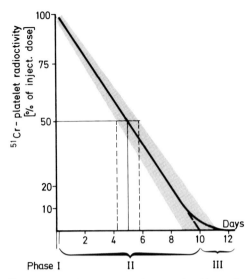

Fig. 7.7. ^{51}Cr-platelet disappearance in normal subjects showing the half-life of disappearance (T_{50}) and mean life span, estimated as the point where the nearly straight extrapolated line of platelet radioactivity crosses the abscissa. The activity of the terminal curve accounts for ~10% of the total platelet radioactivity injected.

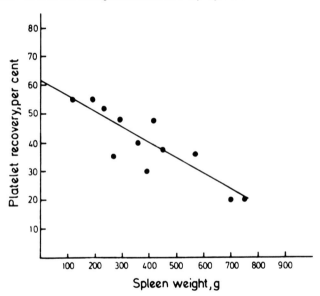

Fig. 7.8. ^{51}Cr platelet recovery in relation to spleen weight in 12 patients with Hodgkin's disease ($p < 0.001$). (Reproduced by permission from Abrahamsen, 1972.)

Even within a narrow range of spleen weights between 110 and 730 g (mean 390 g; $n = 12$), a highly significant correlation between platelet recovery and spleen weight has been described in patients with Hodgkin's disease (Fig. 8; Abrahamsen, 1972). Since the mean platelet recovery was possibly as low as 38%, in Hodgkin's disease the splenic platelet pool is especially large in proportion to the size of the spleen. Toghill and Green (1983) investigated 20 biopsy-proven cases with ^{111}In platelets: Mean platelet recovery at 1 h postinfusion was 33%, with a range of 4 to 90%, despite a relatively moderate degree of enlargement (mean 325 g, with a range of 118–893 g).

In most older patients with sickle cell anemia, the spleen becomes infarcted and atrophic, and therefore loses its platelet pool. Some subjects show a paradoxical situation, with a spleen of normal size that is unable to pool platelets.

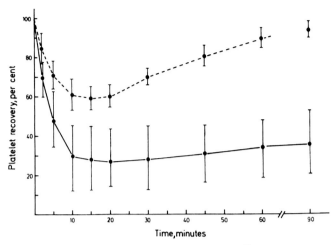

Fig. 7.9. Postinfusion clearance of autologous ^{51}Cr-platelets in 12 patients with Hodgkin's disease. Mean and range before splenectomy:——. Mean and range after splenectomy: -----. (Reproduced with permission from Abrahamsen, 1972.)

Table 7.2
Platelet Recovery in Thrombocytopenic Purpura[a]

| | | Platelet recovery (%) | | | |
| | | Presplenectomy | | Postsplenectomy | |
Authors	Platelet label	n	Mean	n	Mean
Baldini (1966)	^{51}Cr	3	(2–26)		
Solomon and Clatanoff (1967)	^{51}Cr	9	14 (3–54)		
Aster and Keene (1969)	^{51}Cr	15	42	7	93
Harker (1970)	^{51}Cr	14	61(SD 7)	7	93 (77–98)
Ries and Price (1974)	^{51}Cr	16	49 (1–75)		
Branehög (1975)	^{51}Cr	18	30 (SD 3)	18	74 (47–99)
Heyns et al. (1980a)	^{111}In	10	51 (SD 21)		
Gugliotta et al. (1981)	^{51}Cr	197	40 (SD 12)		
Schmidt and Rasmussen (1985)	^{111}In	26	46.5		
Heyns et al. (1986)	^{111}In	10	55 (SD 25)		
Total subjects and mean values:		318	41%	32	82%

[a]Results of platelet recovery are expressed as mean values for each series; in one instance (Baldini, 1966), only a range is given. In four instances, a range is available in addition to means.
SD values are given in six instances.

In the presence of splenomegaly, the splenic platelet pool may contain as much as 95% of the total platelet mass (Kotilainen et al., 1971). Consequently, a low platelet concentration in the peripheral blood may occur without a decrease in total platelet mass; in such cases, the thrombocytopenia results from maldistribution, rather than premature destruction or diminished production. However, in many instances (especially in myeloid metaplasia and the chronic leukemias), reduced platelet production also contributes to the thrombocytopenia, with an increase in the probability of serious clinical sequelae.

7.3.3. SPLENIC PLATELET POOL IN IMMUNE THROMBO-CYTOPENIC PURPURA The question of platelet pooling is of special interest in immune thrombocytopenic purpura (ITP). Table 2 presents published results of platelet recovery in ITP: As ex-

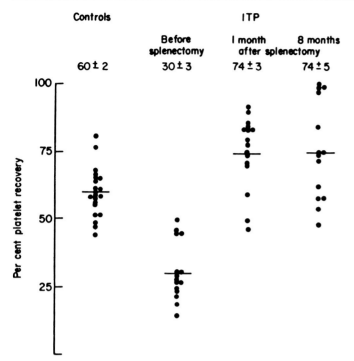

Fig. 7.10. Platelet recovery in 21 healthy controls and in ITP patients before splenectomy, 1 mo after and 8 mo after splenectomy. (Reproduced with permission from Branehög, 1975.)

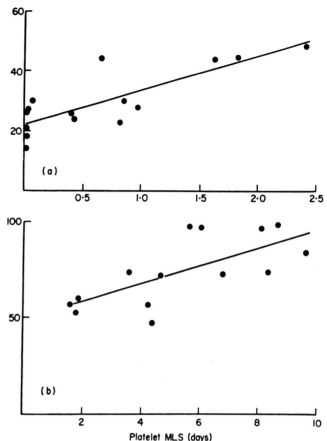

Fig. 7.11. (A) Upper panel: The relationship between platelet recovery 15 min after platelet infusion and mean platelet life-span (MLS) in nonsplenectomized patients with ITP. Ordinate: Platelet recovery as percentage of the infused platelets present in general circulation 15 min after the infusion. Abscissa: MLS in days. **(B)** Lower panel: The relationship between platelet recovery 15 min after platelet infusion and platelet MLS in patients with ITP, 8 mo after splenectomy. Ordinate and abscissa: as for upper panel (A). (Reproduced with permission from Branehög, 1975.)

pected, the majority of cases had spleens of normal size. In a few instances, studies were repeated in the same ITP patients before and after splenectomy (Branehög, 1975). The mean values for platelet recovery vary considerably in the different studies, and individual variation is high (Ries and Price, 1974). Platelet recovery and, indirectly, the splenic platelet pool, in untreated patients with ITP was considered to be normal by Harker (1970), and Ries and Price (1974) obtained a mean value of 49%, which is slightly less than than the normal, but calculated that this was not in fact significantly different from normal. In splenectomized ITP patients, the mean recovery values were found to be close to those of the post-splenectomy state in other conditions (Aster and Keene, 1969; Harker, 1970).

The results obtained by Branehög et al. (1973) were somewhat different: in six patients with ITP, they found a mean ^{51}Cr platelet recovery of 38% (with a range of 23–49%), which was significantly less than in five healthy controls (mean 59%, range 58–60). Likewise, Kutti and Weinfeld (1971a) found a higher platelet recovery in five splenectomized ITP patients (mean 80% SD 3.2, range 65–100), compared to platelet recovery in young and middle-aged normal subjects, and those with cardiovascular disorders. Branehög et al. (1973) infused adrenaline into healthy controls and ITP patients, and showed that the mean values of released, platelet-bound ^{51}Cr radioactivity for the two groups, were equal (40%), but, in nonthrombocytopenic splenomegalic patients, there was a two-fold increase in peripheral platelet radioactivity (Fig. 4).

The apparent abnormalities of splenic pooling in ITP seem most probably related to the rapid rates of destruction to which the labeled platelets are subjected (Figs. 10 and 11). Branehög (1975) demonstrated a positive relationship between recovery values and the platelet life-span, both before and after splenectomy ($r = +0.80$ and $+0.70$, respectively). Consequently, platelet recovery is probably of little value in ITP as an indirect measure of platelet pooling in

the spleen, because a steady state may not be achievable. This also vitiates dynamic and recurrent static imaging for the purpose (Peters et al., 1985).

7.3.4. SPLENIC PLATELET POOL IN MYELOPROLIFERATIVE DISORDERS
Kotilainen (1969) investigated seven patients with polycythemia vera (four with and three without a palpable spleen): Platelet recovery was found to be equal in the two groups, at 58%. Two patients with essential thrombocythemia had platelet recovery of about 44%, compared to 58% in the controls. Kutti and Weinfeld (1972) investigated 20 patients with polycythemia vera in steady-state conditions. In eight lacking a palpable spleen, the mean platelet recovery was 39%; in 12 patients with splenomegaly, it was 26%, and in 16 controls, 53%. As expected, the recoveries were inversely related to the spleen size, but appeared to be independent of the peripheral hematocrit values (Kutti and Weinfeld, 1971b). From these limited studies, platelet recovery appears to decrease even in the absence of splenomegaly.

7.3.5. SURVIVAL OF BLOOD PLATELETS
Clearly, the platelet has a special relationship to the spleen, even in normal circumstances. The molecular basis for the normal pooling phenomenon is still undefined, but a major factor in pathological platelet pool-

ing appears simply to be the total mass of the spleen, which suggests that there may be an affinity between the platelet and structural components, probably endothelium cells, the reticulum cells, and macrophages. A second factor of possible significance is the effect of pooling on platelet survival. Overtly abnormal platelets, such as those sensitized by autoantibody in ITP, can be shown to be destroyed by macrophages in the spleen and elsewhere. A related question is whether otherwise apparently normal platelets are adversely affected by prolongation of the fraction of their life-span that is spent in the environment of the enlarged spleen.

7.3.5.1. Definition and Principles Platelet survival time customarily refers to the total time spent in the blood after the platelet is delivered from the bone marrow or other site of production. The true life-span is in fact longer, because it includes the additional time spent by the platelet in the bone marrow before delivery into the peripheral blood.

Platelets obtained from circulating blood, labeled in vitro and reinjected into the circulation, are heterogeneous with respect to age and size, and their subsequent disappearance from the blood provides an estimate of the mean survival of platelets in the peripheral circulation. In vivo labeling of a cohort of platelets has also been used, but the labels available have proved to be expensive, or to have unsatisfactory physical properties. Consequently, tritiated diisopropyl fluorophosphate (Adelson et al., 1965), ^{75}Se-methionine (Burger and Schmelczer, 1973), and [35]S (Vodopick and Kniseley, 1963) are now seldom used. DF[32]P was frequently used in the period between 1955 and 1967 (Leeksma and Cohen, 1955; Pollycove et al., 1958; Zucker et al., 1961; Bithell et al., 1967; Cooney and Smith, 1968), but the label is unsatisfactory, in that it is, to some extent, reutilized. [51]Cr was, for many years, the preferred in vitro label. For human studies, it was introduced by Aas and Gardner (1958), and, since then, the method has been gradually improved and applied widely (Aster and Jandl, 1964; Abrahamsen, 1968a,b; Kotilainen, 1969; Aster, 1969; Gardner, 1972; Branehög et al., 1974; Harker, 1977). Recommendations for standardized ^{51}Cr-platelet survival studies were published by the International Committee for Standardization in Hematology in 1977, and have recently been further detailed by Snyder et al. (1986).

[111]In is now considered to be the best available platelet label (Heaton et al., 1979; Hawker et al., 1980). Subjects investigated by both ^{51}Cr and ^{111}In have shown comparable estimates of platelet survival time (PST) (Heaton et al., 1979; Schmidt et al., 1983; Schmidt et al., 1985). However, Joist and Baker (1981) showed that the loss of ^{111}In might be less than that of ^{51}Cr in antibody-induced, complement-mediated platelet injury. ^{111}In-platelet survival studies in 91 healthy subjects showed a mean platelet survival of 8.4 d.

A few nonradioisotopic techniques for the estimation of platelet survival have had limited use, in circumstances such as pregnancy (Hirsch and Gardner, 1951; Stouart et al., 1975; Wallenburg and van Kessel, 1978; Catalano et al., 1981).

7.3.5.2. Survival Curves Rate of platelet clearance from the blood can be calculated in radionuclide studies, by plotting the concentration of platelet radioactivity against time (Fig. 11). After complete early mixing (2–3 min) and equilibrated splenic pooling of the labeled platelets (up to 90 min: phase I), the disappearance curve is mainly rectilinear in arithmetic or semilogarhythmic plot (phase II), and ends in a terminal tail of 2–3 d duration (phase III). The tail probably represents the small portion of the youngest and largest of the platelets labeled, and corresponds to about 10% of the total platelet radioactivity injected.

Table 7.3
Mean Platelet Survival Time (^{111}In): Review of Results in Normal Subjects

Authors	n	Mean(days)
Heaton et al. (1979)	10	8.8 ± 0.2
Hawker et al. (1980)	4	8.4 ± 0.2
Heyns et al. (1980a)	6	9.0 ± 0.7
Robertson et al. (1981)	5	8.3 ± 0.3
Scheffel et al. (1982)	9	8.8 ± 1.1
Bautista et al. (1984)	12	8.1 – 10.4
Schmidt et al. (1985)	25	7.7 (5.9–9.4)
Hill-Zobel et al. (1986)	12	8.4 ± 0.8
Vallabhajosula et al. (1986)	8	9.5 ± 0.8
Total subjects and mean platelet life-span (d)	91	8.4

Platelet survival is often expressed as the T_{50} (Fig. 11), which is the time at which platelet radioactivity falls to 50% of the initial (maximum) platelet activity; the mean platelet survival is read as the time at which the extrapolation of the clearance curve crosses the abscissa. Mean platelet survival shows little variation between subjects, but Abrahamsen (1968a) demonstrated that platelet survival decreases with age. Kotilainen (1969) tabulated experimental results obtained up to 1968, which indicated the mean ^{51}Cr platelet survival time in healthy subjects to be 9.0 ± 0.3 d. His own work showed [51]Cr T_{50} to be 4.01 ± 0.48 d. Mean values of the survival times of the ^{111}In platelets are shown in Table 3.

7.3.5.3. Platelet Survival in ITP In ITP, most work has shown platelet survival to be much diminished, often being <1 h to ~1 d (Harker and Finch, 1969; Aster, 1971). However, many studies have not used autologous platelets, because of the difficulty of obtaining sufficient numbers from thrombocytopenic subjects, and it remains to be shown conclusively that autologous platelets behave in a manner identical to that of allogenic platelets.

Platelet production is generally estimated to be increased, sometimes to as much as 8× normal (Harker, 1970). The platelets are removed and destroyed in the reticuloendothelial system, predominantly in the spleen (Firkin et al., 1969), but also in the liver and bone marrow. Platelet clearance curves are usually linear or exponential, but they may be complex and often curvilinear, or even biphasic. If linear in an arithmetic or semilogarithmic plot, the mean survival time is read on the abscissa, where it is cut by the extrapolated disappearance curve. If the plot is curvilinear, survival is read at the point where the abscissa is cut by the extrapolated tangent to the initial slope.

Baldini (1966) demonstrated a positive correlation between the platelet count and platelet survival. Aster (1969) showed that, normally, during the 8 d in which ^{51}Cr platelets are removed from the blood, splenic radioactivity, determined by estimation at the body surface, increased by only 5%, and hepatic activity increased by 21%. Aster (1971) later demonstrated that, in moderately severe ITP, the spleen plays the dominant role in the destruction of platelets; significant hepatic destruction occurs in patients with more severe ITP, in which the platelet T_{50} is very low. That study also emphasized that body surface scanning, after the injection of ^{51}Cr platelets, relates closely to the severity of the ITP, but does not precisely predict the benefit of splenectomy. Nevertheless, other investigators have concluded that the surface pattern of the sites of

Table 7.4
Organ Localized ^{51}Cr-platelet Activity
in Patients with ITP, Who Benefited from Splenectomy

Authors	n	Spleen	Liver	Liver + spleen
		Positive results of splenectomy on thrombocytopenia in relation to site of platelet destruction		
Gehrmann and Bleifeld (1968)	50	27/31	2/9	4/10
Kotilainen (1969)	11	2/7	0/1	2/2
Seidl and Holtz (1970)	10	5/6		2/4
Najean and Ardaillou (1971)	359	90%		60%
Cooper et al. (1972)	111	78%		20%
Gugliotta et al. (1981)	197	58%	6%	17%
Total subjects	738			

nuclide uptake is a useful predictor: About 90% of 540 ITP patients with a hepatic pattern responded (Table 4). However, it is also apparent that the hepatic pattern does not preclude improvement by splenectomy; conversely, even a pronounced splenic pattern may not be followed by a good response to removal of the spleen. In general, there is a tendency for younger subjects to show a splenic pattern of platelet destruction, and these patients often respond well to corticosteroids or splenectomy.

7.3.5.4. Sequential Quantitation in Sites of Platelet Destruction When ^{111}In-labeled platelets are combined with computerized dynamic γ camera imaging, it is possible to follow the fate of ^{111}In platelets from the time of equilibrium to the end of their lifespan. Radionuclide accumulation permits platelet destruction to be followed in various organs, while the radioactivity decreases to zero both in the blood and the platelet pool. Klonizakis et al. (1980) showed, in normal subjects, that, at equilibrium, the injected ^{111}In platelet activity was distributed in blood, spleen, and liver in portions of 58, 35, and 12%, respectively (Fig. 6). Subsequently, decline of the splenic platelet pool was confirmed to be accompanied by transfer of the splenic platelet ^{111}In to the splenic reticulum cells. By sequential determination of ^{111}In, it was possible to show that, at the end of normal platelet survival, the ^{111}In activity in the spleen and liver did not differ appreciably from the values found at equilibrium, and that the bone marrow reticuloendothelial system plays a hitherto unsuspected role in platelet destruction (Klonizakis et al., 1980, 1981; Heyns et al., 1982; Heyns et al., 1982; Scheffel et al., 1982; Hill-Zobel et al., 1983; Hill-Zobel et al., 1986). In ITP, platelet destruction is accelerated, so that the circulating ^{111}In platelets have frequently disappeared from the blood within 1 d. Consequently, splenic ^{111}In activity consists, from an early stage, of a combination of activity from pooled platelets and ^{111}In platelets already destroyed (Klonizakis et al., 1981; Peters et al., 1984; Peters et al., 1985).

7.3.5.5. Platelet Survival in Cases with Splenomegaly Bleifeld (1967) investigated three splenomegalic patients with thrombocytopenia. All had normal platelet survival. De Gabriele and Penington (1967) found that values of the ^{51}Cr T_{50}, in normal, splenectomized, and splenomegalic Wistar rats, were almost identical (4.5, 4.5, and 4 d, respectively). Cooney and Smith (1968) found in 20 normal, 10 splenomegalic, and 9 splenectomized humans, that mean platelet survival times were 11.5, 8.4, and 10.3 d respectively. Aster (1969) demonstrated that the clearance rate of autologous ^{51}Cr platelets from the blood was the same in 10 healthy and

7 asplenic subjects. Kotilainen (1969) found that the autologous ^{51}Cr T_{50} values were lower in six patients with congestive splenomegaly (2.8 d) and in eight with proliferative splenomegaly (2.5 d), compared with the 4.0 d in 10 healthy individuals. Harker (1971, 1977) found the ^{51}Cr T_{50} to be 4.8 d in normal and asplenic subjects, and slightly shorter in splenomegalics (4.4 d). Kummer and Bucher (1971) investigated 23 splenomegalic patients, and concluded that the size of the splenic platelet pool did not influence the ^{51}Cr- survival time. Abrahamsen (1972) studied the ^{51}Cr T_{50} before and after splenectomy in 10 patients with Hodgkin's disease: mean value was 3.2 d in both instances, which was lower than normal. Kutti and Weinfeld (1972) found a slightly reduced ^{51}Cr platelet survival time in 14 patients with polycythemia vera and splenomegaly (4.6 d). Eight patients without splenomegaly showed a mean platelet survival of 5.3 d, compared to 6.4 d in 16 healthy men matched in age. Toghill and Green (1983) found 12/20 patients with chronic liver disease to have a reduced ^{111}In platelet mean survival. Bautista et al. (1984) demonstrated that 11 patients with primary, and 5 with secondary, thrombocythemia had mean ^{111}In platelet life-spans that were significantly decreased by comparison with normal values. Schmidt et al. (1985) demonstrated a shortened ^{111}In platelet mean survival (5.6 d) in 16 patients with various hepatic disorders with splenomegaly and secondary thrombocytopenia, compared to an age-matched normal value of 7.7 d. Hill- Zobel et al. (1986) found a mean ^{111}In platelet survival of 8.4 d for normals, 9.2 d for asplenic subjects, and 6.2 d for splenomegalics.

In conclusion it appears that platelet mean survival time was, for a considerable period, found to be nearly identical in normal subjects, individuals with splenomegaly, and after splenectomy. However, results of later studies have shown convincing evidence that, in the presence of splenomegaly, the platelet survival time is significantly reduced. The pathogenesis of the thrombocytopenia, which so often accompanies splenomegaly, is complex: The distributional effect of the increased splenic platelet pool is usually the major factor; a reduced platelet survival time plays a lesser and less frequent role. In some cases, reduced platelet production is an additional etiological factor.

7.4. GRANULOCYTE POOLING IN THE SPLEEN

The third form of cytopenia associated with disorders of the spleen is granulopenia: there is strong evidence for the spleen being the site of significant granulocyte pooling (Peters et al., 1985; Allsop et al., 1992). It also appears that the total circulating granulocyte pool declines with enlargement of the spleen (Bishop et al., 1971; Dresch, 1975); the marginating pool of granulocytes is reduced in asplenic subjects (Brubaker and Johnson, 1978).

Studies with nuclide-labeled granulocytes have shown that intravenous adrenaline leads to a simultaneous fall in the granulocyte population of the spleen and an increase in circulating granulocyte numbers (McMillan and Scott, 1968). Similar effects have also been demonstrated for granulocytes, as well as for red blood cells and platelets, after the stimulus of severe physical exercise, the changes in the populations of red blood cells being much more rapid than with the platelets and granulocytes (Allsop et al., 1992). Adrenaline, given into the splenic artery, produces an increase in the granulocyte count of arterial blood, and later in hepatic vein blood (Bierman et al., 1953). Peters et al. (1985) have studied granulocytes labeled with ^{111}In-tropolonate, and introduced into the circulation. Hepatic uptake of labeled granulocytes rapidly reaches a plateau; splenic uptake is in slow monoexponential form, and requires 20–40 min to reach a plateau. The activity curves were consistent with a dynamically exchanging splenic pool, with an intrasplenic transit time of 9.3 ± SE 0.6 min.

The splenic granulocyte pool has often been described as a major component of the marginating granulocyte pool (Athens et al., 1961; Fieschi and Sacchetti, 1964; Scott et al., 1971). However, Peters (1997) has observed that "margination," as usually understood, appears to have the characteristics of a pathological process: The tendency of part of the intravascular granulocyte population to roll along the endothelial surface is dependent on endothelial adhesion molecules, such as E-selectin (Chapman and Haskard, 1995), essentially in areas of inflammation.

Nevertheless, labeled granulocyte studies confirm that there are physiological granulocyte pools in specific organs, comparable to those described for platelets. Although especially prominent in the spleen, they are also present in the liver and bone marrow. The pool turnover time appears to be accelerated in inflammatory disease, and Loreal et al. (1990) have used this property as a means to assess the activity of inflammatory bowel disease.

REFERENCES

Aas, K. and Gardner, F. H. (1958) Survival of blood platelets labeled with chromium-51. *J. Clin. Invest.* **37,** 1257–1268.

Abrahamsen, A. F. (1968a) Survival of 51Cr-labelled human platelets. Methodological and clinical studies. *Scand. J. Haematol.* **5(Suppl. 3),** 9–53.

Abrahamsen, A. F. (1968b) A modification of the technique of 51Cr labelling of blood platelets giving increased circulating platelet radioactivity. *Scand. J. Haematol.* **5,** 53–63.

Abrahamsen, A. F. (1970) Platelet survival in Hodgkin's disease. *Scand. J. Haematol.* **7,** 309–313.

Abrahamsen, A. F. (1972) Effects of an enlarged splenic platelet pool in Hodgkins's disease. *Scand. J. Haematol.* **9,** 153–158.

Adelson, E., Kaufman, R. M., Berdeguez, C., Lear, A. A., and Rheingold, J. J. (1965) Platelet tagging with tritium labeled diisopropyl fluorophosphate. *Blood* **26,** 744–750.

Allsop, P., Peters, A.M., Arnot, R. N., et al. (1992) Intrasplenic blood cell kinetics in man before and after brief maximal exercise. *Clin. Sci.* **83,** 47–54.

Aster, R. H. (1965) Splenic platelet pooling as a cause of "hypersplenic" thrombocytopenia. *Trans. Assoc. Am. Physicians* **78,** 362–373.

Aster, R. H. (1966) Pooling of platelets in the spleen: role in the pathogenesis of "hypersplenic" thrombocytopenia. *J. Clin. Invest.* **45,** 645–647.

Aster, R. H. (1967) Studies of the mechanism of "hypersplenic" thrombocytopenia in rats. *J. Lab. Clin. Med.* **70,** 736–751.

Aster, R. H. (1969) Studies of the fate of platelets in rats and man. *Blood* **34,** 117–128.

Aster, R. H. (1971) Sites of platelet destruction in ITP. In: *Platelet Kinetics* (Paulus, J. M., ed.), North-Holland, Amsterdam, pp. 268–273.

Aster, R. H. and Jandl, J. H. (1964) Platelet sequestration in man. I. Methods. *J. Clin. Invest.* **43,** 843–855.

Aster, R. H. and Keene, W. R. (1969) Sites of platelet destruction in idiopathic thrombocytopenic purpura. *Br. J. Haematol.* **16,** 61–73.

Athens, J. W., Haab, O. P., Raab, S. O., et al. (1961) Leukokinetic Studies. IV. The total blood, circulating and marginal granulocyte pools and the granulocyte turnover rate in normal subjects. *J. Clin. Invest.* **40,** 989–995.

Baldini, M. (1966) Idiopathic thrombocytopenic purpura. *N. Engl. J. Med.* **274,** 1245–1251.

Bautista, A. P., Buckler, P. W., Towler, H. M., Dawson, A. A., and Bennett, B. (1984) Measurement of platelet life-span in normal subjects and patients with myeloproliferative disease with indium oxine labelled platelets. *Br. J. Haematol.* **58,** 679–687.

Bierman, H. R., Byron, R. L., and Kelly, K. H. (1953) The role of the spleen in the leukocytosis following the intra-arterial administration of epinephrine. *Blood* **8,** 153–164.

Binet, L. and Kaplan, M. (1923) Mobilization des plaquettes par l'adrenaline. Plaquettose par spleno-contraction adrenalinique. *Compt. Rend. Soc. Biol.* **97,** 1659,1660.

Bishop, C. R., Rothstein, G., Ashenbrucker, H. E., and Athens, J. W. (1971) Leukokinetic studies. XIV. Blood neutrophil kinetics in chronic, steady-state neutropenia. *J. Clin. Invest.* **50,** 1678–1689.

Bithell, T. C., Athens, J. W., Cartwright, G. E., and Wintrobe, M. M. (1967) Radioactive diisopropyl fluorophosphate as a platelet label: an evaluation of in vitro and in vivo technics. *Blood* **29,** 354–372.

Björkman, S. E. (1946) The splenic circulation with special reference to the function of the spleen sinus wall. *Acta Med. Scand.* **128(Suppl. 191),** 7–97.

Bleifeld, W. (1967) Pathogeneses der Thrombozytopenie beim Hypersplenismus. *Dtsch. Med. Wochenschr.* **92,** 2149–2154.

Bowdler, A. J. (1962) Theoretical considerations concerning measurement of the splenic red cell pool. *Clin. Sci.* **23,** 181–195.

Bowdler, A. J. (1963) Dilution anemia corrected by splenectomy in Gaucher's disease. *Ann. Int. Med.* **58,** 664–669.

Bowdler, A. J. (1966) *Annals of Internal Medicine* **65,** 763.

Bowdler, A. J. (1969) Regional variations in the proportion of red cells in the blood in man. *Br. J. Hematol.* **16,** 557–571.

Bowdler, A. J. (1983) Splenomegaly and hypersplenism. *Clin. Haematol.* **12,** 467–488.

Branehög, I. (1975) Platelet kinetics in idiopathic thrombocytopenic purpura (ITP) before and at different times after splenectomy. *Br. J. Haematol.* **29,** 413–426.

Branehög, I., Kutti, J., and Weinfeld, A. (1974) Platelet survival and platelet production in idiopathic thrombocytopenic purpura (ITP). *Br. J. Haematol.* **27,** 127–143.

Branehög, I., Weinfeld, A., and Roos, B. (1973) The exchangeable splenic platelet pool studied with epinephrine infusion in idiopathic thrombocytopenic purpura and in patients with splenomegaly. *Br. J. Haematol.* **25,** 239–248.

Brubaker, L. H. and Johnson, C. A. (1978) Correlation of splenomegaly and abnormal neutrophil pooling (margination). *J. Lab. Clin. Med.* **92,** 508–515.

Burger, T. and Schmelczer, M. (1973) Comparative study of platelet kinetics with 75Se-methionine and 51Cr in ITP and congestive splenomegaly. *Folia Haematol.* **100,** 278–289.

Catalano, P. M., Smith, J. B., and Murphy, S. (1981) Platelet recovery from aspirin inhibition in vivo: differing patterns under various assay conditions. *Blood* **57,** 99–105.

Chapman, P. T. and Haskard, D. O. (1995) Leukocyte adhesion molecules. *Br. Med. Bull.* **51,** 296–311.

Christensen, B. E. (1971) A new method for estimating splenic erythrocyte and plasma volumes combined with quantitation of splenic iron incorporation. *Scand. J. Haematol.* **8,** 245–249.

Christensen, B. E. (1973) Erythrocyte pooling and sequestration in enlarged spleens. Estimations of splenic erythrocyte and plasma volume in splenomegalic patients. *Scand. J. Haematol.* **10,** 106–119.

Christensen, B. E. (1975) Red cell kinetics. *Clin. Haematol.* **4,** 393–405.

Cooney, D. P. and Smith, B. Z. (1968) The pathophysiology of hypersplenic thrombocytopenia. *Arch. Intern. Med.* **121,** 332–337.

Cooper, M. R., Hansen, K. S., Maynard, C. D., Elrod, I. W., and Spurr, C. L. (1972) Platelet survival and sequestration patterns in thrombocytopenic disorders. *Radiology* **102,** 89–100.

Dameshek, W. (1955) Hypersplenism. *Bull NY Acad. Med.* **31,** 113–126.

Dameshek, W. and Estren, I. (1947) *The Spleen and Hypersplenism.* Grune and Stratton, New York.

Danpure, H. J., Osman, S., and Brady, F. (1982) The labelling of blood cells in plasma with 111In-tropolonate. *Br. J. Radiol.* **55,** 247–249.

Dawson, A. A. and Ogston, D. (1969) Exercise-induced thrombocytosis. *Acta Haematol. (Basel)* **42,** 241–246.

DeGabriele, G. and Penington, D. G. (1967) Regulation of platelet production: "hypersplenism" in the experimental animal. *Br. J. Haematol.* **13,** 384–393.

Doan, C. A. (1949) Hypersplenism. *Bull. NY Acad. Med.* **25,** 625–650.

Doan, C. A. and Wright, C. T. (1946) Primary congenital and secondary acquired splenic panhematopenia. *Blood* **1,** 10–26.

Dresch, C., Najean, Y., and Bauchet, J. (1975) Kinetic studies of ^{51}Cr and DF^{32}P labelled granulocytes. *Br. J. Haematol.* **29,** 67–80.

Ferrant, A. (1983) The role of the spleen in hemolysis. *Clin. Haematol.* **12,** 489–504.

Fieschi, A. and Sacchetti, C. (1964) Clinical assessment of granulopoie-sis. *Acta Haematol. (Basel)* **31,** 150–162.

Firkin, B. G., Wright, R., Miller, S., and Stokes, E. (1969) Splenic macro-phages in thrombocytopenia. *Blood* **33,** 240–245.

Fredén, K., Lundborg, P., Vilén, L., and Kutti, J. (1978) The peripheral platelet count in response to adrenergic alpha- and beta-1-receptor stimulation. *Scand. J. Haematol.* **21,** 427–432.

Fredén, K., Olsson, L. B., Suurkula, M., and Kutti, J. (1978) The exchang-eable platelet pool in response to intravenous infusion of isoprena-line. *Scand. J. Haematol.* **20,** 335–340.

Freedman, M. L. and Karpatkin, S. (1975a) Heterogeneity of rabbit plate-lets. IV. Thrombocytosis with absolute megathrombocytosis in phe-nylhydrazine-induced hemolytic anemia in rabbits. *Thromb. Diath. Hemorrh.* **33,** 335–340.

Freedman, M. and Karpatkin, S. (1975b) Heterogeneity of rabbit plate-lets. V. Preferential splenic sequestration of megathrombocytes. *Br. J. Haematol.* **31,** 255–262.

Freedman, M., Altszuler, N., and Karpatkin, S. (1977) Presence of a non-splenic platelet pool. *Blood* **50,** 419–425.

Gardner, F. H. (1972) Platelet kinetics and life span. *Clin. Haematol.* **1,** 307–324.

Gehrmann, G. and Bleifeld, W. (1968) Lebensdauer und abbauort men-schlicher Thrombozyten bei unterschiedlichen Thrombopenieformen. *Blut* **17,** 266–275.

Gehrmann, G. and Elbers, C. (1970) Thrombopenischer Hypersplenie-syndrom. *Dtsch. Med. Wochenschr.* **95,** 1429–1432.

Glass, H. T., De Garreta, A. C., Lewis, S. M., Grammaticos, P., and Szur, L. (1968) Measurement of splenic red-blood-cell mass with radio-active carbon monoxide. *Lancet* **1,** 669–670.

Gray, S. J. and Sterling, K. (1950) Tagging of red cells and plasma pro-teins with radioactive chromium. *J. Clin. Invest.* **29,** 1604–1613.

Gugliotta, L, Isacchi, G., Guarini, A., Ciccone, F., Motta, M. R., Lattarini, C., et al. (1981) Chronic idiopathic thrombocytopenic purpura (ITP): site of platelet sequestration and results of splenectomy. A study of 197 patients. *Scand. J. Haematol.* **26,** 407–412.

Harker, L. A. (1969) Platelet kinetics in splenomegaly. *Blood* **34,** 528 (Abstr.).

Harker, L. A. (1970) Thrombokinetics in idiopathic thrombocytopenic purpura. *Br. J. Haematol.* **19,** 95–104.

Harker, L. A. (1971) The role of the spleen in thrombokinetics. *J. Lab. Clin. Med.* **77,** 247–253.

Harker, L. A. (1977) The kinetics of platelet production and destruction in man. *Clin. Haematol.* **6,** 671–693.

Harker, L. A. and Finch, C. A. (1969) Thrombokinetics in man. *J. Clin. Invest.* **48,** 963–974.

Harris, I. M., McAlister, J. M., and Prankerd, T. A. J. (1958) Splenom-egaly and the circulating red cell. *Br. J. Haematol.* **4,** 97–102.

Hawker, R. J., Hawker, L. M., and Wilkinson, A. R. (1980) Indium (111In)-labelled human platelets: optimal method. *Clin. Sci.* **58,** 243–248.

Heaton, W. A., Davis, H. H., Welch, M. J., et al. (1979) Indium-111: a new radionuclide label for studying human platelet kinetics. *Br. J. Haematol.* **42,** 613–622.

Heyns, A. D., Lotter, M. G., Badenhorst, P. N., van Reenen, O. R., Pieters, H., Minnaar, P. C., and Retief, F. P. (1980a) Kinetics, distribution and sites of destruction of 111Indium-labelled human platelets. *Br. J. Haematol.* **44,** 269–280.

Heyns, A. D., Lotter, M. G., Badenhorst, P. N., et al. (1980b) Kinetics and fate of (111)Indium-oxine labelled blood platelets in asplenic sub-jects. *Thromb. Hemost.* **44,** 100–104.

Heyns, A. D., Lotter, M. G., Badenhorst, P. N., de Kock, F., Pieters, H., Herbst, C., et al. (1982) Kinetics and sites of destruction of 111In-dium-oxine labelled platelets in idiopathic thrombocytopenic pur-pura. A quantitative study. *Am. J. Hematol.* **12,** 167–177.

Heyns, A. D., Lotter, M. G., Kotze, H. F., Pieters, H., and Wessels, P. (1982) Quantification of in vivo distribution of platelets labelled with Indium-111-oxine. *J. Nucl. Med.* **23,** 943–944.

Heyns, A. du P., Badenhorst, P. N., Lotter, M. G., Pieters, H., Wessels, P., and Kotze, H. F. (1986) Platelet turnover and kinetics in immune thrombocytopenic purpura: results with autologous 111In-labeled platelets and homologous 51Cr-labeled platelets differ. *Blood* **67,** 86–92.

Hill-Zobel, R. L., Scheffel, U., McIntyre, P. A., and Tsan, M. F. (1983) 111In-oxine-labeled rabbit platelets: in vivo distribution and sites of destruction. *Blood* **61,** 149–153.

Hill-Zobel, R. L., McCandless, B., Kang, S. A., Chikkappa, G., and Tsan, M. F. (1986) Organ distribution and fate of human platelets: studies of asplenic and splenomegalic patients. *Am. J. Hematol.* **23,** 231–238.

Hirsch, E. O. and Gardner, F. H. (1951) The life span of transfused human blood platelets. *J. Clin. Invest.* **30,** 649–650.

International Committee for Standardization in Hematology (1977) Rec-ommended methods for radioisotope platelet survival studies. *Blood* **50,** 1137–1144.

Jandl, J. H. and Aster, R. H. (1967) Increased splenic pooling and the pathogenesis of hypersplenism. *Am. J. Med. Sci.* **253,** 383–397.

Joist, J. H. and Baker, R. H. (1981) Loss of 111Indium as indicator of platelet injury. *Blood* **58,** 350–353.

Karpatkin, S. (1983) The spleen and thrombocytopenia. *Clin. Haematol.* **12,** 591–604.

Kiefel, V., Becker, T., Mueller-Eckhardt, G., Grebe, S., and Mueller-Eckhardt, C. (1985) Platelet survival determined with 51Cr versus 111In. *Klin. Wochenschr.* **63,** 84–89.

Klonizakis, I., Peters, A. M., Fitzpatrick, M. L., Kensett, M. J., Lewis, S. M., and Lavender, J. P. (1980) Radionuclide distribution following injection of 111Indium-labelled platelets. *Br. J. Haematol.* **46,** 595–602.

Klonizakis, I., Peters, A. M., Fitzpatrick, M. L., Kensett, M. J., Lewis, S. M., and Lavender, J. P. (1981) Spleen function and platelet kinetics. *J. Clin. Pathol.* **34,** 377–380.

Kotilainen, M. (1969) Platelet kinetics in normal subjects and in hae-matological disorders; with special reference to thrombocytopenia and to the role of the spleen. *Scand. J. Haematol.* **6(Suppl. 5),** 9–97.

Kotilainen, M., Harker, L. A., and Aster, R. H. (1971) Increased platelet pooling. In: *Platelet Kinetics* (Paulus, J. M., ed.), North-Holland, Amsterdam, pp. 300–306.

Kummer, H. and Bucher, U. (1971) Thrombokinetik. Einführung Klini-sche Anvendung. *Schw. Med. Wochenschr.* **101,** 1520–1524.

Kutti, J. and Safai-Kutti, S. (1985) In vitro labelling of platelets: an experimental study in healthy asplenic subjects using two different incubation media. *Br. J. Haematol.* **31,** 57–64.

Kutti, J. and Weinfeld, A. (1971a) Platelet survival in man. *Scand. J. Haematol.* **8,** 336–346.

Kutti, J. and Weinfeld, A. (1971b) Platelet survival in active polycythe-mia vera with reference to the hematocrit level. *Scand. J. Haematol.* **8,** 405–414.

Kutti, J. and Weinfeld, A. (1972) Platelet production and platelet sur-vival in polycythemia vera with special reference to the spleen size. *Scand. J. Haematol.* **9,** 97–105.

Kutti, J., Weinfeld, A., and Westin, J. (1972) The relationship between splenic platelet pool and spleen size. *Scand. J. Haematol.* **9,** 351–354.

Kutti, J., Fredén, K., Melberg, P. E., and Lundborg, P. (1977) The ex-changeable splenic platelet pool in response to selective adrenergic beta-I-receptor blockade. *Br. J. Haematol.* **37,** 277–282.

Leeksma, C. H. W. and Cohen, J. A. (1955) Determination of the life of human blood platelets using labelled diisopropylfluorophosphate. *Nature* **175,** 552,553.

Loreal, O., Moisan, A., Bretagne, J. F., et al. (1990) Scintigraphic assess-ment of indium-111-labeled granulocyte splenic pooling: a new ap-proach to inflammatory bowel disease activity. *J. Nucl. Med.* **31,** 1470–1473.

McAfee, J. G. and Thakur, M. D. (1976) Survey of radioactive agents for in-vitro labelling of phagocytic leukocytes. I. Soluble agents. *J. Nucl. Med.* **17,** 480–487.

McMillan, R. and Scott, J. L. (1968) Leukocyte labeling with [51]chromium. Technique and results in normals. *Blood* **32,** 738–754.

Mollison, P. L., Engelfriet, C. P., and Contreras, M. (1987) *Blood Transfusion in Clinical Medicine,* 8th ed. Blackwell, Oxford, pp. 80–94.

Motulsky, A. G., Casserd, F., Giblett, E. R., Broun, G. O., and Finch, C. A. (1958) Anemia and the spleen. *N. Engl. J. Med.* **259,** 1164–1169, and 1215–1219.

Murphy, J. R. (1967) The influence of pH and temperature on some physical properties of normal erythrocytes and erythrocytes from patients with hereditary spherocytosis. *J. Lab. Clin. Med.* **69,** 758–775.

Najean, Y. and Ardaillou, N. (1971) The sequestration site of platelets in idiopathic thrombocytopenic purpura: its correlation with the results of splenectomy. *Br. J. Haematol.* **21,** 153–164.

Olsson, L.-B., Kutti, J., Lundborg, P., and Fredén, K. (1976) The peripheral platelet count in response to intravenous infusion of isoprenaline. *Scand. J. Haematol.* **17,** 213–216.

Pearson, H. A., Spencer, R. P., and Cornelius, E. A. (1969) Functional asplenia in sickle cell anemia. *N. Eng. J. Med.* **281,** 923–926.

Penny R., Rozenberg, M. C., and Firkin, B. G. (1966) The splenic platelet pool. *Blood* **27,** 1–16.

Peters, A. M. (1997) Just how big is the pulmonary granulocyte pool? *Clin. Sci.* **94,** 7–19.

Peters, A. M. and Lavender, J. P. (1982) Factors controlling the intrasplenic transit of platelets. *Eur. J. Clin. Invest.* **12,** 191–195.

Peters, A. M. and Lavender, J. P. (1983) Platelet kinetics with Indium-111 platelets: comparison with chromium-51 platelets. *Semin. Thromb. Hemost.* **9,** 100–114.

Peters, A. M., Saverymuttu, S. H., Wonke, B., Lewis, S. M., and Lavender, J. P. (1984) The interpretation of platelet kinetic studies for the identification of sites of abnormal platelet destruction. *Br. J. Haematol.* **57,** 637–649.

Peters, A. M., Saverymuttu, S. H., Keshavarzian, A., Bell, R. N., and Lavender, J. P. (1985a) Splenic pooling of granulocytes. *Clin. Sci.* **68,** 283–289.

Peters, A. M., Saverymuttu, S. H., Bell, R. N., and Lavender, J. P. (1985b) The kinetics of short-lived Indium-111 radio-labelled platelets. *Scand. J. Haematol.* **34,** 137–145.

Pollycove, M., Dal Santo, G., and Lawrence, J. H. (1958) Simultaneous measurements of erythrocyte, leukocyte, and platelet survival in normal subjects with diisopropylfluorophosphate (DFP32). *Clin. Res.* **6,** 45–6(Abstr.).

Rasmussen, J. W., Christensen, B. E., Holm, H. H., Kardel, T., Stigsby, B., and Larsen, M. (1973) Spleen volume determination by ultrasonic scanning. *Scand. J. Haematol.* **10,** 298–304.

Ries, C.A. and Price, D. C. (1974) [51Cr] platelet kinetics in thrombocytopenia. Correlation between splenic sequestration of platelets and response to splenectomy. *Ann. Intern. Med.* **80,** 702–707.

Robertson, J. S., Dewanjee, M. K., Brown, M. L., Fuster, V., and Casebro, J. H. (1981) Distribution and dosimetry of 111In-labelled platelets. *Radiology* **140,** 169–176.

Rolovic, Z. and Baldini, M. (1970) Megakaryocytopoiesis in splenectomized and "hypersplenic" rats. *Br. J. Haematol.* **18,** 257–268.

Sarajas, H. S. S., Konttinen, A., and Frick, M. H. (1961) Thrombocytosis evoked by exercise. *Nature* **192,** 721–722.

Schaffner, A., Augustini, N., Otto, R. C., and Fehr, J. (1985) The hypersplenic spleen. A contractile reservoir of granulocytes and platelets. *Arch. Int. Med.* **145,** 651–654.

Scheffel, U., Tsan, M. F., Mitchell, T. G., Camargo, E. E., Braine, H., Ezekowitz, M. D., et al. (1982) Human platelets labeled with IN-111-8-hydroxyquinoline: kinetics, distribution, and estimates of radiation dose. *J. Nucl. Med.* **23,** 149–156.

Schlichter, S. J. and Harker, L. A. (1976) Preparation and storage of platelet concentrates. I. Factors influencing the harvest of viable platelets from whole blood. *Br. J. Haematol.* **34,** 395–402.

Schmidt, K. G. and Rasmussen, J. W. (1984) Exercise-induced changes in the in vivo distribution of 111In-labelled platelets. *Scand. J. Haematol.* **32,** 159–166.

Schmidt, K. G. and Rasmussen, J. W. (1985) Kinetics and distribution in the vivo of 111In-labelled autologous platelets in idiopathic thrombocytopenic purpura. *Scand. J. Haematol.* **34,** 47–56.

Schmidt, K. G., Rasmussen, J. W., and Rasmussen, A. D. (1985) Kinetics of 111In-labelled platelets in healthy subjects. *Scand. J. Haematol.* **34,** 370–377.

Schmidt, K. G., Rasmussen, J. W., Rasmussen, A. D., and Arendrup, H. (1983a) Comparative studies of in vivo kinetics of simultaneously injected 111In-and 51Cr-labelled human platelets. *Scand. J. Haematol.* **30,** 465–478.

Schmidt, K. G., Rasmussen, J. W., Rasmussen, A. D., Arendrup, H., and Lorenzen, M. (1983b) Comparative studies of the function and morphology of 111In- and 51Cr-labelled human platelets. *Scand. J. Haematol.* **31,** 69–77.

Schmidt, K. G., Rasmussen, J. W., Bekker, C., and Madsen, P. E. (1985) Kinetics and in vivo distribution of 111In-labelled autologous platelets in chronic hepatic disease: mechanisms of thrombocytopenia. *Scand. J. Haematol.* **34,** 39–46.

Schwartz, A. D. (1972) The platelet reservoir in sickle cell anemia. *Blood* **40,** 678–683.

Scott, J. L., McMillan, R., Davidson, J. G., and Marino, J. V. (1971) Leukocyte labelling with 51-Chromium. II. Leukocyte kinetics in chronic myelocytic leukemia. *Blood* **38,** 162–173.

Seidl, S. and Holtz, G. (1970) Bestimmung der Thrombozyten-Uberlebenszeit und Oberflächenaktivität bei Patienten mit idiopatisch thrombopenischer Purpura. *Dtsch. Med. Wochenschr.* **95,** 266–275.

Shulman, N. R., Weinrach, R. S., Libre, E. P., and Andrews, H. L. (1965) The role of the reticuloendothelial system in the pathogenesis of idiopathic thrombocytopenic purpura. *Trans. Assoc. Am. Physicians* **78,** 374–390.

Shulman, N. R., Watkins, S. P. Jr., Itscoitz, S. B., and Students, A. B. (1968) Evidence that the spleen retains the youngest and hemostatically most effective platelets. *Trans. Assoc. Am. Physicians* **81,** 302–313.

Snyder, E. L., Moroff, G., Simon, T., and Heaton, A. (1986) Recommended methods for conducting radiolabeled platelet survival studies. *Transfusion* **26,** 37–42.

Solomon, A. K. (1953) The kinetics of biological processes. Special problems connected with the use of tracers. In: *Advances in Biological and Medical Physics, III* (Lawrence, J. H. and Tobias, C. A., eds.), Academic, New York, pp. 65–75.

Solomon, R. B. and Clatanoff, D. V. (1967) Platelet survival studies and body scanning in idiopathic thrombocytopenic purpura. *Am. J. Med. Sci.* **254,** 777–784.

Stouart, M. J., Murphy, S., and Oski, F. A. (1975) A simple nonradioisotopic technic for the determination of platelet life-span. *N. Engl. J. Med.* **292,** 1310–1313.

Stutte, H. J. (1970) Pathologische Anatomie der roten Milzpulpa. Quantitative Analyse mit fermentcytochemischen Methoden. In: *Die Milz* (Lennart, K. and Harms, D., eds.), Springer Verlag, Berlin, pp. 53–56.

Toghill, P. J. (1964) Red cell pooling in enlarged spleens. *Br. J. Haematol.* **10,** 347–357.

Toghill, P. J. and Green, S. (1973) Factors influencing red cell pooling of erythrocytes in the myelo- and lympho-proliferative syndromes. *Acta Haematol. (Basel)* **49,** 215–222.

Toghill, P. J. and Green, S. (1983). Platelet dynamics in chronic liver disease using the 111In-oxine label. *Gut* **24,** 49–52.

Vallabhajosula, S. Machac, J., Goldsmith, S. J., et al. (1986) Indium-111 platelet kinetics in normal human subjects: tropolone versus oxine methods. *J. Nucl. Med.* **27,** 1669–1674.

Vilén, L., Fredén, K., and Kutti, J. (1980) Presence of a non-splenic platelet pool in man. *Scand. J. Haematol.* **24,** 137–141.

Vodopick, H. A. and Kniseley, R. M. (1963) Sulfur-35 studies in man: platelet survival and urinary radioactivity assayed by beta liquid scintillation spectrometry. *J. Lab. Clin. Med.* **62,** 109–120.

Wallenburg, H. S. C. and van Kessel, P. H. (1978) Platelet lifespan in normal pregnancy as determined by nonradioisotopic technique. *Br. J. Obstet. Gynecol.* **85,** 33–36.

Watson, H. H. K. and Ludlam, C. A. (1986) Survival of 111-Indium platelet subpopulations of varying density in normal and postsplenectomized subjects. *Br. J. Haematol.* **62,** 117–124.

Weed, R. I. and Bowdler, A. J. (1966) Metabolic dependence of the critical hemolytic volume of human erythrocytes: relationship to osmotic fragility and autohemolysis in hereditary spherocytosis and normal red cells. *J. Clin. Invest.* **45,** 1137–1149.

Wessels, P., Heyns, A. D., Pieters, H., Lotter, M. D., and Badenhorst, P. N. (1985) An improved method for the quantification of the in vivo kinetics of a representative population of 111In-labelled human platelets. *Eur. J. Nucl. Med.* **10,** 522–527.

Weiss, L. (1974) A scanning electron microscopic study of the spleen. *Blood* **43,** 665–691.

Wichmann, H. E. and Gerhardts, M. D. (1981) Platelet survival curves in man considering the splenic pool. *J. Theor. Biol.* **88,** 83–101.

Wright, C.-S., Doan, C. A., Bouroncle, B. A., and Zollinger, R. M. (1951) Direct splenic arterial and venous blood studies in the hypersplenic syndrome before and after epinephrine. *Blood* **6,** 195–212.

Zucker, M. D., Ley, A. B., and Mayer, K. (1961) Studies on platelet lifespan and platelet depots by use of DFP32. *J. Lab. Clin. Med.* **58,** 405–416.

8 Dilutional Anemia

Abnormalities of Blood Volume in Disorders of the Spleen*

ANTHONY J. BOWDLER, MD, PhD, FRCP, FRCPATH, FACP
AND FRANK GARY RENSHAW, DO

8.1. INTRODUCTION

The major components of blood volume are the red cell mass (RCM) and plasma volume (PV), which adapt responsively to a variety of demands. Very short-term stresses, such as hemorrhage and hypoxia, can be met by temporary volume shifts in the circulation, from the "autologous splanchnic blood bank," and by transmural capillary fluid exchange (Isbister, 1997). Longer-term requirements are often met by variation in the circulating volumes of red blood cells and plasma. For a normal individual, the former is the more stable, and is governed by the need for oxygen transport; plasma volume is more labile, and, in teleological terms, it changes according to the need to maintain blood pressure and to fill the vascular space. The mechanisms whereby normal control of volume is achieved are therefore different for the two components. Of clinical importance is the fact that anemia, defined as a hemoglobin or hematocrit level less than that normal for the sex and age of the individual, may result either from a decrease in RCM or an increase in plasma volume, or from a combination of both effects.

8.1.1. ANEMIA AND THE SPLEEN Conditions associated with enlargement of the spleen are frequently accompanied by anemia, contributing to which are several distinct mechanisms varying in importance, depending on the etiology of the splenomegaly. The anemia is often polyfactorial. The principal factors are summarized in Table 1.

Spleen-dependent hemolysis occurs with shortened red blood cell survival, often in well-defined syndromes, which may be corrected or improved by splenectomy. These are discussed in more detail in Chapters 2, 7, and 12, and are also extensively covered elsewhere (McFadzean et al., 1958a; Prankerd, 1963; Pryor, 1967a; Richmond et al., 1967). Less-severe shortening of red blood cell life-span is also a common finding in the presence of splenomegaly, of a degree insufficient to produce anemia if the normal compensatory capacity of erythropoiesis were intact (splenopathic anemia).

Impaired or ineffective erythropoiesis is frequently found in conditions showing enlargement of the spleen, but this usually results from a co-morbidity, such as myelophthisic or infiltrative impairment of marrow function, rather than as a secondary consequence of the specific disorder of the spleen; in other cases, an impaired compensatory bone marrow responsiveness results from hepatocellular dysfunction or folate deficiency. Consequently, there is diminished output of red blood cells and relatively poor compensation for red blood cell loss by hemorrhage and hemolysis.

Splenic red blood cell pooling (*see* Chapter 7) occurs in many conditions with splenomegaly, and consequently may result in a significant diversion of red blood cells from the general circulation, which is especially significant when total red blood cell production is limited (Harris et al., 1958; Motulsky et al., 1958; Bowdler, 1962; Prankerd, 1963; Toghill, 1964; McFadzean and Todd, 1967; Pryor, 1967a).

Expansion of plasma volume is, overall, the commonest factor contributing to anemia in the presence of an enlarged spleen, and results in what is essentially a dilutional anemia: it is to be distinguished from the simple volume expansion that occurs as a reactive compensation for a reduction in RCM, and is usually considerably in excess of the volume required for simple compensation. Consequently, the total blood volume is usually increased above normal. Reviews of the phenomenon include those of Hess et al. (1976), Videbaek et al. (1982), and Bowdler (1983). This chapter further examines the evidence for this, the mechanisms by which it is produced, and its clinical significance.

8.2. BLOOD VOLUME MEASUREMENT AND THEORETICAL CONSIDERATIONS

The measurement of the components of blood volume has been discussed in detail by Mollison (1983) and Mollison et al. (1997). Detailed recommendations have been made for standardization of methodology by the International Committee for Standardization in Hematology (ICSH, 1980a; Pearson et al., 1995).

8.2.1. RED CELL MASS RCM can be accurately measured by the radioactive sodium chromate (^{51}Cr) red blood cell labeling method (Sterling and Gray, 1950; ICSH, 1980b), which has been most widely used.

Other methods include red blood cell labeling with ^{99m}Tc and ^{111}In (Mollison et al., 1997). The nucleide dilution principle is used in all, in which:

From: *The Complete Spleen: A Handbook of Structure, Function, and Clinical Disorders* Edited by: A. J. Bowdler © Humana Press Inc., Totowa, NJ

Table 8.1
Contributing Factors to Anemia Related to Splenomegaly

Factor	Notes
Hemolysis	*See* Chapter 12.
Immune	
Nonimmune	
Impaired responsiveness of erythropoiesis	Often caused by co-morbidity.
Maldistribution	Splenic pooling. *See* Chapter 7.
Blood loss	Portal hypertension; gastric and esophageal varices.
Folate deficiency	Secondary to proliferative disorders or hepatic dysfunction.
Dilutional anemia	Expansion of plasma volume; a common finding.

$$RCM = \frac{\text{Total }^{51}\text{Cr Radioactivity Injected}}{^{51}\text{Cr Radioactivity/mL red blood cell}}$$

The accuracy of the estimation depends on the precise measurement of the volume injected intravenously of the labeled red blood cell sample suspended in autologous plasma. This is obtained by the difference in weight in grams of the syringe, before and after the injection of the labeled blood, and is converted to the volume in milliliters, by dividing the weight by the specific gravity (*SG*) of the blood sample, which can be estimated from the hematocrit of the sample (H_S), as follows:

$$SG = [(H_S/100) \times 1.1] + [(100 - H_S) / 100) \times 1.02]$$

A second important factor is the interval between injection and the time of blood sampling. In normal subjects, mixing of the labeled sample in the circulation in vivo is virtually complete in ~3 min, but, in patients with abnormal red blood cells, with massive splenomegaly or in cardiac decompensation, this may still be incomplete after 30–45 min, or more, because of slow perfusion of some segments of the circulation. Delayed mixing related to splenomegaly can be demonstrated by continuous monitoring of the surface radioactivity over the spleen, and reflects splenic pooling of red blood cells (Bowdler, 1962; Prankerd, 1963; Toghill, 1964; *see* Chapter 7).

Likewise, in appropriate circumstances, it may be advisable to draw several timed blood samples, to establish the volume of distribution of the labeled cells at its stable and maximal expansion.

8.2.2. PLASMA VOLUME   Plasma volume changes more acutely than RCM in response to physiological requirements, and is subject to variation with posture and physical activity (Besa, 1975). In most studies, plasma volume has been standardized, by measurement with the subject recumbent for a specified prior period.

The commonly used method employs radioactive [131]I- or ^{125}I-labeled human serum albumin (HSA): This is simple and accurate, and with ^{131}I has the advantage of permitting surface counting for the determination of regional hematocrit (*see* below). However, it is somewhat dependent on the quality of the albumin preparation, since denatured labeled albumin is rapidly lost from the circulation, giving falsely high estimations; satisfactory preparations, giving consistent results, are available commercially (Takeda and Reeve, 1963; Swan and Nelson, 1971). Recommendations for measurement of plasma volume by this method have been published

extensively elsewhere (ICSH 1980a; Mollison et al., 1997). Radioactivity attached to albumin carrier protein declines steadily in the plasma after injection at a rate variously estimated at between 3 and 20% in the first hour. This is usually ascribed to a slow leak of albumin into the extravascular space, and consequently the preferred method for obtaining the volume of distribution at zero time is by estimating the activity of the label at several timed intervals following intravenous injection (usually at 10, 20, and 30 min), with subsequent calculation of the zero-time value by extrapolation back to the zero time of injection (Mollison et al., 1997; Pearson et al., 1995).

Early work on estimating plasma volume employed albumin-binding dyes, using the dilution principle. The blue azo-dye, Evans blue, or T-1824, has long been known to be satisfactory (Dawson et al., 1920), and is still used. It has the advantages of being usable when the use of a radioactive marker is unacceptable, and also, the dye can be injected directly, which avoids potential errors arising from denaturation of the radioactive albumin during preparation in vitro. It binds to plasma albumin promptly, and leaves the circulation slowly (Gibson and Evans, 1937; Rawson, 1943), and the zero-time value can easily be obtained by extrapolation from sequential values. Some investigators have found the decline in plasma-bound dye to be sufficiently predictable for the plasma volume to be calculated acceptably from a single 10-min sample in normal subjects, with a time-related correction factor (Mollison, 1983). Estimates of plasma volume using T-1824 in normal subjects, are very close to those obtained with ^{131}I-albumin (Fraenkel et al., 1953; Andersen, 1962). Thus, Retzlaff et al. (1969) estimated normal plasma volumes by the dye method, to be 39.8 mL/kg in men and 38.9 mL/kg in women, which are very close to the estimate of 39.8 mL/kg found with ^{131}I-labeled albumin for normal adults (Bowdler, 1970). Although early studies using dye-dilution methods have provided valuable insights, and resolved many of the technical problems of blood volume measurement, radiolabeled albumin has proved in general to be more convenient.

Limited studies with other labeled protein carriers have tended to give slightly lower estimates of plasma volume. Andersen (1962) found ^{131}I-immunoglobulin to give plasma volumes 2.5% lower than T-1824. Likewise, Andersen and Gabuzda (1964) found ^{131}I-myeloma proteins, whether macroglobulin or 6S-proteins, to give volumes 4.7% lower than with T-1824. Baker (1963) also found ^{131}I-fibrinogen to give slightly lower values for plasma volume than T-1824, in dogs. These findings presumably reflect slight differences in the volumes of distribution of different plasma proteins, and are slightly lower, with larger protein molecular sizes than albumin. On the other hand, when [113]In-labeled transferrin ([113]InTF) is used, the plasma volume is overestimated by ~6%, compared with that using ^{125}I-HSA (Zhang and Lewis, 1987). However, it does provide some improvement in surface-scanning characteristics.

8.2.3. INTERPRETATION OF BLOOD VOLUME DATA   The most commonly used expression of normal blood volume values has been in relation to the subject's body weight. Representative values for normal adults are given in Table 2. A significant source of error, using weight alone as the standard, arises from variability in the amount of body fat, since adipose tissue has a relatively low blood content of approx 11–22 mL/kg; that of the lean body mass is about 92 mL/kg. Consequently, a weight-related standard is inappropriate for obese individuals, and, for a population with a high proportion of overweight individuals, other means are to be preferred.

Table 8.2
Blood Volumes of Normal, Splenomegalic and Postsplenectomy Subjects[a]

	No.	H_V	Weight-related volumes (mL/kg)			Height-related volumes (mL/cm)			Formula-related volumes[b] (%)		
			RCM	PV	TBV	RCM	PV	TBV	RCM	PV	TBV
Normal	25	46.8	29.7	39.8	69.5	12.1	16.0	28.1	107	103	105
±		3.3	2.7	7.0	8.7	2.0	2.4	4.1	14	16	14
Splenomegaly	28	32.8	28.1	60.4[c]	88.5[c]	10.1	21.5[c]	31.6[d]	105	151[c]	131[c]
±		7.7	9.3	11.9	18.0	3.4	3.6	5.9	36	25	24
Postsplenectomy	15	38.1	25.2[c]	52.0[e]	77.2[d]	9.7[c]	19.2[e]	28.9	98	135[c]	120[e]
±		7.0	4.4	14.3	14.3	2.6	4.8	5.8	19	30	17

[a]Adapted with permission from Bowdler, A. J. (1970).
[b]Formula-related volumes are those compared to values derived from the formulae of Nadler et al. (1962).
Significant differences from normal control values expressed as probability levels: [c]$p < 0.001$, [d]$p < 0.05$, [e]$p < 0.01$.
Standard deviations are identified by ± , on line below mean values.
No., number of cases investigated; H_V, venous hematocrit; RCM, red cell mass; PV, plasma volume; TBV, total blood volume.

As an alternative, Allen et al. (1956) introduced standards related to the body weight and the cube of the subject's height; others have proposed relating blood volumes to lean body mass (Hyde and Jones, 1962; Muldowney, 1957). However, the measurement of lean body mass optimally requires additional technology, and has not received wide acceptance. A further approach has been to estimate blood volumes and establish formulae empirically to find the best relationship to height and weight (Wennesland et al., 1959; Nadler et al., 1962; Retzlaff et al., 1969; Hurley, 1975). These have been reviewed by Pearson et al. (1995), and each has been found to have some deficiency in design. For example, the RCM predictions of Nadler et al. (1962) are probably too high, compared to measured values (Hall and Malia, 1991), and reviewing reliability data is important when using formulae of this type. Nevertheless, errors are more likely to be significant in relation to assessment of abnormality for individuals, than in the comparison of grouped data expressed as derivatives. The equations given by Nadler et al. (1962) are as follows:

$$\text{For men: } BV = 0.3669 \, H^3 + 0.03219 \, W + 0.6041$$
$$\text{For women: } BV = 0.3561 \, H^3 + 0.03308 \, W + 0.1833$$

where BV is the blood volume in liters, H is the subject's height in meters, and W the weight in kg.

Pearson et al. (1995) recommend the following standards, based on body surface area:

For adult males: Mean normal $RCM = (1486 \times S) - 825$
Mean normal $PV = 1578 \times S$
For adult females: Mean normal $RCM = (1.06 \times \text{age}) + (822 \times S)$
Mean normal $PV = 1395 \times S$

where RCM is the red cell mass in mL, PV is the plasma volume in mL, age = age in years, and S = surface area in $m^2 = W^{0.425} \times h^{0.725} \times 0.007184$, and W is weight in kg, and h is height in cm.

The normal ranges about these mean values are wide, being 25% for the 98–99% limits. These formulae have not been widely used to the present time, and await independent validation.

8.2.4. WHOLE-BODY, REGIONAL, AND VENOUS HEMATOCRITS The proportions of red blood cells in the circulation and its components have customarily been compared with the proportion in the venous hematocrit (H_V), which has required significant refinement in the methodology for determining the hematocrit.

Most earlier work required mechanical centrifuging of anticoagulated blood in glass tubes, usually the Wintrobe tube or the microhematocrit tube (ICSH, 1980b). It is important to measure only the red blood cell column in the tube, and to exclude the leukocyte layer from the measured column: Increased accuracy can be obtained with the microhematocrit method, by making the measurements with the Vernier scale under a low-power microscope. The most important correction is for the residual plasma in the red blood cell column after centrifuging: Correction factors for the hematocrit, obtained by the Wintrobe method, are given by Chaplin and Mollison (1952), and for the microhematocrit technique by England et al. (1972). In samples with morphologically abnormal red blood cells, the amount of plasma trapped may be higher than for normal cells, and, with deoxygenated sickle cells, this may amount to 20% of the packed cell column; with pathological samples, an independent estimate by an alternative method may be necessary. Bowdler (1980) standardized both methods against 100 normal blood samples, for which the packed cell volume was estimated by measuring the plasma content of the sample after labeling with ^{59}Fe, which does not enter the cells. The relationships of the observed hematocrits to the radionuclide-based estimates were as follows:

Microhematocrit method: $H_O = 1.0255 \, H_N + 0.1354$
Wintrobe method: $H_O = 1.0374 \, H_N - 0.2399$

where H_O is the observed hematocrit, H_R is the radionuclide-based packed cell volume, and the hematocrits are expressed as percentages.

The values of hematocrits, as estimated by particle counting, have not been exhaustively evaluated in this context. However, Guthrie and Pearson (1982) identified a tendency for the particle counter to underestimate the hematocrit in blood samples from polycythemics, with some deficits as high as 7%.

The independent measurement of red blood cell and plasma volumes showed that the H_V does not represent the fraction of red blood cells in the total blood volume. That is, the RCM occupies a smaller fraction of the total blood volume than the proportion of red blood cells in the H_V. Consequently, the total blood volume cannot be calculated accurately from the plasma volume and the H_V alone. Mollison (1961) suggested that there was a rapid but unrecognized loss of albumin to the extravascular space, carrying the T-1824 dye out from the circulation, but this was discounted by the studies of Barnes et al. (1948a,b).

The alternative explanation, which accounts for the major part of the discrepancy, is that the difference results from the uneven distribution of red blood cells and plasma in the circulation. One source of this is an effect produced by the flow characteristics of blood: The hematocrit of venous blood is representative of large-vessel blood; in small blood vessels, the axial streaming of red blood cells produces a shorter transit time for red blood cells than for plasma, which is marginalized to a peripheral still-space, so that the fraction of the blood volume occupied by red blood cells is reduced in small vessels, compared to large (Fahraeus, 1929).

The difference between the whole-body hematocrit (H_B) and the H_V is usually expressed as the ratio H_B/H_V, which is normally less than unity. Chaplin et al. (1953) reported an average H_B/H_V ratio of 0.910 (SD 0.026), and noted its remarkable constancy in normal subjects, with a wide range of H_V values produced by anemia and polycythemia. Numerous additional studies have confirmed a normal value of 0.91–0.92 for H_B/H_V in humans. However, in normal dogs, the ratio was found to be much more variable, and Reeve et al. (1958) showed that the principal source of variation in H_B/H_V (which they termed "F_{CELLS}") was the size of the storage spleen, and that, in the splenectomized animal, the ratio remained fairly constant at ~0.87 (SD 0.027) across a wide range of anemia, polycythemia, and hemodilution. In the intact animal, the ratio might be as high as 1.1, when the spleen was relaxed and enlarged.

Rothschild et al. (1954) anticipated the findings of much later work, in seven patients with splenomegaly, for whom they showed, in the human, as in the dog, an increased mean H_B/H_V, in this series, reaching 1.035, compared to their normal value of 0.943. The mixing times of labeled red blood cells in the circulation of four of these subjects was prolonged, although there was no mixing delay for labeled albumin. Plasma volumes were elevated in all the patients with splenomegaly, and, in three, anemia resulted from plasma expansion in the presence of a normal RCM (see Subheading 4.1.).

Likewise, Fudenberg et al. (1961) found a normal mean ratio of 0.896, but in patients with splenomegaly, the H_B/H_V ratio differed significantly from this, with values between 0.986 and 1.156, depending on the degree of enlargement of the spleen. Marked deviations of the H_B/H_V ratio from the normal range were recognized as introducing potentially large errors into the estimation of total blood volume from measurements of RCM or plasma volume alone (Najean and Deschrymer, 1984).

Bowdler (1969) studied 24 subjects with splenomegaly, and found that the H_B/H_V, based on the blood volume estimate at 6 min, was within the normal range (0.92, SD 0.037), but the ratio was increased when estimated from the volume of distribution at 45 min (0.98, SD 0.09), indicating that the increased H_B/H_V in the presence of splenomegaly results from the slowly interchanging splenic red blood cell pool. It further indicates that the red blood cell concentration of the pool must be high. Direct measurement of the hematocrit of splenic blood, during and following splenectomy, has not contributed to an understanding of this phenomenon, because the spleen undergoes contraction and loses blood upon surgical manipulation (McFadzean and Todd, 1967), and the splenic pool comprises only one component of the total blood content of the organ.

The ratio between RCM and plasma volume *in situ*, at various sites related to organs beneath the body surface, has been determined. Using surface counting of ^{51}Cr-labeled autologous red blood cells and ^{131}I-HSA, Bowdler (1969) calculated regional hematocrits (H_R) in normal subjects, and found them to be highest at the pre-

cordium and lowest in the region of the liver. This is consistent with the Fåhraeus model, reflecting, respectively, the large vessels of the mediastinum and the capillaries and sinusoids of the liver. Expressed as H_R/H_V, mean normal values were 0.95 (SD 0.15) for the precordium, 0.75 (SD 0.13) for the hepatic region, 0.84 (SD 0.08) over the site of the spleen, and 0.87 (SD 0.04) over the lumbar spine. In patients with splenomegaly, the mean H_R/H_V over the spleen was higher than the normal value for this site, at 1.26 (SD 0.39), and correlated significantly with the late raised H_B/H_V ratio ($r = +0.66$, $p < 0.001$), showing that the incremental increase in cell concentration in the splenic pool is a significant variable contributing to the increased H_B/H_V. In subjects after splenectomy, the early and late H_B/H_V ratios were 0.87 (SD 0.05) and 0.88 (SD 0.04), respectively, both being significantly less than normal ($p < 0.001$), and comparable to those found in the splenectomized dog. Likewise, the splenic H_R/H_V after splenectomy was 0.79 (SD 0.13). Christensen (1973), employing similar techniques, reported comparable values, with a mean splenic H_R/H_V ratio of 1.41 (SD 0.25) in patients with splenomegaly. Subsequently, Zhang and Lewis (1987), using [113]In-transferrin, which provides better quantitative scanning of plasma within the spleen, and ^{99m}Tc-labeled autologous red blood cells, reported a mean splenic H_B/H_V ratio of 1.30 (SD 0.30) in 12 patients with splenomegaly. These studies provide further direct evidence of plasma-poor, red blood cell-rich blood in enlarged spleens.

8.3. RED BLOOD CELL CONTENT OF THE SPLEEN IN HUMANS

The normal spleen in humans contains only 20–30 mL of red blood cells or <2% of the total RCM (Prankerd, 1963). Therefore, the red blood cell storage function may be regarded as insignificant, and, in this respect, it differs from that of mammals such as horse, dog, and sheep. However, in massive splenomegaly, up to 40% of the total RCM may be in the splenic blood volume (Bowdler, 1967). During gastrointestinal bleeding, or at splenectomy in cryptogenic splenomegaly (Cook et al., 1963), or after exercise in tropical splenomegaly (Pryor, 1967a), the spleen diminishes in volume, and discharges much of its blood into the general circulation. In these disorders, histological examination of the spleen reveals marked hyperplasia and dilatation of the sinuses (Cook et al., 1963; Pitney, 1968; Marsden and Crane, 1976); it is probable that most of the red blood cells expelled are derived from the red pulp. The remarkable ability of an enlarged spleen to discharge red blood cells can be readily demonstrated by infusion of noradrenaline or adrenaline under controlled conditions (Prankerd, 1963; Toghill and Prichard, 1964; Pryor, 1967a), and suggests an atavistic preservation of the vascular structures essential to the storage function.

There is good correlation between the spleen size, as measured by its extension below the costal margin or the surface area of an ultrasound scan, with the actual splenic blood volume as measured by quantitative radioisotope scan with [^{11}C]carbon monoxide (Glass et al., 1968). Likewise, there is correlation between the size of the spleen and the elevation in H_B/H_V ratio, at least among enlarged spleens of like etiology (Motulsky et al., 1958; Bowdler, 1969; Christensen, 1973). Other studies (Blendis et al., 1970; Toghill, 1964; see also Chapter 7) have shown red blood cell pooling to be increased in conditions with morphologically abnormal red blood cells, such as thalassemia and hereditary spherocytosis. Some variation in splenic red blood cell content is related to the etiology of the splenic enlargement, rather than simply to the size of the spleen: for example, in many lymphoproliferative disorders, the spleen contains fewer red blood cells than in myeloproliferative disorders with a comparable increase in the size of the spleen, because splenomegaly in the former is the result of proliferation of lymphoid cells, with effacement of the structure of the splenic cords and sinuses, which results in a diminution of the pulp space accommodation for red blood cells (Pettit et al., 1971).

8.4. SPLENOMEGALY AND PLASMA VOLUME

8.4.1. PLASMA VOLUME IN THE PRESENCE OF AN EN-LARGED SPLEEN
Observations over many years have shown that the plasma volume is increased in many patients with enlargement of the spleen (Rowntree et al., 1929). Rothschild et al. (1954) found plasma volume to be expanded in seven patients with splenomegaly, together with a normal or increased RCM, despite the H_V being depressed. Furthermore, there was prolongation of the mixing time of 51-Cr-labeled red blood cells and the H_B/H_V ratio was above normal, indicating the presence of a volume of red blood cell-rich blood in the spleen. In a larger series of patients with cryptogenic splenomegaly, McFadzean et al. (1958b) reported that there was a consistent increase in plasma volume which contributed to the anemia. Following splenectomy in such patients, the H_V rose, mainly as a result of the decrease in plasma volume, and showing that the anemia was, to a large extent, caused by hemodilution by the excessive plasma volume. Similar observations were reported by Bowdler (1963) in a detailed study of a patient with Gaucher's disease and massive splenomegaly. In these and subsequent reports shown in Tables 2, 4, and 6, there is confirmation of the presence of increased plasma volume and dilutional anemia in patients with moderate-to-massive splenomegaly. That this increase in plasma volume occurs across a broad spectrum of pathological causes for splenomegaly is evident from Table 4. Because anemia itself is associated with a compensatory increase in the plasma volume, so that total blood volume is only slightly reduced (Mollison, 1983), individual patients with a low RCM have been excluded from this table. Also excluded are patients with polycythemia vera and those with thalassemia major, because (with some exceptions) plasma volume is within the normal range in the former, and there is a large increase in the volume of the vascular bone marrow space contributing to the higher plasma and blood volumes in the latter (see Subheading 4.2.). In the series of patients reported by Bowdler (1970), there was a 31% expansion in blood volume, mostly because of the 50% increase in plasma volume above that predicted by the Nadler formulae. The contribution of the splenic red blood cell pool was a minor factor: The mean splenic pool was 7.4% of the circulating RCM, and contributed an average of only 2.4% to the total blood volume.

8.4.2. POSTSPLENECTOMY STUDIES
Blood volume changes, before and after splenectomy, have been reported in patients with enlarged spleens associated with cryptogenic and tropical splenomegaly (McFadzean et al., 1958b; Hamilton et al., 1967; McFadzean and Todd, 1967; Pryor, 1967b; Crane et al., 1972), Gaucher's disease (Bowdler, 1963), primary splenic hyperplasia (Weinstein, 1964), myelo- and lymphoproliferative diseases, other blood dyscrasias and congestive splenomegaly (Bowdler, 1967, 1970; Blendis et al., 1969; Donaldson et al., 1970; Toghill and Green, 1971; Hess et al., 1971; Hess et al., 1976; see also Tables 4 and 5).

When individual patients, in whom the RCM was initially normal, are considered, the plasma volume was high in 77/83 patients (93%); following splenectomy, P.V. decreased to normal levels in 21 (25%); decreased, but remained higher than normal in 47; and was unchanged, or even increased, in 9 (Table 3). In the majority, the hemoglobin concentration and/or the H_V of the peripheral blood rose, and the high H_B/H_V ratio fell, following the disappearance of the splenic pool of red blood cells. Because the red blood cell pool was not large in many of these patients, the improvement in the anemia after splenectomy can be ascribed in most cases to the decrease in the plasma volume.

These changes may be related to a reduction in liver blood flow and portal hypertension following removal of the vascular spleen (Williams, 1966; Hess et al., 1971; Hess et al., 1976), with a resulting decrease in efferent renal sympathetic nerve activity and renal sodium retention (see below). When postsplenectomy studies have been performed serially, the plasma volume has tended to decrease further with time, but often may still remain above normal (McFadzean et al., 1958b; Crane et al., 1972). Consequently, in the series cited above, in many cases, the plasma volume reduction would have been significantly greater, if the volumes had been followed to their nadir. Conversely, when hepatic enlargement increases in the course of relapse or extension of the underlying disease, as in Bowdler (1963), the plasma volume may again tend to expand.

On the other hand, in patients with splenomegaly palpable at less than 4 cm below the costal margin, plasma volume often remained unchanged after splenectomy, and the H_V did not rise. This was also observed in patients with cirrhosis of the liver with relatively minor splenic enlargement (McFadzean and Todd, 1967; Bowdler, 1970), and in several patients in whom the RCM fell after splenectomy, as a result of the associated blood dyscrasia (Table 5).

From Tables 2 and 3, it can be seen that, before splenectomy, the RCM was often above normal, despite a low hemoglobin or H_V value. In many patients, the RCM fell to normal following splenectomy (Table 5). This may be attributable to the diminished need for augmented red blood cell production to maintain a large volume of cells in the expanded vascular bed related to the spleen, and possibly to a diminished stimulus to erythropoiesis with correction of the dilutional anemia (Prankerd, 1963; Pryor, 1967a,b; Bowdler, 1970).

The low hemoglobin and H_V levels in patients with splenomegaly are therefore commonly and mostly the result of hemodilution, with the result that the plasma volume falls and the peripheral hemoglobin concentration and H_V tend to rise after splenectomy (Table 5). With the exception of patients with cirrhosis of the liver, there is a positive correlation between the magnitude of splenomegaly and the increase in plasma volume, and an inverse relationship between the peripheral hematocrit level and plasma volume (Table 3).

However, there is no evidence that the excess plasma is contained exclusively in the enlarged spleen (Rothschild et al., 1954; Pryor, 1967a; Blendis et al., 1970). Because of variability in plasma volume expansion, the customary correlation between the H_V and RCM is lost (Bowdler, 1970).

8.5. DILUTIONAL ANEMIA

Dilutional anemia (dilution, hemodilutional, hypervolemic anemia; pseudoanemia) occurs when the plasma volume expands without a proportionate increase in the RCM, which may be normal, below normal, or increased. Consequently, there is a tendency for the total blood volume to be above normal. The appelation

Table 8.3
Plasma Volume and Splenic Red Cell Pooling in Patients with Splenomegaly[a]

Author	No. patients	Cause of splenomegaly	Spleen size	Low Hb or Hv	Increased PV	RCM above normal	Splenic red cell pool (% RCM)	$H_B{:}H_V$ >1.0	Correlation with spleen size	Correlation with H_V
Rothschild et al. (1954)	7	Myelo- and lymphoproliferative disorders; hepatic cirrhosis	6–25 cm	5/7	7/7	2/7	n/a	5/7	n/a	n/a
McFadzean et al. (1958b)	17	Cryptogenic	15 ± 3	+[b]	+	–				
Bowdler (1963, 1967)	14	Various	2–25 cm	+	+	7/14	7% (13), 40% (1)			(–)
Weinstein (1964)	3	Hyperplasia	1.0–2.8 kg	3/3	3/3	n/a	n/a	0/3	n/a	spleen size
McFadzean and Todd (1967)	30	Cryptogenic with cirrhosis of liver	1–18 cm	+	24/30	n/a	59–458 mL	21/30	(+) PV, (+) $H_B{:}H_V$ (+) Pool	n/a
Pryor (1967a)	62	Tropical splenomegaly	"Massive"	+	62/62	+	3.2–44%	1.23,1.34, (means)	(+) PV	(–) PV, (nil) RCM
Richmond et al. (1967)	13	Tropical splenomegaly	15–31 cm	11/13	12/13	n/a	6–39%, (15–850 mL)	1.07 (mean)	(+) PV, (+) Pool, (–) VH	(nil) RCM, (nil) Pool
Blendis et al. (1969)	39	Myelo- and lymphoproliferative, Gaucher's, Felty's, Idiopathic	0.12–4.68 kg	31/39	30/39	19/39	9–39%	11/39	(+) PV, (+) RCM, (–) Pool	(–) PV
Blendis et al. (1970)	46	Cirrhosis of liver	0.3–1.4 kg	15/46	33/46	23/46	n/a	7/46	(nil) PV, (nil) RCM	(nil) PV
Bowdler (1970)	13	Myelo- and lymphoproliferative	~15 ± 6 cm	+	+	n/a	7.4 ± 5% (includes 7 with hemolytic anemia	n/a	(+) PV	n/a
Bowdler (1970)	3	Hepatic	11 ± 5 cm	+	+	n/a	n/a	n/a	n/a	n/a
Donaldson et al.(1970)	21	Myelo- and lymphoproliferative Felty's	12–34 cm	19/21	19/21	4/21	10% (0–540 mL)	7/21	(+) PV, (–) Pool, Pool size correlates with PV	PV
Donaldson et al. (1970)	8	Idiopathic, Cirrhosis of liver	1–20 cm	5/8	7/8	1/8	6.3% (0–265 mL)	4/8		
Hess et al. (1971,1976)	11	Myelo- and lymphoproliferative	1.5–4.2 kg	11/11	11/11	1/11	n/a	9/11		
Toghill and Green (1971)	8	Myelo- and lymphoproliferative	4–8 cm	n!a	4/8	1/8	13.1%		(+) PV, (+) Pool, (nit) RCM	
Crane et al. (1972)	11	Tropical splenomegaly	Massive	11/11	11/11	5/11	31.7%			(–) PV
Christensen (1973)	5	Myelo-lymphoproliferative	960–3273 mL		4/5	0/5	21.1%		(+) PVI (+) Pool	
Pengelly (1977)	18	Myelo- and lymphoproliferative	1–25+ cm	7/18	16/18	7/18		3/18	(+) PV, (+) RCM	
Lewis et al. (1977)	4	Hairy cell leukemia	7–10 cm	4/4	3/4	0/4	28.1% (211–726 mL)			
Castro-Malaspina et al. (1979)	29	Hairy cell leukemia	Moderate to massive	28/29	25/29				(+) PVI (+) Pool	
Kesteven et al. (1985)	53	Myelo- and lymphoproliferative	Mild to massive		53/53				(+) PV	1

[a] Hb, hemoglobin g/dL; H_V, venous hematocrit; PV, plasma volume; RCM, red cell mass; H_B, whole body hematocrit; Pool, splenic red cell pool.
[b] Mean value significantly different from controls.
Correlations: (+) positive; (–) negative; (nil) none.

"pseudoanemia" is inappropriate, and arises from an implicit expectation that low values in the hemoglobin concentration or the hematocrit in the peripheral blood indicate a subnormal RCM. However, anemia is recognized in practice when these values are below those accepted as normal for the individual's age and sex, and they are rarely confirmed as related to abnormalities of blood volumes, except in the context of the dilutional states, which are summarized in Table 7.

8.5.1. THE CAUSES OF DILUTIONAL ANEMIA

8.5.1.1. Pregnancy

Pregnancy is the commonest cause of dilutional anemia (Chesley, 1972): A healthy woman increases plasma volume by approx 50% (or ~1250 mL, depending partly on the size of the conceptus) during the course of a normal pregnancy, usually between wk 12 and 34 wk. The effect tends to be greater in multi-gravida. The increase in plasma volume is associated with an increase in extracellular fluid volume, total body water, and sodium.

Table 8.4
Blood Volumes in Splenomegaly by Category of Disease [a,b,c]

Disorder	No. Patients	Mean H_V (%)	Mean RCM	Mean PV
Myeloproliferative	16	32.5	114 ± 49	157 ± 24
Lymphoproliferative	6	26.4	99 ± 59	172 ± 26
Hepatic disorders	10	38.6	119 ± 28	150 ± 26
Hereditary spherocytosis	5	35.3	100 ± 4	137 ± 18
Autoimmune hemolysis	7	33.4	89 ± 27	124 ± 11
Thalassemia	7	23.1	77 ± 11	163 ± 2
Miscellaneous	11	36.9	107 ± 5	148 ± 23

[a]Adapted with permission from Bowdler (1967).
[b]Volumes expressed as percentage of predicted volumes from Nadler et al. (1962).
[c]H_V, venous hematocrit; RCM, red cell mass; PV, plasma volume.

Table 8.5
Postsplenectomy Changes in Plasma Volume [a]

Authors	Diagnosis	Presplenectomy increase in plasma volume (PV)	Postsplenectomy PV normal	Postsplenectomy PV decreased but still high	Postsplenectomy PV unchanged	Postsplenectomy H_V or Hb	Remarks
McFadzean et al. (1958b)	Cryptogenic splenomegaly	10/10[a]		10 (at 1 mo)		Increased	PV further reduced at 5 mo
Bowdler (1963)	Gaucher's disease	1/1		1 (at 6 mo)		Increased	RCM reduced and PV further reduced after splenectomy
Weinstein (1964)	Splenic hyperplasia	3/3		3 (at 6–18 wk)		Increased	RCM reduced after splenectomy
Bowdler (1967)	Congestive splenomegaly, and myeloproliferative disease	3/3		3 (at 6–17 wk)		2/3 Increased[c]	
Hamilton et al. (1967)	Tropical splenomegaly	5/5	1 (at 15 mo)	4 (at 15 mo)		Increased	
McFadzean and Todd (1967)	Cryptogenic splenomegaly with cirrhosis	11/14	5 (at 2 yr)	4 (at 2 yr)	5	10/14 Increased	PV unchanged or increased in patients with minor splenomegaly
Pryor (1967b)	Tropical splenomegaly	8/8		8 (at 2–18 mo)		6 Increased	
Blendis et al. (1969)	Blood dyscrasia	5/5	3	2			RCM reduced after splenectomy
Donaldson et al. (1970)	Idiopathic splenomegaly, myeloproliferative disease	3/3	2 (at 2–4 mo)		1 (at 2–4 mo)	2/3 Increased[c]	
Hess et al. (1971)	Myelo- and lymphoproliferative disease	4/4	1	3	1	Increased	
Toghill and Green (1971)	Myelo- and lymphoproliferative disease	5/8	7		1		Chemotherapy or radiotherapy only
Crane et al. (1972)	Tropical splenomegaly	111/11	1 (at 9–41 mo)	10 (at 9–41 mo)		Increased	
Hess et al. (1976)	Myelo- and lymphoproliferative disease	8/8	1 (at 2–4 mo)	5 (at 2–4 mo)	2 (at 2–4 mo)	6/8 Increased[c]	

[a]H_V, venous hematocrit; Hb, hemoglobin; PV, plasma volume; RCM, red cell mass.
[b]Denominator, number of patients.
[c]Of these, a total of four patients showed a marked decrease in red blood cell mass following splenectomy.

Blood volumes usually return to normal within 1–2 wk of delivery. During pregnancy, metabolic rate and heat production are increased: hemodilution decreases blood viscosity, and increases blood flow, heat dissipation through the skin, and excretion by the kidneys. The RCM increases proportionately less, usually by 250–450 mL, depending mostly on the adequacy of iron intake. The excess plasma volume increase leads to a typical fall in H_V from ~40 to ~33% before term (Hytten, 1985).

The effect is related to the increased estrogen production, which arises as a secondary response to the increased estrogen substrate generated by the fetal adrenal, the estrogen in turn stimulating hepatic renin substrate: This results in increased renal sodium resorption and water retention, caused by increased aldosterone production via the renin–angiotensin axis. The effect of arteriovenous shunting in the placenta may also be important (Longo, 1983), but the role of the latter has been questioned (Hytten, 1985). Plasma

Table 8.6
Blood Volumes Before and After Splenectomy in Cryptogenic or Tropical Splenomegaly[a]

Authors	No. Patients	Spleen size (cm)	PV before splenectomy (mL/kg)	PV after splenectomy (mL/kg)	RCM before splenectomy (mL/kg)	Remarks
McFadzean et al. (1958b)	10	15 ± 2	92.3 ± 11.5	75.5 ± 11.9[b]		Patients with hepatic cirrhosis excluded
	Controls	0	45.2 ± 3.4			
Pryor (1967b)	8	Grossly enlarged	94.1 ± 13.6	70.3 ± 12.0	35.5 ± 7.3	
	Controls	0	40–50		25.1 ± 30.3	
Richmond et al. (1967)	13	15–31	68.3 ± 21.2	Decreased when calculated from H_V	31.2 ± 5.6	2 patients with low RCM excluded
	Controls	0	37.0–45.4		27.4–33.6	

[a]PV, plasma volume; RCM, red cell mass; H_V, venous hematocrit.
[b]1 mo after splenectomy. Further decreased when studied 5 mo after splenectomy.

Table 8.7
Causes of Dilutional Anemia

Pregnancy
Hepatic cirrhosis
Paraproteinemias
Expansion of extravascular space
   Splanchnic
   Bone marrow
Sports anemia

expansion is therefore independent of the stimulus to erythropoiesis, which appears to be mediated by the effect of placental chorionic somatomammatrophin, progesterone, and possibly prolactin (Longo, 1983).

8.5.1.2. Hepatic Cirrhosis Hepatic cirrhosis commonly leads to expansion of the plasma volume which, in this case, is not usually closely related to the degree of splenic enlargement (Bateman et al., 1949; Eisenberg, 1956; McFadzean and Todd, 1967; Blendis et al., 1970; Donaldson et al., 1970). With moderate-to-massive splenomegaly, the effect on plasma volume is not totally independent of spleen size, which does play a role, as shown by the decrease in plasma volume that often follows splenectomy, although not necessarily with a return to normal values (McFadzean and Todd, 1967). Eisenberg (1956) demonstrated a significant expansion of blood and plasma volumes in 20 patients with Laennec's cirrhosis, the increase being especially present in patients with esophageal varices and/or cyanosis. The hypervolemia was suggested to be the passive consequence of an expanded vascular bed, and, in one patient, pulmonary arteriovenous shunting was demonstrated. Among the many different factors contributing to anemia in such patients, it was concluded that "in many instances the low hemoglobin values represent an expansion of the plasma volume rather than an actual shrinkage of the RCM."

Lieberman and Reynolds (1967) studied 140 patients with hepatic cirrhosis, and 10 with noncirrhotic portal hypertension, and confirmed the tendency to hypervolemia with a disproportionately greater increase in plasma volume than RCM. In 36 patients studied, there was a demonstrable correlation between plasma volume and wedged hepatic venous pressure ($r = 0.5$, $p < 0.05$), indicating that portal hypertension is responsible for the plasma volume expansion. Likewise, Levy (1974) showed hepatic venous congestion stimulated aldosterone secretion and renal retention of sodium in dogs. Better and Schrier (1983) supported a concept of "underfilling," implying a discrepancy between the circulating blood volume and the vascular capacity. This was held to result from the raised hydrostatic pressure in the portosplanchnic vascular bed, diverting blood volume from the systemic circulation, with a consequent stimulus to the renal retention of sodium and water. However, Anderson et al. (1976) suggested that there are both volume-dependent and volume-independent mechanisms acting as stimuli to avid renal sodium retention.

In moderate cirrhosis, hepatic venous congestion and portal hypertension increase wedged hepatic venous pressure, which acts as a stimulus to the renin–angiotensin–aldosterone axis. In advanced cirrhosis, patients show high levels of plasma catecholamines, which correlate closely with sodium retention. Hendrikson et al. (1984) measured high levels of norepinephrine in the renal vein plasma of cirrhotics; it has been proposed that receptors detecting raised intrahepatic sinusoidal pressure activate an autonomic hepatorenal reflex arc, the efferent limb of which stimulates renal tubular sodium reabsorption (DiBona, 1977, 1984), with secondary expansion of the plasma and extravascular fluid volume. These may not be the exclusively involved mechanisms of the plasma expansion: Other contributory factors probably include arteriovenous shunting, increased levels of antidiuretic hormone, and abnormalities in the renal prostaglandin and kinin systems (Better and Schrier, 1983; Di Bona, 1984; Rocco and Ware, 1986).

8.5.1.3. Paraproteinemias Paraproteinemias have also been shown to be associated with hypervolemic anemia: Herreman et al. (1968) demonstrated this in macroglobulinemia, and Kopp et al. (1969) found an increased total blood volume in all four patients investigated with macroglobulinemia: in these patients, the plasma volume was increased and the RCM normal, showing that their anemia was dilutional in origin. Total blood volume was above normal in 9/11 patients with myelomatosis, and resulted from expanded plasma volume in seven of these. In the majority, the RCM was normal, and their anemia consequently dilutional. The blood volumes correlated poorly with the concentrations of paraproteins. The recognition of dilutional anemia in these conditions is of importance, since the blood volume, when sufficiently expanded, can result in high output cardiac failure, and blood transfusion may be inappropriate, because the red blood cells increase blood viscosity, and may worsen the condition. Conversely, it may be relieved by plasma exchange therapy, provided that the need is recognized.

8.5.1.4. Increased Plasma Volume in Patients with Splenomegaly This has been investigated extensively, especially with respect to factors found to be of significance in other disorders. The increase in plasma volume has been regarded as arising from expansion of the intravascular space, especially in the portosplanchnic vasculature, consequent upon the development of splenomegaly (Bowdler, 1963, 1970), in circumstances in which the capacity for additional erythropoiesis is limited. This may be the result of a diminished erythropoietic capacity, concurrent hemolysis, and a high proportion of circulating red blood cells being pooled in the enlarged spleen. The increased plasma volume then fills that portion of the increased intravascular space that erythropoiesis is unable to maintain (Bowdler, 1967). In support of this concept is the frequent finding of a greater-than-normal RCM in these patients. This increase in RCM suggests a productive stress on erythropoiesis, and may be related to an increased basal oxygen consumption related to the spleen, and to basal metabolic rate, which is found to fall after splenectomy (Hess et al., 1976). In keeping with this view is the finding that, when the decrease in plasma volume following splenectomy is most pronounced, the RCM commonly declines as well (Bowdler, 1963, 1970; Weinstein, 1964; Blendis et al., 1969).

Experimental induction of splenomegaly in rats, by the intraperitoneal injection of methylcellulose, has been shown to result in anemia in the majority of animals, by dilution of the normal red blood cell volume by expansion of plasma volume. The increase of blood volume and extrasplenic blood volume correlated well with the size of the spleen. The expanded blood volume was not generalized throughout the circulation, but was mostly localized to the portal bed comprising the spleen, liver, and the gastrointestinal tract (Ooyirilangkumaran, 1973).

Garnett et al. (1969) investigated 19 patients with moderate to massive splenomegaly: total splenic blood flow in 17/19 showed a mean of 1.6 L/min, with a range of 0.5 to 4.0 L/min, which was between 8.5 and 55% of the cardiac output, and more than 20% in five of the patients. The high splenic blood flow was reflected in a bruit, audible over the spleen in eight subjects, of whom five also showed a raised jugular venous pressure. Cardiac output measured in 13 patients was 3.7–10.6 L/min, and the cardiac index in nine patients was 2.3–7.7 L/min/m², with the normal being 3.2 L/min/m². It was concluded that increased blood flow through an enlarged spleen acts as a functional arteriovenous shunt, the increased venous return to the heart causing a high cardiac output, together with an increase in the blood volume, by analogy with the increased blood volume that may accompany traumatic arteriovenous fistulae (Warren, Nickerson, et al., 1951; Warren, Elkin, et al., 1951). Williams et al. (1968) measured spleen blood flows up to 910 mL/min, which they regarded as a contributory factor to portal hypertension. Hess et al. (1976) studied 20 patients with anemia and massive splenomegaly, finding elevated splenic blood flow in 4/4 subjects investigated; portal blood pressure elevation, which was corrected by splenectomy, in 12/12 subjects investigated, but no evidence of

formal arteriovenous shunting in three subjects tested by dye dilution study.

In patients with cirrhosis of the liver, there is a demonstrated correlation between plasma volume and wedged hepatic venous pressure (Lieberman and Reynolds, 1967; *see* Subheading 5.1.2.). There is evidence that intrahepatic hypertension plays an important role in activating hepatic baroreceptors, leading in turn to increased renal sodium reabsorption and plasma volume expansion (Di Bona, 1984). Hepatic sinusoidal hypertension also augments hepatic lymph formation, and results in ascites formation, with a decrease in the effective vascular volume.

Increased splenic and portal blood flow, with elevation of the portal venous pressure and wedged hepatic vein pressure, have been demonstrated in noncirrhotic patients with splenomegaly (Leather, 1961; Rosenbaum et al., 1966; Williams., 1966; Blendis et al., 1970; Hess et al., 1971; Hess et al., 1976). Williams (1966) reported that increased blood flow through the enlarged spleen and liver of patients with tropical splenomegaly, together with an unexplained increase in presinusoidal resistance, accounted for the portal hypertension. Similar observations have been made in patients with blood dyscrasias and splenomegaly (Blendis et al., 1970; Hess et al., 1971; Hess et al., 1976), in whom the degree of portal hypertension was closely related to the magnitude of splenomegaly and the accompanying increase in splenic blood flow. In general, there was significant correlation of both the increased intrasplenic and wedged hepatic venous pressures with the expansion in plasma volume. Thus, in patients with enlarged and vascular spleens, flow-induced portal and intrahepatic hypertension appear to play an important role in renal sodium retention and increase in the plasma volume, as in patients with cirrhosis of the liver. The expansion of the anatomical portal vascular bed, with portal venous blood pooling, contributes to activation of the renin–angiotensin–aldosterone system, which may also be augmented by the decrease in systemic peripheral resistance that accompanies the hypermetabolic state of massive splenomegaly (Hess et al., 1976).

An alternative suggestion, considered in some depth, has been that an increase in plasma oncotic pressure may underlie the hypervolemia in patients with increased levels of serum globulins (Weinstein, 1964; Pryor, 1967a). However, these levels are usually not abnormal in nontropical splenomegaly, and Blendis (1970) found no correlation between the plasma volume and the serum albumin, globulin, or total protein concentrations, in a large series of patients with splenomegaly. The poor correlation between serum globulin concentration and the increased plasma volume in patients with macroglobulinemia and myelomatosis, found by Kopp et al. (1969; *see* Subheading 5.1.3.), does not argue for a close causal relationship. Hess et al. (1976) reported that the intravascular pool of albumin was increased in their patients with splenomegaly, and decreased only slowly in most patients after splenectomy, so that this may have been one factor contributing to the slow return of plasma volume to normal values in these circumstances (McFadzean and Todd, 1967; Crane et al., 1972). Increased albumin synthesis is, therefore, to be considered a secondary consequence of augmented plasma volume rather than a primary causative factor.

Apparently, as the spleen enlarges, there is expansion of the vascular bed, both in the spleen and elsewhere in the portal circulation. Plasma volume expands to fill this enlarged intravascular space. However, as splenomegaly further increases, flow-induced portal hypertension initiates renal sodium retention, with possibly a later augmentation by efferent renal sympathetic nerve activity.

Suggestions that plasma expansion may be caused by an intrinsic splenic hormone have not been supported experimentally; on the contrary, Kaubman and Deng (1999) obtained an extract of rat spleen, which produced a decrease in plasma volume, an increase in urine flow and glomerular filtration rate, and a fall in arterial pressure.

8.5.1.5. Sports Anemia   This is a dilutional anemia that may arise in endurance-trained athletes, including swimmers (Nichols, 1999), and is related to the tendency for regular physical training to result in a 10–20% increase in plasma volume (Bartsch et al., 1998). Iron deficiency and other forms of anemia do not appear to be more common in athletes than in the general population (Weight et al., 1992).

8.6. PLASMA VOLUME IN SPECIFIC DISORDERS

8.6.1. CRYPTOGENIC AND TROPICAL SPLENOMEGALY

Splenomegaly of uncertain origin occurs in a variety of different forms, and, where commonly present, is frequently designated in relation to the geographical area in which the disorder is found. Associated findings often include chronic infection, such as malaria, excessive immunoglobulin production, macrophage hyperplasia (Fakunle, 1981), and a decrease in suppressor T-lymphocytes (Hoffman et al., 1984). The spleen is often grossly enlarged and the hematological sequelae severe (Kirk, 1957; Cook et al., 1963; Pitney, 1968, Marsden and Crane, 1976; Fakunle, 1981). Relatively homogeneous groups of patients have been studied, and the effect of splenectomy on the associated anemia and blood volume changes defined.

Anemia is often accompanied by a moderate shortening of red blood cell survival, red blood cell pooling in the spleen (Table 3), increased values of H_B/H_V, and normal values of RCM despite a reduction of hemoglobin and hematocrit levels. Significant improvement in these abnormalities usually follows splenectomy (McFadzean et al., 1958a; Pryor, 1967a; Richmond et al., 1967; McFadzean and Todd, 1967). In most instances, the plasma volume in the unsplenectomized subject is significantly and consistently increased, and falls following splenectomy, although it may not return to normal values (Table 6).

In general, there is a reasonable correlation between the magnitude of splenomegaly and the increase in plasma volume, and an inverse correlation between the H_V and the plasma volume. Conversely, there is no correlation between the H_V and the volume of the splenic red blood cell pool.

8.6.2. THALASSEMIA MAJOR

In thalassemia major with splenomegaly, the PV is markedly expanded, and this may occur despite a normal RCM (Blendis et al., 1974). In a series of six patients with thalassemia major and one with HbE/thalassemia, plasma volumes were 1.4–1.7 ×greater than predicted. 4/5 studied before splenectomy showed moderate to severe anemia and shortened red blood cell life-span. The splenic pool was between 9 and 39% of the RCM, and the corresponding values of H_B/H_V between 1.0 and 1.26. In only two was the RCM less than normal. After splenectomy, the red blood cell life-span increased significantly, the RCM increased by 18–170% in three patients, but fell in a fourth. However, the plasma volume remained grossly expanded: of the five investigated both before and after splenectomy, the plasma volume decreased by about 15 mL/kg in three, was unchanged in one, and increased slightly in one. This suggests that the plasma volume expansion differed from that of most patients with splenomegaly, in that it was virtually unaffected by removal of the spleen. A major abnormality in thalassemia major is the expansion of the bone marrow, and evidence suggests that the marrow could be acting as a vascular shunt, and so act as a source of plasma expansion. This is supported by observations that maintenance blood transfusion therapy, which impairs bone marrow expansion, also suppresses expansion of the plasma volume. A parallel circumstance appears to be present in patients with sickle cell anemia uncomplicated by splenomegaly; Erlandson et al. (1960) measured plasma volumes of 61.7–73.2 mL/kg in patients who did not show splenomegaly, this being a greater expansion than they had found in other chronic anemias.

8.6.3. POLYCYTHEMIA VERA

In this disorder, there is an uncontrolled production of red blood cells and, when splenomegaly is slight or moderate, the plasma volume is usually normal in association with a high RCM (Verel, 1961; Donaldson et al., 1970). This differs from other splenomegalic states, in which the expanded intravascular volume is associated with structural or hyperkinetic changes in the portal circulation, and the increased volume requirement is met principally by plasma volume. Earlier work had suggested that plasma volume was reduced in this condition, possibly as a compensatory phenomenon limiting the expansion of total blood volume. This was not confirmed by Bowdler (1972), in a study of 23 patients with polycythemia vera, of whom 15 showed splenomegaly. Seven of the patients with the larger spleens also showed evidence of red blood cell pooling: Similarly, subjects with splenomegaly showed significantly higher values for the RCM than those without splenic enlargement (for weight-related volumes, $t = 2.95, 0.01 > p > 0.001$; Nadler-predicted volumes, $t = 2.74, 0.02 > p > 0.01$). H_B/H_V values were not elevated above those of controls, regardless of the presence of splenomegaly or of a red blood cell pool; likewise, H_R values, expressed as H_R/H_V in the region of the spleen were not elevated. Apparently, the high red blood cell content of circulating blood does not prevent the pooling of red blood cells in the spleen, but there is a limiting level of H_V above which the splenic mechanism for concentrating red blood cells is ineffective in producing a further increase above the H_V of large vessel blood. Donaldson et al. (1970) likewise found a mean value for H_B/H_V of 0.915, in eight polycythemic patients with splenomegaly. The mean plasma volume for the series of 23 polycythemics did not differ from normal, at 42.9 (SD 7.7) mL/kg, but, for the subgroup with the greatest enlargement of the spleen and showing red blood cell pooling, the plasma volume was significantly increased at 48.3 (SD 7.1) mL/kg (when compared with controls, weight-related volumes showed $t = 2.82, 0.01 > p > 0.02$; Nadler-predicted volumes, $t = 2.38, 0.05 > p > 0.0l$), showing that the size of the spleen affects plasma volume despite the total volume expansion produced by the RCM (Bowdler, 1972).

8.7. CLINICAL CONSIDERATIONS

The circumstances of splenic enlargement involve the development of symptomatology from several sources, namely, the local effects of the enlarged organ, the underlying symptoms of the disorder of etiology, such as the hematological malignancies, and the cytopenias and their sequelae, as outlined in Chapter 9. Dilutional anemia adds its own additional morbid burden.

The clinical importance of the dilutional anemia and splenic pooling of red blood cells lies, first, in their recognition; otherwise, inappropriate therapy for the anemia may be selected. In conditions other than pregnancy, in which the expansion of plasma volume is highly predictable, the recognition of dilutional anemia requires the accurate measurement of both the RCM and plasma volume; in conditions associated with organomegaly, there should preferably be organ volume and scintillation surface-counter studies for assessing the distribution of blood components related to the principal relevant organs.

Jonsson et al. (1992) have discussed the parallels between the organs capable of developing plasma volume expansion with high arteriovenous blood flows, and which have an interposed small vessel vasculature capable of skimming plasma-rich blood. These are the spleen, in which skimming is necessary for hemoconcentration and the diversion of plasma-soluble antigens to the sites of immune processing. Second, there is the bone marrow in which plasma skimming provides a washout mechanism for newly formed cells. Third, there is the uteroplacental complex, in circumstances in which the high plasma content of the blood may beneficially increase the blood flow to the myometrium, kidneys, and skeletal musculature.

The disordered circulatory physiology associated with the dilutional anemias has the potential for adding an additional burden to the need for an augmented cardiac output: In severe anemias, the diminished oxygen-carrying capacity of the blood is compensated by the increase in cardiac output produced both by increasing stroke volume and cardiac rate. Ultimately, this may result in high-output cardiac failure, despite the reduction in required cardiac work provided by the fall in blood viscosity as the hematocrit declines. The high transsplenic and portal venous blood flow produced by splenomegaly (*see* Subheadings 5.1.2. and 5.1.4.) has the potential for increasing the venous return to the heart, and adding an additional increment to the obligatory cardiac output, and reducing cardiac reserve, as indicated by the clinical observations of Garnett et al. (1969). The correction of these sequelae of splenomegaly requires splenectomy, an equivalent procedure, or an appropriate pharmacological means of diminishing spleen size.

The longer-term effects of chronic plasma expansion with hemodilution do not appear to have been explored experimentally, but the effects of acute hemodilution with plasma expansion in the dog have been described by Levy et al. (1996), and suggest its complexity. They showed that isovolemic hemodilution, to a H_V of 20 mL/dL, increased the cardiac index by 35% in normal, control dogs, despite which there was significant reduction in regional oxygen delivery to splanchnic organs. Animals with experimentally impaired coronary circulation showed reduced splanchnic oxygen delivery at higher hematocrits, indicating that, in these circumstances, conditions limiting cardiac reserve may significantly compromise the splanchnic circulation. Therefore, it is therefore important to evaluate cardiac function in the circumstances of hemodilution, to determine the tolerance to increased cardiac output, and especially so in those disorders, such as the myeloproliferative syndromes, which are more common in older age groups.

Whether dilutional anemia constitutes an effective stimulus to erythropoiesis is not yet clear. In the specific case of pregnancy, Cotes et al. (1983) found that serum erythropoietin increased at some time after 8 wk of gestation, but this was not shown to vary with the degree of anemia or hemodilution. However, there was a highly significant correlation between serum erythropoietin and placental lactogen. In the dilutional anemia related to splenomegaly, the finding that, in some cases, there is a reduction in the RCM after splenectomy may indicate the loss of a stimulus to erythropoiesis, probably because of correction of the anemia. However, if it proves possible to translate this into a potential therapy for increasing the RCM and hematocrit, the effects of increasing the blood viscosity on cardiac output and regional perfusion will need careful definition.

REFERENCES

Allen, T. H., Peng, M. T., Chen, K. P., Huang, T. F., Chang, C. and Fang, H. S. (1956) Prediction of blood volume and adiposity in man from body weight and cube of height. *Metabolism* **5**, 328–345.

Andersen, S. B. (1962) Simultaneous determination of plasma volume with ^{131}I-labelled gamma globulin, ^{131}I-labelled albumin and T-1824. *Clin. Sci.* **23**, 221–228.

Andersen, S. B. and Gabuzda, T. G. (1964) Simultaneous determination of plasma volume with T-1824 and ^{131}I-labelled autologous and homologous paraprotein. *Clin. Sci.* **26**, 41–45.

Anderson, R. J., Cronin, R. E., McDonald, K. M. and Schrier, R. W. (1976) Mechanisms of portal hypertension-induced alterations in renal hemodynamics, renal water excretion, and renin secretion. *J. Clin. Invest.* **58**, 964–970.

Baker, C. H. (1963) Cr51-labeled red cell, ^{131}I-fibrinogen and T-1824 dilution spaces. *Am. J. Physiol.* **1**, 176–180.

Barnes, D. W. H., Loutit, J. F., and Reeve, E. B. (1948a) Observations on the estimate of the circulating red blood cell volume in man given by T 1824 and the haematocrit, with special reference to uncorrected dye loss from the circulation. *Clin. Sci.* **7**, 135–154.

Barnes, D. W. H., Loutit, J. F., and Reeve, E. B. (1948b) A comparison of estimates of circulating red blood cell volume given by the Ashby marked red cell method and the T 1824-haematocrit method in man. *Clin. Sci.* **7**, 155–173.

Bartsch, P., Mairbaurl, H., and Friedmann, B. (1998) [Pseudo-anemia caused by sports.] *Ther. Umsch.* **55**, 251–255.

Bateman, J. C., Shorr, H. M., and Elgvin, T. (1949) Hypervolemic anemia in cirrhosis. *J. Clin. Invest.* **28**, 539–547.

Besa, E. C. (1975) Physiological changes in blood volume. *CRC Crit. Rev. Clin. Lab. Sci.* **6**, 67–79.

Better, O. S. and Schrier, R. W. (1983) Disturbed volume homeostasis in patients with cirrhosis of the liver. *Kidney Int.* **23**, 303–311.

Blendis, L. M., Clarke, M. B., and Williams, R. (1969) Effect of splenectomy on the haemodilutional anaemia of splenomegaly. *Lancet* **i**, 795–798.

Blendis, L. M., Ramboer, C., and Williams, R. (1970) Studies on the haemodilution anaemia of splenomegaly. *Eur. J. Clin. Invest.* **1**, 54–64.

Blendis, L. M., Banks, D. C., Ramboer, C., and Williams, R. (1970) Spleen blood flow and splanchnic haemodynamics in blood dyscrasia and other splenomegalies. *Clin. Sci.* **38**, 73–84.

Blendis, L. M., Modell, C. B., Bowdler, A. J., and Williams R. (1974) Some effects of splenectomy in thalassaemia major. *Br. J. Haematol.* **28**, 77–87.

Bowdler, A. J. (1962) Theoretical considerations concerning measurement of the splenic red cell pool. *Clin. Sci.* **23**, 181–195.

Bowdler, A. J. (1963) Dilution anaemia corrected by splenectomy in Gaucher's disease. *Ann. Intern. Med.* **58**, 664–669.

Bowdler, A. J. (1967) Dilution anaemia associated with enlargement of the spleen. *Proc. R. Soc. Med.* **60**, 44–47.

Bowdler, A. J. (1969) Regional variations in the proportion of red cells in the blood in man. *Br. J. Haematol.* **16**, 557–571.

Bowdler, A. J. (1970a) Blood volume changes in patients with splenomegaly. *Transfusion* **10**, 171–181.

Bowdler, A. J. (1970b) The clinical significance of chronically expanded blood volume. *Lab. Management* **8**, 22–25.

Bowdler, A. J. (1972) Plasma volume and splenomegaly in polycythaemia vera. *Br. J. Haematol.* **22**, 331–340.

Bowdler, A. J. (1983) Splenomegaly and hypersplenism. *Clin. Haematol.* **12**, 467–488.

Castro-Malaspina, H., Najean, Y., and Flandrin, G. (1979) Erythrokinetic studies in hairy-cell leukaemia. *Br. J. Haematol.* **42**, 189–197.

Chaplin, H. Jr. and Mollison, P. L. (1952) Correction for plasma trapped in the red cell volume of the hematocrit. *Blood* **7**, 1227–1238.

Chaplin, H. Jr., Mollison, P. L., and Vetter, H. (1953) The body/venous hematocrit ratio: its constancy over a wide hematocrit range. *J. Clin. Invest.* **32**, 1309–1316.

Chesley, L. C. (1972), Plasma and red cell volumes during pregnancy. *Am. J. Obstet. Gynecol.* **112**, 440–450.

Christensen, B. E. (1973) Erythrocyte pooling and sequestration in enlarged spleens. Estimations of splenic erythrocyte and plasma volume in splenomegalic patients. *Scand. J. Haematol.* **10**, 106–119.

Cook, J., McFadzean, A. J. S., and Todd, D. (1963) Splenectomy in cryptogenetic splenomegaly. *Br. Med. J.* **2**, 337–344.

Cotes, P. M., Canning, C. E., and Lind, T. (1983) Changes in serum immunoreactive erythropoietin during the menstrual cycle and normal pregnancy. *Br. J. Obstet. Gynaecol.* **90**, 304–311.

Crane, G. G., Pryor, D. S., and Wells, J. V. (1972) Tropical splenomegaly syndrome in New Guinea. 11. Long term results of splenectomy. *Trans. R. Soc. Trop. Med. Hyg.* **66**, 733–742.

Dawson, A. B., Evans, H. M., and Whipple, G. H. (1920) Blood volume studies. 111. Behavior of a large series of dyes introduced into the circulating blood. *Am. J. Physiol.* **51**, 232–257.

DiBona, G. F. (1977) Neurogenic regulation of renal tubular sodium reabsorption. *Am. J. Physiol.* **233**, F73–F81.

Di Bona, G. F. (1984) Renal neural activity in hepatorenal syndrome. *Kidney Int.* **25**, 841–853.

Donaldson, G. W., McArthur, M., Macpherson, A. I., and Richmond, J. (1970) Blood volume changes in splenomegaly. *Br. J. Haematol.* **18**, 45–55.

Eisenberg, S. (1956) Blood volume in patients with Laennec's cirrhosis of liver as determined by radioactive chromium tagged red cells. *Am. J. Med.* **17**, 189–195.

Erlandson, M. E., Schulman, I., and Smith, C. H. (1960) Studies on congenital hemolytic syndromes. III Rates of destruction and production of erythrocytes in sickle cell anemia. *Pediatrics* **25**, 629–644.

England, J. M., Walford, D. M., and Waters, D. A. W. (1972) Re-assessment of the reliability of the haematocrit. *Br. J. Haematol.* **23**, 247–256.

Fahraeus, R. (1929) The suspension stability of the blood. *Physiol. Rev.* **9**, 241–274.

Fakunle, Y. M. (1981) Tropical splenomegaly. Part 1: Tropical Africa. *Clin. Haematol.* **10**, 963–975.

Freinkel, N., Schreiner, G. E., and Athens, J. W. (1953) Simultaneous distribution of T-1824 and ^{131}I-labelled human serum albumin in man. *J. Clin. Invest.* **32**, 138.

Fudenberg, H. H., Baldini, M., Mahoney, J. P., and Dameshek, W. (1961) The body hematocrit/ venous hematocrit ratio and the 'splenic reservoir'. *Blood* **17**, 71–82.

Garnett, E. S., Goddard, B. A., Markby, D., and Webber, C. E. (1969) The spleen as an arteriovenous shunt. *Lancet* **i**, 386–388.

Gibson, J. G. and Evans, W. A. Jr. (1937) Clinical studies of the blood volume. 1. Clinical application of a method employing the azo-dye 'Evans Blue' and the spectrophotometer. *J. Clin. Invest.* **16**, 301–306.

Glass, H. I., De Garreta, A. C., Lewis, S. M., Grammaticos, P., and Szur, L. (1968) Measurement of splenic red-blood-cell mass with radioactive carbon monoxide. *Lancet* **i**, 669–670.

Hall, R. and Malia, R. G. (1991) *Medical Laboratory Haematology,* 2nd ed., Butterworth-Heinemann, Oxford.

Hamilton, P. J., Richmond, J., Donaldson, G. W., Williams, R., Hutt, M. S., and Lugumba, V. (1967) Splenectomy in "big spleen disease." *Br. Med. J.* **3**, 823–825.

Harris, I. M., McAlister, J. M., and Prankerd, T. A. J. (1958) Splenomegaly and the circulating red cell. *Br. J. Haematol.* **4**, 97–102.

Henriksen, J. H., Ring-Larsen, H., Kanstrup, I. L., and Christensen, N. J. (1984) Splanchnic and renal elimination and release of catecholamines in cirrhosis. Evidence of enhanced sympathetic nervous activity in patients with decompensated cirrhosis. *Gut* **25**, 1034–1043.

Herreman, G., Piguet, H., Zittoun, R., Bilski-Pasquier, G., and Bousser, J. (1968) L'hypervolemie de la macroglobulinemie de Waldenstrom. *Nouv. Rev. Franc. Hemat.* **8**, 209–226.

Hess, C. E., Ayers, C. R., Wetzel, R. A., Mohler, D. N., and Sandusky, W. R. (1971) Dilutional anemia of splenomegaly: an indication for splenectomy. *Ann. Surg.* **173**, 693–699.

Hess, C. E., Ayers, C. R., Sandusky, W. R., Carpenter, M. A., Wetzel, R. A., and Mohler, D. N. (1976) Mechanism of dilutional anemia in massive splenomegaly. *Blood* **47**, 629–644.

Hoffman, S. L., Piessens, W. F., Ratiwayanto, S., et al. (1984) Reduction of suppressor T-lymphocytes in the tropical splenomegaly syndrome. *N. Engl. J. Med.* **310**, 337–341.

Hurley, P. J. (1975) Red cell and plasma volumes in normal adults. *J. Nucl. Med.* **16**, 46–52.

Hyde, R. D. and Jones, N. F. (1962) Red cell volume and total body water. *Br. J. Haemat.* **8**, 283–289.

Hytten, F. (1985) Blood volume changes in normal pregnancy. *Clin. Haematol.* **14**, 601–612.

International Committee for Standardization in Haematology (1980a) Recommended methods for measurement of red-cell and plasma volume. *J. Nucl. Med.* **21**, 793–800.

International Committee for Standardization in Haematology (1980b) Recommendation for reference method for determination by centrifugation of packed cell volume of blood. *J. Clin. Pathol.* **33**, 1–2.

Isbister, J. P. (1997) Physiology and pathophysiology of blood volume regulation. *Transfusion Sci.* **18**, 409–423.

Jepson, J. H. and Friesen, H. G. (1968) The mechanism of action of human placental lactogen on erythropoiesis. *Br. J. Haematol.* **15**, 465–471.

Jonsson, V., Bock, J. E., and Nielsen, J. B. (1992) Significance of plasma skimming and plasma volume expansion. *J. Appl. Physiol.* **72**, 2047–2051.

Kaufman, S. and Deng, Y. (1999) Effect of splenic extract on plasma volume and renal function in the rat. *Life Sci.* **65**, 2653–2662.

Kesteven, P. J. L., Pullan, J. M., and Wetherly-Mein, G. (1985) Hypersplenism and splenectomy in lymphoproliferative and myeloproliferative disorders. *Clin. Lab. Haematol.* **7**, 297–306.

Kirk, R. (1957) The pathogenesis of some tropical splenomegalies. *Ann. Trop. Med. Parasitol.* **51**, 225–234.

Kopp, W. L., MacKinney, A. A. Jr., and Wasson, G. (1969) Blood volume and hematocrit value in macroglobulinemia and myeloma. *Arch. Intern. Med.* **123**, 394–396.

Leather, H. M. (1961) Portal hypertension and gross splenomegaly in Uganda. *Br. Med. J.* **1**, 15–18.

Levy, M. (1974) Renal function in dogs with acute selective hepatic venous outflow block. *Am. J. Physiol.* **227**, 1073–1083.

Levy, P. S., Quigley, R. L., and Gould, S. A. (1996) Acute dilutional anemia and critical left anterior descending artery stenosis impairs end organ oxygen delivery. *J. Trauma* **41**, 416–423.

Lewis, S. M., Catovsky, D., Hows, J. M., and Ardalan, B. (1977) Splenic red cell pooling in hairy cell leukaemia. *Br. J. Haematol.* **35**, 351–357.

Lieberman, F. L. and Reynolds, T. B. (1967) Plasma volume in cirrhosis of the liver: its relation to portal hypertension, ascites and renal failure. *J. Clin. Invest.* **46**, 1297–1308.

Longo, L. D. (1983) Maternal blood volume and cardiac output during pregnancy: a hypothesis of endocrinologic control. *Am. J. Physiol.* **245**, R720–R729.

Lowdon, A. G. R., Stewart, R. H. M., and Walker, W. (1966) Risk of serious infection following splenectomy. *Br. Med. J.* **1**, 446–450.

McFadzean, A. J. S. and Todd, D. (1967) The blood volume in postnecrotic cirrhosis of the liver with splenomegaly. *Clin. Sci.* **32**, 339–350.

McFadzean, A. J. S., Todd, D., and Tsang, K. C. (1958a) Observations on the anemia of cryptogenetic splenomegaly. I. Hemolysis. *Blood* **13**, 513–523.

McFadzean, A. J. S., Todd, D., and Tsang, K. C. (1958b) Observations on the anemia of cryptogenetic splenomegaly. II. Expansion of the plasma volume. *Blood* **13**, 524–532.

Manasc, B. and Jepson, J. (1969) Erythropoietin in plasma and urine during human pregnancy. *Can. Med. Assoc. J.* **100**, 687–691.

Marsden, P. D. and Crane, G. G. (1976) The tropical splenomegaly syndrome. A current appraisal. *Rev. Inst. Med. Trop. Sao Paulo* **18**, 54–70.

Mollison, P. L. (1961) *Blood Transfusion in Clinical Medicine,* 3rd ed., Blackwell, Oxford.

Mollison, P. L. (1983) *Blood Transfusion in Clinical Medicine,* 7th ed., Blackwell, Oxford.

Mollison, P. L., Engelfriet, C. P., and Contreras, M. (1997) *Blood Transfusion in Clinical Medicine,* 10th ed., Blackwell, Oxford. Appendices 2–5.

Motulsky, A. C., Casserd, F., Giblett, E. R., Broun, G. O., and Finch, C. A. (1958) Anemia and the spleen. *N. Engl. J. Med.* **259**, 1164–1169.

Muldowney, F. P. (1957) The relationship of total red cell mass to lean body mass in man. *Clin. Sci.* **16,** 163–169.

Nadler, S. B., Hidalgo, J. U., and Bloch, T. (1962) Prediction of blood volume in normal human adults. *Surgery* **51,** 224–232.

Najean, Y. and Deschrymer, F. (1984) The body/venous haematocrit ratio and its use for calculating total blood volume from fractional volumes. *Eur. J. Nucl. Med.* **9,** 558–560.

Nichols, A. W. (1999) Nonorthopaedic problems in the aquatic athlete. *Clin. Sports Med.* **18,** 395–411.

Ooyirilangkumaran, T. (1973) The blood volume changes in the anaemia of experimental splenomegaly. *Br. J. Haematol.* **25,** 547.

Pearson, T. C., Guthrie, D. L., Simpson, J., et al. (1995) Interpretation of measured red cell mass and plasma volume in adults: Expert Panel on Radionuclides of the International Council for Standardization in Haematology. *Br. J. Haematol.* **89,** 748–756.

Pengelly, C. D. R. (1977) The influence of splenomegaly on red cell and plasma volume. *J. R. Coll. Physicians Lond.* **12,** 61–66.

Pettit, J. E., Williams, E. D., Glass, H. I., Lewis, S. M., Szur, L., and Wicks, C. J. (1971) Studies of splenic function in the myeloproliferative disorders and generalized malignant lymphomas. *Br. J. Haematol.* **20,** 575–586.

Pitney, W. R. (1968) The tropical splenomegaly syndrome. *Trans. R. Soc. Trop. Med. Hyg.* **62,** 717–728.

Prankerd, T. A. J. (1963) The spleen and anaemia. *Br. Med. J.* **ii,** 517–524.

Pryor, D. S. (1967a) The mechanism of anaemia in tropical splenomegaly. *Q. J. Med.* **36,** 337–356.

Pryor, D. S. (1967b) Splenectomy in tropical splenomegaly. *Br. Med. J.* **3,** 825–828.

Rawson, R. A. (1943) The binding of T-1824 and structurally related diazo dyes by plasma proteins. *Am. J. Physiol.* **138,** 708–717.

Retzleff, J., Newlon Tauxe, W., Kiely, J., and Stroebel, C. (1969) Erythrocyte volume, plasma volume and lean body mass in adult men and women. *Blood* **33,** 649.

Richmond, J., Donaldson, G. W., Williams, R., Hamilton, P. J., and Hutt, M. S. (1967) Haematological effects of the idiopathic splenomegaly seen in Uganda. *Br. J. Haematol.* **13,** 348–363.

Rocco, V. K. and Ware, A. J. (1986) Cirrhotic ascites: pathophysiology, diagnosis and management. *Ann. Intern. Med.* **105,** 573–585.

Rosenbaum, D., Murphy, G. W., and Swisher, S. N. (1966) Hemodynamic studies of the portal circulation in rnyeloid metaplasia. *Am. J. Med.* **41,** 360–368.

Rothschild, M. A., Bauman, A., Yalow, R. S., and Berson, S. A. (1954) Effect of splenomegaly on blood volume. *J. Appl. Physiol.* **6,** 701–706.

Rowntree, L. G., Brown, G. D., and Roth, G. M. (1929) *The Volume of the Blood and Plasma in Health and Disease.* Mayo Clinic Monograph, Philadelphia.

Sterling, K. and Gray, S. J. (1950) Determination of the circulating red cell volume in man by radiochromium. *J. Clin. Invest.* **29,** 1614–1619.

Swan, H. and Nelson, A. W. (1971) Blood volume, 1. Critique: spun vs. isotope hematocrit, 125RIHSA vs. 51CrRBC. *Ann. Surg.* **173,** 481–495.

Takeda, K. and Reeve, E. B. (1963) Clinical and experimental studies of the metabolism and distribution of albumin with autologous 1311 albumin in healthy man. *J. Lab. Clin. Med.* **61,** 183–202.

Toghill, P. J. (1964) Red-cell pooling in enlarged spleens. *Br. J. Haematol.* **10,** 347–357.

Toghill, P. J. and Green, S. (1971) The influence of spleen size on the distribution of red cells and plasma. *J. Clin. Pathol.* **25,** 570–573.

Toghill, P. J., and Prichard, B. N. C (1964) A study of the action of noradrenaline on the splenic red cell pool. *Clin. Sci.* **26,** 203–212.

Verel, D. (1961) Blood volume changes in cyanotic congenital heart disease and polycythemia rubra vera. *Circulation* **23,** 749–753.

Videbaek, A., Christensen, B. E., and Jonsson, V. (1982) *The Spleen in Health and Disease.* Year Book, Chicago.

Warren, J. V., Nickerson, J. L., and Elkin, D. C. (1951) The cardiac output in patients with arteriovenous fistulas. *J. Clin. Invest.* **30,** 210–214.

Warren, J. V., Elkin, D. C., and Nickerson, J. L. (1951) The blood volume in patients with arteriovenous fistulas. *J. Clin. Invest.* **30,** 220–225.

Weight, L. M., Klein, M., Noakes, T. D., and Jacobs, P. (1992) 'Sports anemia': a real or apparent phenomenon in endurance-trained athletes? *Int. J. Sports Med.* **13,** 344–347.

Weinstein, V. E. (1964) Haemodilution anaemia associated with simple splenic hyperplasia. *Lancet* **ii,** 218–223.

Wennesland, R., Brown, E., Hopper, J., Hodges, J. L., Guttentag, O. E., Scott, K. G., Tucker, I. N., and Bradley, B. (1959) Red cell, plasma and blood volume in healthy men measured by radiochromium cell tagging and hematocrit: influence of age, somatotype and habits of physical activity on the variance after regression of volumes to height and weight combined. *J. Clin. Invest.* **38,** 1065–1077.

Williams, R. (1966) Portal hypertension in idiopathic tropical splenomegaly. *Lancet* **i,** 329–333.

Zhang, B. and Lewis, S. M. (1987) Splenic haematocrit and the splenic plasma pool. *Br. J. Haematol.* **66,** 97–102.

CLINICAL ASPECTS OF DISORDERS OF THE SPLEEN

III

9 The Clinical Significance of the Spleen

ANTHONY J. BOWDLER, MD, PhD, FRCP, FRCPATH, FACP

Occam's Razor: "We are to admit no more causes of natural things than such as are both true and sufficient to explain their appearances. To this purpose the philosophers say that Nature does nothing in vain, and more is in vain when less will serve; for Nature is pleased with simplicity, and affects not the pomp of superfluous causes."

Isaac Newton,
Philosophia Naturalis Principia Mathematica

9.1. THE EVOLUTION OF CONCEPTS OF THE HUMAN SPLEEN

The role of the spleen in human disease has been slow to emerge from the shadow of Galen's aphorism describing the spleen as "an organ full of mystery." Anatomical accuracy was achieved by Aristotle in classical times (Lewis, 1983): One surprising, but long-persisting, speculation concerning its dysfunction was that the spleen impaired athletic prowess. Pliny stated, "This member hath a proprietie by itself sometimes, to hinder a man's running." It may well be that the ancients were referring to the pathologically enlarged organ. They were also aware that it might be removed and the subject survive: "They say that the spleen may be taken out of the body by way of incision, and yet the creature live nevertheless" (Moynihan, 1921).

This was confirmed by anecdotal accounts of uncertain value describing traumatic or surgical removal of the spleen before the days of anesthesia. The clinical and biological importance of the spleen has attracted little attention over the intervening years. Conditions involving splenomegaly, sometimes of severe degree, must have affected a significant proportion of the human race: These have included thalassemia major, leishmaniasis (Kala-azar), and especially malaria, which formerly extended over a much wider area of the temperate world than is presently the case. Indeed, the increased severity and special hazards of malaria to the hyposplenic subject suggest that a defensive spleen may have been a necessary requirement for the widespread geographic expansion of primates and humans during evolution.

With the advent of appropriate surgical technique, splenectomy was in large part reserved initially for cases of trauma to the organ. In the absence of clearly defined physiological functions for the human spleen, the study of the effects of splenectomy provided an essentially empirical insight into its functions and the effects of pathological disorder in the organ. Specific disorders were recognized in which splenectomy was shown to be therapeutically effective, including idiopathic (immune) thrombocytopenic purpura and hereditary spherocytosis. Conversely, in other disorders, such as acute leukemia, the operation was found to carry a high and early mortality (Collier, 1882), and, at various times, special risks were described in association with specific disorders. Hickling (1937, 1953), for example, at one time discouraged splenectomy in cases of primary myeloid metaplasia with myelosclerosis, in the expectation that such cases became dependent on the spleen for hematopoiesis, a concept which was not subsequently substantiated.

9.1.1. THE SPLEEN AND THE CIRCULATION
An insight into the special relationship between circulating blood and the spleen was evident in the work of van Leeuwenhoeck (1632–1723 AD), who suggested that the spleen plays a role in the "elaboration and purification" of the blood. Likewise, Stukely, in his Goulstonian lecture of 1722, showed remarkable prescience, when, relying essentially on macroscopic structure, he rejected the classical concept of a secretory function for the organ, and proposed that it was a diverticulum of the systemic circulation, filling and emptying with blood, and acting as a controller of blood volume.

9.1.2. COMPARATIVE STUDIES OF THE SPLEEN
Comparative studies have shown a wide diversity of splenic functions in different species, and one of the principal barriers to developing an understanding of the physiology of the human spleen has been the considerable interspecies variability of both function and structure.

In lower vertebrate species, splenic hematopoiesis is, in many cases, prominent, and, in some, the spleen is the dominant organ for erythropoiesis. In mammals, blood cell production, especially splenic erythropoiesis, is variable between species, and is often restricted to fetal life as an atavism or phylogenic reminiscence (Tischendorf, 1985). The adult human spleen retains some capacity for supporting hematopoiesis as a compensatory or a pathological process.

In mammals, two principal functional types of spleen can be identified in different species, namely, the "storage" spleen and the "defensive" spleen. The storage spleen matches the concept of Stukely and other investigators, including Cooper, Winslow, Heister, and Hodgkin, as an organ modifying the composition and volume of the blood. Gray (1854) described extensive researches

From: The Complete Spleen: A Handbook of Structure, Function, and Clinical Disorders Edited by: A. J. Bowdler © Humana Press Inc., Totowa, NJ

into the comparative anatomy of the spleen, and was especially impressed by the variable size of the equine spleen, relating this to the activity and hydration of the animal before death. He was also aware of the reservoir function of the spleen in diving mammals. He concluded that the spleen functions "to regulate the quantity and quality of the blood."

Other species with a storage spleen include dog, cat, bovine, and goat. Such a spleen is characterized, in the resting state, by a high content of erythrocytes; it is structurally rich in trabeculae and smooth muscle, and may produce profound circulatory effects on the red blood cell content and packed cell volume of blood in the extrasplenic circulation by its degree of contraction. Such a spleen is large, compared to the size of the animal.

The control of the quantity of circulating red blood cells by the spleen has received more attention than the qualitative effects. Researches by Barcroft et al. between 1923 and 1927, identified many of the factors influencing quantitative control in small mammals (Barcroft and Barcroft, 1923; Barcroft, 1925; Barcroft and Poole, 1927). Studies relevant to this function were also performed by Scheunert, Cannon, Cruickshank, and others. Unfortunately, it was many years before the physiological storage of red blood cells was recognized as not a significant function of the human spleen: The average red blood cell content of the spleen in man is 30–50 mL, which does not offer a significant potential for augmenting the circulating red blood cell mass. Sympathomimetic drugs may, however, raise the packed cell volume of the blood, but this does not appear to be exclusively because of the spleen, being probably a more widely distributed shift of red blood cells away from the splanchnic area (Schaffner et al., 1985; Schaffner and Fehr, 1981; Toghill and Green, 1973).

The defensive spleen is relatively smaller in relation to body weight, and is phylogenetically more primitive than the storage spleen: trabeculae and capsulotrabecular muscle are less prominent, and lymphoid development is of greater degree. The human spleen is essentially a representative of the defensive type, and is relatively small in relation to body size. Detailed understanding of the defensive spleen necessarily awaited insight into the functions of the lymphocyte, the lymphatic system, and the splenic microvasculature. Consequently, the storage concept was long accepted, erroneously, as the model for the physiology of the human spleen.

9.1.3. CLINICAL EXPERIENCE AND THE SPLEEN
Uncertainty with respect to the validity of animal models led clinicians to organize their clinical experiences conceptually, in terms of postulated or apparently necessary splenic functions. Once the operation of splenectomy had been shown to be a reasonably safe procedure, by experience gained mainly in the context of trauma to the organ, it was widely applied to conditions showing enlargement of the spleen. Before the end of the nineteenth century, Spencer Wells (1888) summarized the use of the operation for conditions such as the wandering spleen and splenic cysts of various etiologies, as well as for "simple hypertrophy," "malarial hypertrophy," and "hypertrophy with leukaemia."

Conditions now identified as hereditary spherocytosis (formerly better known as "acholuric family jaundice") and idiopathic thrombocytopenic purpura were treated successfully by removal of the spleen. In a discussion of hereditary spherocytosis, Chauffard (1907) introduced the concept of "hypersplenism," which implied that the anemia of the condition resulted from excessive activity of the spleen, in a manner analogous to hyperthyroidism, with thyroid enlargement and its correction by thyroidectomy. The concept of hypersplenism and its present clinical usage are developed further in Subheading 5.

9.2. FUNCTIONS OF THE SPLEEN

The defensive spleen of humans is a highly specialized structure, organized predominantly around a unique microvasculature (*see* Chapter 2), capable of filtering out inappropriate particles from the bloodstream, and producing an immune response to particles such as microorganisms, as well as to soluble antigens. The principal function of the defensive spleen is protection against infection; an extensive speculative literature relating the spleen to this function had emerged by the beginning of the twentieth century, but the association was effectively demonstrated by three landmark observations.

1. Moris and Bullock (1919) showed that splenectomized rats had a higher mortality than orchiectomized rats, when both were exposed to endemic laboratory infection with "rat plague bacillus."
2. In humans, the relationship was given significance by King and Shumaker (1952), describing fulminant sepsis in five infants, following splenectomy for hereditary spherocytosis.
3. Furthermore, it became apparent that the postsplenectomy state involved susceptibility to a highly lethal septicemia, identified as "overwhelming postsplenectomy infection," and that this was not limited to early childhood (Diamond, 1969; Chaikoff and McCabe (1985); Singer, 1973; Franke and Neu, 1981; Shaw and Print, 1989; Rebentish and Bernstein, 1993).

The activities of the spleen contributing to defense against infection include efficient particulate filtration, removing microorganisms from the bloodstream (Scher et al., 1983), a slow-flowing circulation through the red pulp, providing prolonged contact between abnormal particulates and a densely populated reticulum of macrophages, opsonization of microorganisms, which becomes impaired in the absence of the spleen (this may in part result from the synthesis of properdin, and also from the synthesis of tuftsin, which acts as a stimulant to phagocytosis). Antibody production is also a significant function of the spleen, which is a site for the interaction of memory B-cells and helper T-cells in the primary response producing specific immunoglobulin M (IgM) antibodies. Absence of splenic activity also impairs the normal subsequent switch to IgG-class antibodies (Sullivan et al., 1978).

9.2.1. PARTICULATE FILTRATION
Approximately 5% of the cardiac output normally flows through the spleen. Removal of abnormal particulates, such as microorganisms, immune complexes, senescent blood cells, and red blood cells of abnormal shape or membrane flexibility, occurs mainly in the red pulp compartment. The vasculature in the human spleen has few direct structural connections between the arterioles and the splenic sinuses (the "closed" route), and the greater part of the splenic blood flow in humans (probably more than 90%) enters the open circulation of the cords of Billroth, and must traverse the interendothelial slits of the sinus walls to return to the splenic veins and the general circulation. Dynamic adaptation of the pulp structure permits close apposition of the arterioles to the sinus walls, so that the high volume of flow can be accommodated.

Filtration depends, first, on the relatively slow flow of the blood through the macrophage-rich red pulp, which potentiates contact with macrophages, and enhances the phagocytosis of opsonized particles, and which may initiate an immune response. The second major factor in filtration occurs at the walls of the splenic sinuses, where particles meet the barrier of the interendothelial slits. Normal red blood cells are usually sufficiently flexible for penetration of this barrier. At this level, the nonopsonized encapsulated microorganism, or other particle, may be held in the red pulp. This constitutes an important mechanism for pathological hemolysis because nondeformable red blood cells including spherocytes, sickle cells, acanthocytes, and senescent red blood cells may also be prevented from reentering the extrasplenic circulation (culling). Intraerythrocytic inclusions may be removed during passage of cells through the sinus wall (pitting): Debris, such as Howell-Jolly bodies, Pappenheimer bodies, Heinz bodies, and vesicles, may be expressed back into the trailing aspect of the cell during interendothelial passage, and a tail of membrane enclosing the particles discarded on the red pulp aspect of the endothelium. Consequently, the presence of these intracellular bodies in the circulating red blood cells may provide an indication of impaired or absent splenic function.

9.2.2. LYMPHOID COMPONENT The spleen is a major element of the lymphatic system, containing about 25% of the total exchangeable T-cell population and 15% of the B-cell population. Approximately 50% of lymphocytes entering the spleen gain access to the white pulp, which is organized as an irregular cuff around the arterioles. The T-cells are the principal constituent of these periarteriolar sheaths. T-cells remain in the spleen for several hours before returning to the extrasplenic circulation; B-cells may remain for 24 h or longer.

This system is capable of rapid generation of specific antibody early after exposure to antigens presenting in the bloodstream: As a primary response, the antibodies consist principally of IgM, of which the spleen is a major source. Memory cells are also generated in the spleen, and, in some circumstances, impaired secondary responses have been observed with functional asplenia.

Macrophages in both the liver and spleen appear to be the principal source of components of complement, and the spleen also appears to have a role in maintaining the alternative (properdin) pathway in humans.

9.2.3. TUFTSIN SYNTHESIS The spleen is the site of significant synthetic activity, and, following splenectomy, there are commonly reduced levels of properdin, IgM and tuftsin (Lancet editorial, 1985). Tuftsin is a tetrapeptide (threonyl-lysyl-prolyl-arginine) derived from the CH2 domain of the Fc segment of the heavy chain of molecules of IgG. γ-globulin is bound to the surface of blood cells as erythrophilic, thrombophilic, and leukophilic globulin, the last being known as "leukokinin," which can stimulate phagocytic activity of blood granulocytes, monocytes, and tissue macrophages. The tuftsin peptide is released from the carrier leukokinin by two enzymes: One is the spleen-derived tuftsin-endocarboxypeptidase, and the other a membrane-bound leukokininase (Najjar, 1975, 1983).

Following splenectomy in dogs, the tuftsin level falls for several months, and phagocytosis becomes defective; similar findings have been made in hyposplenic humans (Spirer et al., 1977a; Spirer et al., 1977b; Spirer et al., 1980). Tuftsin stimulates phagocytosis, pinocytosis, phagocyte motility, antigen processing, bactericidal activity, and, experimentally in mice, tumoricidal activity (Fridkin and Najjar, 1989).

9.3. THE ENLARGED SPLEEN

The principal clinical indicator of disease or disorder in the spleen is enlargement of the organ; nevertheless, not all diseases significantly related to the spleen, cause its enlargement. For example, idiopathic (immune) thrombocytopenia is not usually associated with splenomegaly, and, if an enlarged spleen is demonstrated, an alternative cause for the thrombocytopenia should be sought. Conversely, a palpable spleen in an adult should lead to a comprehensive review and investigation for its cause, although, occasionally, it may be regarded as a benign finding (Arkles et al., 1986). The principal clinical conditions associated with splenomegaly are summarized in Table 1, and the pathological processes involved are shown in Table 2.

9.3.1. PATHOGENESIS OF SPLENOMEGALY
9.3.1.1. Splenic Hyperplasia The spleen responds to a wide variety of stimuli by an increase in cellularity and vascularity of the organ. This does not require intact connection to the portal venous system, since hyperplasia can be demonstrated experimentally in the transplanted organ lacking such connection.

1. Hyperplasia secondary to hemolysis. Jacob et al. (1963) showed that intravenous administration of autologous red blood cell debris will induce splenic hyperplasia, involving both lymphoid cells and pulp macrophages. Prolonged stimulation can result in an autonomous, partially irreversible hyperplasia (Jandl et al., 1965). These investigators also estimated the nucleated cell content of the human spleen by measurements of DNA content, and found normal-sized spleens to have nucleated cell contents of $70-230 \times 10^9$ cells. Spleens from patients with hereditary spherocytosis showed values of $720-2020 \times 10^9$ cells, and intermediate values were found in other spleens with slight to moderate enlargement. The 10-fold increase above normal in hereditary spherocytosis is significant, in that it appears to be a work-induced hyperplasia secondary to hemolysis and phagocytosis, in the absence of an immune component.

   Hyperplasia of this type appears to be a significant contributor to splenomegaly in numerous other hemolytic disorders, including the hemolytic cases of hereditary ovalocytosis, thalassemia major, hemoglobinopathies, including juvenile sickle-cell disease, and some cases of paroxysmal nocturnal hemoglobinuria.

2. Hyperplasia secondary to infection is common, probably as a response to phagocytic overload. An immune process does not appear to be required. Experimentally, splenic enlargement can be stimulated by injections of macromolecular substances, such as methylcellulose, zymosan, and endotoxin (Palmer et al., 1953; Heuper, 1944; Benacerraf and Sebastyen, 1957; Gorstein and Benacerraf, 1960). The principal infections associated with splenomegaly are summarized in Table 3.

3. Hyperplasia secondary to immune and autoimmune disorders commonly leads to splenomegaly, in conditions including rheumatoid arthritis and Felty syndrome, systemic lupus erythematosus, serum sickness, collagen vascular disorders, angioimmunoblastic lymphadenopathy, immune hemolytic anemias and cytopenias, and thyrotoxicosis.

9.3.1.2. Congestive Splenomegaly Chronic passive venous congestion in the portal system or splenic vein leads to enlargement of the spleen. The height of the venous pressure is not itself the major determinant of the size of the spleen, which in this condition averages 900 g, but occasionally may exceed 3 kg. Venous congestion alone usually does not produce a spleen palpable below the

Table 9.1
Principal Causes of Splenomegaly

Infections
  Acute
    Infectious mononucleosis; viral hepatitis; septicemia (including tuberculous); salmonelloses; relapsing fever; tularemia; splenic abscess; cytomegalovirus infection; toxoplasmosis.
  Subacute and chronic
    Chronic septicemias; tuberculous splenomegaly; leprosy; Yersinia; subacute bacterial endocarditis; brucellosis; syphilis; malaria; leishmaniasis; schistosomiasis; systemic fungal disease; inflammatory pseudotumor.
  Immune proliferations and noninfectious granulomatous disorders
    Angioimmunoblastic lymphadenopathy; angiofollicular hyperplasia; systemic lupus erythematosus; rheumatoid arthritis; Still's disease; rheumatic fever; Behcet's syndrome; serum sickness; sarcoidosis; berylliosis; necrotizing splenic granulomas.
  Vasculitides
    Polyarteritis nodosa; leukocytoclastic angiitis; peliosis.
Congestive splenomegaly
  Intrahepatic
    Portal cirrhois; postnecrotic scarring; biliary cirrhosis; Wilson's disease; hemochromatosis; veno-occlusive disease; congenital fibrosis; bilharziasis.
  Portal vein obstruction
    Thrombosis, stenosis, atresia; cavernous malformation; arteriovenous aneurysm; obstructive lesions at porta hepatis.
  Splenic vein obstruction
    Thrombosis, stenosis, atresia; cavernous malformation; obstruction by pancreatic disease, splenic arterial aneurysm, and retroperitoneal fibrosis.
  Hepatic vein occlusion
    Budd-Chiari syndrome.
  Cardiac
    Acute, chronic, or recurrent congestive cardiac failure; constrictive pericarditis.
Hematological disorders
  Hemolytic disorders
    Hereditary red blood cell membrane disorders; thalassemia; sickle-thalassemia; sickle cell disease (early stages); hemoglobin-SC disease.
  Myeloproliferative disorders
    Primary (agnogenic) myeloid metaplasia; polycythemia vera (variable); essential thrombocythemia (variable).
  Miscellaneous
    Primary splenic hyperplasia; megaloblastic anemias; iron deficiency.
Neoplasm
  Hematological
    Acute leukemias; chronic lymphatic and myelogenous leukemias; prolymphocytic leukemia; hairy cell leukemia; malignant lympho-mata; malignant histiocytosis; systemic mastocytosis; myelomatosis.
  Intrinsic
    Primary lymphosarcoma; plasmacytoma; fibrosarcoma; angiosarcoma; endothelial cell sarcoma; lymphangiosarcoma; malignant fibrous histiocytoma.
  Metastatic
    Carinoma, especially lung and breast; melanoma; neuroblastoma; malignant teratoma; choriocarcinoma.
  Benign
    Hamartoma (single, multiple); hemangioma (capillary, cavernous); lymphangioma; lipoma.
Miscellaneous
  Storage diseases
    Gaucher's disease; Neimann-Pick disease; Histiocytosis X; ceroid histiocytosis; Tangier disease; Hurler's syndrome; Hunter's syndrome.
  Cysts
    Pseudocyst; epidermoid (epithelial) cyst; echinococcal (hydatid) cyst.
  Others
    Amyloidosis; Albers-Schönberg disease; hereditary hemorrhagic telangiectasia; hyperthyroidism.

Table 9.2
Processes Leading to Enlargement of Spleen

Splenic hyperplasia
  Primary
    Idiopathic splenomegaly:
      Nontropical[a]
      Tropical[a]
  Secondary to
    Hemolysis
    Acute and chronic infections
    Immune and autoimmune disorders
    Congestive splenomegaly
      Intrahepatic obstruction
      Extrahepatic obstruction
      Cardiac decompensation
      Hyperkinetic portal hypertension
Red blood cell pooling
  Intrinsic red blood cell defects, usually with abnormal cell shape
  Structural splenic defects in pathways of flow
Myeloid metaplasia
  Primary (pathological)[a]
  Compensatory (reactive)
Cellular proliferative disorders
  Lymphoproliferative disorders
    Hodgkin's disease
    Non-Hodgkin's lymphoma
    Primary splenic lymphoma
    Acute lymphoblastic leukemia
    Chronic lymphocytic leukemia
    Lymphoma with prominent splenomegaly
    Hairy cell leukemia
  Nonlymphoproliferative neoplasms
    Hemangioma
    Splenic lymphangioma[b]
    Hemangioendothelioma
    Angiosarcoma
    Malignant fibrous histiocytoma
    Myeloproliferative disorders
  Secondary (metastatic) neoplasms
  Hamartomata
  Splenic cysts
Macrophage and storage disorders
  Hereditary
  Acquired
Infiltrative disorders
  Sarcoidosis
  Amyloidosis

[a] Has potential for massive splenomegaly.
[b] Benign neoplasm.

costal margin: Westaby et al. (1978) found no correlation between spleen size and portal pressure, which confirmed an earlier study by Krook (1956), showing no significant difference in hepatic wedge pressures between cirrhotic patients with and without splenomegaly. The duration of the condition is a more important determinant of spleen size than the level of venous pressure. Secondary splenic hyperplasia is thus responsible in major degree for the splenic enlargement.

The principal causes of congestive splenomegaly include:

1. Intrahepatic obstructive portal hypertension, most commonly caused by portal obstructive cirrhosis, postnecrotic scarring, and biliary cirrhosis. Other causes include Wilson's disease, hemochromatosis, occlusion of the hepatic veins, and sarcoidosis.

Table 9.3
Infections Associated with Splenomegaly

Viral:	viral hepatitis, infectious mononucleosis, acquired immunodeficiency syndrome, cytomegalovirus
Bacterial:	subacute bacterial endocarditis, bacterial septicemias, splenic abscess, chronic septicemias (including tuberculous) salmonelloses, brucellosis, congenital syphilis
Protozoal:	malaria, leishmaniasis, trypanosomiasis
Fungal:	histoplasmosis, paracoccidioidomycosis

2. Extrahepatic obstructive portal hypertension caused by venous malformation, thrombosis, atresia, or extrinsic pressure with compression or occlusion of the portal vein or splenic vein. Note that the classic observation, that splenomegaly in the presence of obstructive jaundice is a sign of carcinoma of the pancreas, relates to occlusion of the splenic vein by local extension of the tumor.
3. Chronic passive congestion caused by cardiac decompensation (rarely).

Williams (1966) has shown that total splenic blood flow tends to be higher than normal in these cases, despite the element of venous obstruction. The increased flow may result in an incremental increase in portal hypertension (i.e., hyperkinetic portal hypertension).

The capacity to remove heat-treated autologous red blood cells from the circulation is preserved, and may increase with the degree of enlargement of the spleen (Holzbach et al., 1964). Cytopenias are not uncommon: Leukopenia or thrombocytopenia have been estimated to occur, in various series, in 10–55% of cases (Ferrara et al., 1979; Toghill and Green, 1979; Muchnik et al., 1975; Fegiz et al., 1983; Soper and Rikkers, 1986).

The relationship of cytopenias to specific disorders is also variable and controversial. Cytopenias were present in 17/21 patients with portal hypertension secondary to extrahepatic obstruction (Stathers et al., 1968). A low incidence was found with cases of isolated splenic vein thrombosis (Sutton et al., 1970), and a relative infrequency was found in chronic active hepatitis (Gramlich et al., 1970; Toghill and Green, 1975). The principal determinant of cytopenias in the presence of splenomegaly is the size of the spleen (el-Khishen et al., 1985; Soper and Rikkers, 1986).

The spleen contributes only in minor degree to the anemia associated with liver disease. Measurable red blood cell pooling is usually present in congestive splenomegaly, but rarely comprises more than 15% of the total circulating red blood cell mass. Moderate reductions in red blood cell life-span have been demonstrated, but red blood cell destruction in the spleen does not appear to be active.

9.3.1.3. Red Blood Cell Pooling   In pathological circumstances, it is frequently possible to demonstrate a pool of red blood cells in the spleen, which only very slowly exchanges with the red blood cell population of the general extrasplenic circulation. This pool must be distinguished clearly from the blood component of the normal blood supply to the parenchyma of the spleen, which is comparable to the blood content of other solid organs.

The red blood cell pool can be studied by following the time course of the surface-detectable radioactivity over the spleen after the intravenous injection of ^{51}Cr- labeled autologous red blood cells. The rise in detectable radioactivity to a stable maximum, with a non-pooling spleen, is similar in pattern to that found over the liver, heart, or thigh, or elsewhere at the body surface, with a single rapid component to the rise having a mean half-life (T_{50}) of 24 ± 12 s.

In the presence of a red blood cell pool, the initial rapid phase of increasing radioactivity is followed by a prolonged slow rise in accumulating radioactivity with a (T_{50}) of 2.6–29 min. The fraction of the surface radioactivity attributable to the pool may be as high as 72% of the total surface detectable radioactivity. The percentage of the total circulating red blood cells present in the pool may be greater than 50%, although the mean value for diverse disorders is 12.6 ± 8.4% of all red blood cells.

Pooling appears to result from two distinct pathological phenomena:

1. Abnormality of the red blood cells, especially in shape. It may thus appear with spherocytosis, whether hereditary or acquired, ovalocytosis, thalassemia, and pernicious anemia.
2. Structural distortion of the pathways of flow though the spleen, especially in the open circulation of the red pulp between the arteriolar capillaries and the walls of the splenic sinuses. This is likely to occur, e.g., in the enlarged spleens of hairy cell leukemia and myeloproliferative disorders. Normal ^{51}Cr-labeled red blood cells will also accumulate in structurally distorted spleens, showing that the pooling is not dependent on abnormal properties of the red blood cells in these cases.

The turnover time of the red blood cell pool is usually between 5 and 45 min, indicating an extremely slow flow of red blood cells through the pooling compartment of the spleen. This leads to recurrent prolonged exposure of cells to a metabolic environment unfavorable to red blood cells, which will be in competition with other cells of the splenic pulp with higher metabolic rates. Second, the slow flow and prolonged contact with lymphoid cells and macrophages increases the probability of antibody attachment and phagocytosis (*see also* Chapter 7, Subheading 4.2).

Under pathological circumstances, the human spleen can show a pattern of cell accumulation similar to that of the mammalian storage spleen, despite having no related physiological role in this respect. These radionucleide studies describe a stable exchanging red blood cell pool: Otherwise, the labeled cells would not gain access to the splenic pool from the larger red blood cell pool of the extrasplenic circulation. Consequently, they do not measure irreversibly trapped cells in the spleen, which cannot be exchanged. Nor does the stable exchanging pool have kinetic similarity to the unidirectional sequestration, which can produce acute anemic crises in sickle cell disease when the spleen is still intact: The latter is an acute pooling phenomenon, in which the inflow, often quite suddenly, exceeds the outflow from the pool.

9.3.1.4. Myeloid Metaplasia   The environment provided by the human spleen has the properties necessary for supporting hematopoiesis. As a classic example of ontogeny recapitulating phylogeny, the human fetus shows hematopoietic cells in numerous sites, including the spleen, until ~20 wk of gestation. In the spleen, this is most evident between the second and the sixth month, despite which the liver continues to be the dominant site during this period. The productive activity of the spleen is, however, debatable (*see* Chapter 13, Subheading 2).

Extramedullary hematopoiesis with blood cell formation elsewhere than in the bone marrow may appear in later life under the

Table 9.4
Reports of Patients with Idiopathic Nontropical Splenomegaly

Author	Title of syndrome	No cases*	Subsequently developed lymphoma
Hayhoe and Whitby (1955)	Primary hypersplenic pancytopenia	5	No follow-up
Gevirtz et al. (1962)	Primary hypersplenism	1	0 (2 yr)
Weinstein (1964)	Simple splenic hyperplasia	5 (1)	No follow-up
Dacie et al. (1979)	Nontropical idiopathic splenomegaly	10 (2)	4 (1–7 yr after Sx)
Goonwardene et al. (1979)	None given (abstracted from a series of 13)	5 (2)	1 (2 yr after Sx)
Ellis and Damashek (1975)	Primary hypersplenism	12 (NS)	3 (Incomplete follow-up)
Knudson et al. (1982)	None given (abstracted from a series of 28)	2 (2)	1 (2 yr)
Manoharan et al. (1982)	Nontropical idiopathic splenomegaly	5 (3)	2 (2 and 6 yr after Sx)

NS, Not stated; Sx, Splenectomy.
*Males in parentheses.

stimulus of inadequate production by the bone marrow. This appears most prominently in long-standing hemolytic anemias, including the thalassemias, sickle cell disease, hereditary spherocytosis, and pernicious anemia. The liver and spleen are the most common sites to show this, although, in some degree, many other organs may be involved, and sometimes prominent aggregates of hematopoietic tissue are found in the mediastinum and in retroperitoneal sites. The expression of extramedullary hematopoiesis shows much individual variation, but it rarely constitutes a major contribution to red blood cell production (Symmers, 1948; Wiland and Smith 1956; Dacie, 1985).

Pathological extramedullary hematopoiesis occurs as a clonal disorder of the hematopoietic stem cells, and usually affects both liver and spleen in primary (agnogenic) myeloid metaplasia. Active erythropoiesis can frequently be detected in the spleen, by sequential estimates of surface-detectable radioactivity from the organ, following intravenous injection of transferrin-bound ^{59}Fe: The pattern of uptake and release during erythropoiesis is often obscured by the radioactivity of circulating labeled red blood cells in the same detection field, following the initial phase of uptake (Bowdler, 1961; Szur and Smith, 1961; Pribilla and Oettgen, 1968; Christensen, 1975). Ferrant et al. (1982) showed, in a study using ^{52}Fe, that Fe uptake by the spleen increased with increasing size of the spleen, and marrow Fe uptake diminished as splenic Fe uptake increased, so that the spleen acted as a competitive Fe sink in these cases. The role of the spleen in myeloproliferative disorders is considered further in Chapter 13, Subheading 3.

9.3.1.5. Cellular Proliferations, Neoplastic and Non-Neoplastic Neoplastic disorders of the spleen are predominantly examples of malignant lymphoproliferative disorders, most commonly as part of a generalized disease, usually lymphomas or acute or chronic lymphocytic leukemias. Metastatic tumors from elsewhere are relatively uncommon, and seldom result in clinical splenomegaly.

9.3.1.5.1. Lymphoproliferative Disorders The lymphoproliferative disorders affecting the spleen include:

1. Hodgkin's disease, in which the spleen is often not clinically enlarged at the time of diagnosis. Splenectomy for staging purposes provided unexpected information, in that it was found that the spleen can be affected by Hodgkin's lymphoma without being enlarged, and that an enlarged spleen may show no histological involvement. The frequency of splenic disease at the time of diagnosis is given by Warnke et al. (1995), as follows: in cases with lymphocyte predominance, 11–23%; nodular sclerosing disease, 39%; mixed cellularity, 63%; and

lymphocyte depletion, 67%. Involvement of the spleen indicates advancing disease, and suggests hematogenous spread: Rarely does hepatic or bone marrow involvement occur without the spleen being affected.

Diagnostic splenectomy for splenomegaly with no apparent cause showed none with Hodgkin's disease in 28 instances in a series in the United States (Knudson et al., 1982), but 13/34 patients showed the disease in a United Kingdom series (Mitchell and Morris, 1985). Lymphomas, developing in patients with idiopathic nontropical splenomegaly, have not been of the Hodgkin's type (Table 4).

2. Non-Hodgkin's lymphomas show splenomegaly and hypersplenism more frequently, the cell deficits being related to cell pooling, accelerated cell destruction, and plasma volume expansion. Involvement is especially common with the low-grade lymphomas. Warnke et al. (1995) give frequencies at diagnosis of 60–100% of splenomegaly in small lymphocytic lymphomas (well-differentiated lymphocytic lymphoma), 57% for lymphoplasmacytoid and mantle cell lymphoma, and the incidence for diffuse large-cell lymphoma is 6–38%.

3. Primary splenic lymphoma is uncommon, probably comprising 0.5–1.0% of all lymphomas, in which the lymphoma is confined to the spleen and its hilar lymph nodes, although Falk and Stutte (1992) found it to have an incidence of 3% of lymphomas affecting the spleen. It is usually non-Hodgkin in type: Primary Hodgkin's disease of the spleen is distinctly rare. Patients with primary splenic lymphoma are usually adult, presenting with upper abdominal pain, pyrexia, and evidence of splenic enlargement. Primary large-cell lymphoma may be aggressive, with invasion of local structures, including the stomach, pancreas, and colon (Hall et al., 1993).

4. Acute lymphoblastic leukemia in children frequently results in splenomegaly, although this is infrequent in adults.

5. Chronic lymphocytic leukemia of B-cell-type frequently shows splenic enlargement. Hansen (1973) found palpable enlargement at the apparent onset of the disorder, in approx 50% of patients, with the spleen more than 5 cm from the costal margin in 20–30%. There is progressive enlargement, as the duration of the condition increases. The related prolym-phocytic leukemia usually shows massive splenomegaly (Galton et al., 1974). Videbaek et al. (1982) have also described a splenomegalic aleukemic CLL with splenomegaly and slight lymphocytosis in the bone marrow, but without lymphocytosis in the blood. The rare, phenotypically T-cell variant of chronic lymphocytic leukemia may show marked splenomegaly (Brouet et al., 1975).

6. Lymphoma with prominent splenomegaly occurs in some uncommon variants of lymphoma: Hepatosplenic T-cell lymphoma is rare, and usually occurs in young adults. Lymphocytoplasmoid lymphoma (immunocytoma) is sometimes splenomegalic in presentation, and the splenic B-cell lymphoma with circulating villous lymphocytes also may show gross splenomegaly: Both of the latter disorders occur mainly in older age groups. Marginal zone cell lymphoma may also show prominent splenomegaly.

7. Hairy cell leukemia is a lymphoproliferative disorder, usually of B-cell lineage, in which splenomegaly is common, although it is possible for the disease to present with cytopenias, before splenomegaly is evident. The spleen pulp typically shows an intense and extensive infiltration with mononuclear cells. Red blood cell pooling is often prominent, and blood lakes (pseudosinuses) are frequently found. Involvement of the red pulp is a characteristic feature of hairy cell leukemia, distinguishing it from the lymphomata, which essentially involve the white pulp, with the red pulp only involved secondarily and later. Further consideration of the spleen in lymphoproliferative disorders is given in Chapter 14.

9.3.1.5.2. Nonlymphoproliferative Neoplasms A small number of histologically distinct tumors arises in the spleen, mostly originating from cells of the lymphatic and blood vessels. These are mostly benign, with the exception of angiosarcoma and rare cases of nonvascular sarcomas of the spleen.

1. Primary neoplasms include the following: Hemangioma, which is the commonest, and is usually an incidental finding clinically, but has the potential for producing major splenomegaly. It may be associated with consumption coagulopathy, portal hypertension, microangiopathic anemia, and thrombocytopenia. It may also be one component of extensive angiomatosis. Splenic lymphangioma may be solitary or multiple, and other viscera may be involved simultaneously. It may better be regarded as one form of splenic hamartoma. Hemangioendothelioma is also a primary tumor of blood vessels, with characteristics intermediate between those of the benign hemangioma and the malignant angiosarcoma. Angiosarcoma of the spleen is a rare malignant tumor. Hematologic complications include consumption coagulopathy, microangiopathic hemolysis, and thrombocytopenia. Hematogenous dissemination is common, and survival of short duration, usually of less than 1 yr. Other sarcomas of the spleen are rare. Malignant fibrous histiocytoma is an aggressive tumor that may result in massive splenomegaly. Leiomyosarcoma and fibrosarcoma have also been described.

2. Secondary malignant disease of the spleen may arise from either nonmetastatic invasion or by hematogenous spread from distant tumors. Contiguous spread may occur from tumors of adjacent sites, including the pancreas, stomach, colon, adrenal and left kidney. Spread to the spleen may also occur from splenic hilar lymph nodes through lymphatic vessels, and tumor may also enter the spleen through the splenic veins (Willis, 1973). Hematogenous spread is usually part of a widespread metastatic process affecting many organs. It is rare for splenic metastases to present an isolated clinical problem; they are usually apparent as an incidental radiological or autopsy finding. Most cases arise from carcinoma of the lung or breast, or are caused by malignant melanoma.

There has been a long-standing impression that splenic metastasis is relatively uncommon, and even the speculation that there may be an antineoplastic process that diminishes the incidence of discoverable splenic metastasis (Harman and Dacorso, 1948). However, careful comparisons of the frequency of bloodborne metastasis to various organs has not confirmed this impression, especially when allowance is made for the relatively small size of the spleen (Willis, 1973; Berge, 1974).

3. Chronic myelogenous leukemia usually involves the spleen, the normal architecture being largely obliterated by myeloid cells at various stages of maturation. Anecdotal cases have been encountered in which early splenectomy led to prolonged remission, suggestive of early interdiction of the primordial pathological clone. However, in most cases, splenectomy does not affect the course of the disease significantly, and is not useful as a general intervention (*see also* Chapter 13).

9.3.1.5.3. Splenic Hamartoma (Splenoma) The hamartoma is an uncommon benign mass, usually presenting as an incidental finding after splenectomy or autopsy. Some cause abdominal discomfort, and others are found following evaluation for blood cytopenias. Most are solitary, spherical lesions composed of vascular tissue resembling the pulp cords.

9.3.1.5.4. Cysts of the Spleen Splenic cysts are true cysts in 20% of cases, but 80% are false cysts. True cysts are most commonly epithelial (epidermoid) cysts, and arise from embryonic tissue inclusions. Usually asymptomatic, they may produce local pressure symptoms. Malignant transformation is possible. False cysts lack the epithelial lining of the true cyst, and may become calcified and visible radiographically. Many appear to result from previous trauma to the spleen leading to hematoma formation, which later liquefies; others may arise by cystic degeneration of a benign tumor or hamartoma.

Other cysts include the rare dermoid cyst and parasitic cysts, which may be ecchinococcal (hydatid), or caused by *Cysticercus* or *Pentastoma*.

9.3.1.6. Macrophage and Storage Disorders This is a heterogeneous group of disorders, some hereditary and others acquired, having in common proliferation of the macrophage system. The spleen is of significance because of the dense population of macrophages in the organ, and the consequent frequency of splenomegaly or hepatosplenomegaly, often as an early sign of the disorder. Secondary hypersplenism is common.

9.3.1.6.1. Hereditary Storage Disorders These arise from the excessive storage of lipids or mucopolysaccharides in macrophages. The essential defect in most instances is deficiency in the activity of an enzyme necessary for the catabolism of the stored substance. Examples of well-investigated disorders of this group include:

1. Gaucher's disease (glucosyl ceramide lipidosis) is a familial sphingolipidosis. Three clinical forms are recognized: Hepatosplenomegaly occurs in all three. Type 1 is the most common: It has a predilection for Ashkenazi Jews, and is known as the "adult" form. This is, however a misnomer, since the condition may be recognized in childhood, and even in infancy, often because of the splenomegaly and protruding abdomen. Inheritance is autosomal-recessive, with variable penetrance (Brady,1978). Splenomegaly frequently leads to

hypersplenism, with thrombocytopenia and leukopenia. Microcytic anemia is common: Fe is diverted from erythropoiesis by storage in Gaucher cells. The infantile type 2 and juvenile type 3 show predominantly neurological deficits. All types have subnormal activity of the enzyme glucocerebrosidase. Anemia in the adult form has been extensively investigated, and is usually multifactorial: Marrow infiltration with Gaucher cells reduces effective erythropoiesis, and some cases show extramedullary erythropoiesis and leukoerythroblastosis. Erythrocyte glucocerebroside is increased 2/3-fold, and red blood cell life-span is reduced, often without frank evidence of hemolysis (Bowdler, 1963; Lee et al., 1967). Hemolytic anemia with spherocytosis has been described (Mandelbaum et al., 1942). Portal hypertension is another complication, probably caused by hepatic portal infiltration, and esophageal varices occur, sometimes resulting in lethal hemorrhage (Aderka et al., 1984).

2. Niemann-Pick disease (sphingomyelin lipidosis) is a group of disorders characterized by hepatosplenomegaly and tissue accumulations of sphingomyelin and other lipids. It is a genetic disorder inherited as an autosomal recessive, and resulting in deficient activity of the enzyme sphingomyelinase, which degrades sphingomyelin, derived from cell membranes and subcellular particles, to ceramide and phosphoryl choline. There are five clinical types, A–E.

Type A is the classical infantile form, and the commonest: Hepatosplenomegaly usually appears early in infancy, and characteristic neurological deficits include defects of motor function and failure of learning. Types B and E show visceral involvement, but no neurological disease, type B becoming evident in childhood, and E being an adult variant. Type C also occurs in early childhood, with visceral involvement, followed by later progressive neurological deterioration. Type D is similar to C, but appears to be a variant geographically confined to Nova Scotia.

The spleen is extensively disordered in structure in this condition, with masses of foam cells present in the pulp and about the pulp arteries. Hematologic abnormalities are usually of moderate degree, with a microcytic anemia that does not appear closely related to the size of the spleen (Crocker and Farber, 1958). Thrombocytopenia and leukopenia may be present.

3. Wolman's disease is an invariably fatal disorder with widespread tissue accumulations of cholesteryl esters and glycerides. Hepatosplenomegaly is present, and sometimes appears in the neonate; splenomegaly may be massive. Clinically, the condition resembles Niemann-Pick disease, but adrenal calcification is characteristic. There is deficiency of an acid-hydrolase-catalyzing hydrolysis of cholesteryl esters and triglycerides.

4. Hurler's syndrome is a rare, familial, inherited mucopolysaccharide storage disease caused by a deficiency of α-L-iduronidase. Clinically, it shows marked skeletal abnormalities (dysostosis multiplex), mental retardation, corneal clouding, and, usually, hepatosplenomegaly, although the last is not invariable. The enzyme is required for the degradation of heparan sulfate and dermatan. The spleen may show marked enlargement and vacuolated cells in the pulp. Peripheral blood leukocytes may show metachromatic Reilly granules. The condition is usually evident after infancy and is progressive during early childhood.

5. The sea-blue Histiocyte syndrome is a systemic histiocytosis, occurring as a primary familial disorder, and presenting at almost any age, but most commonly in young adults. The defining cells are granulated histiocytes with sea-blue coloration when stained by Wright-Giemsa. They contain a ceroid material identifiable as sphingomyelin, and leukocytes and fibroblasts show a deficiency of sphingomyelinase activity. Splenomegaly is usual, and hepatomegaly common. Skin pigmentation and pulmonary infiltration may be present, and neurological disorders occur, especially in younger subjects. The affected tissues have a high lipid content, especially sphingolipids, and the condition appears to have characteristics overlapping with Niemann-Pick disease. In some instances, splenomegaly is exaggerated and gives rise to the "big spleen syndrome"; splenectomy may be necessary.

A nonfamilial acquired form of the condition also occurs, usually secondary to disorders with a high turnover rate of hematopoietic cells, including immune thrombocytopenic purpura, chronic myelogenous leukemia and hemolytic anemias. It may also be associated with hyperlipemia, chronic granulomatous disease, and Takayasu arteritis.

6. Langerhans cell histiocytosis (histiocytosis X) is a complex of mostly sporadic conditions of unknown etiology, pathologically demonstrating proliferation of histiocytes, granuloma formation, cholesterol containing foam cells, xanthoma formation, and fibrosis. The most localized form of the disorder is solitary eosinophilic granuloma of bone, which is benign and usually confined to a single skeletal site. Chronic systemic histiocytosis (Hand-Schuller-Christian disease) usually involves multiple foci of eosinophilic granuloma of bone, classically involving the orbit, calvarium, and sella turcica, with which diabetes insipidus and exophthalmos may be associated. Widespread lesions of other tissues also occur, including pulmonary, skin, and central nervous system lesions. Lymphadenopathy and hepatosplenomegaly also occur. Acute systemic histiocytosis (Lettere-Siwe's disease) is an acutely progressive form usually appearing in children under the age of 3 yr. The lesions are pathologically less developed than in the chronic forms.

7. Familial hemophagocytic histiocytosis is a familial disorder usually appearing before the age of 2 yr, and frequently in siblings. Most cases show hepatosplenomegaly and pancytopenia is common as the disease progresses. Lymphohistiocytic infiltration of the liver, spleen, lymph nodes, and bone marrow is present, with engorgement of macrophages with phagocytosed blood cells. An acquired form of hemophagocytic histiocytosis also shows hepatosplenomegaly, especially in children. Severe cytopenias occur. The condition appears as an exaggerated response to infection, usually viral, but is sometimes related to malignancy, connective tissue disorder, or drug therapy.

8. Familial lipoprotein lipase deficiency results in a rare syndrome characterized by massive chylomicronemia and type-1 hyperlipoproteinemia. Chylomicrons accumulate in macrophages which may lead to hepatosplenomegaly, and which can regress with dietary fat restriction. Splenomegaly can also occur with the secondary chylomicronemia of diabetes or alcoholism.

9. Tangier disease (Familial high-density lipoprotein deficiency) is a rare disease characterized by deficiency of high

density lipoprotein and accumulation of cholesteryl esters in many tissues, including the liver, spleen, lymph nodes, and skin. Prominent features are hyperplasia of the nasopharyngeal tonsils, and palatine tonsils, which have a characteristic orange-yellow streaking. Polyneuropathies are common. Foamy macrophages are seen in the spleen; hypersplenism has occurred, and thrombocytopenia is common.

9.3.1.7. Infiltrative Disorders   Infiltrative disorders, affecting the spleen, may produce splenomegaly during a phase of active enlargement, leading to hypersplenism, or ultimately to hyposplenism, when organ structure has been sufficiently comprom-ised. Such a progression may occur in chronic granulomatous diseases, such as sarcoidosis; hyposplenism is more probable in amyloidosis.

Sarcoidosis is a multisystem granulomatous disorder most frequently involving the lungs, skin, eyes, and the reticuloendothelial system. Despite the frequency with which lymph nodes are palpably enlarged (in about one-third of affected subjects) and the liver involved (liver biopsy showing granulomata in more than 85%), splenomegaly, which is uncommon (Scadding, 1967), is usually slight to mild. Overt splenomegaly is mostly associated with extensive disease and constitutional symptoms (Kataria and Whitcomb, 1980). Cytopenias are not uncommon, however, and frank hemolysis may occur (Partenheimer and Meredith, 1950; Davis et al., 1954; Garcia et al., 1959; Maycock et al., 1963; Thadani et al., 1975) and also thrombocytopenia (Dickerman et al., 1972; Edwards et al., 1952; Kunkel and Yesner, 1950). Rarely, massive splenomegaly may be an early manifestation (Peter, 1986). The spleen size declines with resolution of the disorder. Functional hyposplenism has been described in some patients during the course of the disease (Stone et al., 1986).

Amyloidosis comprises a diverse group of disorders characterized by deposition in connective tissue and blood vessels of amorphous fibrillar materials derived from a variety of precursor proteins present in serum. The pattern of organ involvement differs with the underlying protein. Amyloid AL gives rise to primary amyloidosis, in which palpable splenomegaly occurs in 5% of cases. The protein arises from the variable portion of the light chains of immunoglobulins. The condition can be difficult to distinguish from amyloidosis associated with myelomatosis. Cytopenias are uncommon, except in the presence of myeloma, and the prognosis depends essentially on the functional impairment of other systems, especially congestive heart failure and renal failure.

Secondary amyloidosis (AA amyloidosis) is usually associated with chronic inflammatory and infectious disorders, especially rheumatoid disease, chronic suppuration and tuberculosis, and, less commonly, malignant disorders. The organs involved are usually the kidney, liver, and spleen. Splenomegaly, in the presence of a disorder with the potential for inducing amyloidosis, raises the possibility of amyloid as a secondary diagnosis.

Hyposplenic changes in the peripheral blood, with Howell-Jolly bodies, target cells, and Pappenheimer bodies, may provide a diagnostic clue to the diagnosis of amyloidosis (Boyko et al., 1982; Selby et al., 1987). Amyloid tissue in the splenic pulp is presumed to induce sufficient reticuloendothelial blockade to interfere with the culling role of the spleen, and sufficient rigidity of the sinusoidal clefts to interfere with pitting. The extent to which this impairs resistance to infection is uncertain, but 8% of deaths in amyloidosis result from sepsis (Kyle and Bayrd, 1975).

9.4. CLINICAL DETECTION OF THE ENLARGED SPLEEN

9.4.1. CLINICAL EXAMINATION OF THE SPLEEN   Clinical examination of the spleen in the adult is principally directed toward detecting enlargement of the organ, which is almost invariably an abnormal finding, and in all cases indicates the need for detailed review and an explanation, especially as it may be the principal clinical evidence of underlying infection, hepatic disease, malignancy, or connective tissue disorder.

The normal spleen is an oblong, flattened organ, with its long axis following the line of the left tenth rib in the left hypochondrium and epigastrium. In shape, it conforms closely to surrounding structures; it occupies a position between the fundus of the stomach and the left dome of the diaphragm. The posteromedial pole is directed toward the vertebral column, and reaches the level of the twelfth thoracic vertebra. The lower (anterior) pole is close to the midaxillary line, and the medial surface relates to the stomach, the left kidney, the tail of the pancreas, and the splenic flexure of the colon. Its weight is usually 250 g or less, and varies with race, sex, and age, declining in size, as with other lymphoid structures, in the elderly.

A spleen of normal size in the adult is almost entirely protected by the rib cage, and normally cannot be palpated. A widely accepted rule of thumb is that the palpable spleen is abnormal and enlarged, although exceptions have been demonstrated (Arkles et al., 1986). Nevertheless, the clinical examination is necessarily the customary screen that determines whether splenomegaly is a feature to be further evaluated: There is at present no suitable surrogate examination with equivalent significance.

The enlarging spleen is limited in its expansion by its relationship to the vertebral column, the diaphragm, and the left lower ribs. However, it can displace the stomach and the colon, and the principal direction of enlargement is inferomedially, approximately following the line of the left tenth rib, toward the umbilicus and the right iliac fossa. In some cases, the axis of enlargement lies more vertically, and the spleen expands into the left lumbar region (loin) and left iliac fossa, and, in others, it enlarges medially to occupy, principally, the epigastrium. These can be significant variables in exploring the possibility of splenomegaly by clinical signs. Likewise, the relationships of the superior aspect of the organ limit movement, on inspiration, to descent, making the enlarged spleen one of the abdominal masses that descend on inspiration.

The grossly enlarged spleen may extend predominantly along its long axis, or enlarge more symmetrically, to become an irregular spheroidal body: Shape may therefore determine the projection of the organ on the body surface, in addition to the increase in size.

9.4.1.1. The Technique of Clinical Examination   Inspection of the abdomen may show alteration of the abdominal contour and abdominal distention, in patients with moderate or marked enlargement of the spleen, which is usually most evident in the left upper quadrant of the abdomen. Inspection is a test of low sensitivity, because the majority of enlarged spleens in adults do not distort the abdominal wall. Furthermore, other enlarged organs, such as an abnormal left lobe of the liver, a polycystic kidney, or gastric carcinoma, may be found in the same region of the abdomen. Occasionally, in the presence of a chronically enlarged spleen, a corona of small radiating stretch marks may be seen in the skin surrounding the point where the anterior pole of the spleen impinges on the anterior abdominal wall.

Diagnostic palpation of the abdomen requires a firm but gentle technique by the examining hand, which should be warm and applied essentially with the flat of the hand, rather than the tips of the fingers. The patient's abdomen needs to be relaxed, which is sometimes facilitated by moderate flexion of the hips and knees over a soft support.

Palpation of the spleen is directed not only to establishing the presence of the organ, but also to identifying features that confirm a palpable mass as the spleen: The upper border of the spleen lies above the costal margin, behind the lower rib cage, and so cannot be reached by the examining fingers; and the notches normally found on the superior border of the spleen may become palpable on the enlarged spleen, usually on the medial border, proximal to the anterior (lower) pole of the organ.

Many techniques have been recommended for palpating the spleen; three that have been carefully evaluated are as follows (Grover et al., 1993):

1. One-handed method with patient supine. The examiner stands to the right of the supine patient, and, with the right hand, presses below the patient's left costal margin, while the patient takes long, deep breaths. Some examiners find it useful to draw the lowermost portion of the rib cage forward, by lifting it from behind with the left hand. If no mass is felt, the procedure is repeated progressively, with the right hand approaching the umbilicus and the right iliac fossa. Alternatively, the process may be started in the right lower quadrant, and progressively approaches the left costal margin. When the spleen is identified, information may be obtained on the consistency of the spleen and the smoothness of its surface and contour.

2. Two-handed method; right lateral decubitus position. The patient is placed in the right lateral decubitus position. The examiner stands to the right of the patient, and places his left hand around the left lower thorax, to lift the rib cage anteromedially; the right hand palpates below the left costal margin, while the patient takes deep breaths. The spleen is sought progressively, as in the one-handed method.

3. The hooking maneuver of Middleton. The patient lies supine, with the left fist supporting the left lower chest posteriorly. The examiner stands to the patient's left side, facing toward the feet, with the fingers of both hands curled over the left costal margin. The spleen may become palpable as the patient takes long, deep breaths.

A clinical method for recording the degree of splenic enlargement is to identify the lower most dextrad point of the palpable spleen, usually the anterior pole, and measuring its distance from the left costal margin along a line perpendicular to the costal margin, known as the "splenic axis." Although not providing precise values of weight or volume, this may be accurately performed, and provides sequential assessment of enlargement for the individual patient.

Percussion is a useful additional means for detecting splenomegaly, especially when the degree of enlargement is limited. Its value lies in detecting the dullness to percussion of the spleen, by contrast with the resonance of air- or gas-filled surrounding viscera (lung, stomach, and colon). Three methods have been proposed and evaluated (Grover et al., 1993).

1. Nixon's method. With the patient in the right lateral decubitus position, the examiner percusses at the midpoint of the left costal margin, and continues proximally in a direction perpendicular to the costal margin. Splenomegaly is indicated if the border of dullness above the costal margin is met at less than 8 cm from the margin (Nixon, 1954; Sullivan and Williams, 1976).

2. Castell's method. With the patient supine, percussion is performed in the lowermost left intercostal space, usually the eighth or ninth, in the anterior axillary line, continuing with the patient in full inspiration and expiration. Normally, there is resonance at this site, even in full inspiration. Dullness to percussion at this site or dullness induced by inspiration is evidence of splenomegaly (Castell, 1967).

3. Percussion of Traube's space. Traube's space is an approximately triangular area of the left lower chest, bounded below by the left costal margin, superiorly by the sixth rib, and laterally by the mid-axillary line. With the patient supine, it is percussed across its mediolateral extent: Splenomegaly converts the normal resonance to percussive dullness, but this is not the exclusive cause of dullness at this site, because pleural effusion can also produce dullness in this area (Grover et al., 1993; Barkun et al., 1991; Barkun et al., 1989).

Auscultation rarely contributes significantly to the examination of the spleen. However, with perisplenitis or the localized perisplenitis of splenic infarction, a splenic rub may become audible. It resembles the pleural rub in characteristics, except that it is heard best over the affected surface of the spleen.

9.4.1.2. The Significance of Clinical Detection of the Spleen

The usefulness of recognizing enlargement of the spleen depends on how effectively the clinical methods described will detect the spleen when enlarged, and whether the finding of the palpable spleen is necessarily a sign of immediate clinical significance.

Grover et al. (1993) reviewed seven studies of the accuracy of palpation: Two studies assessed the accuracy of routine examination, by comparing the record of examination for splenomegaly to the assessment of spleen size at autopsy, or by scintillation scanning (Riemenschneider and Whalen, 1965; Halpern et al., 1974). These studies showed a low sensitivity for routine clinical examination (at 27%), but high specificity (95%), with a low rate for false-positive reporting. In specifically directed studies, sensitivity was higher and specificity lower. Sullivan and Williams (1976) compared the results of palpation and percussion performed in both the supine and right lateral positions with the results of ^{99m}Tc sulfur colloid scintillation scanning, and concluded that 88% of enlarged spleens were detectable clinically. Palpation was false-positive in two cases, one because of enlargement of the left hepatic lobe, and a second because of a "large intra-abdominal tumor." Arkles et al. (1986) also used posterior spleen length on radionuclide scanning as the standard against which to compare the effectiveness of palpation.

As shown in Table 5, the effectiveness of palpation improves with increasing spleen size, but tends to be problematic with spleens not greatly enlarged. However, not all clinicians have confirmed such accuracy in the palpation of the large spleen. In a study of 4000 patients, Fischer (1970) found that 50% of moderately enlarged spleens weighing 600–750 g, and 20% of greatly enlarged spleens, weighing 900–1600 g, were not palpable. Riemenschneider and Whalen (1965), however, found that, in some circumstances with gross splenomegaly, palpation could be more accurate than radiological assessment. Grover et al. (1993) showed percussion to be compromised by two principal factors, recent food intake and obesity. Recent food intake tended to produce false-positive re-

Table 9.5
The Relationship of Palpability
of the Spleen to Size Estimated by Radionucleide Scanning

Posterior spleen length (cm) on radionuclide scan	Proportion of subjects with spleen palpable (%)
13	0
14	30
16	42
18	68
20	80
>20	100

In this study a posterior scan length of less than 13 cm is regarded as within normal limits.
(Adapted with permission from Arkles et al., 1986.)

sults, and increased the discrepancies of observation between multiple observers. Better concordance was obtained when patients were examined no earlier than 2 h after eating. Obesity, on the other hand, tended to increase false-negative observations. Experienced gastroenterologists nevertheless showed good concordance, with an intraclass correlation coefficient of 0.81. Comparison of the Nixon and Castell techniques for percussion showed the Castell method to have a significantly higher sensitivity (82 vs 59%), but lower specificity. Likewise, the Castell method was rather more sensitive than palpation, which was the original objective of the method (Castell, 1967).

Furthermore, it was shown that all three methods of palpation are similar in their capacity to discriminate between "no detectable spleen" and "splenomegaly," with discriminating abilities of 73–79%. Likewise, palpation is a better discriminator when the percussion test is positive, and percussion identifies those subjects in which palpation is most useful; false negatives are frequent, when percussion is not positive.

In addition to a relatively small degree of enlargement, there are several factors that reduce the effectiveness of palpation, including:

1. There is a wide range of size to the normal spleen: the age, ethnicity, and sex of the subject influence the size of the normal spleen, which tends to atrophy with age. This has been established by several autopsy studies (Krumbhaar and Lippincott, 1939; Deland, 1970; Myers and Segal, 1974). Median values of weight are about 90 g in black women and 170 g in young white males.
2. The degree of enlargement may be sufficiently great to prevent the borders of the organ from being recognized by the examining hand, at the customary margins of palpation.
3. The spleen may be in an abnormal or unstable position. A spleen with a long vascular pedicle may vary its position, even to the extent of being found in the pelvis (Hunter and Haber, 1977; Vermylen et al., 1983). Absence or laxity of the phrenicocolic ligament, poor development of the lienorenal and lienogastric ligaments, and loss of tone of the abdominal wall, may all contribute to what has been termed the "wandering spleen syndrome." Torsion of the long splenic pedicle may lead to ischemia or infarction of the spleen (Simpson and Ashby, 1965). Anomalous orientation of the spleen may also allow it to be palpated more easily, although, in reports of the "upside-down spleen," no abdominal mass was detected (Westcott and Krufky, 1972).

4. Ascites may obscure the organ, making it difficult to palpate, e.g., in the presence of portal hypertension.
5. Pathological changes in the spleen, such as infarction or perisplenitis, may make the organ tender to the touch, and the patient resistant to palpation and other examinations.

In the absence of such exceptional circumstances, careful clinical examination will detect enlargement of the spleen in the majority of cases, although imaging will still be required for greater precision, qualitative evaluation, and a long-term, objective record. A small number of studies have found exceptions to the general rule that the enlarged spleen indicates significant disease, either of a local or generalized nature. Ebaugh and McIntyre (1967) detected splenomegaly in 3% of U.S. college freshmen, and found no significant clinical disorder on follow-up (McIntyre and Ebaugh, 1979). Hesdorffer et al. (1986) identified 10 young males with mild splenomegaly for which no significant cause was found, although five had IgG antibodies specific for cytomegalovirus. Berris (1966) found 12% of normal postpartum women to have palpable spleens. Nevertheless, it is clear that the detection of splenomegaly in adults is a finding that can provide an entry into the recognition of serious and sometimes life-threatening disease, and the clinical skill required is a necessary part of the clinical armamentarium.

9.4.1.3. Gross Enlargement of the Spleen   The spleen may become slightly enlarged in a wide range of conditions, but there are some in which gross enlargement may occur. When this is found, there is a considerable narrowing of the diagnostic field of possibilities. In temperate climates, massive splenomegaly extending into the lower abdominal quadrants is most commonly caused by:

1. Myeloproliferative disorders, especially chronic myelogenous leukemia, primary (agnogenic) myeloid metaplasia, and secondary myelofibrosis.
2. Chronic myelomonocytic leukemia.
3. Gaucher's disease.
4. Thalassemia major and intermedia.
5. Hemoglobinopathies, especially double heterozygotes of sickle cell disease: (Sickle thalassemia, SC disease).
6. Lymphoproliferative disorders (Hairy cell leukemia, Chronic lymphocytic leukemia, subacute lymphocytic leukemia, Lymphoplasmacytoid lymphoma, splenic lymphoma with circulating villous lymphocytes, hepatosplenic T-cell lymphoma, and marginal zone cell lymphoma).

In tropical areas, massive splenomegaly is associated with idiopathic tropical splenomegaly, malaria, and leishmaniasis (Kala-azar).

9.5. HYPERSPLENISM

The term "hypersplenism" has been broadly applied to situations in which enlargement of the spleen is associated with one or more deficits of the cell lines that exist in the peripheral blood (anemia, leukopenia, and thrombocytopenia). Implicit underlying assumptions have been that a single mechanism underlies such deficits, and that the causal mechanism becomes increasingly active whenever the spleen enlarges. Two opposing concepts of such hypothetical mechanisms produced a prolonged debate in the literature: Dameshek (1955) was the proponent of a controlling inhibitory humoral influence of the spleen on blood cell production by the bone marrow; Doan (1949) proposed that cell deficits, such as anemia and thrombocytopenia, were caused by cell destruction mediated by the spleen *in situ*, a position supported by evidence of the phagocytic and filtering activity of the spleen in such disorders (Crosby, 1962a,b).

Clearly, there are several mechanisms related to the spleen, which can diminish the populations of circulating blood cells, including the following.

9.5.1. THE CAUSES OF CYTOPENIAS RELATED TO THE SPLEEN

9.5.1.1. Abnormalities of Cell Distribution Red blood cells may be pooled in the red pulp of the spleen, either because they are abnormal, especially in shape, and are delayed in leaving the spleen, or because pathological structural abnormalities of the vascular pathways of the organ obstruct red blood cell egress. Although such cells are in dynamic equilibrium with the cells in the extrasplenic circulation, they represent a population of cells diverted from the general circulation, which must be maintained by a sometimes limited proliferative potential of the bone marrow (Bowdler, 1962).

Platelets are also pooled normally in the spleen, and the proportion of the total population pooled increases as the spleen enlarges (Aster, 1966; Aster and Jandl, 1964; Penny et al., 1966). In a markedly enlarged spleen, more than 90% of circulating platelets may be intrasplenic.

The margination of granulocytes is abnormally high in the blood vessels of the spleen, so that the apparent population included in the blood count is diminished as the spleen enlarges. (Fieschi and Sacchetti, 1964; Scott et al., 1971).

9.5.1.2. Blood Cell Destruction Red blood cells and platelets may both be destroyed in the spleen itself, and in some circumstances red blood cells may be conditioned, especially by prolonged delay in a splenic red blood cell pool, to be released to premature destruction elsewhere in the circulation, for example in the liver (Bowdler, 1962).

9.5.1.3. Antibody Production The spleen may also be a significant site of antibody production, as in autoimmune hemolysis and thrombocytopenia, aggravating or enhancing splenic or extrasplenic destruction of cells (Corrigan et al., 1983).

9.5.1.4. Blood Volume Expansion Enlargement of the spleen is commonly accompanied by expansion of blood volume, which is principally related to an obligatory increase in intravascular space, chiefly related to the organ itself and the expansion of the splanchnic intravascular volume (Hoffbrand and Pettit, 1988; Blendis et al., 1970). In many conditions associated with splenomegaly, the bone marrow is unable to adapt by increasing cell output sufficiently to maintain normal peripheral blood values. When red blood cell output is insufficient to maintain normal packed cell volume in the circulation, the volume deficit is compensated by expansion of the plasma volume, resulting in dilutional anemia (Bowdler, 1963, 1967, 1970; Hess et al., 1971; Hess et al., 1976; Weinstein, 1964; Pryor, 1967; Blendis et al., 1970).

9.5.2. HYPERSPLENISM: DEFINITION Earlier hypotheses identifying the spleen as a source of inhibitors to hematopoiesis have not received convincing experimental support.

Clearly, when the causes of cytopenias which may accompany enlargement of the spleen are identified in detail, they are found to be complex, and often multiple in individual cases. Consequently, hypersplenism does not describe a unified mechanism operative in all instances of splenic enlargement, as required by the Doan-Dameshek models, which imply a hypothetical uniform mechanism of localized destruction in the spleen *in situ* or humoral suppression of cell production. The concept of hypersplenism has therefore required a fundamental paradigm shift.

In a restricted syndromatic sense, the term "hypersplenism" retains a clinical usefulness. Many alternative uses of the term have been offered; e.g., Crosby (1962) regarded it simply as a state in which the patient is improved by losing the spleen.

A useful definition as a clinical descriptor is recommended, as follows: Hypersplenism is a syndrome in which there is enlargement of the spleen, accompanied by a deficit in one or more of the circulating cell lines of the peripheral blood (anemia, thrombocytopenia, and granulopenia), together with demonstrated active hematopoiesis of the affected cell line(s) in the bone marrow. Retrospectively, the syndrome is justified by correction of the deficit by splenectomy. By convention, hereditary spherocytosis and idiopathic thrombocytopenic purpura are no longer regarded as examples of hypersplenism, despite the high proportion of cases corrected by splenectomy.

9.5.3. VARIANTS OF HYPERSPLENISM

9.5.3.1. Primary Hypersplenism Syndromatic hypersplenism may occur with moderate-to-gross enlargement of the spleen without evidence of underlying disease: Although uncommon, it is not excessively rare. This condition has been described as nontropical idiopathic splenomegaly (Dacie et al., 1969; Manoharan et al., 1982), but it is probable that conditions variously described as primary splenic neutropenia (Wiseman and Doan, 1942), primary hypersplenic pancytopenia (Hayhoe and Whitby, 1955), and simple splenic hyperplasia (Weinstein, 1964) are variants of the same syndrome (*see also* Table 4).

Slight and unremarkable histological changes from normal were found in the excised spleens from Dacie's series (1969). There was variation in the lymphoid follicles, with an abnormal configuration of the germinal centers. Some patients had dilatation of the splenic sinuses, with an increase in the nucleated cells in the red pulp, and erythrophagocytosis was prominent. Four of the patients in the original series died from non-Hodgkin's lymphoma, but the histological findings in the previously removed spleens did not differ from those of other patients who remained well after splenectomy.

The hematological changes in this syndrome have shown variable degrees of anemia, neutropenia and thrombocytopenia, with no specific diagnostic features in blood films. In Dacie's patients, 4/10 had positive direct antiglobulin (Coombs') tests. Radionuclide studies to define the factors responsible for the anemia have shown variable results, with red blood cell life-span varying from normal to markedly reduced, but with no excessive splenic uptake of ^{51}Cr-labeled cells by liver or spleen (Dacie et al., 1969; Goonewardene et al., 1979). A major factor contributing to the anemia, in many cases, was expansion of the plasma volume (Weinstein, 1964; Goonewardene et al., 1979), but the hemoglobin levels in the peripheral blood were further reduced by significant splenic red blood cell pooling, reaching levels of up to 28% of the total red blood cell mass. Little evidence is available regarding leucocyte and platelet kinetics, but excessive splenic pooling seems the likely major factor responsible for the leucopenia and thrombocytopenia.

This is a syndrome in which the response to splenectomy is likely to be gratifying, and, although most authors recommend splenectomy, Coon (1985) has sounded a note of caution, suggesting that, in some younger patients, a decision regarding splenectomy should be deferred. Such caution has to be set against the possibility of the spleen being the initiating site of non-Hodgkin's lymphoma, in which case, diagnostic splenectomy may be advisable (Long and Aisenberg, 1974). Statistics available for this syndrome suggest that approx 20% of patients eventually develop non-Hodgkin's lymphoma (Manoharan et al., 1982). It has been suggested, on the evidence of the conversion to frank lymphoma, that some of these cases result from low-grade small cell lymphoma *ab initio*, either of B-cell small lymphocytic lymphoma type or marginal cell lymphoma.

The following case history shows the typical findings seen in nontropical idiopathic splenomegaly:

> *A 45-year-old farmer presented with a 3-mo history of tiredness and night sweats. Examination revealed pallor and gross splenomegaly. A blood count showed hemoglobin 5.3 g/dL, leukocytes 1.9 × 10⁹/L, and platelets 52 × 10⁹/L. Blood cell appearances were within normal limits. Bone marrow aspiration and trephine biopsy showed active hematopoiesis. Investigations, including lymphangiography, yielded no evidence of disease elsewhere. Radionucleide studies, using ⁵¹Cr-labeled autologous cells, revealed a red blood cell mass of 13.8 mL/kg (normal 25–35 mL/kg), splenic red blood cell pool 28% of red blood cell mass, red blood cell survival (T₁/₂ ⁵¹Cr) 22 d (normal 24–28 d), plasma volume 60 mL/kg (normal 38–42 mL/kg). Surface counting studies showed no excess splenic or hepatic uptake. Following splenectomy, histopathology of the excised spleen (1570 g) revealed no specific features. At last review, 17 years later, the blood count was normal, with hemoglobin 15.7 g/dL, leukocytes 8.3 × 10⁹/L, and platelets 350 × 10⁹/L. The patient has remained well, apart from the development of insulin-dependent diabetes.*

The etiology of the syndrome of nontropical idiopathic splenomegaly remains unknown. The similarities between the histological features of the spleen and those of tropical splenomegaly and Felty syndrome led Dacie et al. (1969) to consider the possibility of its arising from an exaggerated or abnormal reaction to an as-yet-unknown antigenic stimulus. In the 20% of patients who progress to lymphoma, no features were found to distinguish the excised spleen from the spleen in patients not progressing to malignancy. Table 4 summarizes reports of cases comparable to idiopathic nontropical splenomegaly.

9.5.3.2. SECONDARY HYPERSPLENISM Cytopenias associated with splenomegaly, in which the origin of the splenic disease is identifiable, are the hallmark of secondary hypersplenism. The majority of disorders with splenomegaly may result in syndromatic hypersplenism, with some minor variations, depending on the underlying cause.

1. Acute and chronic infections are rarely associated with true hypersplenism in temperate climates. Jandl et al. (1961) described hypersplenism in viral hepatitis, endocarditis, mononucleosis, and psittacosis, but the cytopenias in these were predominantly low-grade spleen-related hemolysis, without consistent accompanying leukopenia or thrombocytopenia. More typical hypersplenism occurs with the occasional case of tuberculosis showing gross splenomegaly (Engelbreth-Holm, 1938), including cases of septicemic tuberculosis. Kala-azar, which is not necessarily confined to the tropics, shows progressive pancytopenia, with increasing spleen size (Cartwright et al., 1948). Hematological findings remained close to normal in a patient previously splenectomized (Bada et al., 1979; *see also* Subheading 3.1.1.2.

2. Tropical splenomegaly is a common finding in tropical regions, and the etiology in many instances remains obscure. Geary et al. (1980) have said, "Most patients in the tropics have enlarged spleens; some are just larger than others." The tropical splenomegaly syndrome (TSS) has emerged as a distinct syndromatic entity, with a close relationship to malaria (Fakunle, 1981; Crane, 1981). Appropriate findings are immunity to malaria, a response to antimalarial drugs, high levels of serum IgM, and lymphocytic infiltration of the hepatic sinusoids on liver biopsy. Not all cases of splenomegaly of obscure origin in the tropics justify this diagnosis, however.

   Hypersplenism is a common although not invariable, feature of this syndrome, and becomes progressively more common as the spleen enlarges. The underlying pathophysiology has been shown to include red blood cell pooling, splenic hemolysis, and plasma volume expansion, together with granulocytopenia and thrombocytopenia, in cases in East Africa (Richmond et al., 1967), Nigeria (Watson Williams and Allan, 1968), and Oceania (Crane, 1981). Cook et al. (1963) have described a similar syndrome as "Cryptogenetic splenomegaly," in cases from south China; this syndrome is often secondary to severe liver disease.

   Hypersplenism in TSS is often severe, especially with respect to neutropenia, which may impair responses to bacterial infections (Crane, 1973).

3. Congestive splenomegaly, most commonly secondary to hepatic cirrhosis, is a common cause of syndromatic hypersplenism. The granulocytopenia and thrombocytopenia are seldom sufficiently severe to be symptomatic, and splenectomy is rarely indicated (*see also* Subheading 3.2).

4. Other causes of secondary splenomegaly, arising from a widely diverse etiology, both localized disease and as part of a systemic disorder, may be associated with hypersplenism.

9.5.3.3. Occult Hypersplenism This occurs when there is an imbalance between the levels of cell production by the bone marrow and the effect of the spleen in reducing circulating cell populations. Thus, the cell deficits associated with splenomegaly are sometimes masked by active compensatory regeneration by the bone marrow. Consequently, the cytopenias are uncovered and recognized only when the activity of the bone marrow is impaired by factors such as infection or chemotherapy. A second rare form is evident following splenectomy, when the spleen has masked a high proliferative state of the bone marrow, which then becomes apparent in the absence of splenic activity (Barosi et al., 1984). Occult hypersplenism may occur both in primary and in secondary hypersplenism.

9.6. SEQUELAE OF SPLENIC ENLARGEMENT

9.6.1. SYMPTOMATIC SPLENOMEGALY The enlarged spleen is frequently asymptomatic, but discomfort is common, even with a relatively mild degree of enlargement. Gross enlargement may result in an especially unpleasant "dragging pain" in the left upper quadrant; pressure on the stomach may produce gastrointestinal reflux and "early satiety," with a feeling of epigastric discomfort and fullness after meals. Pressure on the colon produces disturbances of bowel habit. Extreme degrees of splenomegaly may result in the spleen descending into the pelvis, sometimes resulting in vaginal or rectal prolapse.

Pain in the enlarged spleen may be severe. One significant cause is splenic infarction, which may be either embolic or nonembolic. Embolic infarction occurs in septicemic conditions, such as bacterial endocarditis, in which mild enlargement of the spleen occurs. Painful perisplenitis may supervene, and the condition becomes clinically more insistent if it progresses to splenic abscess formation.

Nonembolic infarction tends to occur in spleens that are markedly or grossly enlarged: Consequently, the spleen in primary myeloid metaplasia and chronic myeloid leukemia is especially at risk of infarct. The spleen in these cases may enlarge, without its vasculature increasing proportionately. In chronic myelogenous leukemia at autopsy, secondary adhesions, between the spleen and surrounding structures, are present in about one-third of cases, and indicate prior infarction (Krumbhaar and Stangel, 1942). Recurrent infarction may be sufficiently symptomatic to justify splenectomy.

Severe pain may also arise from rupture of the spleen, and is felt either in the abdomen or referred to the region of the left shoulder.

9.6.2. BIG SPLEEN SYNDROME　　Given that there is no single effect generated by the enlarging spleen that encompasses all the sequelae of splenomegaly, these have been combined under the term "big spleen syndrome," which has several components, as follows:

1. Cytopenias, whether caused by cell destruction, abnormal distribution, or the dilutional effect of high plasma volume.
2. Hyperkinetic portal hypertension, caused by the enlarged spleen acting as a shunt, with increased blood flow. This may be added to the intrahepatic obstructive effects of hepatic disease concomitant with the disorder of the spleen. There is, consequently, expansion of the splanchnic intravascular space, as was formerly frequently demonstrable by portal venography. The expanded intravascular volume of the spleen itself, of the splanchnic vasculature, and, in some cases, the vasculature of the bone marrow may exceed the compensatory capacity of the bone marrow, producing the dilutional effect associated with expansion of total blood plasma volumes.
3. Secondary consequences may include increased renin secretion, salt and water retention, and increased extravascular fluid volume.
4. Hypermetabolism, resulting from the metabolic activity of the massively enlarged spleen, especially when highly cellular, as in lymphomata, leading to increased cutaneous blood flow and cardiac output (Hess et al., 1976).

9.6.3. HYPOSPLENISM　　The processes leading to splenomegaly may in some cases lead to sufficiently disordered organ structure that its function is significantly impaired: Examples include amyloidosis of the spleen, the later stages of sickle cell disease, and essential thrombocythemia. Therapeutic strategies, including splenectomy and radiation therapy, are, of course, additional hazards to splenic function (*see also* Chapter 10, Subheading 3.1, 3.2.6.1, and Table 1).

REFERENCES

Aderka, D., Garfinkel, D., Rothem, A., and Pinkhas. J. (1984) Fatal bleeding from esophageal varices in a patient with Gaucher's disease. *Am. J. Gastroenterol.* **77,** 838–839.

Arkles, L. B., Gill, C. D., and Molan, M. P. (1986) A palpable spleen is not necessarily enlarged or pathological. *Med. J. Aust.* **45,** 15–18.

Aster, R. H. (1966) Pooling of platelets in the spleen: role in the pathogenesis of 'hypersplenic' thrombocytopenia. *J. Clin. Invest.* **45,** 645–657.

Aster, R. H. and Jandl, J. H. (1964) Platelet sequestration in man. II Immunological and clinical studies *J. Clin. Invest.* **43,** 856–869.

Bada, J. L., Arderiu, A., Gimenez, J., and Gumez-Acha, J. A. (1979) Kala-azar of longstanding evolution in an asplenic patient. *Trans. R. Soc. Trop. Med. Hyg.* **73,** 347–348.

Barcroft, J. (1925) Recent knowledge of the spleen. *Lancet* **i,** 319–322.

Barcroft, J. and Barcroft, H. (1923) Observations on the taking up of carbon monoxide by the haemoglobin in the spleen. *J. Physiol. Lond.* **58,** 138–144.

Barcroft, J. and Poole, L. T. (1927) The blood in the spleen pulp. *J. Physiol. Lond.* **64,** 23–29.

Barkun, A. N., Camus, M., Meagher, T., et al. (1989) Splenic enlargement and Traube's space: how useful is percussion? *Am. J. Med.* **87,** 562–566.

Barkun, A. N., Camus, M., Green, L., et al. (1991) Bedside assessment of splenic enlargement. *Am. J. Med.* **91,** 512–518.

Barosi, G., Baraldi, A., Cazzola, M., et al. (1984) Polycythaemia following splenectomy in myelofibrosis with myeloid metaplasia. A reorganization of erythropoiesis. *Scand. J. Haematol.* **32,** 12–18.

Benacerraf, B. and Sebastyen, M. M. (1957) Effect of bacterial endotoxins on the reticuloendothelial system. *Fed. Proc.* **16,** 860–867.

Berge, T. (1974) Splenic metastases. Frequencies and Patterns. *Acta Path. Microbiol. Scand. [A]* **82,** 499–506.

Berris, B. (1966) The incidence of palpable liver and spleen in the postpartum period. *Can. Med. Assoc. J.* **95,** 1318–1319.

Blendis, L. M., Banks, D. C., Ramboer, C., and Williams, R. (1970) Spleen blood flow and splanchnic haemodynamics in blood dyscrasia and other splenomegalies. *Clin. Sci.* **38,** 73–84.

Blendis, L. M., Ramboer, C., and Williams, R. (1970) Studies on the haemodilution anaemia of splenomegaly. *Eur. J. Clin. Invest.* **1,** 54–64.

Bowdler, A. J . (1961) Radioisotope investigations in primary myeloid metaplasia. *J. Clin. Pathol.* **14,** 595–602.

Bowdler, A. J. (1962) Theoretical considerations concerning measurement of the splenic red cell pool. *Clin. Sci.* **23,** 181–195.

Bowdler, A. J. (1963) Dilution anemia corrected by splenectomy in Gaucher's disease. *Ann. Int. Med.* **58,** 664–669.

Bowdler, A. J. (1967) Dilution anaemia associated with enlargement of the spleen. *Proc. Roy. Soc. Med.* **60,** 44–47.

Bowdler, A. J. (1970) Blood volume changes in patients with splenomegaly. *Transfusion* **10,** 171–181.

Bowdler, A. J. (1983) Splenomegaly and hypersplenism. *Clin. Haematol.* **12,** 467–488.

Boyco, W. J., Pratt, R., and Wass, H. (1982) Functional hyposplenism. A diagnostic clue in amyloidosis. *Am. J. Clin. Pathol.* **77,** 745–748.

Brady, R. O. (1978) Glucosyl ceramide lipidosis: Gaucher's disease. In: *The Metabolic Basis of Inherited Disease,* 4th ed. (Stanbury, J. B., Wyngaarden, J. B., and Fredrickson, D. S., eds.), McGraw-Hill, New York, pp. 731–746.

Brouet, J. C., Sasportes, M., Flandrin, G., Preud-Homme, J. L., and Seligman, M. (1975) Chronic lymphocytic leukemia of T-cell origin. An immunological and clinical evaluation in eleven patients. *Lancet* **ii,** 890–893.

Burt, R. W. and Kuhl, D. E. (1971) Giant splenomegaly in sarcoidosis demonstrated by radionuclide scintiphotography. *JAMA* **215,** 2110, 2111.

Cartwright, G. E., Chung, H.-L., and Chang, A. (1948) Studies on kala-azar. *Blood* **3,** 249–275.

Castell, D. O. (1967) The spleen percussion sign. A useful diagnostic technique. *Ann. Intern. Med.* **67,** 1265–1267.

Chaikoff, E. L. and McCabe, C. J. (1985) Fatal overwhelming postsplenectomy infection. *Am. J. Surg.* **149,** 534–539.

Chauffard, M. A. (1907a) Pathogene de l'ictere congenitale de l'adulte. *Sem. Med. Paris* **27,** 25.

Christensen, B. E. (1975) Red cell kinetics. *Clin. Haematol.* **4,** 393–405.

Collier, H. (1882) *Lancet* **i,** 219. Quoted by Moynihan, B., *loc cit,* p. 14.

Cook, J., MacFadzean, A. J. S., and Todd, D. (1963) Splenectomy in cryptogenic splenomegaly. *Br. Med. J.* **ii,** 337–344.

Coon, W. W. (1985) Splenectomy for splenomegaly and secondary hypersplenism. *World J. Surg.* **3,** 437–443.

Corrigan, J. J., Van Wyck, D. B., and Crosby, W. H. (1983) Clinical disorders of splenic function: the spectrum from asplenism to hypersplenism. *Lymphology* **16,** 101–106.

Crane, G. G. (1981) Tropical splenomegaly: Oceania. *Clin. Haematol.* **10,** 976–982.

Crocker, A. C. and Farber, S. (1958) Niemann-Pick disease: a review of eighteen patients. *Medicine* **37,** 1–96.

Crosby, W. H. (1962a) Hypersplenism. *Annu. Rev. Med.* **13,** 127–146.

Crosby, W. H. (1962b) Is hypersplenism a dead issue? *Blood* **20,** 94–99.

Dacie, J. F. (1985) *The Haemolytic Anaemias: Vol. 1. Part I,* 3rd ed. Churchill, London, pp. 93,94.

Dacie, J. V., Brain, M. D., Harrison, C. V., Lewis, S. M., and Worlledge, S. M. (1969) 'Non-tropical idiopathic splenomegaly' ('primary hypersplenism'): a review of ten cases and their relationship to malignant lymphomas. *Br. J. Haematol.* **17,** 317–333.

Dameshek, W. (1955) Hypersplenism. *Bull. NY Acad. Med.* **31,** 113.

Davis, A. E., Belber, J. P., and Movitt, E. R. (1954) The association of hemolytic anemia with sarcoidosis. *Blood* **9,** 379–383.

DeLand, F. H. (1970) Normal spleen size. *Radiology* **97,** 589–592.

Diamond, L. K. (1969) Splenectomy in childhood and the hazard of overwhelming infection. *Pediatrics* **43,** 886–889.

Dickerman, J. D., Holbrook, P. R., and Zinkham, W. H. (1972) Etiology and therapy of thrombocytopenia associated with sarcoidosis. *J. Pediatr.* **81,** 758–764.

Doan, C. A. (1949) Hypersplenism. *Bull. NY Acad. Med.* **25,** 625.

Doan, C. A. and Wright, C. S. (1946) Primary congenital and secondary acquired splenic pancytopenia. *Blood* **1,** 10–26.

Ebaugh, F. G. Jr., and McIntyre, O. R. (1979) Palpable spleens: ten-year follow-up. *Ann. Intern. Med.* **90,** 130,131.

Edwards, M. H., Wagner, J. A., and Krause, L. A. M. (1952) Sarcoidosis with thrombocytopenia. Report of a case. *Ann. Intern. Med.* **37,** 803–812.

el-Khishen, M. A., Henderson, J. M., Millikan, W. J. Jr., Kutner, M. H., and Warren, W. D. (1985) Splenectomy is contraindicated for thrombocytopenia secondary to portal hypertension. *Surg. Gynecol. Obst.* **160,** 233–238.

Engelbreth-Holm, J. (1938) Study of tuberculous splenomegaly and splenogenic controlling of the cell emission from the bone marrow. *Am. J. Med. Sci.* **195,** 32–40.

Fakunle, Y. M. (1981) Tropical splenomegaly. Part 1: Tropical Africa. *Clin. Haematol.* **10,** 963–975.

Fegiz, G., Bracci, F., Cesarini, C., Capuano, G., Cozzolino, E., and Isacchi, G. (1983) La valutazione della sopravivenza piastrinica prima e dopo shunt porto-cavale latero-laterale. *Minerva Med.* **74,** 205–208.

Ferrant, A., Rodhain, J., Cauwe, F., Cogneau, M., Beckers, C., Michaux, J. L., Verwilghen, R., and Sokal, G. (1982) Assessment of bone marrow and splenic erythropoiesis in myelofibrosis. *Scand. J. Haematol.* **29,** 373–380.

Ferrara, J., Ellison, E. C., Martin, E. W. Jr., and Cooperman, M. (1979) Correction of hypersplenism following distal splenorenal shunt. *Surgery* **86,** 570–573.

Fieschi, A. and Sacchetti, C. (1964) Clinical assessment of granulopoiesis. *Acta Haematol. (Basel)* **31,** 150–162.

Fischer, J. (1970) Spleen scanning as a method of functional analysis of the spleen. In: *The Spleen* (Lennerts, K. and Harms, D., eds.), Springer, Berlin, pp. 11–13.

Franke, E. L. and Neu, H. C. (1981) Postsplenectomy infection. *Surg. Clin. N. Am.* **61,** 135–136.

Galton, D. A., Goldman, J. M., Wiltshaw, E., Catovsky, D., Henry, K., and Goldenberg, G. J. (1974) Prolymphocytic leukaemia. *Br. J. Haematol.* **27,** 7–23.

Garcia, E. L., Garrido, T. A., Lorenzo, E. M., and Guedes, J. R. (1959) Sarcoidosis con anemia hemolytica sintomatica. *Rev. Clin. Esp.* **72,** 183–186.

Geary, G. C., Clough, V., and MacIver, J. E. (1980) Tropical splenomegaly. *Br. J. Hosp. Med.* **24,** 417–421.

Goonewardene, A., Bourke, J. B., Ferguson, R., and Toghill, P. J. (1979) Splenectomy for undiagnosed splenomegaly. *Br J. Surg.* **66,** 62–65.

Gorstein, F. and Benacerraf, B. (1960) Hyperactivity of the reticuloendothelial system and experimental anemia in mice. *Am. J.Pathol.* **37,** 569–582.

Gramlich, F., et al (1970) The spleen in liver disease, In: *The Spleen* (Lennerts, K. and Harms, D., eds.), Springer, Berlin, pp. 336–346.

Green, J. B., Schackford, S. R., and Fridlund, P. (1986) Late septic complications in adults following splenectomy for trauma: a prospective analysis in 144 patients. *J. Trauma* **26,** 999–1004.

Gray, H. (1854) *On the Structure and Use of the Spleen.* Astley Cooper Prize Essay. J. W. Parker, London.

Grover, S. A., Barkun, A. N., and Sackett, D. L. (1993) Does this patient have splenomegaly? *JAMA* **270,** 2218–2221.

Halpern, S., Coel, M., Ashburn, W., Alazraki, N., Littenberg, R., Hurwitz, S., and Green, J. (1974) Correlation of liver and spleen size: determinations by nuclear medicine studies and physical examination. *Arch. Intern. Med.* **134,** 123–124.

Hansen, M. M. (1973) Chronic lymphocytic leukemia.Clinical studies based on 189 cases followed for a long time. *Scand. J. Haematol.* **18(Suppl.),** 3–286.

Harman, J. W. and Dacorso, P. (1948) Spread of carcinoma to the spleen. Its relation to generalized carcinomatous spread. *Arch. Pathol.* **45,** 179–186.

Hayhoe, F. G. J. and Whitby, L. (1955) Splenic function. *Q. J. Med.* N.S. **XXIV, 96,** 365–391.

Hesdorffer, C. S., Macfarlane, B. J., Sandler, M. A., Grant, S. C., and Ziady, F. (1986) True idiopathic splenomegaly: a distinct clinical entity. *Scand. J. Haematol.* **37,** 310–315.

Hess, C. E., Ayers, C. R., Sandusky, W. R., Carpenter, M. A., Wetzel, R. A., and Mohler, D. N. (1976) Mechanism of dilutional anemia in massive splenomegaly. *Blood* **47,** 629–644.

Hess, C. E., Ayers, C. R., Wetzel, R. A., Mohler, D. N., and Sandusky, W. R. (1971) Dilutional anemia of splenomegaly:an indication for splenectomy. *Ann. Surg.* **173,** 693–699.

Heuper, W. C. (1944) Reactions of the blood and organs of dogs after intravenous injections of solutions of methyl celluloses of graded molecular weights. *Am. J. Pathol.* **20,** 737–771.

Hickling, R. A. (1937) Chronic non-leukaemic myelosis. *Q. J. Med.* **6,** 253–275.

Hickling, R. A. (1953) Treatment of patients with myelosclerosis. *Br. Med. J.* **ii,** 411–413.

Hoffbrand, A. V. and Pettit, J. E., eds. (1988) *Clinical Hematology.* Gower Medical, London.

Holzbach, R. T., Shipley, R. A., Clark, R. E., and Chudzik, E. B. (1964) Influence of spleen size and portal pressure on erythrocyte sequestration. *J. Clin. Invest.* **43,** 1125–1135.

Hunter, T. B. and Haber, K. (1977) Weight of the spleen. *Arch. Pathol.* **98,** 33–35.

Jacob, H. S, MacDonald, R. A., and Jandl, J. H. (1963) Regulation of spleen growth and sequestering function. *J. Clin. Invest.* **42,** 1476–1490.

Jandl, J. H., Files, N. M., Barnett, S. B., and MacDonald, R. A. (1965) Proliferative response of the spleen and liver to hemolysis. *J. Exp. Med.* **122,** 299–326.

Jandl, J. H., Jacob, H. S., and Daland, G. A. (1961) Hypersplenism due to infection: a study of 5 cases manifesting hemolytic anemia. *N. Engl. J. Med.* **264,** 1063–1071.

Kararia, Y. F. and Whitcomb, M. E. (1980) Splenomegaly in sarcoidosis. *Arch. Intern. Med.* **140,** 35–37.

King, H. and Shumaker, H. B. (1952) Susceptibility to infection after splenectomy performed in infancy. *Ann. Surg.* **136,** 239–242.

Knudson, P., Coon, W., Schnitzer, B., and Liepman, M. (1982) Splenomegaly without an apparent cause. *Surg. Gyn. Obst.* **155,** 705–708.

Krook, H. (1956) Circulatory studies in liver cirrhosis. *Acta Med. Scand.* **156(Suppl. 318),** 6–134.

Krumbhaar, E. B. and Lippincott, S. W. (1939) The post-mortem weight of the 'normal' human spleen at different ages. *Am. J. Med. Sci.* **197,** 344–430.

Krumbhaar, E. B. and Stengel, A. (1942) The spleen in leukemias. *Arch. Pathol.* **34,** 117–132.

SECTION III / CLINICAL ASPECTS OF DISORDERS OF THE SPLEEN

Kunkel, P. and Yesner, R. (1950) Thrombocytopenic purpura associated with sarcoid granulomas of the spleen. *Arch. Pathol.* **50**, 778–786.

Kyle, R. A. and Bayrd, E. L. (1975) Amyloidosis. Review of 236 cases. *Medicine* **54**, 271–299.

Editorial (1985) Splenectomy: risk of infection, long-term. *Lancet* **ii,** 928,929.

Lee, R. E., Balcerzak, S. P., and Westerman, M. P. (1967) Gaucher's disease: a morphologic study and measurements of iron-metabolism. *Am. J. Med.* **42**, 891–898.

Lewis, S. M. (1983) The spleen: mysteries solved and unresolved: historical perspective. *Clin. Haematol.* **12**, 363–373.

Long, J. C. and Aisenberg, A. C. (1974) Malignant lymphoma diagnosed at splenectomy and idiopathic splenomegaly: a clinico-pathologic comparison. *Cancer* **33**, 1054–1061.

Mandelbaum, H.,Berger, L., and Lederer, M. (1942) Gaucher's disease: I. A case with hemolytic anemia and marked thrombocytopenia; improvement after removal of spleen weighing 6822g. *Ann. Intern. Med.* **16**, 438–446.

Manoharan, A., Bader, L. V., and Pitney, W. R. (1982) Non-tropical idiopathic splenomegaly (Dacie's syndrome). Report of 5 cases. *Scand. J. Haematol.* **28**, 175–179.

McIntyre, R.R. and Ebaugh, F. G. Jr. (1967) Palpable spleens in college freshmen. *Ann. Intern. Med.* **66**, 301–306.

Mitchell, A. and Morris. P. J. (1985) Splenectomy for malignant lymphomas. *World J. Surg.* **9**, 444–448.

Moris, D. H. and Bullock, F. D. (1919) The importance of the spleen in resistance to infection. *Ann. Surg.* **70**, 513–521.

Moynihan, B. (1921) *The Spleen and some of its Diseases.* W.B. Saunders, Philadelphia.

Mutchnik, M. G., Lerner, E., and Conn, H. O. (1975) Effect of portacaval anastomosis on hypersplenism in cirrhosis. A prospective controlled evaluation. *Gastroenterology* **68**, 1070 (Abstract).

Myers, J. and Segal, R. J. (1974) Weight of the spleen. *Arch. Pathol.* **98**, 33–35.

Najjar, V. A. (1975) Defective phagocytosis due to deficiencies involving the tetrapeptide Tuftsin. *J. Pediatr.* **87**, 1121–1124.

Najjar, V. A. (1983) Tuftsin, a natural activator of phagocytic cells: an overview. In: *Antineoplastic, Immunogenic and Other Effects of the Tetrapeptide Tuftsin: a Natural Macrophage Activator* (Najjar, V. A. and Fridkin, M., eds.), *Ann. NY Acad. Sci.* **419**, 1–11.

Nixon, R. K. Jr. (1954) The detection of splenomegaly by percussion. *N. Engl. J. Med.* **250**, 166,167.

Notter, D. T., Grossman, P. L., Rosenberg, S. A., and Remington, J. S. (1980) Infection in patients with Hodgkin's disease. A clinical study of 300 consecutive adult patients. *Rev. Infect. Dis.* **2**, 761–800.

Palmer, J. G., Eichwald, E. J., Cartwright, G. E., and Wintrobe, M. M. (1953) Experimental production of splenomegaly,anemia and leukopenia in albino rats. *Blood* **8**, 72–80.

Partenheimer, R. C. and Meredith, H. C. (1950) Splenomegaly with hypersplenism due to sarcoidosis. *N. Engl. J. Med.* **243**, 810–812.

Penny, R., Rozenberg, M. C., and Firkin, B. G. (1966) The splenic platelet pool. *Blood* **27**, 1–16.

Peter, S. A. (1986) Massive splenomegaly as the presenting manifestation of sarcoidosis. *JAMA* **78**, 243,244.

Pribilla, W. and Oettgen, H. F. (1968) Isotopenuntersuchungen bei Osteomyelofibrose. *Blut* **8**, 72–80.

Pryor, D. S. (1967) Splenectomy in tropical splenomegaly. *Br. Med. J.* **ii**, 825–828.

Rebentish, A. and Bernstein, J. M. (1993) Postsplenectomy sepsis. *Postgrad. Gen. Surg.* **5**, 166–168.

Richmond, J., Donaldson, G. W., Williams, R., Hamilton, P. J., and Hutt, M. S. (1967) Haematological effects of the idiopathic splenomegaly seen in Uganda. *Br. J. Haematol.* **13**, 348–363.

Riemenschneider, P. A. and Whalen, J. P. (1965) The relative accuracy of estimation of enlargement of the liver and spleen by radiologic and clinical methods. *Am. J. Roentgenol.* **94**, 462–468.

Scadding, J. G. (1967) *Sarcoidosis.* Eyre and Spottiswood, London. p. 253.

Schaffner, A., Augustiny, N., Otto, R. C., and Fehr, J. (1985) The hypersplenic spleen. A contractile reservoir of granulocytes and platelets. *Arch. Int. Med.* **145**, 651–654.

Scher, K. S., Wroczynski, A. F., and Jones, C. W. (1983) Protection from post-splenectomy sepsis: effect of prophylactic penicillin and pneumococcal vaccine on clearance of type 3 pneumococcus. *Surgery* **93**, 792–797.

Schaffner, A. and Fehr, J. (1981) Granulocyte demargination by epinephrine in evaluation of hypersplenic states. *Scand. J. Haematol.* **27**, 225–230.

Scott, J. L., McMillan, R., Davidson, J. G., and Marino, J. V. (1971) Leukocyte labelling with ^{51}Chromium. II. Leukocyte kinetics in chronic myelocytic leukemia. *Blood* **38**, 162–173.

Selby, C. D., Sprott, V. M. A., and Toghill, P. J. (1987) Impaired splenic function in systemic amyloidosis. *Postgrad. Med. J.* **63**, 357–360.

Shaw, J. H. F. and Print, C. G. (1989) Postsplenectomy sepsis. *Br. J. Surg.* **76**, 1074–1081.

Singer, D. B. (1973) Postsplenectomy sepsis. *Perspect. Pediatr. Pathol.* **1**, 285–311.

Simpson, A. and Ashby, E. C. (1965) Torsion of the wandering spleen. *Br. J. Surg.* **52**, 344–346.

Soper, N. J. and Rikkers, L. F. (1986) Cirrhosis and hypersplenism. Clinical and haemodynamic correlates. *Curr. Surg.* **43**, 21–24.

Spencer Wells D.B. (1888) Remarks on splenectomy,with a report of a successful case. *Medico-chirurg. Trans.* **71**, 255–263.

Spirer, Z., Zakuth,V., Bogair, N., and Fridkin, M. (1977a) Radioimmunoassay of the phagocytosis-stimulating peptide tuftsin in normal and splenectomized subjects. *Eur. J. Immunol.* **7**, 69–74.

Spirer, Z., Zakuth,V., Diamant, S., Mondorf, W., Stefanescu, T., Stabinsky,Y., and Fridkin, M. (1977b) Decreased tuftsin concentrations in patients who have undergone splenectomy. *Br. Med. J.* **ii**, 1574–1576.

Spirer, Z., Weisman,Y., Zakuth, V., Fridkin, M., and Bogair, N. (1980) Decreased serum tuftsin concentration in sickle cell disease. *Arch. Dis. Child.* **55**, 566,567.

Stathers, G. M., Ma, M. H., and Blackburn, C. R. B. (1968) Extra-hepatic portal hypertension: the clinical evaluation, investigation and results of treatment of 28 patients. *Aust. Ann. Med.* **17**, 12–19.

Stone, R. W., McDaniel, W. R., Armstrong, E. M., and Young, R. C. Jr. (1986) Acquired functional asplenia in sarcoidosis. *J. Natl. Med. Assoc.* **930**, 935–936.

Sullivan, J. L., Ochs, H. D., Schiffman, G., Hammerschlag, M. R., Miser, J., Vichinsky, E., and Wedgwood, R. J. (1978) Immune response after splenectomy. *Lancet* **i**, 178–181.

Sullivan, S. and Williams, R. (1979) Reliability of clinical techniques for detecting splenic enlargement. *Br. Med. J.* **2**, 1043,1044.

Sutton, J. P.,Yarborough, D. Y., and Richards, J. T. (1970) Isolated splenic vein occlusion. Review of literature and report of additional case. *Arch. Surg.* **100**, 623–626.

Symmers, D. (1948) Splenomegaly. *Arch. Pathol.* **45**, 385–409.

Szur, L. and Smith, M. D. (1961) Red cell production and destruction in myelosclerosis. *Br . J. Haematol.* **7**, 147,148.

Thadani, U., Aber, C. P., and Taylor, J. J. (1975) Massive splenomegaly,pancytopenia and haemolytic anaemia in sarcoidosis. *Acta Haematol.* **53**, 230–240.

Tischendorf, F. (1985) On the evolution of the spleen. *Experientia* **41**, 145–152.

Toghill, P. J. and Green, S. (1973) Factors influencing splenic pooling of erythrocytes in the myelo- and lympho-proliferative syndromes. *Acta Haematol.* **49**, 215–222.

Toghill, P. J. and Green, S. (1975) Haematological changes in active chronic hepatitis with reference to the role of the spleen. *J. Clin. Pathol.* **28**, 8–11.

Toghill, P. J. and Green, S. (1979) Splenic influences on the blood in chronic liver disease. *Q. J. Med.* **48**, 613–625.

Vermylen, C., Lebecque, P., Claus, D., Otte, J. B., and Cornu, G. (1983) The wandering spleen. *Eur. J. Pediatr.* **140**, 112–125.

Videbaek, A., Christensen, B. E., and Jonsson, V., eds. (1982) *The Spleen in Health and Disease.* Yearbook, Copenhagen.

Warnke, R. A., Weiss, L. M., Chan, J. K. C., Cleary, M. L., and Dorfman, R. F. (1995) *Atlas of Tumor Pathology (Third series, Fascicle 14) Tumors of the Lymph Nodes and Spleen.* Armed Forces Institute of Pathology, Washington, DC.

Watson Williams, E. J. and Allan, N. C. (1968) Idiopathic tropical splenomegaly syndrome in Ibadan. *Br. Med. J.* **iv,** 793–796.

Weinstein, V. F. (1964) Haemodilution anaemia associated with simple splenic hyperplasia. *Lancet* **ii,** 218–223.

Westcott, J. L. and Krufky, E. L. (1972) The upside-down spleen. *Radiology* **105,** 517–521.

Westaby, S., Wilkinson, S. P., Warren, R., and Williams, R. (1978) Spleen size and portal hypertension in cirrhosis. *Digestion* **17,** 63–68.

Wiland, E. K. and Smith, E. B. (1956) The morphology of the spleen in congenital hemolytic anemia (hereditary spherocytosis). *Am. J. Clin. Pathol.* **26,** 619–629.

Williams, R. (1966) Portal hypertension in idiopathic tropical splenomegaly. *Lancet* **i,** 329–333.

Willis, R. A. (1973) *The Spread of Tumors in the Human Body,* 3rd ed. Butterworths. London, pp. 203–206.

Wiseman, B. K. and Doan, C. A. (1942) Primary splenic neutropenia; a newly recognized syndrome closely related to congenital hemolytic icterus and essential thrombocytopenic purpura. *Ann. Int. Med.* **16,** 1097–1117.

10 Hyposplenism*

*MONTY SEYMOUR LOSOWSKY, MD, FRCP
AND PETER NIGEL FOSTER, PhD, BM, FRCP*

10.1. INTRODUCTION

The term "hyposplenism" was introduced to describe the condition that follows splenectomy (Eppinger, 1913), and its use was extended subsequently to include states of impaired splenic function, regardless of etiology (Schilling, 1924; Dameshek, 1955). Although hyposplenism is most commonly caused by splenectomy, it may also result from agenesis or atrophy of the spleen, or may be functional. The concept of functional hyposplenism arose from the observation that Howell-Jolly bodies can occur in the red blood cells of the peripheral blood of patients with no prior history of splenectomy, and whose spleens are of normal size or even enlarged (Pearson et al., 1969). Furthermore, in some conditions, the hematological features are transient, indicating that hyposplenism may be reversible (Lockwood et al., 1979). Customarily, hyposplenism has been detected by hematological, rather than immunological, methods, the principal hallmark of the hyposplenic state being the presence of Howell-Jolly bodies in the red blood cells of the peripheral blood (*see* Subheading 2.1).

10.2. ASSESSMENT OF SPLENIC FUNCTION

10.2.1. PERIPHERAL BLOOD FILM
Evidence for hyposplenism is most easily obtained by light microscopy of a peripheral blood film, the most characteristic feature being the presence of Howell-Jolly bodies, which are small intraerythrocytic inclusions consisting of nuclear remnants, ordinarily removed by the spleen's pitting process; other red blood cell abnormalities include the presence of acanthocytes and target cells (Fig. 1). None of these abnormalities is individually diagnostic, but their appearance together is virtually pathognomonic of hyposplenism. When the presence of these features was compared with the clearance of heat-damaged erythrocytes in patients with hyposplenism and celiac disease (Robertson et al., 1983a), Howell-Jolly bodies were found to occur only when splenic function was markedly impaired; acanthocytes and target cells were found with milder degrees of hyposplenism. Absence of Howell-Jolly bodies in the blood film cannot be taken as evidence of normal splenic histology (Seo and Li 1995). Other abnormalities of red blood cells, which are not diagnostic, but have been observed in association with hyposplenism, include circulating siderocytes and cells containing Heinz bodies (Acevedo and Mauer 1963).

*Submitted for publication July 1997.

From: *The Complete Spleen: A Handbook of Structure, Function, and Clinical Disorders* Edited by: A. J. Bowdler © Humana Press Inc., Totowa, NJ

10.2.2. PITTED ERYTHROCYTES
Differential interference contrast microscopy gives red blood cells a three-dimensional appearance, which allows detailed examination of the cell surface: Indentations in the surface membrane, with the appearance of craters or pits, were observed in two thalassemic patients after splenectomy (Nathan and Gunn, 1966), but were not found in unsplenectomized subjects (Fig. 2). Similar membrane changes had been noted previously, using chromium shadowing techniques (Koyama et al., 1962). Further detailed examination of these pits, using transmission and scanning electron microscopy, has revealed that they are in fact vacuoles containing the so-called "intracellular rubbish," including ferritin, hemoglobin, and remnants of mitochondria or membranes (Schnitzer et al., 1971; Nathan, 1969). Removing these pits appears to be a normal function of the spleen: Normal erythrocytes acquire pits when transfused into an asplenic subject; pits disappear from erythrocytes of a splenectomized subject when transfused into a normal recipient (Holroyde and Gardner, 1970; Buchanan et al., 1987). The number of erythrocytes with pits begins to rise a few days after splenectomy, reaching about 50% of their maximum numbers by the postsplenectomy d 20, and a constant level after 2–3 mo (Zago et al., 1986). The red blood cells of some families with hereditary spherocytosis exhibit impaired formation of pits after splenectomy, possibly because of a specific membrane defect that limits the cells' ability to form vacuoles; this has also been postulated to explain the reduction in drug-induced vacuole formation in such families (O'Grady et al., 1984a; Kvinesdal and Jensen, 1986; Schrier et al., 1974). The pitted erythrocyte count is determined on red blood cells from fresh venous blood, fixed with 3% glutaraldehyde buffered to pH 7.4, and examined as a wet preparation, using an interference phase microscope fitted with Nomarski optics (Holroyde and Gardner, 1970). The counts are reproducible, provided that sufficient cells are examined: 2000 has been recommended (Corazza et al., 1981). In the majority of series, less than 2% of erythrocytes from normal subjects have been found to bear surface pits, which are usually single. The simplicity of the technique has led to the widespread use of counting pitted erythrocytes to study residual splenic function after splenectomy, and in the quantitative assessment of the functional hyposplenism associated with a variety of disorders.

10.2.3. ARGYROPHILIC INCLUSIONS
A new technique has been described, which utilizes silver staining of erythrocytes (Tham et al., 1996). This shows up erythrocytic inclusions, such as Howell-Jolly bodies, Pappenheimer bodies, and intracellular organelles awaiting disposal. Such inclusions are presumed to be removed by the spleen, much as happens for the structures counted as pits. The

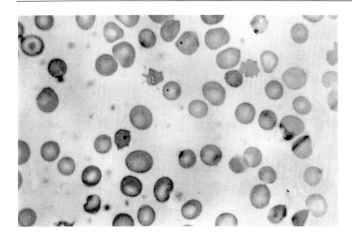

Fig. 10.1. Peripheral blood film showing the typical features of hyposplenism: Howell-Jolly bodies, acanthocytes and target cell.

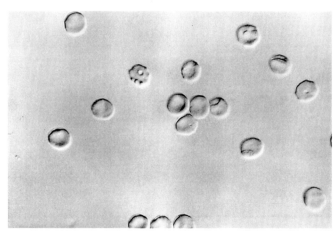

Fig. 10.2. Erythrocytes from a splenectomised subject viewed with direct interference contrast microscopy, showing surface craters or pits.

advantage of this method is that an ordinary microscope is used, and thus no special equipment is required.

Experience of this technique in other clinical situations is required. For example, the authors point out that it is not established whether an increased reticulocyte count affects the result. The authors provide sufficient information to suggest that the technique will prove comparable to counting pitted erythrocytes in detecting and quantitating hyposplenism.

10.2.4. CLEARANCE OF RADIOLABELED, DAMAGED ERY-THROCYTES The ability of the spleen to recognize damaged erythrocytes, and to remove them from the circulation, is utilized to provide a sensitive and quantitative measure of splenic function, in which the clearance of radiolabeled, damaged red blood cells is determined (Marsh et al., 1966a; Armas, 1985).

Erythrocytes can be damaged chemically, thermally, or immunologically, but, regardless of the method used, insufficient damage results in little or no splenic uptake; excessive damage causes hemolysis or sequestration in the liver. Controlling erythrocyte damage is the most difficult and critical step in the preparation of a spleen-specific probe. All the methods are laborious and require meticulous attention to detail. Heating is probably the most widely used physical agent; mercury-based sulphydryl-blocking compounds are effective chemical agents. The uptake of chemically damaged cells by the spleen is slower than that of heat-damaged cells. Methods in which cells sensitized with immunoglobulin G (IgG) anti-Rh(D) antibody are employed provide a probe for splenic Fc-receptor-specific phagocytic function. In normal volunteers, infusion of IgG-sensitized erythrocytes is followed by progressive clearance of the cells from the circulation. Specific radionuclide counting over the liver and spleen shows that these cells are cleared by the spleen and phagocytosed, never reappearing in the circulation. If this experiment is performed with the F(ab)$_2$ antibody fragment, with the Fc portion of the molecule removed, there is no clearance whatsoever, demonstrating that clearance depends on the interaction of the IgG Fc-fragment with the receptor on phagocytic cells specific for that fragment of the molecule (Frank et al., 1983). [51]Cr and technetium-99m (^{99m}Tc) sodium pertechnetate are the isotopes most commonly used as red blood cell labels. Technetium is more widely used, because the radiation dose to the spleen is less, but some investigators have claimed that the technetium

label is unstable and inferior to ^{51}Cr for quantitative work (Desai and Thakur, 1985).

The method used in our lab is as follows: Autologous red blood cells are labeled with 52 MBq (1.4 mCi) ^{99m}Tc sodium pertechnetate (Dacie and Lewis, 1975), then incubated at 50°C for exactly 20 min. The cells are reinjected intravenously, and samples of blood obtained at intervals. After saponin lysis, the radioactivity of the samples is measured in an automatic well scintillation counter. The time to reach 50% remaining radioactivity in normal subjects (the clearance half-life) ranges between 10 and 18 min, which is in accordance with values obtained by others using similar methods (Marsh et al., 1966a; Ryan et al., 1978).

10.2.5. SCINTISCANS Radiolabeled colloids are phagocytosed by reticuloendothelial cells throughout the body, the site of uptake being dependent in part on the size of the particles. [99m]Tc sulfur colloid, with a particle size of approx 1 μ, is the most widely used for scanning the spleen. Following an intravenous dose, about 10% localizes in the spleen, and images may be obtained using a γ camera positioned to view the posterior left upper quadrant of the abdomen (Armas, 1985; Desai and Thakur, 1985). The uptake of radiocolloid provides an index of the spleen's phagocytic activity, and the failure of an anatomically present organ to accumulate sulfur colloid indicates functional hyposplenism (Spencer et al., 1978a). Because of the uniform distribution of reticuloendothelial cells within the spleen, scintiscans provide information about splenic morphology, and, if appropriate images are obtained, estimates of splenic volume may be made (Roberts et al., 1976; Robinson et al., 1980).

10.2.6. CORRELATION OF FUNCTIONS Each of the above methods assesses different aspects of splenic function. The presence of Howell-Jolly bodies and surface pits reflects impaired pitting function, prolongation of the clearance of damaged erythrocytes indicates a reduction in the spleen's ability to cull cells from the circulation, and the uptake of radiolabeled sulfur colloid provides an index of phagocytic activity. Generally, there is a good correlation between these various functions (Traub et al., 1987); an increased pitted erythrocyte count is associated with prolonged clearance times and reduced splenic volume, as determined by scintigraphy (Corazza et al., 1981; Robinson et al., 1980), and estimates of splenic volume correlate with clearance times (Robinson et al.,

1980; Smart et al., 1978). Occasionally, dissociation of functions may occur: For example, cases have been described in which Howell-Jolly bodies were observed in the peripheral blood, but the spleen retained the ability to take up sulfur colloid normally (Spencer and Pearson, 1974; Spencer et al., 1984). Some of these patients show a significant reticulocytosis, and thus it has been suggested that the spleen's pitting function may have been overloaded by the large number of cells presented for the clearance of intracellular inclusions (Spencer and Pearson, 1974). The converse, in which there is failure to accumulate radiocolloid by the spleen and no features of hyposplenism in the peripheral blood, has been described in patients with acute occlusion of the splenic artery (Dhawan et al., 1977). Other patients have been reported in whom the spleen was invisible by scintigraphy, following injection of ^{99m}Tc sulfur colloid, but was visualized with ^{99m}Tc-labeled heat-damaged red blood cells (Armas, 1985). However, the normal spleen accumulates only about 10% of an injected dose of sulfur colloid, but it traps up to 90% of injected damaged erythrocytes. Thus, if splenic function is reduced to 10% of normal, the spleen will receive only 1% of an injected sulfur colloid dose, which is insufficient for visualization; however, it will still trap 9% of damaged cells, which may be enough to allow differentiation from the blood-pool background. Nevertheless, studies in animals emphasize that different mechanisms exist for the clearance of colloidal particles and erythrocytes by the spleen, and illustrate that these functions are subject to different influences. For example, corticosteroids inhibit the clearance of colloidal particles, but have no effect on the removal of red blood cells (Klausner et al., 1975).

The new technique of counting erythrocytes with argyrophilic inclusions has been compared with the counting of pitted erythrocytes (Tham et al., 1996). The absolute correlation of the counts is highly significant, although not extremely good ($r = 0.65$), but the categorization of patients as having normal or abnormal splenic function by the two methods agrees very well.

10.2.7. ULTRASOUND AND COMPUTERIZED TOMOGRAPHY These noninvasive imaging techniques will detect the presence or absence of the spleen, and estimates of the organ size may be made, but it cannot be assumed that this correlates with function.

10.2.8. IMPROVEMENT IN SPLENIC FUNCTION Improvement in splenic function can occur after splenectomy for trauma, presumably as a consequence of subsequent splenosis (Pearson et al., 1978; and *see* Subheading 3), after transfusion in sickle-cell anemia, presumably resulting from "unblocking" of the reticuloendothelial system or the related pathways of blood flow (Pearson et al., 1970; and *see* Subheading 3), after hyposplenism secondary to a delayed transfusion reaction (Hill and Bowdler, 1988), following bone marrow transplantation in sickle-cell anaemia (Ferster et al., 1993), by the use of hydroxyurea in sickle-cell anaemia (Claster and Vichinsky, 1996) and on treatment of celiac disease and inflammatory bowel disease (*see* Subheading 3). Cessation of alcohol intake may be accompanied by improved splenic function (Muller and Toghill, 1994).

Disappearance of Howell-Jolly bodies from the blood has been reported in single patients with congenital heart disease (Pearson et al., 1971) and chronic aggressive hepatitis (Dhawan et al., 1979).

10.3. CAUSES OF HYPOSPLENISM

10.3.1. SPLENECTOMY Some 35,000 patients undergo splenectomy each year in the United States (Dickerman, 1979), but surgical removal of the spleen does not invariably result in the complete absence of functioning tissue. Using the noninvasive methods of isotope scanning and counting pitted erythrocytes, residual splenic function has been detected in between one-fourth and two-thirds of patients after splenectomy following trauma (Livingston et al., 1983; Kiroff et al., 1983), and in 16% of patients who had undergone splenectomy for hematological disorders (Nielsen et al., 1981; Spencer et al., 1981).

The frequent finding of residual splenic tissue after splenectomy for trauma is the result of splenosis, which occurs when fragments of splenic tissue are seeded into the peritoneal cavity. These autotransplanted nodules range in size from a few millimeters to ~3 cm in diameter. The implants do not have a true vascular pedicle of their own, with a branching arterial system; rather, they depend on new vessels to grow in from the peritoneal surface on which they are implanted. There are usually no associated surrounding reactive tissue changes. Implants have been found most often on the serosal surface of the small bowel, the greater omentum, the parietal peritoneum, the serosal surface of the colon, and under the diaphragm. They have also been described in extraperitoneal locations, such as the pleural cavity, pericardium, and in the subcutaneous tissue of old scars; these result from splenic injury, especially gunshot wounds (Widmann and Laubscher, 1971).

Splenosis should be differentiated from the accessory spleens, which have been observed in 10% of the population at necropsy (Bowdler, 1982). Accessory splenic tissue is supplied by branches of the splenic artery, there is usually a well-developed hilar region, and the capsule has both muscle and elastic fibers. Rarely are more than five accessory spleens found in any one subject. The pattern of distribution is determined by embryonic development, and includes the splenic hilum and pedicle, the retroperitoneum, and the greater omentum. Probably, splenic tissue persisting after elective splenectomy results, at least in part, from the presence of accessory spleens, which, because of their small size, have been missed at laparotomy.

The presence of an accessory spleen can result in significant splenic function after splenectomy, but the effect of splenosis is less clear. Certainly the pitting function of the spleen can be restored (Corazza et al., 1984), and the ability to accumulate radiocolloid indicates some phagocytic function, but whether the spleen's immune functions are preserved is uncertain. The low incidence of serious infection in patients splenectomized for trauma may result from a partial return of splenic function consequent on splenosis (Pearson et al., 1978); however, there are reports of fatal infections in patients with significant residual tissue (Rice and James, 1980), and experimentally induced splenosis offers little protection against infection.

10.3.2. NONSURGICAL HYPOSPLENISM Hyposplenism not caused by surgical removal of the spleen occurs in a wide variety of conditions (Table 1). In some disorders, such as sickle-cell disease and celiac disease, hyposplenism is a frequent association; in others, hyposplenism is observed only in isolated cases.

10.3.2.1. Splenic Function and Age Developmental immaturity is characteristic of the neonate, so that impaired splenic function is to be expected in premature and term infants (Holroyde et al., 1969; Freedman et al., 1980). In normal individuals, the spleen reaches a maximum weight early in adult life, and, after 65 yr, there is a rapid loss in the weight of the spleen, because of the aging process, to which an increasing atherosclerotic vascular obstruction and fibrosis of the spleen may contribute (Krumbhaar and

Table 10.1
Causes of Nonsurgical Hyposplenism

Congenital
  Asplenia
    Ivemark syndrome
    Isolated anomaly
  Cyanotic heart disease
Hematological
  Sickle-cell disorders
  Essential thrombocythaemia
  Hodgkin's and non-Hodgkin's lymphoma
  Fanconi's syndrome
Autoimmune
  Systemic lupus erythematosus
  Mixed connective tissue disease
  Rheumatoid arthritis
  Sjögren's syndrome
  Thyroid disease
  Chronic active hepatitis
Gastrointestinal
  Coeliac disease
  Dermatitis herpetiformis
  Ulcerative colitis
  Crohn's disease
  Idiopathic ulcerative enteritis
  Tropical sprue
  Whipple's disease
  Intestinal lymphangiectasia
  Alcoholic liver disease
Circulatory
  Occlusion of splenic artery or vein
  Thrombosis of coeliac artery
Miscellaneous
  Irradiation
  Thorotrast
  Amyloidosis
  Sarcoidosis
  Allogeneic bone marrow transplantation
  Graft-vs-host disease
  Breast cancer
  Haemangiosarcoma
  Methyldopa administration
  Acquired immune deficiency syndrome (AIDS)
  Long-term intravenous nutrition
  Selective IgA deficiency

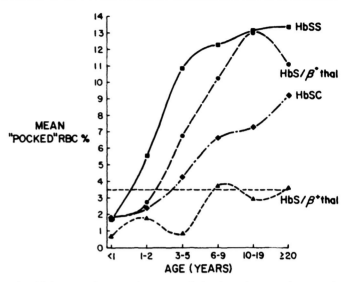

Fig. 10.3. Developmental pattern of pitted erythrocytes in several sickle haemoglobinopathies. (Reproduced by permission of Pediatrics, from Pediatrics, Vol. 76, p. 392, 1985.)

Lippincot, 1939). In addition, old age is accompanied by splenic hypofunction, as judged by increased numbers of pitted erythrocytes and delayed clearance of heat-damaged red blood cells (Zago et al., 1985). 50% of individuals over 60 years of age have pit counts above the upper limit observed in young adults.

10.3.2.2. Congenital Absence or Hypoplasia of the Spleen

Congenital absence of the spleen is often associated with severe malformations of the heart and great vessels, partial situs inversus, and symmetrical three-lobed lungs, a combination of abnormalities that led to the recognition of a syndrome now known as the asplenia or Ivemark syndrome (Polhemus and Schafer, 1952; Ivemark, 1955; Rose et al., 1975). In addition to the cardiovascular and pulmonary abnormalities, a variety of other malformations has been reported in the gastrointestinal, respiratory, genitourinary, and musculoskeletal systems (Freedom, 1972; Mishalany et al., 1982). A few patients with congenital cyanotic heart disease and

typical features of hyposplenism in the peripheral blood, but anatomically normal spleens, have been observed (Pearson et al., 1971); these patients with functional hyposplenism should be distinguished from those with the asplenia syndrome. Estimates of the incidence of the asplenia syndrome range from 1/40,000 to 1/1750 (Rose et al., 1975; Majeski et al., 1978), and it is generally agreed that the syndrome occurs about twice as often in males; however, in one study, this incidence was reversed (Majeski and Upshur, 1978). Possible factors in the pathogenesis of the asplenia syndrome include a developmental disturbance, occurring before the fifth week, and affecting the heart, lungs, spleen, and other viscera. The syndrome has been observed in a child born to a mother given warfarin during the first 6 wk of pregnancy (Cox et al., 1977), and may be the expression of bilateral right-sidedness, leading to absent or abnormal left-sided structures and organs (Van Mierop et al., 1972). In addition, vascular abnormalities may lead to agenesis of the spleen (Monie, 1982). More rarely, congenital asplenia occurs as an isolated anomaly (Waldman et al., 1977), and, in some cases, there appears to be an hereditary basis (Kevy et al., 1968).

10.3.2.3. Hyposplenism in Disorders of Blood and Reticuloendothelial System

10.3.2.3.1. Splenic Function in Sickle-Cell Diseases Splenomegaly is present consistently in the early years of life in sickle-cell anemia, and is followed by atrophy of the spleen, which reduces it to a fibrotic nodule, as the result of repeated episodes of infarction. Functional hyposplenism occurs when the spleen is still clinically enlarged (Pearson et al., 1969). Analysis of pitted erythrocyte data from over 2000 patients has revealed differences between several sickling disorders in the development of splenic hypofunction (Pearson et al., 1985; Fig. 3). In general, the pattern of dysfunction parallels the expected rates of intravascular sickling and clinical severity, and correlates with the epidemiology of severe bacterial meningitis and sepsis in these diseases. The functional hyposplenism may be reversed transiently by the transfusion of normal red blood cells. The high viscosity of sickle-cell blood has been proposed to cause diversion of splenic blood flow through intrasplenic shunts, thus bypassing the phagocytic elements of the organ and producing functional asplenia; when sickle-cells are replaced by normal red blood cells, splenic circulation and function are temporarily restored (Pearson et al., 1970).

10.3.2.3.2. Essential Thrombocythemia In a study of eight patients with essential thrombocythemia, three were found to have delayed clearance of damaged red blood cells, and Howell-Jolly bodies in the peripheral blood (Marsh et al., 1966b). Splenic atrophy was noted in 3/23 cases described in the literature (Hardisty and Wolff, 1955). It has been proposed that splenic atrophy results from infarction caused by platelet-initiated vascular occlusion (Crosby, 1963).

10.3.2.3.3. Malignant Lymphoma Hyposplenism following splenic irradiation in patients with Hodgkin's disease and non-Hodgkin's lymphomas is well-recognized (*see* below). There are also reports of hyposplenism in patients who have not received irradiation, which are presumed to reflect infiltration of the spleen by neoplastic tissue (Pettit et al., 1971; Balchandran et al., 1980; Gross et al., 1982).

10.3.2.3.4. Other Disorders Splenic atrophy has been identified as a feature of the familial form of aplastic anemia, Fanconi's syndrome, and Garriga and Crosby (1959) have suggested that it results from a generalized dystrophy of mesenchymal tissue. Isolated cases of hyposplenism in patients with combined immunodeficiency (Spencer et al., 1978b), malignant mastocytosis (Roth et al., 1985), and selective IgA deficiency (Ramsahoye et al., 1994) have been reported.

10.3.2.4. Hyposplenism and Autoimmune Disorders Both splenic atrophy and functional hyposplenism occur in association with a variety of autoimmune diseases; it is not clear whether the abnormalities of splenic function are a consequence of, or contribute to, the development of autoimmunity.

10.3.2.4.1. Systemic Lupus Erythematosus The reported frequency of hyposplenism in systemic lupus erythematosus has varied according to the method used to assess splenic function. 5/70 patients (7.1%) had Howell-Jolly bodies in the peripheral blood (Dillon et al., 1982) and a similar portion (4.6%) was found using counts of pitted erythrocytes in 44 patients (Neilan and Berney, 1983). However, prolongation of the clearance of IgG-sensitized erythrocytes was detected in 13/15 (87%) patients (Frank et al., 1979). Impaired splenic Fc-receptor function was observed in most patients with active disease and there was a significant correlation between clinical improvement, improvement of Fc-specific clearance, and decreased levels of immune complexes (Frank et al., 1979; Frank et al., 1983). Prolonged clearance of heat-damaged red blood cells, which may be improved by plasmapheresis, was found in patients with active nephritis, but was unusual in patients without renal involvement, despite high levels of circulating immune complexes (Lockwood et al., 1979; Elkon et al., 1980). These observations suggest that, in some patients, there is reversible blockade of splenic phagocytic function. Histological examination of atrophic spleens, removed at autopsy from two patients, revealed marked depletion of lymphoid tissue, but no evidence of involvement by vasculitis (Dillon et al., 1982; Foster et al., 1984).

10.3.2.4.2. Mixed Connective Tissue Disease This condition exhibits features of systemic lupus erythematosus, polymyositis, and scleroderma. It is distinguished by the presence of high titers of antibody to extractable nuclear antigen, a ribonucleoprotein moiety. Clinically significant renal disease is uncommon. Defective splenic reticuloendothelial Fc-specific function, as measured by clearance of IgG-sensitized erythrocytes, was found in 4/18 patients

studied, the majority having normal reticuloendothelial function, despite high levels of circulating immune complexes (Frank et al., 1983). In addition, we have seen a patient with mixed connective tissue disease who developed the typical features of hyposplenism in the peripheral blood and an increased number of pitted erythrocytes, and had a small spleen on computerized tomography (Losowsky and Foster). A case is described by Guertler and Carter (1996).

10.3.2.4.3. Rheumatoid Arthritis There have been several studies of the clearance of heat-damaged red blood cells in patients with active rheumatoid arthritis. The number of patients investigated was small in each series, and the frequency of prolonged clearance ranged from 21 to 85% (Williams et al., 1979; Gordon et al., 1981; Henderson et al., 1981). In one study, there was a significant correlation between the level of circulating immune complexes and the clearance time, but this was not observed in the other series. Fc-receptor specific clearance was measured using IgG-coated erythrocytes, in 50 patients with rheumatoid arthritis, and mild or moderate impairment was found in 65% (Frank et al., 1983). There was no correlation with disease activity, titer of rheumatoid factor, immunoglobulin levels, or circulating immune complexes. Atrophy of the spleen has been reported by Parr et al. (1953), in a patient with juvenile chronic arthritis (Still's disease).

10.3.2.4.4. Sjögren's Syndrome Sjögren's syndrome is characterized by xerophthalmia (with or without lachrymal gland enlargement), xerostomia (with or without salivary gland enlargement), and the presence of various connective tissue disorders. Defective clearance of heat-damaged and IgG-sensitized erythrocytes has been found in patients with this syndrome, but almost invariably in patients with extraglandular disease (Hersey et al., 1983; Hamburger et al., 1979).

10.3.2.4.5. Other Disorders Reports of hyposplenism in autoimmune thyroid disease are confined to isolated cases (Wardrop et al., 1979; Brownlie et al., 1975; Jellinek and Ball, 1976). Reversible functional hyposplenism has been described in a patient with autoimmune chronic active hepatitis (Dhawan et al., 1979).

10.3.2.5. Hyposplenism in Gastrointestinal Disorders This subject has been reviewed by Muller and Toghill (1995).

10.3.2.5.1. Celiac Disease The association of splenic atrophy with intestinal malabsorption was first recognized more than 60 yr ago (Blumgart, 1923). Subsequently, further cases were reported (Engel, 1939; Martin and Bell, 1965), and, for many of these patients, the malabsorption was probably caused by celiac disease, which more-recent studies have shown to be frequently associated with hyposplenism.

There are two components to the impaired splenic function associated with celiac disease: functional hyposplenism and splenic atrophy. The functional hyposplenism fluctuates with disease activity, and improves after withdrawal of gluten from the diet (Palmer et al., 1979; Corazza et al., 1983; O'Grady et al., 1984b). It appears to be closely related to the morphological state of the jejunal mucosa, whereas splenic atrophy results in irreversible loss of splenic function (Robinson et al., 1980; Trewby et al., 1981). The reported incidence of hyposplenism in celiac disease varies with the diagnostic method used. Splenic atrophy was found in 10/24 patients at autopsy (Thompson, 1974); evidence of hyposplenism on a peripheral blood film has been found in 16–36% of patients (McCarthy et al., 1966; Marsh and Stewart, 1970; Bullen et al., 1981; Trewby et al., 1981), and elevated pitted erythrocyte counts in 32 and 79% of patients (Corazza et al., 1981; O'Grady et al., 1984b); prolonged clearance of heat-damaged red blood cells occurred in 28–77% of patients studied (Trewby et al., 1981; Robinson et al., 1980; Marsh and Stewart, 1970), and reduction in splenic volume, computed from isotope scintigrams, was observed in 34–43% (Robinson et al., 1980; Trewby et al., 1981). Differences in the sensitivity of the methods explain some of this variation, but another important factor is the effect of gluten withdrawal and the intensity of treatment among the patients studied. The frequency and severity of hyposplenism increases with advancing age and duration of exposure to dietary gluten (Corazza et al., 1981; O'Grady et al., 1984b); hyposplenism does not appear to be a common feature of celiac disease in childhood, despite autopsy-based case reports of splenic atrophy in children believed to have celiac disease (Corazza et al., 1982; Macrae and Morris, 1931; Meyer, 1932). It is not clear whether splenic atrophy is a consequence of prolonged functional hyposplenism or is an independent development. There are also reports of hyposplenism progressing despite gluten withdrawal (Szur et al., 1972; Trewby et al., 1981).

The mechanism leading to hyposplenism in celiac disease remains obscure. The original reports of splenic atrophy in association with severe malabsorption raised the possibility that hyposplenism might be a consequence of malnutrition, but atrophy of the spleen was not observed among severely malnourished inmates of the concentration camps of World War II (de Jongh, 1948), and the presence of hyposplenism in celiac disease does not correlate with nutritional disturbances (Ferguson, 1976). Rats rendered deficient in folate develop splenic atrophy that can be reversed by administration of the vitamin (Asenjo, 1948). However, the impaired splenic function associated with celiac disease is not correlated with folate deficiency, nor does it improve following folic acid administration (Ferguson et al., 1970; McCarthy et al., 1966). There may be an hereditary component. Marked abnormalities of splenic Fc-receptor function have been found in association with the HLA-B8 antigen (Lawley et al., 1981), which is commonly found in patients with celiac disease, but the results of several studies suggest that splenic hypofunction in celiac disease is independent of the presence of this antigen (Bullen et al., 1981; O'Grady et al., 1984b). However, the observation of increased numbers of pitted erythrocytes in first-degree relatives of patients with celiac disease, and with normal small bowel morphology (O'Grady, Stevens and McCarthy, 1985a), is another pointer to a genetic influence on splenic function in celiac disease. Considerable interfamily variation has been found, and the pattern tends to run true within families, and is compatible with a recessive mode of inheritance.

In some patients with celiac disease, splenic atrophy occurs in association with atrophy or cavitation of peripheral and mesenteric lymph nodes (McCarthy et al., 1966; Matuchansky et al., 1984), and it has been suggested that hyposplenism is a manifestation of a more widespread atrophy of the lympho-reticuloendothelial system. However, this concept is not supported by the finding of normal Kupffer cell function in patients with hyposplenism (Palmer et al., 1983).

Increased levels of circulating immune complexes, which could lead to functional blockade of the splenic reticuloendothelial system, have been detected, especially in untreated celiac disease (Doe et al., 1973), but no significant difference in the levels of C1q-binding activity has been found in adult celiac patients with or without hyposplenism (Bullen et al., 1980). Furthermore, very high levels of immune complexes are insufficient to induce splenic hypofunction in childhood celiac disease (Corazza et al., 1983).

By analogy with animal models, it has been suggested that hyposplenism in celiac disease results from lymphocyte depletion caused by chronic loss into the gut (Bullen and Losowsky, 1978). Chronic drainage of the thoracic duct in calves produces lymphoreticular atrophy, and cessation of lymph drainage results in repopulation of the spleen with lymphocytes (Fish et al., 1970). The absolute lymphocyte count and T-cell numbers are reduced in untreated celiac disease, and tend to return to normal after treatment (Bullen and Losowsky, 1978).

10.3.2.5.2. Dermatitis Herpetiformis Dermatitis herpetiformis is known to be closely related to celiac disease. It is linked to the same histocompatibility antigens, and in most cases gluten-sensitive jejunal lesions are present, similar to those of celiac disease, but usually less severe and extensive. Impaired splenic function has been detected by prolonged clearance of heat-damaged erythrocytes in 7/24 patients with dermatitis herpetiformis (Pettit et al., 1972), and in 3/7 patients, using the pitted cell count (Corazza et al., 1981). Splenic reticuloendothelial function in dermatitis herpetiformis has also been studied by antibody-coated autologous red blood cell clearance, which was delayed in half the cases studied, indicating abnormal Fc-receptor function of splenic macrophages (Lawley et al., 1981). The presence of circulating immune complexes may be a significant factor in the development of hyposplenism in this disease (Mowbray et al., 1973).

10.3.2.5.3. Inflammatory Bowel Disease Functional hyposplenism is well-recognized to be associated with active ulcerative colitis, and tends to improve, or even to return to normal, as the inflammation declines with medical treatment, or after colectomy (Ryan et al., 1974, 1978; Palmer et al., 1981; Jewell et al., 1981); irreversible atrophy also occurs (Ryan et al., 1978; Foster et al., 1982). In a survey of 65 patients with ulcerative colitis, hyposplenism was detected by prolonged clearance of heat-damaged erythrocytes, or typical features on a peripheral blood film, in 29% of patients (Palmer et al., 1981). In another, smaller study, delayed clearance of heat-damaged red blood cells was observed in 13/16 patients with ulcerative colitis (Jewell et al., 1981). Hyposplenism is detected more frequently in patients with extensive disease. It appears to be less common in patients with Crohn's disease. Delayed clearance of heat-damaged red blood cells was found in 11/42 and 4/17 patients, in two separate studies (Palmer et al., 1981; Jewell et al., 1981), and we observed increased pitted erythrocyte counts in only 2/34 patients with Crohn's disease (Losowsky and Foster). Impaired splenic function seems to occur only in those patients with colonic involvement, although, in a recent study of splenic size in patients who had undergone laparotomy for inflammatory bowel disease, small spleens (<11 cm) were found in 7/36 patients with Crohn's disease affecting only the small bowel (Pereira et al., 1987). The relationship to disease activity is less clear than with ulcerative colitis, but improvement in splenic function has been reported, as the activity of the Crohn's disease abates (Palmer et al., 1981). The mechanisms underlying hyposplenism in inflammatory bowel disease have been less extensively studied than in celiac disease, but, as in that condition, raised levels of circulating immune complexes (Doe et al., 1973) and enteric loss of lymphocytes (Douglas et al., 1976; Segal et al., 1981) have been reported, which may contribute to the development of splenic hypofunction.

10.3.2.5.4. Chronic Idiopathic Ulcerative Enteritis This condition is characterized by small-intestinal ulceration and malabsorption, but probably represents a spectrum of disorders that bears an inconsistent relationship to gluten sensitivity and small-intestinal lymphoma. In two different studies, splenic atrophy or Howell-Jolly bodies were observed in 3/5 and 3/8 patients with small-intestinal ulceration (Mills et al., 1980; Robertson et al., 1983b). In some of these patients, a diagnosis of celiac disease was made, but it is still unclear whether the hyposplenism seen in patients with chronic idiopathic ulcerative enteritis is directly linked to this condition, or whether it reflects pre-existing celiac disease.

10.3.2.5.5. Tropical Sprue Splenic atrophy proved to be a frequent postmortem finding in a series of 16 patients who died from tropical sprue (Suarez et al., 1947). Spleen weight varied between 5 and 140 g, with an average of 75 g. No in vivo measurements of splenic function in tropical sprue have been made, and the relationship between possible reticuloendothelial dysfunction and other immunological changes in this disease is still unknown.

10.3.2.5.6. Whipple's Disease Splenic atrophy and increased pitted cell counts have been observed in cases of Whipple's disease, which often involves the spleen by infiltration or infarction (Plummer et al., 1950; Haeney and Ross, 1978; Corazza et al., 1982).

10.3.2.5.7. Intestinal Lymphangiectasia The characteristic features of intestinal lymphangiectasia are dilated lymphatics, protein-losing enteropathy, and lymphopenia. We have reported a patient with this condition and associated hyposplenism (Foster et al., 1985a). The splenic volume was reduced, and there was progressive development of the typical features of hyposplenism in the peripheral blood, and an increase in the number of pitted erythrocytes. The abnormalities of the red blood cells subsequently returned to normal, suggesting an element of functional hyposplenism, in addition to loss of splenic volume. Thrombocytosis was a prominent feature in this case, and it is unclear whether the increased platelet count reflected impaired splenic function, or contributed to it in a manner analogous to that proposed for essential thrombocythemia (see Subheading 3.2.3.2). In addition to this case, there is a report of splenic atrophy in a patient with lymphangiectasia secondary to lymphoma (Crosby, 1963).

10.3.2.5.8. Alcoholic Liver Disease Hyposplenism in alcoholic liver disease may be more related to a toxic effect of alcohol than to the liver damage (Muller and Toghill, 1994).

10.3.2.6. Miscellaneous Conditions
10.3.2.6.1. Radiation Splenic atrophy has been reported following external radiation (Dailey et al., 1980; Coleman et al., 1982), or the use of the radiocontrast agent, Thorotrast (Bensinger et al., 1970). The histological changes seen in the irradiated spleens included collapse of the architecture from loss of red pulp, vessel wall thickening, and varying degrees of fibrosis with lymphoid depletion. The risk of developing significant splenic atrophy (spleen weight <60 g) has been estimated at 30–40% from the results of a retrospective, necropsy study of patients who had received splenic irradiation for Hodgkin's disease (Dailey et al., 1980), and the majority of patients who have received more than 4000 rads have elevated numbers of pitted erythrocytes (Coleman et al., 1982).

10.3.2.6.2. Amyloidosis In a retrospective study of 91 patients with systemic amyloidosis, the typical features of hyposplenism were observed in the peripheral blood of 24% (Gertz et al., 1983). Palpable splenomegaly was seen in 2/22 patients with hyposplenism. In a smaller series, 6/14 patients had evidence of hyposplenism (Boyko et al., 1982). Histological examination of spleens removed at autopsy revealed extensive amyloid replacement of splenic cords and malpighian follicles.

10.3.2.6.3. Sarcoidosis Although microscopic involvement of the spleen is common in sarcoidosis, evidence of hyposplenism is confined to a single case of functional hyposplenism, based on the presence of Howell-Jolly bodies and failure to accumulate technetium-labeled sulfur colloid, which improved with steroid therapy (Stone et al., 1985). In a case in which the patient died of fulminant pneumococcal sepsis, functional hyposplenism was proposed as a contributory factor, the spleen weighing 300 g and being heavily infiltrated by sarcoid tissue (Guyton and Zumwalt, 1975).

10.3.2.6.4. Other Disorders Impairment of the splenic circulation, caused by occlusion of the splenic artery or vein, or thrombosis of the celiac artery, has been described as a cause of functional hyposplenism (Spencer et al., 1977; Dhawan et al., 1977). Isolated cases of hyposplenism, caused by direct involvement of the spleen by metastatic breast cancer (Costello et al., 1977) and hemangiosarcoma (Steinberg et al., 1983), have been reported.

Reversible hyposplenism occurs in patients with graft-vs-host disease following bone marrow transplantation (Demetrakopolous et al., 1982; Al-Eid et al., 1983). Demetrakopolous et al. (1982) have suggested that splenic hypofunction results from allogeneic killing of the host lymphoid tissue, and that recovery of splenic function results from either repopulation of the spleen with allogeneic lymphocytes or tolerance of the host's lymphocytes by the engrafted population. Functional hyposplenism has been described after allogeneic bone marrow transplantation in the absence of evidence of graft-vs-host disease (Cuthbert et al., 1995).

Delayed clearance of IgG-sensitized erythrocytes has been observed in patients taking methyldopa for more than 1 year and it appears that the drug directly depresses the Fc-receptor specific function of splenic reticuloendothelial cells (Kelton, 1985).

Evidence of defective reticuloendothelial function may occur in the acquired immune deficiency syndrome (AIDS) (Bender et al., 1985), and this may be in association with other evidence of hyposplenism (Corazza et al., 1991). There has been a report of abnormal Fc-receptor specific function in patients with AIDS (Bender et al., 1984), but no evidence of hyposplenism was observed in a series of patients with the syndrome complicated by bacterial pneumonia caused by *Streptococcus pneumoniae* and *Haemophilus influenzae* (Polsky et al., 1986).

Impaired splenic function has been reported in patients with the short-bowel syndrome on long-term parenteral nutrition (Zoli et al., 1993).

10.4. SEQUELAE OF HYPOSPLENISM
10.4.1. BLOOD
10.4.1.1. Erythrocytes Changes in mature erythrocytes after splenectomy have been described above. In addition, there may be a transient normoblastosis, and the reticulocyte count is elevated, as a consequence of displacement to the peripheral blood of the immature red blood cells that normally complete maturation within the spleen (Lipson et al., 1959).

10.4.1.2. Leucocytes Leucocytosis is a well-recognized sequela of splenectomy. Initially, the leucocytosis reflects a neutrophilia, which then diminishes, and is followed by a more persistent lymphocytosis. A monocytosis and a slight-to-moderate rise in basophil and eosinophil counts may also occur (Crosby, 1963; Lipson et al., 1959; McBride et al., 1968). A marked lymphocytosis is also found in association with hyposplenism not caused by splenectomy (Bullen and Losowsky, 1978; Wilkinson et al., 1983), and after splenectomy (Juneja et al., 1995). There is considerable traffic of lymphocytes through the spleen, and splenectomy results in loss of this pool, which presumably contributes to the peripheral blood lymphocytosis. In addition, animal experiments suggest that the spleen exerts an inhibitory influence on lymphocyte production (Ernstrom and Sandberg, 1970). Lymphocyte populations after splenectomy have been examined in several studies using a variety of marker techniques, and no consistent abnormality in the proportion of B-cells, T-cells, and their subsets, has been observed, and, when the absolute numbers of the different types of cell have been calculated, the counts have been normal or increased (Millard and Bannerjee, 1979; Lauria et al., 1981; Grattner et al., 1982; Neilsen et al., 1983b; Foster et al., 1985a,b; Durig et al., 1984).

10.4.1.3. Platelets Thrombocytosis is a well-recognized feature of the early postsplenectomy period. The platelet count increases between two- and six-fold during the first 2 postoperative weeks and tends to return toward normal values after a period of weeks or months; in some patients, the thrombocytosis may persist for years (Laufer et al., 1978; Lipson et al., 1959). Chronic elevation of the platelet count was noted, particularly, in association with continuing anemia and hemolysis (Hirsh and Dacie, 1966), but, clearly, it commonly occurs in splenectomized subjects without anemia (O'Grady et al., 1985; Robertson et al., 1981). Thrombocytosis also occurs in association with splenic atrophy. In some patients with ulcerative colitis or celiac disease, both activity of the inflammatory lesion and hyposplenism contribute to the thrombocytosis (Bullen et al., 1977a). Splenic atrophy secondary to thrombocytosis may further increase the platelet count. Platelet volume is increased after splenectomy (Laufer et al., 1978; O'Grady et al., 1985), and the platelets appear hyperactive, as judged by their tendency to aggregate (Kenny et al., 1980; Zucker and Mielke, 1972). The thrombocytosis is presumed to be mostly caused by the loss of the splenic reservoir of platelets, but, in addition, there is evidence for increased platelet production after splenectomy, and it has been postulated that the spleen produces a factor that suppresses platelet formation (Crosby and Ruiz, 1962; Bessler et al., 1978).

10.4.1.4. Viscosity Blood viscosity increases within a few weeks of splenectomy, and remains elevated. The hyperviscosity does not appear to be related to thrombocytosis, but rather is consequent on decreased deformability of the red blood cell (Robertson et al., 1981).

10.4.1.5. Thrombosis Venous thrombosis complicating splenectomy was first described by Rosenthal (1925). Subsequently, there have been case reports confirming the association and studies of the incidence of postsplenectomy thrombosis; however, these have been the subject of a critical review (Dawson et al., 1981), in which imperfections in the information have been emphasized. The data have usually been collected without regard for the disorder for which splenectomy was performed, and both benign and malignant disorders, in which the incidence of deep vein thrombosis might be expected to differ, have been included. Most studies are retrospective, and the methods for detection of venous thrombosis have varied from clinical signs to venography and isotope techniques. Finally, the majority of studies have not included an appropriate or adequately described control group. In the two studies that avoided many of these deficiencies (Butler et al., 1977; Dawson et al., 1981), no significant increase in deep vein thrombosis was observed after splenectomy. Furthermore, no increase in mortality caused by venous thromboembolism was observed in a study of veterans of the Second World War, who had undergone

splenectomy for trauma (Robinette and Fraumeni, 1977). However, this latter study did reveal an excess mortality from ischemic heart disease, principally myocardial infarction, which raises the possibility that the increase in platelet numbers and activity and hyperviscosity, observed after splenectomy, may predispose to coronary artery thrombosis.

10.4.2. IMMUNITY

10.4.2.1. Immunoglobulins Immunoglobulin levels after splenectomy have been widely studied, with conflicting results, which probably result from important differences in age, time after splenectomy, and the presence of associated disease in the patients investigated. Generally, in older children and adults, compared with preoperative values, or with levels in matched control subjects, IgM levels are significantly lower after splenectomy, IgG levels remain constant or increase, and IgA and IgE levels increase (Schumacher, 1970; Claret et al., 1975; Andersen et al., 1976; Chaimoff et al., 1978; Constantoulakis et al., 1978; Westerhausen et al., 1981; Chelazzi et al., 1985). Low IgM levels have been found in patients with sickle-cell disease and splenic atrophy (Gavrilis et al., 1974), but in the few patients with celiac disease and hyposplenism studied, immunoglobulin levels were normal (Wardrop et al., 1975). There is long-standing evidence of an impaired response to intravenously administered antigens (Rowley, 1950).

The switch from IgM to IgG production, during the secondary response to an intravenous antigen, is impaired after splenectomy (Sullivan et al., 1978), and a similar defect has been observed in patients with hyposplenism associated with celiac disease and inflammatory bowel disease (Baker et al., 1975; Bullen et al., 1977b; Ryan et al., 1981). There is increasing evidence that the spleen is necessary for the generation of a normal response to immunization with pneumococcal polysaccharides, and that splenectomy results in impaired antipneumococcal antibody production (Hosea et al., 1981; Di Padova et al., 1985). Absence of the spleen appears to cause a long-lasting B-cell defect characterized by a limited capacity of circulating B-cells to differentiate into antibody-secreting cells (Di Padova et al., 1983; Drew et al., 1984; Muller et al., 1984).

10.4.2.2. Complement After splenectomy, defective function of the alternative pathway or low levels of particular components of complement have been recorded by some investigators (Carlisle and Saslaw, 1959; Polhill and Johnston, 1975; Corry et al., 1979), but not others (Winkelstein and Lambert, 1975; Ciuttis et al., 1978; Nielsen et al., 1983a). Thus, the spleen appears to make a contribution to maintaining the integrity of the alternative pathway in humans, but the role is not crucial.

10.4.2.3. Tuftsin Tuftsin is a naturally occurring tetrapeptide, threonyl-lysil-prolyl-arginine, which stimulates phagocytosis by neutrophils, macrophages, and monocytes. It originates from the Fc-fragment of IgG, and is released in vivo as the free peptide after enzymatic cleavage, one step of which is believed to occur in the spleen, because splenectomy results in low levels of tuftsin (Spirer et al., 1977).

Hyposplenism in sickle-cell disease is also associated with decreased levels of tuftsin (Spirer et al., 1980b). Low tuftsin levels in the Acquired Immune Deficiency Syndrome (AIDS) have been shown to correlate with impairment of splenic function (Corazza et al., 1991).

10.4.2.4. Neutrophil Function The function of neutrophils after splenectomy has been studied using various methods, and with disparate results (Constantopoulos et al., 1973; Winkelstein and Lambert, 1975; von Fliedner et al., 1980; Deitch and O'Neal,

1982; Cooper et al., 1982; Falcao et al., 1982; Hauser et al., 1983; Foster et al., 1985b; Dahl et al., 1986); there appears to be no intrinsic abnormality of the cells, but rather, in some patients, the serum is deficient in opsonic and chemotactic factors, which results in impaired neutrophil activity.

10.4.2.5. Lymphocyte Function No consistent abnormality of the transformation response of lymphocytes to the plant lectins, phytohemagglutinin, concanavalin A, and pokeweed mitogen, which test T-cell function in vitro, has been observed after splenectomy (Andersen et al., 1976; Nielsen et al., 1983b; Cohen and Ferrante, 1982; Ferrante et al., 1985), but in two studies, suppressor cell activity was reduced (Melamed et al., 1982; Robertson et al., 1982a). Suppressor cell function is impaired in patients with celiac disease, but it is not related to associated hyposplenism (Robertson et al., 1982a). Natural killer cell activity has been found to be normal or increased after splenectomy (Foster et al., 1985b; Ferrante et al., 1985) and is unaffected by hyposplenism in patients with celiac disease. Antibody-dependent, cell-mediated cytotoxicity has been found to be defective in some patients after splenectomy (Kragballe et al., 1981).

10.4.2.6. Reticuloendothelial Function The results of studies of reticuloendothelial function, after splenectomy in animals and humans, suggest that the spleen may have a necessary role in the normal phagocytic activity of other reticuloendothelial cells throughout the body. In the rat, alveolar macrophage function has been found to be impaired after splenectomy (Chaudry, 1982; Shennib et al., 1983), and some workers (Chaudry, 1982), but not others (Nashat et al., 1982), have reported reduced Kupffer cell function after splenectomy. Using the clearance of microaggregated albumin from the circulation as a measure of Kupffer cell function, Palmer et al. (1983) showed significantly reduced rates of clearance in otherwise healthy subjects who had undergone splenectomy, and in patients with hyposplenism associated with celiac disease and ulcerative colitis.

10.4.3. INFECTION Overwhelming infection is a well-recognized complication of splenectomy. Despite occasional dissension (Holdsworth et al., 1991), there is widespread acceptance of this dictum (McMullin and Johnston, 1993). Hyposplenism not caused by surgical removal of the spleen may also be complicated by severe infections (Table 2). The pneumococcus is the most frequently encountered organism (Selby et al., 1987; Kabins and Lerner, 1970; Torres and Bisno, 1973), but infection with other encapsulated bacteria, particularly *H. influenzae* and the meningococcus, is well-described. The clinical course is usually fulminant, and frequently fatal (Balfanz et al., 1976; Gopal and Bisno, 1977). In addition, infection with organisms not usually pathogenic in humans has been seen in hyposplenic subjects (Archer et al., 1979; Findling et al., 1980; Curti et al., 1985; Fish et al., 1985; Morgan and Cruickshank, 1987; Lindquist et al., 1995; Spelman, 1996). The parasitic infection, babesiosis, is more common in asplenic subjects (Rosner et al., 1984), and there have been reports of nonfatal and fatal malaria developing in patients after splenectomy (Boone and Watters, 1995; Coetzee, 1982; Israeli et al., 1987). Some viral infections may be more frequent and severe after splenectomy (Stone et al., 1967; Baumgartner et al., 1982; Langenhuijsen and van Toorn, 1982), and there is a report suggesting that splenectomy predisposes to the development of clinical AIDS in HIV-positive individuals (Barbui et al., 1987).

10.4.4. AUTOIMMUNE PHENOMENA The production of erythrocyte autoantibodies by mice injected with rat red blood cells

Table 10.2
Cases of Severe Infection
Complicating Nonsurgical Hyposplenism

Etiology of Hyposplenism	Refs.
Congenital	Myerson and Koelle, 1956; Kevy et al., 1968; Waldman et al., 1977; Dyke et al., 1991
Sickle-cell disease	Falter et al., 1973
Celiac disease	O'Donaghue, 1986
Ulcerative colitis	Ryan et al., 1978; Foster et al., 1982
Systemic lupus erythematosus	Dillon et al., 1982; Foster et al., 1984
Mixed connective tissue disease	Guertler and Carter, 1996
Sarcoidosis	Guyton and Zumwalt, 1975
Amyloidosis	Frank and Palomino, 1987
Irradiation	Bensinger et al., 1970; Dailey et al., 1980
Still's disease	Parr et al., 1953
Ischemia	Whitaker, 1969; Grant et al., 1970
Thorotrast	Herin et al., 1992
Idiopathic	Bisno and Freeman, 1970; Hatch et al., 1983
Long-term intravenous nutrition	Zoli et al., 1993
Alcoholic liver diease	Muller and Toghill, 1994

is enhanced by splenectomy (Cox and Finley-Jones, 1979). Several studies have shown an increased incidence of autoantibodies in splenectomized subjects, when compared with normal subjects (Spirer et al., 1980a; Nielsen et al., 1982; Robertson et al., 1983c), and autoantibodies have been observed to develop within a few months of splenectomy. One study found no increase in the prevalence of autoantibodies in patients splenectomized following trauma (Aaberge and Gaarder, 1986), but no attempt had been made to assess the degree of splenosis, which has been shown to be associated with a reduced frequency of autoantibodies (Neilsen, Andersen and Ellegaard, 1982). Whether the development of autoantibodies after splenectomy heralds the onset of clinical autoimmune disease is uncertain. There is a single case report of a patient who underwent splenectomy for idiopathic thrombocytopenic purpura, and subsequently developed chronic active hepatitis, antiglobulin-positive hemolytic anemia, and pulmonary fibrosis, and in whom it was suggested that splenectomy might have contributed to the development of these autoimmune disorders (Kleiner-Baumgarten et al., 1983). An increased prevalence of autoantibodies and autoimmune diseases has been reported among celiac patients with splenic atrophy, compared with celiac patients without evidence of hyposplenism (Bullen et al., 1981) and autoimmune thyroid disease occurs more frequently than would otherwise be expected in patients with dermatitis herpetiformis, a condition in which hyposplenism is a frequent association (Cunningham and Zone, 1985; Foster, 1985).

The spleen is a rich source of suppressor cell activity (Sampson et al., 1976), and suppressor cells are believed to play a role in the regulation of immune responses; it is therefore possible that reduced or absent splenic function may lead to impaired suppressor cell activity or an imbalance in immunoregulatory cells, which in turn could explain the increase in autoimmune phenomena associated with hyposplenism. There is some evidence for this hypothesis. Although the numbers of peripheral blood suppressor cells and the ratio of helper-inducer to cytotoxic-suppressor cells appears to be normal in patients with hyposplenism (Foster et al., 1985a), decreased suppressor cell function has been reported in two studies of splenectomized patients (Melamed et al., 1982; Robertson et al., 1982a).

Alternatively, it may be that defective splenic Fc-receptor-specific function, on which the clearance of circulating immune complexes probably depends, contributes to the development of immune-complex-mediated autoimmune disease (Frank et al., 1983). The clearance of IgG-sensitized erythrocytes, which is a function of splenic macrophages bearing a receptor specific to the Fc-fragment of IgG, is abnormal, in a range of autoimmune disorders. This is also the case in normal subjects with HLAB8-DRw3, which is an HLA type associated with an increased incidence of autoimmune disease.

10.4.5. MALIGNANCY AND HYPOSPLENISM IN COELIAC DISEASE
Splenic atrophy has been observed in patients with celiac disease complicated by lymphoma (Thompson, 1974; O'Grady et al., 1985b), and it has been suggested that it may be a contributory factor to the development of malignancy. However, in a retrospective study of 41 cases of celiac disease complicated by malignancy, the proportion with evidence of hyposplenism in a peripheral blood film was no greater than that of patients without malignancy (Robertson et al., 1982b).

10.4.6. LONG-TERM HYPOSPLENISM
10.4.6.1. Severe Infections
In the context of splenectomy, there is ample evidence that severe infections can occur many years postoperatively. In the series by Robinette and Fraumeni (1977), mortality was increased, and significant contributions to this were made by pneumonia and ischemic heart disease. The deaths from pneumonia were at least 4 years, and, in some cases, over 20 years, postsplenectomy.

Late severe infections and deaths are recorded by other authors (Murdoh and Dos Anjos, 1990; Cullingford et al., 1991; Scopes 1991; Hassan et al., 1996).

10.4.6.2. Malignancy
Animal experiments suggest that splenectomy leads to an increase in malignant foci, under some circumstances (Shiratori et al., 1995), although, paradoxically, there may be increased survival, perhaps related to delayed suppressor activity (Meyer et al., 1980).

There is agreement that splenectomy for trauma leads to no increased risk of late malignancy (Robinette and Fraumeni, 1977, Mellemkjoer et al., 1995; Linet et al., 1996).

Splenectomy, in situations other than trauma, is often for conditions such as lymphomas, and the interpretation of the significance of subsequent malignancies is complex. Splenectomy for nontraumatic, nonmalignant conditions may be followed by a significant increase in malignancies at some sites, but the interpretation, here too, is difficult (Linet et al., 1996), and findings in other studies are not convincing (Mellemkjoer et al., 1995).

Splenectomy in Hodgkin's disease has been studied, with various conclusions, including that there is an increased risk of leukemia (Tura et al., 1993), a nonsignificant increase in leukemia (Swerdlow et al., 1993), no increase overall in second cancers (Swerdlow et al., 1993), and a 2–3-fold increase in second cancers (Dietrich et al., 1994).

10.4.6.3. Lipid Metabolism
Evidence is accumulating of a role for the spleen in lipid metabolism, and, hence, possibly in athero-

sclerosis. Two lines of evidence converge in the understanding of the effect of the spleen on lipid metabolism. The first is the correlation of lipid levels with spleen size. Juliusson et al. (1995) found that plasma total cholesterol, low-density lipoprotein (LDL) cholesterol, and triglyceride were inversely correlated with spleen size, but not with other markers of tumor burden; Gilbert et al. (1981) found that, in myeloproliferative disorders, spleen size was the variable that best correlated with the low levels of total cholesterol, LDL cholesterol, and high-density lipoprotein (HDL) cholesterol. The second line of evidence is the effect of splenectomy. Rises in plasma lipid levels after splenectomy have been described in myeloproliferative disorders (Aviram et al., 1986; Gilbert et al., 1981), in hemolytic anemia (Rifkind and Gale, 1967), and in Gaucher's type 1 disease (Ginsberg et al., 1984). In rats, Fatouros et al. (1995) found that splenectomy was followed by a rise in plasma triglyceride, but, paradoxically, there was a fall in HDL cholesterol.

Robinette and Fraumeni (1977) reported an increased risk of death from ischemic heart disease many years after splenectomy, and these changes in lipid metabolism might be invoked in helping to explain this finding.

10.5. MANAGEMENT RECOMMENDATIONS

10.5.1. AVOIDING SPLENECTOMY
Given the long-term risk of infection, the need for splenectomy should be considered carefully. The conventional surgical dogma, that an injured spleen should be removed, has been challenged (Roy, 1984). Alternatives include conservative management, splenic repair, splenorrhaphy, partial splenectomy, and splenic autotransplantation (Cooper and Williamson, 1984; Traub et al., 1987; Williams et al., 1990): Some form of splenic salvage was found to be possible in 56% of 200 patients with splenic injury (Moore et al., 1984). On the basis of animal experiments, procedures conserving the normal blood supply, and more than 25% of normal splenic mass, seem most likely to preserve normal splenic function (Horton et al., 1982; Van Wyck et al., 1980). The value of autotransplantation is controversial (Oakes, 1981; Kiroff et al., 1985; Rice and James, 1980), and there are reports of fatal, overwhelming sepsis occurring in patients with functional autotransplants, as judged by their ability to accumulate radiocolloid (Moore et al., 1983; Tesluk, 1984). Controlled trials, with long-term follow-up, are needed.

10.5.2. PENICILLIN PROPHYLAXIS
The rationale for penicillin prophylaxis in hyposplenic subjects is as follows: The pneumococcus is the most frequently encountered bacterium responsible for overwhelming sepsis in these patients, and has been shown usually to be very susceptible to the concentration of penicillin achieved in the blood by twice-daily oral administration. The mortality of experimentally induced infection with pneumococci can be reduced by penicillin prophylaxis (Dickerman, 1979; Dickerman et al., 1980). The results of a controlled trial in children with sickle-cell disease provide strong evidence for the efficacy of penicillin prophylaxis (Gaston et al., 1986). 215 children, aged between 3 and 36 mo, were randomized to receive either oral penicillin, twice daily, or placebo. The trial was terminated early, when it became clear that the frequency of pneumococcal infections in the children taking placebo was high: 13 infections occurred in 110 subjects, and three of these were fatal. Only 2/105 subjects on oral penicillin produced infections, and neither was fatal. Uncontrolled studies in splenectomized subjects, and anecdotal reports of overwhelming infection occurring in patients soon after cessation of

penicillin prophylaxis, are evidence favoring long-term oral administration of penicillin in this group of patients (Lanzowsky et al., 1976; Lum et al., 1980; Hays et al., 1984). Failure of penicillin prophylaxis to prevent post-splenectomy sepsis has hitherto been rare. In a review of the literature, 14 cases of patients who had undergone splenectomy and developed serious infection, despite penicillin prophylaxis, were identified (Zarrabi and Rosner, 1986). All but one of the patients were under 17 yr old, and most had had their spleens removed during staging laparotomy for Hodgkin's disease. In six patients, the sepsis was caused by bacteria other than the pneumococcus.

The risks of penicillin allergy appear to be relatively small (Anonymous, 1986), but the problem of poor compliance with long-term oral administration of penicillin is real (Buchanan et al., 1982; Buchanan and Smith, 1986). Unfortunately, intramuscular injections of long-acting penicillin are impractical for prolonged use.

Resistant strains of pneumococcus are increasing, perhaps even engendered by penicillin prophylaxis (Wang et al., 1994), and necessitate careful consideration of appropriate treatment for such infections (Friedland, 1993).

10.5.3. PNEUMOCOCCAL VACCINE A 23-valent vaccine, which contains antigens to the pneumococcal types responsible for at least 85% of infections with pneumococcus, has been developed, and replaced the previous octavalent and 14-valent vaccines. There have been no randomized, controlled clinical trials of the efficacy of this pneumococcal vaccine in preventing overwhelming infection in hyposplenic subjects, but in a study of the value of octavalent pneumococcal vaccine in 77 patients with sickle-cell disease, no infections with pneumococci were observed during a 2-yr follow-up period. This contrasts to the nine infections, two of which were fatal, experienced by a group of 106 nonimmunized patients (Ammann et al., 1977). From the results of a study of the distribution of serotypes of pneumococci isolated from patients previously given pneumococcal vaccine, and compared with the distribution of serotypes isolated from unvaccinated persons, the efficacy of vaccination has been calculated to be 85% in adults with hyposplenism caused by splenectomy or sickle-cell disease (Bolan et al., 1986). Use of the vaccine is currently recommended in these patients (Ammann, 1982; Health and Public Policy Committee, 1986). However, the antibody response to pneumococcal antigen is blunted in children under the age of 2 yr (Pedersen et al., 1982; Lawrence et al., 1983), in splenectomized subjects (Hosea et al., 1981; Di Padova et al., 1985), and in patients with concomitant immunodeficiency states (Siber et al., 1978). Appropriate responses to pneumococcal vaccine have been shown to occur in patients with celiac disease, although the duration of response in these patients is not documented (McKinley et al., 1995).

Evidence suggests that pneumococcal vaccine is frequently not administered routinely after splenectomy, and that the proportion of patients vaccinated can be improved by directing attention to the problem (Kinnersley et al., 1993; McDonald et al., 1997). The majority of reports of true vaccine failures have involved patients who were receiving, or had undergone, immunosuppressive therapy (Ammann, 1982). New types of pneumococcal vaccines are showing promise of improved protection (Eskola and Käyhty, 1995).

In practice, we recommend that children under the age of 2 years should receive oral penicillin prophylaxis, which should be continued at least to the age of 5 years and perhaps indefinitely. Pneumococcal vaccine should be administered once the child has reached 2 years. All adults should receive pneumococcal vaccine

and penicillin prophylaxis, probably for life. Whenever elective splenectomy or adjuvant immunosuppressive therapy is considered, the vaccine should be administered at least 1 month beforehand. Revaccination after some years is probably advisable (Davidson et al., 1994).

10.5.4. GENERAL Patients should be advised of the risk of serious infection, and urged to seek medical assistance immediately in the event of illness or fever. There is a case for issuing patients with a splenectomy warning card, to be carried at all times, and a supply of amoxicillin, or an alternative, for self-administration at the first symptoms of illness or fever. The attending physician should be aware of the dangers of fulminant sepsis in these patients, and be willing to prescribe antibiotics appropriately for any symptoms of infection.

Possibilities for the future include the more widespread use of vaccines against other organisms implicated in overwhelming infection, such as the meningococcus and *H. influenzae*, and the administration of tuftsin, which can be prepared synthetically.

Numerous publications have listed recommendations, based on individual studies or on consensus (e.g., *see* McMullin and Johnston, 1993; Lane, 1995; Working Party Guidelines, 1996; Nathwani, 1996; Spelman, 1996; Williams and Kaur, 1996).

REFERENCES

Aaberge, S. I. and Gaarder, P. I. (1986) Autoantibodies in individuals splenectomised because of trauma. *Scand. J. Haematol.* **37,** 296–300.

Acevedo, G. and Mauer, A. (1963) The capacity for removal of erythrocytes containing Heinz bodies in premature infants and patients following splenectomy. *J. Pediatr.* **63,** 61–64.

Al-Eid, M. A., Tutschka, P. J., Wagner, H. N. Jr., Santos, G. W., and Tsan, M. F. (1983) Functional asplenia in patients with graft-versus-host disease. *J. Nucl. Med.* **24,** 1123–1126.

Ammann, A. J. (1982) Current status of pneumococcal polysaccharide immunization in patients with sickle cell disease or impaired splenic function. *Am. J. Pediatr. Hemat. Oncol.* **4,** 301–306.

Ammann, A. J., Addiego, J., Wara, D. W., Lubin, B., Smith, W. B., and Mentzer, W. C. (1977) Polyvalent pneumococcal polysaccharide immunization of patients with sickle cell anemia and patients with splenectomy. *N. Engl. J. Med.* **297,** 897–900.

Andersen, V., Cohn, J., and Sorensen, S. F. (1976) Immunological studies in children before and after splenectomy. *Acta Paed. Scand.* **65,** 409–415.

Anonymous Lancet Editorial (1986) Penicillin prophylaxis for babies with sickle-cell disease. *Lancet* **2,** 1432–1433.

Archer, G. L., Coleman, P. H., Cole, R. M., Duma, R. J., and Johnston, C. L. Jr. (1979) Human infection from an unidentified erythrocyte-associated bacterium. *N. Engl. J. Med.* **301,** 897–900.

Armas, R. R. (1985) Clinical studies with spleen-specific radiolabelled agents. *Semin. Nucl. Med.* **15,** 260–275.

Asenjo, C. F. (1948) Pteroylglutamic acid requirement of the rat and a characteristic lesion observed in the spleen of the deficient animal. *J. Nutr.* **36,** 601–612.

Aviram, M., Brook, J. G., Tatarsky, I., Levy, Y., et al. (1986) Increased low-density lipoprotein levels after splenectomy: a role for the spleen in cholesterol metabolism in myeloproliferative disorders. *Am. J. Med. Sci.* **291,** 25–28.

Baker, P. G., Jones, J. V., Peacock, D. B., and Read, A. E. (1975) The immune response of φX174 in man. III. Evidence for an association between hyposplenism and immunodeficiency in patients with co-eliac disease. *Gut* **16,** 538–542.

Balchandran, S., Kumar, R., and Kuo, T. T. (1980) Functional asplenia in the Sézary syndrome. *Clin. Nucl. Med.* **5,** 149–151.

Balfanz, J. R., Nesbit, M. E. Jr., Jarvis, C., and Krivit, W. (1976) Overwhelming sepsis following splenectomy for trauma. *J. Pediatr.* **88,** 458–460.

Barbui, T., Cortelazzo, S., Minetti, B., Galli, M., and Buelli, M. (1987) Does splenectomy enhance risk of AIDS in HIV positive patients with chronic thrombocytopenia? *Lancet* **2**, 342,343.

Baumgartner, J. D., Glauser, M. P., Burgo-Black, A. L., Black, R. D., Pyndiah, N., and Chiolero, R. (1982) Severe cytomegalovirus infection in multiply transfused splenectomized, trauma patients. *Lancet* **2**, 63–66.

Bender, B. S., Quinn, T. C., and Lawley, T. J. (1984) Acquired immune deficiency syndrome (AIDS): a defect in Fc-receptor specific clearance. *Clin. Res.* **32**, 511A.

Bender, B. S., Frank, M. M., Lawley, T. J., Smith, W. J., Brickman, C. M., and Quinn, T. C. (1985) Defective reticuloendothelial system Fc-receptor function in patients with acquired immunodeficiency syndrome. *J Infect. Dis.* **152**, 409–412.

Bensinger, T. A., Keller, A. R., Merrell, L. F., and O'Leary, D. S. (1971) Thorotrast-induced reticuloendothelial blockade in man. Clinical equivalent of the experimental model associated with patent pneumococcal septicemia. *Am. J. Med.* **51**, 663–668.

Bessler, H., Mandel, E. M., and Djaldetti, M. (1978) Role of the spleen and lymphocytes in regulation of the circulating platelet numbers in mice. *J. Lab. Clin. Med.* **91**, 760–768.

Bisno, A. L. and Freeman, J. C. (1970) The syndrome of asplenia, pneumococcal sepsis and disseminated intravascular coagulation. *Ann. Intern. Med.* **72**, 389–393.

Blumgart, H. L. (1923) Three fatal adult cases of malabsorption of fat with emaciation and anemia, and in two acidosis and tetany. *Arch. Intern. Med.* **32**, 113–128.

Bolan, G., Broome, C. V., Facklam, R. R., Plikaytis, B. D., Fraser, D. W., and Schlech, W. F., III. (1986) Pneumococcal vaccine efficacy in selected populations in the United States. *Ann. Intern. Med.* **104**, 1–6.

Boone, K. E. and Watters, D. A. K. (1995) The incidence of malaria after splenectomy in Papua New Guinea. *Br. Med. J.* **311**, 1273.

Bowdler, A. J. (1982) The spleen in disorders of the blood. In: *Blood and its Disorders* (Hardisty, R. M. and Weatherall, D. J., eds.), Blackwell, Oxford.

Boyko, W. J., Pratt, R., and Wass, H. (1982) Functional hyposplenism: a diagnostic clue in amyloidosis. *Am. J. Clin. Pathol.* **77**, 745–748.

Brownlie, B. E., Hamer, J. W., Cook, H. B., and Hamwood, S. M. (1975) Thyrotoxicosis associated with splenic atrophy. *Lancet* **2**, 1046–1047.

Buchanan, G. R., Siegel, J. D., Smith, S. J., and DePasse, B. M. (1982) Oral penicillin prophylaxis in children with impaired splenic function: a study of compliance. *Pediatrics* **70**, 926–930.

Buchanan, G. R. and Smith, S. J. (1986) Pneumococcal septicemia despite pneumococcal vaccine and prescription of penicillin prophylaxis in children with sickle-cell anemia. *Am. J. Dis. Child.* **140**, 428–432.

Buchanan, G. R., Holtkamp, C. A., and Horton, J. A. (1987) Formation and disappearance of pocked erythrocytes: studies in human subjects and laboratory animals. *Am. J. Hematol.* **25**, 243–251.

Bullen, A.W. and Losowsky, M.S. (1978) Lymphocyte subpopulations in adult coeliac disease. *Gut* **19**, 892–897.

Bullen, A. W., Maini, R. W., and Losowsky, M. S. (1980) Circulating immune complexes in coeliac disease. *Gut* **21**, A915.

Bullen, A. W., Hall, R., Brown, R. C., and Losowsky, M. S. (1977a) Mechanisms of thrombocytosis in coeliac disease. *Gut* **18**, A962.

Bullen, A. W., Hall, R., Cooke, E. M., and Losowsky, M. S. (1977b) Immunity and the hyposplenism of coeliac disease. *Gut* **18**, A961,A962.

Bullen, A. W., Hall, R., Gowland, G., Rajah, S., and Losowsky, M. S. (1981) Hyposplenism, adult coeliac disease, and autoimmunity. *Gut* **22**, 28–33.

Butler, M. J., Matthews, F., and Irving, M. H. (1977) The incidence of postoperative deep vein thrombosis after splenectomy. *Clin. Oncol.* **3**, 51–56.

Carlisle, H. N. and Saslaw, S. (1959) Properdin levels in splenectomized persons. *Proc. Soc. Exp. Biol. Med.* **109**, 150–154.

Chaimoff, C., Douer, D., Pick, I. A., and Pinkhas, J. (1978) Serum immunoglobulin changes after accidental splenectomy in adults. *Am. J. Surg.* **136**, 332,333.

Chaudry, I. H. (1982) Tuftsin restores the depressed reticuloendothelial function after splenectomy and improves survival following splenectomy and sepsis. *J. Reticuloendothel. Soc.* **32**, 53,54.

Chelazzi, G., Pinotti, G., Nicora, C., Rossi, D., and Senaldi, G. (1985) Increased total serum IgE concentration in patients who have undergone splenectomy after trauma. *J. Clin. Pathol.* **38**, 1309,1310.

Ciuttis, A., Polley, M. J., Metakis, L. J., and Peterson, C. M., (1978) Immunologic defect of alternative pathway of complement activation postsplenectomy: a possible relation between splenectomy and infection. *J. Natl. Med. Assoc. NY,* **70**, 667–670.

Claret, I., Morales, L., and Montaner, A. (1975) Immunological studies in the post-splenectomy syndrome. *J. Pediatr. Surg.* **10**, 59.

Claster, S. and Vichinsky, E. (1996) First report of reversal of organ dysfunction in sickle-cell anemia by the use of hydroxyurea: splenic regeneration. *Blood* **88**, 1951–1953.

Coetzee, T. (1982) Clinical anatomy and physiology of the spleen. *S. Afr. Med. J.* **61**, 737–746.

Cohen, R. C. and Ferrante, A. (1982) Immune dysfunction in the presence of residual splenic tissue. *Arch. Dis. Child.* **57**, 523–527.

Coleman, C. N., McDougall, I. R., Dailey, M. O., Ager, P., Bush, S., and Kaplan, H. S. (1982) Functional hyposplenia after splenic irradiation for Hodgkin's disease. *Ann. Intern. Med.* **96**, 44–47.

Constantopoulos, A., Najjar, V. A., Wish, J. B., Necheles, T. H., and Stolbach, L. L. (1973) Defective phagocytosis due to tuftsin deficiency in splenectomized subjects. *Am. J. Dis. Child.* **125**, 663–665.

Constantoulakis, M., Trichopoulos, D., Avgoustaki, O., and Economidou, J. (1978) Serum immunoglobulin concentrations before and after splenectomy in patients with homozygous beta-thalassaemia. *J. Clin Pathol.* **31**, 546–550.

Cooper, M. J. and Williamson, R. C. N. (1984) Splenectomy: indications, hazards and alternatives. *Br. J. Surg.* **71**, 173–180.

Cooper, M. R., DeChatelet, L. R., and Shirley, P. S. (1982) Does tuftsin alter phagocytosis in human polymorphonuclear neutrophils? *Inflammation* **6**, 103–112.

Corazza, G. R., Lazzari, R., and Frisoni, M. (1983) C1q binding activity in childhood coeliac disease. *Ital. J. Gastroenterol.* **15**, 14–16.

Corazza, G. R., Bullen, A. W., Hall, R., Robinson, P. J., and Losowsky, M. S. (1981) Simple method of assessing splenic function in coeliac disease. *Clin. Sci.* **60**, 109–113.

Corazza, G. R., Lazzari, R., Frisoni, M., Collina, A., and Gasbarrini, G. (1982) Splenic function in childhood coeliac disease. *Gut* **23**, 415–416.

Corazza, G. R., Frisoni, M., Vaira, D., and Gasbarrini, G., (1983) Effect of gluten-free diet on splenic hypofunction of adult coeliac disease. *Gut* **24**, 228–230.

Corazza, G. R., Tarozzi, C., Vaira, D., Frisoni, M., and Gasbarrini, G. (1984) Return of splenic function after splenectomy: how much tissue is needed? *Br. Med. J. (Clin. Res. Ed.)* **289**, 861–864.

Corazza, G. R., Zoli, G., Ginaldi, L., Cancellieri, C., Profeta, V., Gasbarrini, G., and Quaglino, D. (1991) Tuftsin deficiency in AIDS. *Lancet* **337**, 12–13.

Corry, J. M., Polhill, R. B. Jr., Edmonds, S. R., and Johnston, R. B. Jr. (1979) Activity of the alternative complement pathway after splenectomy: comparison to activity in sickle-cell disease and hypogammaglobulinaemia. *J. Pediatr.* **95**, 964–969.

Costello, P., Gramm, H. F., and Steinberg, D. (1977) Simultaneous occurrence of functional asplenia and splenic accumulation of diphosphonate in metastatic breast cancer. *J. Nucl. Med.* **18**, 1237–1238.

Cox, D. R., Martin, L., and Hall, B. D. (1977) Asplenia syndrome after fetal exposure to Warfarin. *Lancet* **2**, 1134.

Cox, K. O. and Finlay-Jones, J. J. (1979) Impaired regulation of erythrocyte autoantibody production after splenectomy. *Br. J. Exp. Pathol.* **60**, 466–470.

Crosby, W. H. (1963) Hyposplenism: an inquiry into normal functions of the spleen. *Annu. Rev. Med.* **14**, 349–370.

Crosby, W. H. and Ruiz, F. (1962) Evidence of a myeloinhibitory factor in the spleen. *Blood* **20**, 793.

Cullingford, G. L., Watkins, D. N., Watts, A. D., and Mallon, D. F. (1991) Severe late postsplenectomy infection. *Br. J. Surg.* **78**, 716–721.

Cunningham, M. J. and Zone, J. J. (1985) Thyroid abnormalities in dermatitis herpetiformis. *Ann. Intern. Med.* **102**, 194–196.

Curti, A. J., Lin, J. H., and Szabo, K. (1985) Overwhelming post-splenectomy infection with Plesiomonas shigelloides in a patient cured of Hodgkin's disease. *Am. J. Clin. Pathol.* **83**, 522–523.

Cuthbert, R. J., Iqbal, A., Gates, A., Toghill, P. J., and Russell, N. H. (1995) Functional hyposplenism following allogeneic bone marrow transplantation. *J. Clin. Pathol.* **48,** 257–259.

Dacie, J. V. and Lewis, J. M. (1975) *Practical Haematology*, 5th ed. Churchill Livingstone, London, pp. 438–451.

Dahl, M., Haakansson, L., Kreuger, A., Olsen, L., Nilsson, U., and Venge, P. (1986) Polymorphonuclear neutrophil function and infections following splenectomy in childhood. *Scand. J. Haematol.* **37,** 137–143.

Dailey, M. O., Coleman, C. N., and Kaplan, H. S. (1980) Radiation-induced splenic atrophy in patients with Hodgkin's disease and non-Hodgkin's lymphoma. *N. Engl. J. Med.* **302,** 215–217.

Dameshek, W. (1955) Hyposplenism. *JAMA* **157,** 613.

Davidson, M., Bulkow, L. R., Grabman, J., et al. (1994) Immunogenicity of pneumococcal revaccination in patients with chronic disease. *Arch. Intern. Med.* **154,** 2209–2214.

Dawson, A. A., Bennett, B., Jones, P. F., and Munro, A. (1981) Thrombotic risks of staging laparotomy with splenectomy in Hodgkin's disease. *Br. J. Surg.* **68,** 842–845.

Deitch, E. A. and O'Neal, B. (1982) Neutrophil function in adults after traumatic splenectomy. *J. Surg. Res.* **33,** 98–102.

De Jongh, C. L. (1948) *Malnutrition and Starvation in the Western Netherlands*, 90. General State Printing Office, The Hague.

Demetrakopoulos, G. E., Tsokos, G. C., and Levine, A. S. (1982) Recovery of splenic function after GVHD-associated functional asplenia. *Am. J. Haematol.* **12,** 77–80.

Desai, A. G. and Thakur, M. L. (1985) Radiopharmaceuticals for spleen and marrow studies. *Semin. Nucl. Med.* **15,** 229–237.

Dhawan, V., Spencer, R. P., and Pearson, H. A. (1977) Functional asplenia in the absence of circulating Howell-Jolly bodies. *Clin. Nucl. Med.* **2,** 395–396.

Dhawan, V. M., Spencer, R. P., and Sziklas, J. J. (1979) Reversible functional asplenia in chronic aggressive hepatitis. *J. Nucl. Med.* **20,** 34–36.

Dickerman, J. D. (1979) Splenectomy and sepsis: a warning. *Pediatrics* **63,** 938,939.

Dickerman, J. D., Chalmer, B., and Horner, S. R. (1980) The effect of penicillin on the mortality of splenectomised mice exposed to an aerosol of *Streptococcus pneumoniae* type 3. *Pediatr. Res.* **14,** 1139–1141.

Dietrich, P.-Y., Henry-Amar, M., Cosset, J. M., et al. (1994) Second primary cancers in patients continuously disease-free from Hodgkin's disease: a protective role for the spleen? *Blood* **84,** 1209–1215.

Dillon, A. M., Stein, H. B., and English, R. A. (1982) Splenic atrophy in systemic lupus erythematosus. *Ann. Intern. Med.* **96,** 40–43.

Di Padova, F., Durig, M., Wadstrom, J., and Harder, F. (1983) Role of the spleen in immune response to polyvalent pneumococcal vaccine. *Br. Med. J.* **287,** 1829–1832.

Di Padova, F., Durig, M., Harder, F., DiPadova, C., and Zanussi, C. (1985) Impaired antipneumococcal antibody production in patients without spleens. *Br. Med. J.* **290,** 14–16.

Doe, W. F., Booth, C. C., and Brown, D. L. (1973) Evidence for complement-binding immune complexes in adult coeliac disease, Crohn's disease and ulcerative colitis. *Lancet* **1,** 402–403.

Douglas, A. P., Weetman, A. P., and Haggith, J. W. (1976) The distribution and enteric loss of ^{51}Cr-labelled lymphocytes in normal subjects and in patients with coeliac disease and other disorders of the small intestine. *Digestion* **14,** 29–43.

Drew, P. A., Kiroff, G. K., Ferrante, A., and Cohen, R. C. (1984) Alterations in immunoglobulin synthesis by peripheral blood mononuclear cells from splenectomised patients with and without splenic regrowth. *J. Immunol.* **132,** 191–196.

Durig, M., Landmann, R. M., and Harder, F. (1984) Lymphocyte subsets in human peripheral blood after splenectomy and auto-transplantation of splenic tissue. *J. Lab. Clin. Med.* **104,** 110–115.

Dyke, M. P., Martin, R. P., and Berry, P. J. (1991) Septicaemia and adrenal haemorrhage in congenital asplenia. *Arch. Dis. Child.* **66,** 636–637.

Elkon, K. B., Sewell, J. R., Ryan, P. F., and Hughes, G. R. (1980) Splenic function in non-renal systemic lupus erythematosus. *Am. J. Med.* **69,** 80–82.

Engel, A. (1939) Om sprue och mjaltatrofi. *Nordisk Med.* **1,** 388–392.

Eppinger, H. (1913) Zur pathologie milzfunktion. *Klin. Wochenschr.* **50,** 1509–1512.

Ernstrom, U. and Sandberg, G. (1970) Influence of splenectomy on thymic release of lymphocytes into the blood. *Scand. J. Haematol.* **7,** 342–348.

Eskola, J. and Käyhty, H. (1995) New vaccines for prevention of pneumococcal infections. *Ann Med.* **27,** 53–56.

Falcao, R. P., Voltarelli, J. L., and Bottura, C. (1982) The possible role of the spleen in the reduction of nitro-blue tetrazolium by neutrophils. *Acta Haematol.* **68,** 89–95.

Falter, M. L., Robinson, M. G., Kim, O. K., Go, C., and Taubkin, S. P. (1973) Splenic function and infection in sickle-cell anaemia. *Acta Haematol.* **50,** 154–161.

Fatouros, M., Bourantas, K., Bairaktari, E., Elisaf, M., Tsolas, O., and Cassioumis, D. (1995) Role of the spleen in lipid metabolism. *Br. J. Surg.* **82,** 1675–1677.

Ferguson, A. (1976) Coeliac disease and gastrointestinal food allergy. In: *Immunological Aspects of the Liver and Gastrointestinal Tract* (Ferguson, A. and MacSween, R. N. M., eds.), MTP Press, Lancaster, pp. 153–202.

Ferguson, A., Hutton, M. M., Maxwell, J. D., and Murray, D., (1970) Adult coeliac disease in hyposplenic patients. *Lancet* **1,** 163–164.

Ferrante, A., Kiroff, G. K., Goh, D. H., and Drew, P. A. (1985) Elevated natural killer (NK) cell activity: a possible role in resistance to infection and malignancy in immunodeficient splenectomised patients. *Med. Hypoth.* **16,** 133–146.

Ferster, A., Bujan, W., Corazza, F., Devalck, C., Fondu, P., Toppet, M., Verhas, M., and Sariban, E., (1993) Bone marrow transplantation corrects the splenic reticuloendothelial dysfunction in sickle-cell anemia. *Blood* **81,** 1102–1105.

Findling, J. W., Pohlmann, G. P., and Rose, H. D. (1980) Fulminant gram-negative bacillemia (DF-2) following a dog-bite in an asplenic woman. *Am. J. Med.* **68,** 154–159.

Fish, H. R., Chia, J. K., and Shakir, K. M. (1985) Post-splenectomy sepsis caused by Group B streptococcus (S. agalactiae) in an adult patient with diabetes mellitus. *Diabetes Care* **8,** 608–609.

Fish, J. C., et al. (1970) Circulating lymphocyte depletion: effect on lymphoid tissue. *Surgery* **67,** 658–666.

von Fliedner, V., Salvatori, V., Higby, D. J., Stutzman, L., and Park, B. H. (1980) Polymorphonuclear neutrophil function in malignant lymphomas and the effects of splenectomy. *Cancer* **45,** 469–475.

Foster, K. J., Devitt, N., Gallagher, P. J., and Abbott, R. M. (1982). Overwhelming pneumococcal septicaemia in a patient with ulcerative colitis and splenic atrophy. *Gut* **23,** 630–632.

Foster, P. N. (1985) Thyroid disease, dermatitis herpetiformis and splenic atrophy. *Ann. Intern. Med.* **130,** 157.

Foster, P. N., Hardy, G. J., and Losowsky, M. S. (1984) Fatal salmonella septicaemia in a patient with systemic lupus erythematosus and splenic atrophy. *Br. J. Clin. Pract.* **38,** 434–435.

Foster, P. N., Heatley, R. V., and Losowsky, M. S. (1985a) Hyposplenism and T-lymphocyte sub-populations in coeliac disease and after splenectomy. *J. Clin. Lab. Immunol.* **17,** 75– 77.

Foster, P. N., Heatley, R. V., and Losowsky, M. S. (1985b) Natural killer cells in coeliac disease. *J. Clin. Lab. Immunol.* **17,** 173–176.

Foster, P. N., Bullen, A. W., Robertson, D. A., Chalmers, D. M., and Losowsky, M. S. (1985a) Development of impaired splenic function in intestinal lymphangiectasia. *Gut* **26,** 861–864.

Foster, P. N., Bolton, R. P., Cotter, K. L., and Losowky, M. S. (1985b) Defective neutrophil activation after splenectomy. *J. Clin. Pathol.* **38,** 1175–1178.

Frank, J. M. and Palomino, N. J. (1987) Primary amyloidosis with diffuse splenic infiltration presenting as fulminant pneumococcal sepsis. *Am. J. Clin. Pathol.* **87,** 405–407.

Frank, M. M., Hamburger, M. I., Lawley, T. J., Kimberly, R. P., and Plotz, P. H. (1979) Defective reticuloendothelial system Fc-receptor function in systemic lupus erythematosus. *N. Engl. J. Med.* **300,** 518–523.

Frank, M. M., Lawley, T. J., Hamburger, M. I., and Brown, E. J. (1983) Immunoglobulin G Fc-receptor mediated clearance in autoimmune diseases. *Ann. Intern. Med.* **98,** 206–218.

Freedman, R. M., Johnston, D., Mahoney, M. J., and Pearson, H. A. (1980) Development of splenic reticuloendothelial function in neonates. *J. Pediatr.* **96,** 466–468.

Freedom, R. M. (1972) The asplenia syndrome: a review of significant extracardiac structural abnormalities in twenty-nine necropsied patients. *J. Pediatr.* **81,** 1130–1133.

Friedland, I. R. (1993) Therapy of penicillin and cephalosporin-resistant pneumococcal infections. *Annals of Medicine,* **25,** 451–455.

Garriga, S. and Crosby, W. H. (1959) The incidence of leukemia in families with hypoplasia of the marrow. *Blood* **14,** 1008–1014.

Gaston, M. H., Verter, J. I., Woods, G., Pegelow, C., Kelleher, J., Presbury, G., et al. (1986) Prophylaxis with oral penicillin in children with sickle- cell anemia.A randomized trial. *N. Engl. J. Med.* **314,** 1593–1599.

Gavrilis, P., Rothenberg, S.P., and Roscoe, G. (1974) Correlation of low serum IgM levels with absence of functional splenic tissue in sickle-cell disease syndromes. *Am. J. Med.* **57,** 542–545.

Gertz, M. A., Kyle, R. A., and Griepp, P. R. (1983) Hyposplenism in primary systemic amyloidosis. *Ann. Intern. Med.* **98,** 475–477.

Gilbert, H. S., Ginsberg, H., Fagerstrom, R., and Brown, W. V. (1981) Characterization of hypocholesterolemia in myeloproliferative disease.Relation to disease manifestations and activity. *Am. J. Med.* **71,** 595–602.

Ginsberg, H., Grabowski, G. A., Gibson, J. C., Fagerstrom, R., Goldblatt, J., Gilbert, H. S., and Desnick, R. J. (1984) Reduced plasma concentrations of total, low density lipoprotein and high density lipoprotein cholesterol in patients with Gaucher type I disease. *Clin. Genet.* **26,** 109–116.

Gopal, V. and Bisno, A. L. (1977) Fulminant pneumococcal infections in 'normal' asplenic hosts.*Arch. Intern Med.* **137,** 1526–1530.

Gordon, P. A., Davis, P., Russell, A. S., Coates, J. E., Rothwell, R. S., and LeClercq, S. M. (1981) Splenic reticuloendothelial function in patients with active rheumatoid arthritis. *J. Rheumatol.* **8,** 491–493.

Grant, M. D., Horowitz, H. I., Lorian, V., and Brodman, H. R. (1970) Waterhouse-Friderichsen syndrome induced by pneumococcemic shock. *JAMA* **212,** 1373–1374.

Grattner, H., Gullstrand, P., and Hallberg, T. (1982) Immunocompetence after incidental splenectomy. *Scand. J. Haematol.* **28,** 369–375.

Gross, D.J., Braverman,A.J., Koren,G., Rabinowitz,Y.S., Gordon,R., and Okon,E. (1982) Functional asplenia in immunoblastic lymphoma. *Arch. Intern. Med.* **142,** 2213–2215.

Guertler, A. T. and Carter, C. T. (1996) Fatal pneumococcal septicaemia in a patient with a connective tissue disease. *J. Emerg. Med.* **14,** 33–38.

Guyton, J. R. and Zumwalt, R. E. (1975) Pneumococcemia with sarcoid infiltrated spleen. *Ann. Intern. Med.* **82,** 847–848.

Haeney, M. R. and Ross, I. N. (1978) Whipple's disease in a female with impaired cell mediated immunity unresponsive to cotrimoxazole and levamisol therapy. *Postgrad. Med. J.* **54,** 45–50.

Hamburger, M. I., Moutsopoulos, H. M., Lawley, T. J., and Frank, M. M. (1979) Sjögren's syndrome: a defect in Fc-receptor specific clearance. *Ann. Intern. Med.* **91,** 534–538.

Hardisty, R. M. and Wolff, H. H. (1955) Haemorrhagic thrombocythaemia: a clinical and laboratory study. *Br. J. Haematol.* **1,** 390–405.

Hassan, I. S. A., Snow, M. H., and Ong, E. L. C. (1996) Overwhelming pneumococcal sepsis in two patients splenectomised more than ten years previously. *Scott. Med. J.* **41,** 17–19.

Hatch, J. P., Sibbald, W. J., and Austin, T. W. (1983) Overwhelming pneumococcal infection in a hyposplenic adult. *Can. Med. Assoc. J.* **129,** 851–854.

Hauser, G. J., Zakuth, V., and Spirer, Z. (1983) Normal reduction of nitroblue tetrazolium by neutrophils. *Acta Haematol.* **70,** 142–143.

Hays, D. M., Ternberg, J. L., Chen, T. T., et al. (1984) Complications related to 234 staging laparotomies performed in the Inter-group Hodgkin's Disease in Childhood Study. *Surgery* **96,** 471–478.

Health and Public Policy Committee, American College of Physicians (1986) Pneumococcal vaccine. *Ann. Intern. Med.* **104,** 118–120.

Henderson, J. M., Bell, D. A., Harth, M., and Chamberlain, M. J. (1981) Reticuloendothelial function in rheumatoid arthritis: correlation with disease activity and circulating immune complexes. *J. Rheumatol.* **8,** 486–489.

Herin, M., Hantson, P., Gosseye, S., and Mahieu, P. (1992) Overwhelming septicaemia due to *Streptococcus pneumoniae*: unexpected autopsy findings. *Histopathology* **20,** 84–86.

Hersey, P., Lawrence, S., Prendergast, D., Bindon, C., Benson, W., and Valk, P. (1983) Association of Sjögren's syndrome with C4 deficiency, defective reticuloendothelial function and circulating immune complexes. *Clin. Exp. Immunol.* **52,** 551–560.

Hill, D. B. and Bowdler, A. J. (1988) Transient hyposplenism associated with delayed transfusion reaction due to Anti-Kidd (Jk) antibodies. *South. Med. J.* **81(Suppl. 4),** 29.

Hirsh, J. and Dacie, J. V. (1966) Persistent post-splenectomy thrombocytosis and thromboembolism: a consequence of continuing anaemia. *Br. J. Haematol.* **12,** 44.

Holdsworth, R.J., Irving, A.D., Cuschieri, A. (1991) Postsplenectomy sepsis and its mortality rate: actual versus perceived risks. *Br. J. Surg.* **78,** 103–108.

Holroyde, C. P. and Gardner, F. H. (1970) Acquisition of autophagic vacuoles by human erythrocytes. Physiological role of the spleen. *Blood* **36,** 566–575.

Holroyde, C. P., Oski, F. A., and Gardner, F. H. (1969) The 'pocked' erythrocyte: red cell surface alterations in reticuloendothelial immaturity in the neonate. *N. Engl. J. Med.* **281,** 516– 520.

Horton, J., Ogden, M. E., Williams, S., and Coln, D. (1982) The importance of splenic blood flow in clearing pneumococcal organisms. *Ann. Surg.* **195,** 172–176.

Hosea, S. W., Burch, C. G., Brown, E. J., Berg, R. A., and Frank, M. M. (1981) Impaired immune response of splenectomised patients to polyvalent pneumococcal vaccine. *Lancet* **1,** 804–807.

Israeli, A., Shapiro, M., and Ephros, M. A. (1987) Plasmodium falciparum malaria in an asplenic man. *Trans. R. Soc. Trop. Med. Hyg.* **81,** 233–234.

Ivemark, B. I. (1955) Implications of agenesis of the spleen on the pathogenesis of cono-truncus anomalies in childhood. An analysis of the heart malformations in the splenic agenesis syndrome with fourteen new cases. *Acta Paediatr.* **44(Suppl. 104),** 1–110.

Jellinek, E. H. and Ball, K. (1976) Hashimoto's disease, encephalopathy and splenic atrophy. *Lancet* **1,** 1248.

Jewell, D. P., Berney, J. J., and Pettit, J. E. (1981) Splenic phagocytic function in patients with inflammatory bowel disease. *Pathology* **13,** 717– 723.

Juliusson, G., Vitols, S., Liliemark, J. (1995) Disease-related hypocholesterolemia in patients with hairy cell leukemia. *Cancer* **76,** 423–428.

Juneja, S., Januszewicz, E., Wolf, M., and Cooper, I. (1995) Post-splenectomy lymphocytosis. *Clin. Lab. Haematol.* **17,** 335–337.

Kabins, S. A. and Lerner, C. (1970) Fulminant pneumococcemia and sickle-cell anemia. *JAMA* **211,** 467–471.

Kelton, J. G. (1985) Impaired reticuloendothelial function in patients treated with methyldopa. *N. Engl. J. Med.* **313,** 596–600.

Kenny, M. W., George, A. J., and Stuart, J. (1980) Platelet hyperactivity in sickle-cell disease: a consequence of hyposplenism. *J. Clin. Pathol.* **33,** 622–625.

Kevy, S. F., Tefft, M., and Vawter, G. F. (1968) Hereditary splenic hypoplasia. *Pediatrics* **42,** 752–757.

Kinnersley, P., Wilkinson, C. E., Srinivasan, J. (1993) Pneumococcal vaccination after splenectomy: survey of hospital and primary care records. *Br. Med. J.* **307,** 1398–1399.

Kiroff, G. K., Mangos, A., Cohen, R., Chatterton, B. E., and Jamieson, G. G. (1983) Splenic regeneration following splenectomy for traumatic rupture. *Aust. NZ. J. Surg.* **53,** 431–434.

Kiroff, G. K., Hodgen, A. N., Drew, P. A., and Jamieson, G. G. (1985) Lack of effect of splenic regrowth on the reduced antibody responses to pneumococcal polysaccharides in splenectomised subjects. *Clin. Exp. Immunol.* **62,** 48–56.

Klausner, M. A., Hirsch, L. J., Leblond, P. F., Chamberlain, J. K., Klemperer, M. R., and Segel, G. B. (1975) Contrasting splenic mechanisms in the blood clearance of red blood cells. *Blood* **46,** 965–976.

Kleiner-Baumgarten, A., Schlaeffer, F., and Keynan, A. (1983) Multiple autoimmune manifestations in a splenectomized subject with HLA-B8. *Arch. Intern. Med.* **143,** 1987–1989.

Koyama, S., et al. (1962) Post-splenectomy vacuole: new erythrocyte inclusion body. *Mie. Med. J. (Japan)* **11,** 425–443.

Kragballe, K., Nielsen, J. L., Solling, J., and Ellegaard, J. (1981) Monocyte cytotoxicity after splenectomy. *Scand. J. Haematol.* **27,** 271–278.

Krumbhaar, E. B. and Lippincot, S. W. (1939) The post-mortem weight of the "normal" human spleen at different ages. *Am. J. Med. Sci.* **197,** 344–358.

Kvinesdal, B. B. and Jensen, M. K. (1986) Pitted erythrocytes in splenectomised subjects with congenital spherocytosis and in subjects splenectomised for other reasons. *Scand. J. Haematol.* **37,** 41–43.

Lane, P. A. (1995) The spleen in children. *Curr. Opin. Pediat.* **7,** 36–41.

Langenhuijsen, M. M. and van Toorn, T. W. (1982) Splenectomy and the severity of cytomegalovirus infection. *Lancet* **2,** 820.

Lanzowsky, P., Shende, A., Karayalcin, G., and Aral, I. (1976) Staging laparotomy and splenectomy: treatment and complications of Hodgkin's disease in children. *Am. J. Haematol.* **1,** 393–404.

Laufer, N., Freund, H., Charuzi, I., and Grover, N. B. (1978) The influence of traumatic splenectomy on the volume of human platelets. *Surg. Gynecol. Obstet.* **146,** 889–891.

Lauria, F., Pulvirenti, A., Raspadori, D., and Tura, S. (1981) T-lymphocyte subsets in healthy splenectomised patients. *Boll. Ist. Sieroter. Milan* **60,** 417–420.

Lawley, T. J., Hall, R. P., Fauci, A. S., Katz, S. I., Hamburger, M. I., and Frank, M. M. (1981) Defective Fc-receptor functions associated with HLA-B8/DRw3 haplotype: studies in patients with dermatitis herpetiformis and normal subjects. *N. Engl. J. Med.* **304,** 185–192.

Lawrence, E. M., Edwards, K. M., Schiffman, G., Thompson, J. M., Vaughn, W. K., and Wright, P. F. (1983) Pneumococcal vaccine in normal children. Primary and secondary vaccination. *Am. J. Dis. Child.* **137,** 846–850.

Lindquist, S. W., Weber, D. J., Mangum, M. E., Hollis, D. G., and Jordan, J. (1995) *Bordetella holmesii* sepsis in an asplenic adolescent. *Paed. Inf. Dis. J.* **14,** 813–815.

Linet, M. S., Nyren, O., Gridley, G., et al. (1996) Risk of cancer following splenectomy. *Int. J. Cancer* **66,** 611–616.

Lipson, R. L., Bayrd, E. D., and Watkins, C. H. (1959) The post-splenectomy blood picture. *Am. J. Clin. Pathol.* **32,** 526–532.

Livingston, C. D., Levine, B. A., Lecklitner, M. L., and Sirinek, K. R. (1983) Incidence and function of residual splenic tissue following splenectomy for trauma in adults. *Arch. Surg.* **118,** 617–620.

Lockwood, C. M., Worlledge, S., Nicholas, A., Cotton, C., and Peters, D. K. (1979) Reversal of impaired splenic function in patients with nephritis or vasculitis (or both) by plasma exchange. *N. Engl. J. Med.* **300,** 524–530.

Lum, L. G., Tubergen, D. G., Corash, L., and Blaese, R. M. (1980) Splenectomy in the management of the thrombocytopenia of the Wiskott-Aldrich syndrome. *N. Engl. J. Med.* **302,** 892–896.

Macrae, O. and Morris, N. (1931) Metabolism studies in coeliac disease. *Arch. Dis. Child.* **6,** 75–96.

Majeski, J. A. and Upshur, J. K. (1978) Asplenia syndrome: a study of congenital abnormalities in sixteen cases. *JAMA* **240,** 1508–1510.

Marsh, G. W. and Stewart, J. S. (1970) Splenic function in adult coeliac disease. *Br. J. Haematol.* **19,** 445–447.

Marsh, G. W., Lewis, S. M., and Szur, L. (1966a) The use of 51Cr-labelled heat damaged red cells to study splenic function. I. Evaluation of the method. *Br. J. Haematol.* **12,** 161–166.

Marsh, G. W., Lewis, S. M., and Szur, L. (1966b) The use of 51Cr-labelled heat damaged red cells to study splenic function. II. Splenic atrophy in thrombocythaemia. *Br. J. Haematol.* **12,** 167–171.

Martin, J. B. and Bell, H. E. (1965) The association of splenic atrophy and intestinal malabsorption: report of a case and review of the literature. *Can. Med. Assoc. J.* **92,** 875–878.

Matuchansky, C., Colin, R., Hemet, J., Touchard, G., Babin, P., Eugene, C., et al. (1984) Cavitation of mesenteric lymph nodes, splenic atrophy, and a flat small intestinal mucosa. Report of six cases. *Gastroenterology* **87,** 606–614.

McBride, J. A., Dacie, J. V., and Shapley, R. (1968) The effect of splenectomy on the leucocyte count. *Br. J. Haematol.* **14,** 225–231.

McCarthy, C. F., Fraser, I. D., Evans, K. T., and Read, A. E. (1966) Lym-phoreticular dysfunction in idiopathic steatorrhoea. *Gut* **7,** 140–148.

McDonald, P., Friedman, E. H., Banks, A., Anderson, R., and Carman, V. (1997) Pneumococcal vaccine campaign based in general practice. *Br. Med. J.* **314,** 1094–1098.

McKinley, M., Leibowitz, S., Bronzo, R., Zanzi, I, Weissman, G., and Schiffman, G. (1995) Appropriate response to pneumococcal vaccine in celiac sprue. *J. Clin. Gastroenterol.* **20,** 113–116.

McMullin, M. and Johnston, G. (1993) Long term management of patients after splenectomy. *Br. Med. J.* **307,** 1372,1373.

Melamed, I., Zakuth, V., Tzechoval, E., and Spirer, Z. (1982) Suppressor T-cell activity in splenectomized subjects. *J. Clin. Lab. Immunol.* **7,** 173–177.

Mellemkjoer, M. S., Olsen, J. H., Linet, M. S., Gridley, G., and Mclaughlin, J. K. (1995) Cancer risk after splenectomy. *Cancer* **75,** 577–583.

Meyer, A. (1932) Uber coeliakie. *Zeit. Klin. Med.* **1198,** 667–686.

Meyer, J. D., Argyris, B. F., and Meyer, J. A. (1980) Splenectomy, suppressor cell activity and survival in tumor bearing rats. *J. Surg. Res.* **29,** 537–552.

Millard, R. E. and Banerjee, S. K. (1979) Changes in T and B blood lymphocytes after splenectomy. *J. Clin. Pathol.* **32,** 1045–1049.

Mills, P. R., Brown, I. L., and Watkinson, G. (1980) Idiopathic chronic ulcerative enteritis. Report of five cases and review of the literature. *Q. J. Med.* **49,** 133–149.

Mishalany, H., Mahnovski, V., and Wooley, M. (1982) Congenital asplenia and anomalies of the gastrointestinal tract. *Surgery* **91,** 38–41.

Monie, I. W. (1982) The asplenia syndrome: an explanation for absence of the spleen. *Teratology* **25,** 215–219.

Moore, F. A., Moore, E. E., Moore, G. E., and Millikan, J. S. (1984) Risk of splenic salvage after trauma. *Am. J. Surg.* **148,** 800–803.

Moore, G. E., Stevens, R. E., Moore, E. E., and Aragon, G. E. (1983) Failure of splenic implants to protect against fatal post-splenectomy infection. *Am. J. Surg.* **146,** 413,414.

Mowbray, J. F. Hoffbrand, A. V., Holborow, E. J., Seah, P. P., and Fry, L. (1973) Circulating immune complexes in dermatitis herpetiformis. *Lancet* **1,** 400–401.

Muller, A. F. and Toghill, P. J. (1994) Functional hyposplenism in alcoholic liver disease: a toxic effect of alcohol? *Gut* **35,** 679–682.

Muller, A. F. and Toghill, P. J. (1995) Hyposplenism in gastrointestinal disease. *Gut* **36,** 165–167.

Muller, C., Mannhalter, J. W., Ahmad, R., Zlabinger, G., Wurnig, P., and Eibl, M. M. (1984) Peripheral blood mononuclear cells of splenectomised patients are unable to differentiate into immunoglobulin-secreting cells after pokeweed mitogen stimulation. *Clin. Immunol. Immunopathol.* **31,** 118–123.

Murdoh, I. A. and Dos Anjos, R. (1990) Continued need for pneumococcal prophylaxis after splenectomy. *Arch. Dis. Child.* **65,** 1268–1269.

Myerson, R. M. and Koelle, W. A. (1956) Congenital absence of the spleen in an adult. Report of a case with recurrent Waterhouse-Friderichsen syndrome. *N. Engl. J. Med.* **254,** 1131,1132.

Nashat, K., Triger, D., Underwood, J. C. E., Slater, D. N., and Woods, H. F. (1982) A method for the study of Kupffer cell function. *Clin. Sci.* **63,** 59P.

Nathan, D. G. (1969) Rubbish in the red cell. *N. Engl. J. Med.* **281,** 558–559.

Nathan, D. G. and Gunn, R. B. (1966) Thalassemia: the consequence of unbalanced hemoglobin synthesis. *Am. J. Med.* **41,** 815–830.

Nathwani, D. (1996) Infections in splenectomised patients: how to prevent. *Scott. Med. J.* **41,** 10–11.

Neilan, B. A. and Berney, S. N. (1983) Hyposplenism in systemic lupus erythematosus. *J. Rheumatol.* **22,** 176–178.

Nielsen, J. L., Andersen, P., and Ellegaard, J. (1982) Influence of residual splenic tissue on autoantibodies in splenectomised patients. *Scand. J. Haematol.* **28,** 273–277.

Nielsen, J. L., Ellegaard, J., Marqversen, J., and Hansen, H. H. (1981) Detection of splenosis and ectopic spleens with 99mTc-labelled heat damaged autologous erythrocytes in 90 splenectomised patients. *Scand. J Haematol.* **27,** 51–56.

Nielsen, J. L., Buskjaer, L., Lamm, L. U., Sφlling, J., and Ellegaard, J. (1983a) Complement studies in splenectomised patients. *Scand. J. Haematol.* **30,** 194–200.

Nielsen, J. L., Tauris, P., Johnsen, H. E., and Ellegaard, J. (1983b) The cellular immune response after splenectomy in humans. *Scand. J. Haematol.* **31,** 85–95.

O'Donoghue, D. J. (1986) Fatal pneumococcal septicaemia in coeliac disease. *Postgrad. Med. J.* **62,** 229–230.

O'Grady, J. G., Stevens, F. M., and McCarthy, C. F. (1985a) Genetic influences on splenic function in coeliac disease. *Gut* **26**, 1004–1007.

O'Grady, J. G., Stevens, F. M., and McCarthy, C. F. (1985b) Coeliac disease: does hyposplenism predispose to the development of malignant disease? *Am. J. Gastroenterol.* **80**, 27–29.

O'Grady, J. G., Harding, B., Egan, E. L., Murphy, B., O'Gorman, T. A., and McCarthy, C. F. (1984a) 'Pitted' erythrocytes: impaired formation in splenectomised subjects with congenital spherocytosis. *Br. J. Haematol.* **57**, 441–446.

O'Grady, J. G., Stevens, F. M., Harding, B., O'Gorman, T. A., McNicholl, B., and McCarthy, C. F. (1984b) Hyposplenism and gluten sensitive enteropathy: natural history, incidence and relationship to diet and small bowel morphology. *Gastroenterology* **87**, 1326–1331.

O'Grady, J. G., Harding, B., Stevens, F. M., Egan, E. L., and McCarthy, C. F. (1985) Influence of splenectomy and the functional hyposplenism of coeliac disease on platelet count and volume. *Scand. J. Haematol.* **34**, 425–428.

Oakes, D. D. (1981) Splenic trauma. *Curr. Prob. Surg.* **18**, 346–401.

Orda, R., Barak, J., Baron, J., Spirer, Z., and Wiznitzer, T. (1981) Postsplenectomy splenic activity. *Ann. Surg.* **194**, 771–774.

Palmer, K. R., Sherriff, S. B., and Holdsworth, C. D. (1979) Changing pattern of splenic function in coeliac disease. *Gut* **20**, A920.

Palmer, K. R., Sherriff, S. B., Holdsworth, C. D., and Ryan, F. P. (1981) Further experience of hyposplenism in inflammatory bowel disease. *Q. J. Med.* **50**, 462–471.

Palmer, K. R., Barber, D. C., Sherriff, S. B., and Holdsworth, C. D. (1983) Reticuloendothelial function in coeliac disease and ulcerative colitis. *Gut* **24**, 384–388.

Parr, L. J. A., Shipton, E. A., and Holland, E. H. (1953) A fatal case of Still's disease associated with Waterhouse-Friderichsen syndrome due to pneumococcal septicaemia. *Med. J. Aust.* **1**, 300–304.

Pearson, H. A., Spencer, R. P., and Cornelius, E. A. (1969) Functional asplenia in sickle-cell anemia. *N. Engl. J. Med.* **281**, 923–926.

Pearson, H. A., Schiebler, G. L., and Spencer, R. P. (1971) Functional hyposplenia in cyanotic congenital heart disease. *Pediatrics* **48**, 277–280.

Pearson, H. A., Cornelius, E. A., Schwartz, A. D., Zelson, J. H., Wolfson, S. L., and Spencer, R. P. (1970) Transfusion-reversible functional asplenia in young children with sickle-cell anemia. *N. Engl. J. Med.* **283**, 334–337.

Pearson, H. A., Johnston, D., Smith, K. A., and Touloukian, R. J. (1978) The born-again spleen. Return of splenic function after splenectomy for trauma. *N. Engl. J. Med.* **298**, 1389– 1392.

Pearson, H. A., Gallagher, D., Chilcote, R., et al. (1985) Developmental pattern of splenic dysfunction in sickle-cell disorders. *Pediatrics* **76**, 392–397.

Pedersen, F. K., Henrickson, J., and Schiffman, G. (1982) Antibody response to vaccination with pneumococcal capsular polysaccharides in splenectomised children. *Acta Paediatr. Scand.* **71**, 451–455.

Pereira, J. L. R., Hughes, L. E., and Young, H. L. (1987) Spleen size in patients with inflammatory bowel disease. Does it have any clinical significance? *Dis. Col. Rect.* **30**, 403–409.

Pettit, J. E., Williams, E. D., Glass, H. I., Lewis, S. M., Szur, L., and Wicks, C. J. (1971) Studies of splenic function in the myeloproliferative disorders and generalised malignant lymphomas. *Br. J. Haematol.* **20**, 575–586.

Pettit, J. E., Hoffbrand, A. V., Seah, P. P., and Fry, L. (1972) Splenic atrophy in dermatitis herpetiformis. *Br. Med. J.* **2**, 438–440.

Pines, A., Kaplinsky, N., Olchovsky, D., Holtzman, E., and Frankl, O. (1983) Hyposplenism in systemic lupus erythematosus. *Br. J. Rheumatol.* **22**, 176–178.

Plummer, K., Russi, S., Harris, W. H. Jr., and Carvati, C. M. (1950) Lipophagic intestinal granulomatosis (Whipple's disease). *Arch. Intern. Med.* **86**, 280–310.

Polhemus, D. W. and Schafer, W. B. (1952) Congenital absence of the spleen. Syndrome with atrio-ventricularis and situs inversus. *Pediatrics* **9**, 696–708.

Polhill, R. B. and Johnston, R. B. (1975) Diminished alternative complement pathway activity after splenectomy. *Pediatr. Res.* **9**, 333.

Polsky, B., Gold, J. W., Whimbey, E., Dryjanski, J., Brown, A. E., Schiffman, G., and Armstrong, D. (1986) Bacterial pneumonia in patients with the acquired immunodeficiency syndrome. *Ann. Intern. Med.* **104**, 38–41.

Ramsahoye, B. M., Evely, R., Mumar-Bashi, W., and Lim, S. H. (1994) Case Report. Selective IgA deficiency and hyposplenism. *Clin. Lab. Haematol.* **16**, 375–377.

Rice, H. M. and James, P. D. (1980) Ectopic splenic tissue failed to prevent fatal pneumococcal septicaemia after splenectomy for trauma. *Lancet* **1**, 565,566.

Rifkind, B. M. and Gale, M. (1967) Hypolipidaemia in anaemia. *Lancet* **2**, 640–642.

Roberts, J. G., Wisbey, M. L., Newcombe, R. G., Leach, K. G., and Baum, M. (1976) Prediction of human spleen size by computer analysis of splenic scintigrams. *Br. J. Radiol.* **49**, 151–155.

Robertson, D. A. F., Simpson, F. G., and Losowsky, M. S. (1981) Blood viscosity after splenectomy. *Br. Med. J.* **283**, 573–575.

Robertson, D. A., Bullen, A., Field, H., Simpson, F. G., and Losowsky, M. S. (1982a) Suppressor cell activity, splenic function, and HLA-B8 status in man. *J. Clin. Lab. Immunol.* **9**, 133–138.

Robertson, D. A., Swinson, C. M., Hall, R., and Losowsky, M. S. (1982b) Coeliac disease, splenic function and malignancy. *Gut* **23**, 666–669.

Robertson, D. A., Bullen, A. W., Hall, R., and Losowsky, M. S. (1983a) Blood film appearances in the hyposplenism of coeliac disease. *Br. J. Clin Pract.* **37**, 19–22.

Robertson, D. A. F., Dixon, M. F., Scott, B. B., Simpson, F. G., and Losowsky, M. S. (1983b) Small intestinal ulceration: diagnostic difficulties in relation to coeliac disease. *Gut* **24**, 565–574.

Robertson, D. A., Simpson, F. G., Gowland, G., and Losowsky, M. S. (1983c) Splenectomy causes autoantibody formation. *J. Clin. Lab. Immunol.* **11**, 63–65.

Robinette, C. D. and Fraumeni, J. F. (1977) Splenectomy and subsequent mortality in veterans of the 1939-45 war. *Lancet* **2**, 127–129.

Robinson, P. J., Bullen, A. W., Hall, R., Brown, R. C., Baxter, P., and Losowsky, M. S. (1980) Splenic size and function in adult coeliac disease. *Br. J. Radiol.* **53**, 532–537.

Rose, V., Izukawa, T., and Moes, C. A. F. (1975) Syndrome of asplenia and polysplenia: a review of cardiac and non-cardiac malformations in 60 cases with special reference to diagnosis and prognosis. *Br. Heart J.* **37**, 840–852.

Rosenthal, N. (1925) Clinical and hematological studies on Banti's disease: the platelet factor with reference to splenectomy. *JAMA.* **84**, 1887–1891.

Rosner, F., Zarrabi, M. H., Benach, J. L., and Habicht, G. S. (1984) Babesiosis in splenectomized adults: review of 22 reported cases. *Am. J. Med.* **76**, 696–701.

Roth, J., Brudler, O., and Henze, E. (1985) Functional asplenia in malignant mastocytosis. *J. Nucl. Med.* **26**, 1149–1152.

Rowley, D. A. (1950) The formation of circulating antibody in the splenectomised human being following intravenous injection of heterologous erythrocytes. *J. Immunol.* **65**, 515–521.

Roy, D. (1984) The spleen preserved. *Br. Med. J.* **289**, 70,71.

Ryan, F. P., Smart, R., Preston, F. E., and Holdsworth, C. D. (1974) Hyposplenism in ulcerative colitis. *Lancet* **2**, 318–320.

Ryan, F. P., Smart, R. C., Holdsworth, C. D., and Preston, F. E. (1978) Hyposplenism in inflammatory bowel disease. *Gut* **19**, 50–55.

Ryan, F. P., Jones, J. V., Wright, J. K., and Holdsworth, C. D. (1981) Impaired immunity in patients with inflammatory bowel disease and hyposplenism: the response to intravenous ØX174. *Gut* **22**, 187–189.

Sampson, D., Kauffman, H. M. Jr., Grotelueschen, C., and Metzig, J. (1976) Suppressor activity of the human spleen and thymus. *Surgery* **79**, 393–397.

Schilling, V. (1924) Uber Die Diagnose einer Milzatrophie durch den Befund von Kernkugeln als Teilerscheinung pluriglandular insuffizienz. *Klin. Wochenschr.* **43**, 1960–1962.

Schnitzer, B., Rucknagel, D. L., and Spencer, H. H. (1971) Erythrocytes: pits and vacuoles as seen with transmission and scanning electron microscopy. *Science* **173**, 251–252.

Schrier, S. L., Ben-Bassat, I., Bensch, K., Seeger, M., and Junga, I. (1974) Erythrocyte membrane vacuole formation in hereditary spherocytosis. *Br. J Haematol.* **26**, 59–69.

Schumacher, M. J. (1970) Serum immunoglobulin and transferrin levels after childhood splenectomy. *Arch Dis. Child.* **45,** 114–117.

Scopes, J. W. (1991) Continued need for pneumococcal prophylaxis after splenectomy. *Arch. Dis. Child.* **66,** 750.

Scully, R. E., Galdabini, J. J., and McNeely, B. U. (1975) Case records of the Massachusetts General Hospital. *N. Engl. J. Med.* **293,** 547–553.

Segal, A. W., Munro, J. M., Ensell, J., and Sarner, M. (1981) Indium-111 tagged leucocytes in the diagnosis of inflammatory bowel disease. *Lancet* **2,** 230–232.

Selby, C., Hart, S., Ispahani, P., and Toghill, P. J. (1987) Bacteraemia in adults after splenectomy or splenic irradiation. *Q. J. Med.* **63,** 523–530.

Seo, I. N. and Li, C.-Y. (1995) Hyposplenic blood picture in systemic amyloidosis. *Arch. Pathol. Lab. Med.* **119,** 252–254.

Shennib, H., Chu-Jeng Chiu, R., and Mulder, D. S. (1983) The effects of splenectomy and splenic implantation on alveolar macrophage function. *J. Trauma,* **23,** 7–12.

Shiratori, Y., Kawase, T., Nakata, R., Tanaka, M., Hikiba, Y, Okano, K., et al. (1995) Effect of splenectomy on hepatic metastasis of colon carcinoma and natural killer activity in the liver. *Dig. Dis Sci.* **40,** 2398–2406.

Siber, G. R., Weitzman, S. A., Aisenberg, A. C., Weinstein, H. J., and Schiffman, G. (1978) Impaired antibody response to pneumococcal vac-cine after treatment for Hodgkin's disease. *N. Engl. J. Med.* **229,** 442–448.

Smart, R. C., Ryan, F. P., Holdworth, C. D., and Preston, F. E. (1978) Relationship between splenic size and splenic function. *Gut* **19,** 56–59.

Spelman, D. W. (1996) Postsplenectomy overwhelming sepsis: reducing the risks. *Med. J. Aust.* **164,** 648.

Spencer, G. R., Bird, C., Prothero, D. L., Brown, T. R., Mackenzie, F. A. F., and Phillips, M. J. (1981) Spleen scanning with ^{99m}Tc-labelled red blood cells after splenectomy. *Br. J. Surg.* **68,** 412.

Spencer, R. P. and Pearson, H. A. (1974) Splenic radiocolloid uptake in the presence of circulating Howell-Jolly bodies. *J. Nucl. Med.* **15,** 294,295.

Spencer, R. P., Johnson, P. M., and Sziklas, J. J. (1977) Unusual scan presentation of splenic vasculature occlusion by tumour. *Clin. Nucl. Med.* **2,** 197–199.

Spencer, R. P., Dhawan, V., Suresh, K., Antar, M. A., Sziklas, J. J., and Wasserman, I. (1978a) Causes and temporal sequence of onset of functional asplenia in adults. *Clin Nucl. Med.* **3,** 17,18.

Spencer, R. P., et al. (1978b) 'Reversible' functional asplenia in combined immunodeficiency. *Int. J. Nucl. Med. Biol.* **5,** 125.

Spencer, R.P., et al. (1984) Splenic overload syndrome: possible relationship to a small spleen. *J. Nucl. Med. Biol.* **11,** 291–294.

Spirer, Z., Zakuth, V., Diamant, S., et al. (1977) Decreased tuftsin concentrations in patients who have undergone splenectomy. *Br. Med. J.* **2,** 1574–1576.

Spirer, Z., Hauser, G. J., Hazaz, B., and Joshua, H. (1980a) Autoimmune antibodies after splenectomy. *Acta Haematol.* **63,** 230–233.

Spirer, Z., Weisman, Y., Zakuth, V., Fridkin, M., and Bogair, N. (1980b) Decreased serum tuftsin concentration in sickle-cell disease. *Arch. Dis. Child.* **55,** 566,567.

Steinberg, M. H., Gatling, R. R., and Tavassoli, M. (1983) Evidence of hyposplenism in the presence of splenomegaly. *Scand. J. Haematol.* **31,** 437–439.

Stone, H. H., Stanley, D. G., and DeJarnette, R. H. (1967) Post-splenectomy viral hepatitis. *J. Am. Med. Assoc. NY* **199,** 851–853.

Stone, R. W., McDaniel, W. R., Armstrong, E. M., Young, R. C. Jr., and Higginbotham-Ford, E. A. (1985) Acquired functional asplenia in sarcoidosis. *J. Natl. Med. Assoc.* **77,** 930–936.

Suarez, R. M., Spies, T. D., and Suarez, R. M. Jr. (1947) The use of folic acid in sprue. *Ann. Intern. Med.* **26,** 643–677.

Sullivan, J. L., Ochs, H. D., Schiffman, G., Hammerschlag, M. R., Miser, J., Vichinsky, E., and Wedgwood, R. J. (1978) Immune response after splenectomy. *Lancet* **1,** 178–181.

Swerdlow, A. J., Douglas, A. J., Vaughan Hudson, G., Vaughan Hudson, B., and MacLennan, K. A. (1993) Risk of second primary cancer after Hodgkin's disease in patients in the British National Lymphoma Investigation: relationships to host factors, histology and stage of Hodgkin's disease, and splenectomy. *Br. J. Cancer* **68,** 1006–1011.

Szur, L., Marsh, G. W., and Pettit, J. E. (1972) Studies of splenic function by means of radioisotope-labelled red cells. *Br. J. Haematol.* **23,** 183–199.

Tesluk, G. C. (1984) Fatal overwhelming post-splenectomy sepsis following autologous splenic transplantation in severe congenital osteopetrosis. *J. Pediatr. Surg.* **19,** 269–272.

Tham, K. T., Teague, M. W., Howard, C. A., and Chen, S. Y. (1996) A simple splenic reticuloendothelial function test. Counting erythrocytes with argyrophilic inclusions. *Am. J. Clin. Pathol.* **105,** 548–552.

Thompson, H. (1974) Necropsy studies in adult coeliac disease. *J. Clin. Pathol.* **27,** 710–721.

Torres, J. and Bisno, A. L. (1973) Hyposplenism and pneumococcemia. *Am. J. Med.* **55,** 851–855.

Traub, A., Giebink, G. S., Smith, C., et al. (1987) Splenic reticuloendothelial function after splenectomy, spleen repair, and spleen autotransplantation. *N. Engl. J. Med.* **317,** 1559–1564.

Trewby, P. N., Chipping, P. M., Palmer, S. J., Roberts, P. D., Lewis, S. M., and Stewart, J. S. (1981) Splenic atrophy in adult coeliac disease: is it reversible? *Gut* **22,** 628–632.

Tura, S., Fiacchini, M., Zinzani, P. L., Brusamolino, E., and Gobbi, P. G. (1993) Splenectomy and the increasing risk of secondary acute leukemia in Hodgkin's disease. *J. Clin. Oncol.* **11,** 925–930.

Van Mierop, L. H. S., Gessner, I. H. S., and Schiebler, G. L. (1972) Asplenia and polysplenia syndromes. *Birth Defects: Original Article Series,* **8,** 36–44.

Van Wyck, D. B., Witte, M. H., Witte, C. L., and Thies, A. C. Jr. (1980) Critical splenic mass for survival from experimental pneumococcemia. *J. Surg. Res.* **78,** 14.

Waldman, J. D., Rosenthal, A., Smith, A. L., Shurin, S., and Nadas, A. S. (1977) Sepsis and congenital asplenia. *J. Pediatr.* **90,** 555–559.

Wang, W., Wong, W., Wilimas, J., et al. (1994) Sepsis caused by penicillin-resistant pneumococcus in children with sickle-cell anemia: a report of 8 cases. *Blood* **84,** 410a.

Wardrop, C. A., Dagg, J. H., Lee, F. D., Singh, H., Dyet, J. F., and Moffat, A. (1975) Immunological abnormalities in splenic atrophy. *Lancet* **2,** 4–7.

Westerhausen, M., Worsdorfer, O., Gessner, U., De Giuli, R., and Senn, H. J. (1981) Immunological changes following post-traumatic splenectomy. *Blut* **43,** 345–353.

Whitaker, A. N. (1969) Infection and the spleen: association between hyposplenism, pneumococcal sepsis and disseminated intravascular coagulation. *Med. J. Aust.* **1,** 1213–1219.

Widmann, W. D. and Laubscher, F. A. (1971) Splenosis: a disease or a beneficial condition? *Arch. Surg.* **102,** 152–158.

Wilkinson, L. S., Tang, A., and Gjedsted, A. (1983) Marked lymphocytosis suggesting lymphocytic leukemia in three patients with hyposplenism. *Am. J. Med.* **75,** 1053–1056.

Williams, B. D., Pussell, B. A., Lockwood, C. M., and Cotton, C. (1979) Defective reticuloendothelial system function in rheumatoid arthritis. *Lancet* **1,** 1311–1314.

Williams, M. D., Young, D. H., and Schiller, W. R. (1990) Trend toward nonoperative management of splenic injuries. *Am. J. Surg.* **160,** 588–593.

Williams, D. N. and Kaur, B. (1996) Postsplenectomy care. *Postgrad. Med.* **100,** 195–205.

Winkelstein, J. A. and Lambert, G. H. (1975) Pneumococcal serum opsonizing activity in splenectomized children. *J. Pediatr.* **87,** 430–433.

Working Party of the British Committee for Standards in Haematology Clinical Haematology Task Force (1996) Guidelines for the prevention and treatment of infection in patients with an absent or dysfunctional spleen. *Br. Med. J.* **312,** 430–434.

Zago, M. A., Figueiredo, M. S., Covas, D. T., and Bottura, C. (1985) Aspects of splenic hypofunction in old age. *Klin. Wochenschr.* **63,** 590–592.

Zago, M. A., Covas, D. T., Figueiredo, M. S., and Bottura, C. (1986) Red cell pits appear preferentially in old cells after splenectomy. *Acta Haematol.* **76,** 54–56.

Zarrabi, M. H. and Rosner, F. (1986) Rarity of failure of penicillin prophylaxis to prevent post-splenectomy sepsis. *Arch. Intern. Med.* **146,** 1207,1208.

Zoli, G., Corazza, G. R., Woods, S., and Farthing, M. J. G. (1993) Impaired splenic function in patients with intestinal failure on long term intravenous nutrition. *Gut* **34(Suppl. 1),** S33.

Zucker, S. and Mielke, C. H. (1972) Classification of thrombocytosis based on platelet function tests: correlation with hemorrhagic and thrombotic complications. *J. Lab. Clin. Med.* **80,** 385–394.

11 The Relationship of the Spleen to Infection

THOMAS C. RUSHTON, MD, GEOFFREY J. GORSE, MD, FACP,
AND ANTHONY J. BOWDLER, MD, PHD, FRCP, FRCPATH, FACP

11.1. INTRODUCTION

The predisposition to infection experienced by patients with diminished or absent splenic function is well-documented (Brozovic, 1994). However, the susceptibility to, and severity of, an infection are dependent on many other variables. The virulence of the infecting microorganism is of critical importance. The degree of resistance mustered by the asplenic or hyposplenic patient is determined by the age of the patient and age at the time of splenectomy (or significant splenic dysfunction), duration of asplenism, underlying diseases that may cause further immunosuppression, and therapeutic interventions, including chemotherapy and radiation. A discussion about the relationship of the spleen to infection must include not only attention to splenic dysfunction, both anatomical and functional, but must also incorporate the relationship between the microorganism and its host, the patient.

11.2. HYPOSPLENISM

The commonest cause of hyposplenism is surgical splenectomy, but an increasingly broad range of diseases and disorders is known to be associated with hyposplenism (Eichner, 1979; Foster et al., 1984): These are reviewed in Chapter 10.

Some disorders carry a high probability of hyposplenism: sickle cell disease, radiation therapy to the spleen, chronic graft-vs-host disease, and splenomegaly secondary to amyloid disease (Cuthbert et al., 1995). In these, the prevention of infection is an intrinsic part of management. However, there are many situations in which hyposplenism is sporadic and occasional, e.g., systemic lupus erythematosis (SLE), mixed connective tissue (CT) disorder, and collagenous colitis, and in which the first evidence of hyposplenism may in fact be severe secondary infection (Freeman, 1996; Guertler and Carter, 1996; Liote et al., 1995).

It is therefore important to be alert to the possibility of hyposplenism in severe infections, even when an anatomically intact spleen is present, and to the need for prophylactic (protective) measures in conditions in which hyposplenism is common enough to be suspected, e.g., inflammatory bowel disease and celiac disease (Maehlen et al., 1997).

Bacteremia has been demonstrated to occur during periods of hyposplenism in ulcerative colitis, in which splenic function waxes and wanes in relation to the activity of the colitis (Foster et al.,

1982). In SLE, impaired splenic function is, in part, caused by reticuloendothelial blockade produced by circulating immune complexes, and is reversible by plasmapheresis. Furthermore, splenic atrophy in patients with SLE results from lymphocyte depletion, and overwhelming septicemia has been reported in association with splenic atrophy in this disorder (Foster et al., 1984).

Sickle cell anemia is also associated with severe bacterial infections: The child with sickle cell disease is at greatest risk for pneumococcal sepsis when the spleen is enlarged early in life. At a later stage, when the spleen is atrophic, there has already been the opportunity for an immunological response to various pneumococcal serotypes, and the resulting production of type-specific antibody enhances the clearance of pneumococci by the reticuloendothelial cells of the liver (*see also* Chapter 15.)

This chapter reviews the pathophysiological mechanisms for the increased risk of infection in the patient with impaired splenic function, and the types of organisms that cause these infections. The prevention of infectious complications and appropriate care in patients at risk are also discussed.

Methods for demonstrating impaired splenic function have been described elsewhere (*see* Chapter 10, Subheading 2.). They have contributed in large measure to the recognition of hyposplenism, and have provided insight into its various degrees of intensity of expression. For example, Coleman et al. (1982) showed that patients newly diagnosed with lymphoma had a mean pitted red blood cell count of 0.6%, which rose to 13% after radiation to the spleen of at least 40 gy, and 33.7% after surgical splenectomy. This indicates that splenic radiation diminishes at least some aspects of splenic function, and, practically, such patients should be regarded as having a significantly increased risk of infection.

Dailey et al. (1980) also documented splenic atrophy induced by radiation in patients with lymphoma: The mean postmortem weight of the spleen in radiated subjects was 75 g, and, in subjects not radiated, it was 200 g. During life, there was a demonstrably decreased uptake of technitium-99m sulfur-colloid in spleen scans after radiation; however, the effect of chemotherapy differed in not being accompanied by a reduction in spleen size.

The degree to which splenic function is reduced is variable, even after splenectomy for trauma to the spleen. Pearson et al. (1978) reported a study that showed that subjects splenectomized for trauma could be divided into two disparate groups, based on the proportion of pitted cells in the peripheral blood. 13/22 children showed ≤6%; the remainder had much higher levels of pitted cells, comparable to the 20% found in patients who underwent splenectomy for hematological disorders. Subjects with ≤6% or less of cells with pits

From: *The Complete Spleen: A Handbook of Structure, Function, and Clinical Disorders* Edited by: A. J. Bowdler © Humana Press Inc., Totowa, NJ

showed multiple nodules of regenerate splenic tissue (splenosis) in technitium-99m sulfur-colloid spleen scans. Those authors attributed the difference to the returning splenic function of the regenerated tissue, and ascribed lower rates of infection to these patients.

11.3. OVERWHELMING POSTSPLENECTOMY INFECTION

A distinguishing feature of the postsplenectomy condition and the hyposplenic state is a propensity to a severe, rapidly developing, overwhelming infection, especially, but not exclusively, in the young. The syndrome of overwhelming postsplenectomy infection (OPSI) usually begins with a prodrome of influenza-like symptoms, followed by an abrupt onset of septicemia, with massive bacteremia from an unknown source. The first report of this syndrome was by King and Shumacker (1952), in five infants splenectomized for congenital hemolytic anemia, four of whom developed meningitis or overwhelming meningococcemia 6 wk to 3 yr later.

Bacteria may be identified using Gram's stain on a buffy coat smear of the peripheral blood. Cultures of blood are useful, not only in identification of the organism, but also its susceptibility to specific antibiotics, especially with the recent tendency to increasing patterns of resistance (Leggiadro, 1997). The likelihood of a blood culture detecting bacteremia is increased by the collection of an adequate volume of blood (Mermel and Maki, 1993; Athanasios et al., 1996). The newer systems, which continuously monitor blood cultures, appear to have a significantly higher yield (Kinnunen et al., 1996), and are especially important in a rapidly evolving infection, such as OPSI.

The syndrome commonly comprises fever, chills, abdominal pain, nausea, vomiting, multiple organ failure, disseminated intravascular coagulation (DIC), adrenal hemorrhage and the Waterhouse-Friderichsen syndrome, seizures, and death within 36 h of onset (Bisno and Freeman, 1970; Kingston and MacKenzie, 1979; Singer, 1973). Purpuric skin lesions are commonly distributed on the face and extremities in patients with DIC and overwhelming septicemia (Kingston and MacKenzie 1979). The causative organism can be cultured from aspirates of the purpuric skin lesions. Severe hypoglycemia, electrolyte imbalance, and shock are frequently noted. Waterhouse-Friderichsen syndrome is usually associated with a fatal outcome, but the incidence of other symptoms and signs in OPSI, and their predictive value with respect to outcome, remains incompletely documented. A low fibrinogen level (≤ 1.5 g/L) is clearly associated with a fatal outcome in overwhelming meningococcal purpura; other predictors may include low factor V concentration ($\leq.20$), thrombocytopenia ($\leq 80 \times 10^9$ /L) and cerebrospinal fluid leukocytosis less than 20×10^6/L (Giraud et al., 1991).

11.4. MICROORGANISMS ASSOCIATED WITH POSTSPLENECTOMY INFECTIONS

The most fulminant infections occurring in the postsplenectomy state are caused by encapsulated bacteria (*Streptococcus pneumoniae*, *Haemophilus influenzae* type b (Hib), and *Neisseria meningitidis*). However, nonencapsulated bacteria and nonbacterial pathogens, such as viruses and protozoa, also produce serious and sometimes modified infections (Table 1; Musher, 1992; Rebentish and Bernstein, 1993).

11.4.1. BACTERIAL INFECTIONS Of the bacterial causes of post-splenectomy infection, the most common organism is *S. pneu-*

Table 11.1
Organisms Causing Severe
Infections in Splenectomized Patients

Bacteria
  Streptococcus pneumoniae
  Haemophilus influenzae type b (Hib)
  Neisseria meningitidis
  Pseudomonas aeruginosa
  Escherichia coli
  Capnocytophaga canimorsus (formerly dysgonic fermenter 2 [DF-2])
  Capnocytophaga ochraceus (formerly dysgonic fermenter 1 [DF-1])
  Other bacteria:
    Neisseria gonorrhoea
    Plesiomonas shigelloides
    Other Streptococcal spp.
Viruses
  Cytomegalovirus
  Varicella zoster virus
  Epstein-Barr virus
  Rubeola virus
Protozoa
  Babesia spp.
  Plasmodium spp.

moniae, particularly in patients with OPSI (Table 2; Foss Abrahamsen et al., 1997; Askergren and Björkholm, 1980; Barrett-Connor, 1971; Buchanan et al., 1983; Green et al., 1979; Hitzig 1985; Rosner and Zarrabi, 1983; Singer, 1973; Wählby and Domellöf. 1981). For instance, Askergren and Björkholm (1980) reported that pneumococcal septicemia accounted for 71% of septic episodes among their splenectomized patients, but for only 4.7% of all septic episodes at their institutions. Other bacterial pathogens each account individually for less than 15% of infections reported in splenectomized patients, including other encapsulated organisms (*H. influenzae* and *N. meningitidis*), other streptococcal species, *Pseudomonas aeruginosa*, *Escherichia coli*, and more unusual bacterial pathogens. A splenectomized patient with HbE/β° thalassemia succumbed to *Campylobacter jejuni* infection (Jackson et al., 1997). Patients with sickle cell anemia have a predisposition to Salmonella infections (Wright et al., 1997).

N. meningitidis is a cause of serious postsplenectomy infection (Salzman and Rubin 1996), and has been reported in patients who required splenectomy for underlying disease (King and Shumacker, 1952), as well as abdominal trauma (Holmes et al., 1981). Loggie and Hinchey (1986) reported that intraperitoneal and intravenous (iv) challenge with *N. meningitidis* group B, in a murine model, did not result in greater mortality among splenectomized mice, compared with normal mice. This supports literature review findings that meningococcal infection is less frequent than pneumococcal in patients who have undergone splenectomy (Holmes et al., 1981; Loggie and Hinchey, 1986; Norris et al., 1996).

Recent surveillance has shown an increase in serogroup Y meningococcal disease (Centers for Disease Control [CDC], 1996). Consequently, there may be a role for increased use of the meningococcal polysaccharide vaccine, which includes A, C, Y, and W-135 serogroups.

One case of fulminant septicemia, shock, and adrenal hemorrhage, caused by *Neisseria gonorrhoeae*, was reported by Austin et al. (1980). The patient had been splenectomized during staging

Table 11.2
Etiologic Agents that Cause Sepsis in Patients with Hyposplenia and Asplenia, and Their Relative Frequencies of Isolation

Ref. no.	Reason for hyposplenism or splenectomy	Total no patients in study	*No. episodes of postsplenectomy sepsis caused by the indicated organism (% episodes)*					
			Total	S. pneumoniae	H. influenzae	H. meningitidis	Salmonella spp	E. coli
Green et al. (1979)	Hodgkin's disease	52	8	6(75)	1(12.5)	–	–	–
Rosner and Zarrabi (1983)	Hodgkin's disease	115	13[a]	7(54)	4(31)	2(15)	–	–
Askergren and Bjorkholm (1980)	Hodgkin's disease	76	5	5(100)	–	–	–	–
	All others	1072	9	4(44)	–	–	–	–
Wahlby and Domellof (1981)	Trauma	413	10	4(40)	3(30)	1(10)	–	–
Barrett-Connor (1971)	Sickle cell anemia	166	9	4(44)	1(12)	–	2(22)	2(22)
Singer (1973)	Mainly hematological[b] (*see* text)	2795	72	36(50)	6(8)	9(13)	–	8(11)
Buchanan et al. (1983)	Hemoglobin SC disease	51	6	5(83)	1(17)	–	–	–
TOTALS		4740	132	71(54)	16(12)	12(9)	2(1)	10(8)

[a]Fatal episodes only.
[b]None with sickle cell anemia.

laparotomy for Hodgkin's disease, and later received radiation therapy. As with the pneumococcus, blood isolates of *N. gonorrhoeae*, from persons with disseminated gonococcal infections, are resistant to killing by serum alone (Schoolnik et al., 1976). This may contribute to the mechanism for the development of overwhelming infection with this organism, in the splenectomized patient. A similar patient, with Hodgkin's disease, who underwent splenectomy and radiotherapy, died of fulminant septicemia caused by *Plesiomonas shigelloides*, and developed DIC and adrenal hemorrhage (Curti et al., 1985). *P. shigelloides* is an unusual cause of septicemia in the general population, in which it is most commonly associated only with a mild diarrheal illness.

Another unusual pathogen, first described in 1976, and reported to be the causative agent of severe infections in splenectomized patients, is a slow-growing Gram-negative bacillus, *Capnocytophaga canimorsus*, formerly named "dysgonic fermenter 2" (DF-2) by the CDC (Bobo and Newton 1976; Kullberg et al., 1991). It is sensitive to penicillin and chloramphenicol, as well as to several other antibiotics. The organism can be confused with other fastidious Gram-negative bacilli, but is distinguishable by routine biochemical laboratory testing (Holmes et al., 1995). Infections caused by *C. canimorsus* have, in general, been characterized by septicemia and a history of a dog bite (Pers et al., 1996; Hicklin et al., 1987; Kalb et al., 1985; Martone et al., 1980). *C. canimorsus* is more frequently isolated from blood and cerebrospinal fluid (CSF). DIC has been reported in association with septicemia: fulminant infections and DIC have occurred in 50% of splenectomized patients reported to be septicemic with this organism. Eschariform skin lesions develop at the site of the dog bite. Myocardial infarction may occur; it is hypothesized that this agent may cause endothelial damage, with subsequent coronary thrombosis (Ehrbar et al., 1996). Peripheral blood smears from these patients may show Gram-negative rods (Mossad et al., 1997). Splenectomized patients should be aware of the association of fulminant infection and dog bites. The organism appears to be serum-sensitive, and it has been postulated that the susceptible host may have a defect in the lytic activity of serum, because of a quantitative or qualitative complement abnormality, or possibly because of the presence of nonbactericidal blocking antibodies (Hicklin et al., 1987).

Capnocytophaga ochraceus (formerly "dysgonic fermenter-1" [DF-1]), and other oxidase- and catalase-negative species, can be found as part of normal oral flora. The immuocompromised host may develop local infections, sepsis, and meningitis during granulocytopenia and breakdown of the oral mucosa. Shifts in the normal flora, with acquisition of new organisms, may occur in periods of neu-tropenia, as described in a patient with acute myeloblastic leukemia and *Capnocytophaga gingivalis* meningitis (Kim et al., 1996).

The incidence of Hib invasive disease, in total, occurs in dramatically decreased numbers in the pediatric population, because of the increased use of Hib conjugate vaccines (CDC, 1996). Because there is no natural host, other than humans for Hib, the vaccine appears to be decreasing the rate of nasopharyngeal carriage in children (Barbour and Phil, 1996). The situation in adults is less clear: Heath et al. (1997) describe two cases of invasive Hib infection in nursing home residents, and confirm the relationship via pulsed-field gel electrophoresis. Further surveillance will be required in adult populations, to see if vaccination has any protective effect. In addition to Hib as a cause of serious postsplenectomy infection, type f was reported to cause meningitis in an asplenic patient with biliary cirrhosis (Meier et al., 1985). The strain isolated from the patient's blood cultures was not cleared as rapidly from the bloodstream of splenectomized rats challenged with the organism, compared to clearance from normal rats. These findings indicate that *H. influenzae* strains other than type b have the potential for causing serious infection in splenectomized patients.

Bacteria newly recognized as human pathogens may prove to hold extra risk for the hyposplenic. A recent report describes an infection in an asplenic adolescent with *Bordetella holmesii* (Lindquist et al., 1995).

11.4.2. VIRAL INFECTIONS Viruses that may be associated with increased severity or rates of infection in splenectomized hosts include varicella-zoster virus and cytomegalovirus (CMV). Although reported rates vary, varicella-zoster virus infection occurs in approx 20% of splenectomized patients with Hodgkin's disease, but less frequently in patients splenectomized for nonneoplastic diseases (Green et al., 1979; Green et al., 1986; Monfardini et al., 1975). The question of the incidence of infection is, however, controversial, and other investigators have denied that a higher rate of varicella-zoster occurs after splenectomy (Guinee et al., 1985; Naraqi et al., 1977; Reboul et al., 1978; Schimpff et al., 1972).

The contributions of radiation treatment and chemotherapy to the increased incidence of viral infections are additional factors that are difficult to distinguish from the effect of splenectomy. Splenectomy appeared to be a risk factor for varicella-zoster virus infection independent of Hodgkin's disease in a series of 1130 patients with lymphoma, reported by Goffinet et al. (1972). Monfardini et al. (1975) reported a higher incidence of varicella-zoster in 232 splenectomized patients with Hodgkin's (26/139 patients [19%]) and non-Hodgkin's lymphomas (11/93 patients [12%]), with a 16% incidence overall, compared with 175 nonsplenectomized patients with Hodgkin's (5/45 patients [11%]) and non-Hodgkin's lymphomas (10/130 patients [8%]), with a 9% overall incidence. The incidence of varicella-zoster was significantly higher in splenectomized patients who received combination chemotherapy with Hodgkin's (27%) and non-Hodgkin's (15%) lymphomas (22% for all chemotherapy recipients), compared to the group that was splenectomized, but not treated with chemotherapy: Hodgkin's (8%) and non-Hodgkin's (6%) lymphomas (7% for all who did not receive chemotherapy). Overall, the rate of varicella-zoster in children and adolescents with Hodgkin's disease is reported to be from 12 to 38%; Green et al. (1979) reported a trend toward a higher rate of varicella-zoster among splenectomized patients with Hodgkin's disease. The cumulative percentage of patients who had undergone splenectomy and experienced zoster was 42.8%, compared to 18.3% of Hodgkin's disease patients who had not undergone splenectomy. However, Guinee et al. (1985) reported attack rates of zoster in patients with Hodgkin's disease using univariate and multiple regression analyses, to be the same, whether laparotomy (and presumably splenectomy) had been performed or not.

The varicella vaccine is available, and its use is becoming more universal in childhood. Gershon et al. (1996) showed that either prior infection with, or vaccination against, varicella reduced the risk of subsequent zoster in children with leukemia. There may also be a booster effect for those whose immune systems are waning (Levin and Hayward, 1996). For therapy, several effective antivirals are available, including acyclovir and the newer agents, famciclovir and valaciclovir (Dwyer and Kesson 1997). Experimental agents, such as sorivudine, may prove more efficacious (Wallace et al., 1996).

An association between the postsplenectomy state and clinical CMV infection has not been firmly established. Severe CMV infection, characterized by interstitial pneumonia, high fever, and lymphocytosis with atypical forms, has been reported in patients who underwent splenectomy for trauma and received multiple blood transfusions (Baumgartner et al., 1982). Anti-CMV immunoglobulin M (IgM) antibodies were detected in only one of the three patients in whom tests for these antibodies were done. Those authors postulated that the lack of anti-CMV IgM antibody may have resulted from the postsplenectomy state. Okun and Tanaka (1978) reported a case of CMV mononucleosis with an associated lymphocyte count >100,000/mm^3, and other authors have reported that 4/26 consecutive patients with CMV infection had previously undergone splenectomy, and none of those patients was seriously ill from the CMV infection. Peterson et al. (1980) reported that the incidence of CMV disease was identical in renal allograft recipients with and without a history of splenectomy. An experimental murine model for CMV infection has demonstrated a different effect of

splenectomy; Katzenstein et al. (1983) showed that splenectomized mice had lower mortality rates than mice with intact spleens, when infected with murine CMV. Those authors concluded that early replication of murine CMV in splenic macrophages augmented virus-induced hepatic injury, and thus contributed to the pathogenesis of lethal murine CMV infection. The relevance of these findings to human infection remains to be clarified.

Current therapy for CMV infection includes the antiviral agents, ganciclovir, foscarnet, and cidofovir, and iv immunoglobulin, indicated for CMV pneumonitis. The application of polymerase chain reaction assays for the determination of CMV infection appears promising, and it may also be useful in gaging efficacy of therapy and detection of recurrence (van der Meer et al., 1996).

Epstein-Barr and rubeola virus infections have been reported to show unusual manifestations in splenectomized patients (Baumgartner et al., 1982). Jones et al. (1975) reported a prolonged course of fever and lymphocytosis in a patient with rubeola infection recently splenectomized for trauma. Purtilo et al. (1980) reported severe Epstein-Barr virus infection, characterized by profound lymphocytosis, acquired hypogammaglobulinemia, and severe hepatitis, in a patient who acquired the infection from blood transfusions following splenectomy for trauma. Modification of the immune response to Epstein-Barr virus by splenectomy, because of trauma, may have led to a Kawasaki disease syndrome in a young adult (Barbour et al., 1979).

11.4.3. PROTOZOAL INFECTIONS *Plasmodium* species and *Babesia* species are associated with more severe and frequent infections in patients who have impaired or absent splenic function (*see also* Chapter 2). Human babesiosis is a febrile illness characterized by myalgias, fatigue, hemolytic anemia, and hemoglobinuria caused by tick-borne protozoan agents of the genus *Babesia* (Boustani and Gelfand 1996; Rosner et al., 1984). Frequently, it will mimic malaria, but it is generally milder in severity. In addition to tick-borne spread, it can be acquired by the transfusion of infected blood. The spleen plays an important role in resistance to *Babesia* infections in animals. Mild infections with low levels of parasitemia in animals can be exacerbated by splenectomy. Rosner et al. (1984) summarized 22 previously reported cases of human babesiosis among splenectomized patients, ranging in age from 23 to 70 years. Splenectomy had been performed for various indications, 1 month to 36 years prior to the Babesia infection; most had moderate to severe clinical disease, and 16 (73%) survived. Dammin et al. (1981) reported 57 clinical cases of *Babesia microti* infection, of which 10 (17%) occurred in splenectomized patients; these were acquired on offshore islands of the northeastern United States (Nantucket Island, Martha's Vineyard, and the eastern tip of Long Island) and Cape Cod. None of these infections was fatal. Cases have occurred outside of coastal regions, including Wisconsin, Minnesota, Georgia, California, and Mexico (Boustani and Gelfand, 1996). A new species of *Babesia* was identified in Washington state (Quick et al., 1993) and in Missouri (Herwaldt et al., 1996). Other *Babesia* species have caused infection in splenectomized patients in whom the resultant disease is often more severe than in patients with an intact spleen (Dammin et al., 1981; Rosner et al., 1984; Shute, 1975). There is one case report of babesiosis in a patient with sickle cell anemia (Klein et al., 1997).

Splenectomy is known to predispose to unusually severe clinical malaria, and to reactivation of latent and subclinical malarial infections in both humans and animals (Boone and Watters, 1995; Looaressuway et al., 1993; Hamilton and Pikacha, 1982). Certain experimental animals not normally susceptible to certain species of *Plasmodium* can be rendered susceptible by splenectomy (Wyler et al., 1978). However, the effects of splenectomy are not uniform, since the species of experimental animal, species of the *Plasmodium*, and timing of splenectomy may affect susceptibility to, and severity of, plasmodium infection (Nooruddin and Ahmed 1967). Monkeys, splenectomized 2–3 mo after infection with *Plasmodium inui*, tolerated their infection without effect on mortality, although these animals rapidly developed the same levels of parasitemia that killed monkeys splenectomized prior to infection (Wyler et al., 1977). The spleen limits the magnitude of parasitemia in acute infections and restricts the level of parasitemia in chronic infections (Littman, 1974; Llende et al., 1986; Looareesuwan et al., 1987; Rosner et al., 1987; Shute, 1975; Tapper and Armstrong, 1976; Walzer et al., 1974). The spleen exerts other influences on host defense against the intraerythrocytic, asexual stage of plasmodia: It may be important for clinical tolerance early in infection, and it is required as an effector organ in mediating protection induced by vaccines, but not for sustaining antibody production in response to these vaccines (Wyler et al., 1978).

The spleen is important in the reduction of parasitemia, probably because erythrocytes infected with *Plasmodia* spp. are more susceptible to splenic filtration, as a result of their reduced deformability (Miller et al., 1971). However, the pitting process lacks a recognition system, which would provide for the species-specificity of malaria immunity (Wyler et al., 1978). Sequestration of erythrocytes parasitized with *Plasmodium falciparum* usually limits the observable parasitemia to ring forms and gametocytes. Splenectomy results in the presence of all stages of the intraerythrocytic parasite in peripheral blood smears (Israeli et al., 1987). Splenectomy appears to have no effect on susceptibility to sporozoite-induced infection, or on the development of exoerythrocytic stages (Wyler et al., 1978). During active experimental infection of rats with *Plasmodium berghei*, the efficiency of the splenic removal of parasitized cells, and of heat-treated red blood cells, is much diminished; spontaneous resolution of the parasitemia is associated with a marked increase in rates of clearance (Wyler et al., 1981). Splenectomy may result in overwhelming infection, and the recurrence of acute symptomatic malaria in patients with chronic asymptomatic *Plasmodium malariae* infection is caused by a rapid rise in parasitemia after splenectomy (Wyler et al., 1978). The mechanism for the role of the spleen in the induction of immunity to malaria, other than its nonimmunological parasiticidal effects, are yet to be determined. One possibility is a cytotoxic effect of a spleen cell population on parasitized erythrocytes (Coleman et al., 1975; *see also* Chapter 3).

Patients with splenic hypofunction should be advised about their susceptibility to severe illness caused by *Plasmodia* spp., and advised to avoid endemic regions. If travel plans cannot be altered, then the standard antimalarial prophylaxis regimens, and protective measures against mosquito vectors, should be recommended and adopted meticulously.

A study of the splenic clearance of autologous heat-treated red blood cells in patients with acute malaria caused by *P. falciparum* has been published by Looareesuwan et al. (1987). Clearance was enhanced in patients with splenomegaly, but not in those in whom the spleen was normal in size, indicating that enlargement of the spleen may itself be an effective means of increasing particle filtration rates. However, within a few days of starting antimalarial therapy, the clearance rates were found to be increased above nor-

mal in the patients without splenomegaly, as well; in both groups, normal clearance rates resumed within 6 weeks of treatment (*see also* Chapter 3).

11.5. THE RELATIONSHIP OF MICROORGANISMS, CLINICAL OUTCOME, AND SITE OF INFECTION TO THE UNDERLYING DISEASE

Rosner and Zarrabi (1983) reported on 115 patients with Hodgkin's disease, who experienced 145 episodes of postsplenectomy infection. These infections included pneumonia in 37.2% of 145 episodes, septicemia in 28.3% of episodes, meningitis in 13.8%, urinary tract infection in 27.7%, skin infection in 4.7%, and infection at other sites in 13.2%. Of the 41 (28.3%) patients with an episode of septicemia, 20 had a fulminant course, with DIC and adrenal hemorrhage; 12 of these 20 patients with a fulminant course were under 10 years of age. At least 50/115 patients (43%) died as a result of their infections. Among those patients who developed DIC, only two survived, giving an overall mortality in this group of 90%. For those without clinical DIC, the mortality rate was 35%.

The bacteria associated with postsplenectomy infection included *S. pneumoniae* in 31.7% of episodes, *H. influenzae* in 7.6%, and *P. aeruginosa* in 6.2%; small percentages were caused by other organisms. The pneumococcus was the most common organism associated with fatal infection in these patients. Barrett-Connor (1971) reviewed, retrospectively, the infections in sickle cell anemia patients, occurring during a period of 1 year at two hospitals in Dade County, FL; these were compared to the infections experienced by blacks in the general population living in the same county. The attack rate in patients with sickle cell anemia was higher than in the controls, with respect to bacterial meningitis (18.5 vs 0.06/1000 patient years), and for *H. influenzae* meningitis (3.5 vs 0.03/1000 patient years). Thus, the relative risk for bacterial, pneumococcal, and *H. influenzae*-caused meningitis, in patients with sickle cell anemia, ranged from 116 to 570× higher than in the controls. Other infections, such as salmonellosis, shigellosis, and tuberculosis, were increased in patients with sickle cell anemia, compared to the control group; however, the relative risk was between 7 and 25. Barrett-Connor was uncertain whether this was an artifactual increase or resulted from better case documentation in the sickle cell anemia patients who were subject to closer medical supervision.

Splenectomy and chemotherapy, in patients who are renal transplant recipients, appears to create a risk for infection that is no greater than that of patients undergoing splenectomy for trauma alone. Bourgault et al. (1979) reported five severe pneumococcal infections in 236 patients (2.1%), who were splenectomized in conjunction with renal transplantation. None of the 57 renal transplant patients with an intact spleen developed severe pneumococcal infection during the same follow-up period, which ranged from 1 month to 150 months, with a mean of 34.1 months. Despite administration of immunosuppressive drugs, such as azathioprine and prednisone to these patients, the rate of pneumococcal infection in the splenectomized renal transplant patients was similar to that reported in patients splenectomized because of trauma.

Other authors have reported the rates of postsplenectomy septicemia in various patient groups who underwent splenectomy for hematological and oncological disorders and trauma. The largest series was a literature review by Singer (1973), of 2795 splenectomized patients, the majority of whom were splenectomized for underlying hematological diseases, such as idiopathic thrombocytopenic purpura, hereditary spherocytosis, hemolytic anemia, and thalassemia. Combining the results of studies in these patients with those in reports of sickle cell disease (Overturf et al., 1977), splenectomized patients with Hodgkin's disease (Chilcote et al., 1976), and patients splenectomized for trauma and in association with miscellaneous abdominal surgery (Wara, 1981), the percentage of patients with postsplenectomy septicemia ranged from 1.5%, in those who had suffered trauma, to 25%, in patients who had undergone splenectomy for thalassemia. 10% of patients with Hodgkin's disease, 15% of patients with sickle cell disease, 3.5% of patients with the miscellaneous hematological diseases, and 8.2% of those with portal hypertension were reported to have had episodes of septicemia. Mufson (1981) reported an incidence of pneumococcal infection of 5–10/1000 patients/year in patients splenectomized for trauma. The number of fatalities caused by septicemia ranged from 33 to 71% of those patients who developed septicemia. Among the 2795 patients reported by Singer (1973), 119 cases of fulminant sepsis occurred (4.3%). Of these 71 patients (representing 60% of these 119 cases and 2.5% of the total patients reported) died from the fulminant septicemia. In comparison, estimated rates of culture-confirmed invasive pneumococcal disease in the general U.S. population range from 8 to 16 cases/100,000 population (Istre et al., 1987). A normal nonsplenectomized population would be expected to have an overall mortality of approx 0.01% caused by septicemia (Wara, 1981). From a sizable population of patients with hereditary spherocytosis, Schilling (1995) estimated a mortality rate of 0.73/1000, years after splenectomy. Because four fatal cases occurred prior to the availability of the pneumococcal vaccine, that author was optimistic that the rate might be lower today.

Rates of septicemia and mortality, derived from pooled retrospective clinical series, must, of course, be interpreted with caution. These figures may only broadly reflect the true incidence rate of fulminant sepsis following splenectomy, because many of the series deal principally with infants and children who have undergone splenectomy for hematological disease, and who may be immunologically immature; data were assimilated from a variety of sources, with differing definitions of sepsis and effectiveness of follow-up; the populations were mostly studied at referral hospitals; and the duration of follow-up was not uniform, and was not taken into account in calculating the true incidence of postsplenectomy sepsis.

Schwartz et al. (1982) attempted to document accurate incidence rates of fulminant sepsis in the splenectomized population, through a retrospective report of 193 persons who had undergone splenectomy between 1955 and 1979 in Rochester, MN. The mean duration of follow-up was 5.6 years. Two cases of fulminant septicemia occurred during this period, and only one patient died as a result of fulminant infection. 52 patients had at least one serious infection in the postsplenectomy period: Abscess, bacteremia, and pneumonia accounted for 62/78 infections. Gram-negative enteric bacilli outnumbered Gram-positive cocci as causative agents of infection, with a ratio of 2.3:1. There was only one pneumococcal infection. Additional risk factors associated with serious infections in these splenectomized patients included irradiation therapy, immunosuppression, and chemotherapy. Those authors felt that their study more accurately reflected the prognosis of patients with a history of splenectomy in a primary care practice. The total of 78 infections resulted in an overall incidence of one infection/14 patient-years. The infection rate, expressed as the incidence of serious infections per 100 person-years, in patients with hematological disorders was 6.5, in patients splenectomized for trauma 3.3, in

patients with incidental splenectomy caused by other surgery, 9.6; and, in patients with incidental splenectomy in association with malignant neoplasm, was 16.6. The highest relative risk of serious infection after splenectomy was therefore in the group with an underlying malignant neoplasm, who had undergone an incidental splenectomy. The relative distribution of microorganisms, sites of infection and mortality are radically different in this series, compared with others. Further investigations, including a carefully followed prospective series, will be needed to resolve these differences.

11/5.1. SUBJECT AGE AND RISK OF INFECTION   Among patients with sickle cell anemia, the risk of infection with encapsulated bacteria appears to be highest in early life. Pearson (1977) reported that 10% of 422 patients with sickle cell anemia experienced one or more severe episodes of infection during the first few years of life. The highest number of episodes of meningitis and septicemia occurred before the age of 5 years. However, cases of osteomyelitis appeared to be equally frequent in age groups from birth to age 25 years. Pearson suggested that susceptibility to encapsulated bacteria was greatest during early childhood, because of a relative lack of circulating antibodies to specific serotypes of encapsulated bacteria. The development of humoral immunity to these organisms allows these patients to overcome, at least partially, their functional hyposplenia and opsonophagocytic defects, resulting in a lower rate of infectious episodes.

Heier (1980) summarized the findings of three series of splenectomized patients in the literature, and related the age of the patients to the risk of bacterial infection. Children and infants appeared more susceptible to postsplenectomy septicemia than adults. Splenectomy between the ages of 1 and 16 years was associated with a frequency of serious infections of between 9 and 20%. In one series, 50% of patients splenectomized before the age of 12 months acquired serious bacterial infections, compared with 2.8% of those splenectomized after the age of 12 months (Horan and Colegbatch, 1962). In another series, 8.1% of patients splenectomized before the age of 5 years developed fatal septicemia or meningitis, compared with 3.3% of those splenectomized after the age of 5 years (Eraklis et al., 1967). Singer (1973) found that 21% of patients splenectomized for hereditary spherocytosis, before the age of 12 months acquired serious bacterial infections, compared with 3.5% of those who were splenectomized later in life. Deaths caused by infection also appear to be significantly higher in children after splenectomy. Chaikof and McCabe (1985) reported a retrospective study of patients who had undergone splenectomy between 1962 and 1972. Follow-up was available in 1982 on 637 patients: For adults, 10% of deaths, overall, were caused by infection, and two cases of fatal overwhelming postsplenectomy infection occurred (0.34%). This was significantly lower than the incidence of fatal OPSI among 53 patients who were under the age of 16 yr at the time of splenectomy (3.77%).

11.5.2. RISK OF POSTSPLENECTOMY INFECTION AS A FUNCTION OF INTERVAL AFTER SPLENECTOMY   The risk of fatal overwhelming postsplenectomy infection appears to be greatest in the first 2 years following splenectomy (Hitzig, 1985). However, sepsis can occur more than 2 years after splenectomy. Wählby and Domellöf (1981) reported 10 cases of postsplenectomy sepsis occurring in 413 patients (2.4%), with a mean follow-up period of 5.9 years after splenectomy for blunt abdominal trauma. Three patients developed pneumococcal septicemia more than 5 years after the splenectomy, and two of these three cases had a fatal outcome. One fatal case of meningococcal septicemia occurred 4 years after splenectomy, and two nonfatal cases of septicemia caused by *H. influenzae* occurred at 3 and 4 years after splenectomy.

Zarrabi and Rosner (1984) reviewed 47 published adult cases of serious bacterial infection following splenectomy performed for splenic trauma. The mean interval between splenectomy and serious infection was 7.2 years, with a range of 6 months to 31 years. 11 patients developed serious infection within 2 years of the splenectomy. Four out-patients died of septicemia, despite the presence of ectopic splenic tissue, suggesting that splenosis did not fully protect against subsequent infection. In a review of 145 episodes of postsplenectomy infection in 115 patients (53.1% between ages 10 and 60 years) with Hodgkin's disease, Rosner and Zarrabi (1983) showed that 35.2% had occurred within 2 years of the splenectomy, and 16.6% developed later; the interval following splenectomy was unknown in 48.2%. The median age at the time of occurrence of the postsplenectomy infection was 19.8 years. The median interval between splenectomy and the infectious episode was 21.9 months. Clearly, therefore, the splenectomized patient may develop overwhelming infection long after loss of the spleen, and continues to require prolonged vigilant observation.

11.6. REASONS FOR INCREASED RATES OF INFECTION IN SPLENECTOMIZED SUBJECTS

Opsonization, at least in the absence of serotype specific antibody, and clearance of encapsulated bacteria are abnormal in splenectomized patients, and the underlying reasons have been investigated in both human and animal models.

An initial question is, "What effect does splenectomy have on serum opsonizing activity?" Winkelstein et al. (1975) investigated phagocytosis of *S. pneumoniae* type 25, by normal polymorphonuclear leukocytes in vitro, in the presence of serum obtained from 24 splenectomized children, none of whom had sickle cell anemia, and from 23 age-matched controls. Pneumococcal opsonizing activity in the two groups of children was not significantly different. Nevertheless, three of the subjects who had undergone splenectomy developed pneumococcal septicemia, despite having normal serum-opsonizing activity for pneumococci. The two groups did not have statistically different serum titers of complement factor 3, complement factor 5, and factor B. Those authors concluded that fulminant bacterial sepsis observed in children after surgical splenectomy cannot be attributed to deficient pneumococcal serum-opsonizing activity. Furthermore, they do not report whether or not their subjects were seropositive for the type 25 pneumococcus used in their study. Presumably, they had serum antibody to this pneumococcal serotype, which resulted in the finding of normal opsonization. An interesting corollary to their findings is that the autosplenectomy, which occurs in children with sickle cell anemia probably does not account completely for the decreased pneumococcal serum-opsonizing activity seen in sickle cell anemia patients. This decreased activity results, in part, from defective alternative pathway function (Johnston et al., 1973).

Clearance of bacteremia appears in part to be dependent on an intact alternative complement pathway. In a guinea pig model, Brown et al. (1983) compared the clearance of an intravenous bolus of *S. pneumoniae* type 7 in normal animals that were nonimmune, animals that were complement-factor-4 deficient, and animals that had been treated with cobra venom factor, which causes a consumption of the alternative complement pathway and complement factors 3–9. They found that, in nonimmune animals with an intact spleen, alternative pathway activation played a critical role in host

defense and clearance of pneumococcal bacteremia. Of the three groups, only the animals that had deficient alternative pathway activity were unable to clear the iv pneumococcal challenge.

Intravascular clearance of *S. pneumoniae* was then investigated in normal nonimmune guinea pigs, and those that had been splenectomized. Clearance was significantly impaired in those animals that were splenectomized; however, the clearance deficit was more severe in those animals challenged with a more virulent strain of pneumococcus (serotype 12) than with a less virulent strain (serotype 7). A rough strain of *S. pneumoniae* (unencapsulated) was cleared equally well in those animals that were splenectomized and the normal nonimmune guinea pigs. The better clearance of the less virulent strains, in splenectomized guinea pigs, appears to be related to better hepatic sequestration of the organisms. The more virulent the pneumococcal strain, the more likely was the host to sequester the pneumococcus preferentially in the spleen. Thus, splenectomized animals were less able to clear the most virulent pneumococcal serotype, because the normal host response is to direct the organism to the spleen, for removal from the blood stream by filtration and phagocytosis.

Type-specific humoral immunity affects intravascular clearance patterns. Brown et al. (1983) further compared sequestration patterns in nonimmune guinea pigs and immune guinea pigs, which were intravenously challenged with radiolabeled *S. pneumoniae*. Immunization against the challenge pneumococcal strain resulted in increased hepatic sequestration of the radiolabeled pneumococci in both normal guinea pigs and those deficient in complement factor 4. The change in sequestration patterns, with preferential sequestration in the liver, induced by immunization was blocked by administration of cobra venom factor, which consumed the alternative pathway and C3–C9 complement factors. Other studies by Hosea et al. (1981) have investigated the differential clearance of particles from the blood by liver and spleen, by measuring the half-life of IgG-sensitized erythrocyte clearance in normal human volunteers, splenectomized patients, and splenectomized patients, who received highly sensitized erythrocytes. There was a significant delay in the rate of clearance in splenectomized patients, compared with normal subjects with an intact spleen; however, the use of highly sensitized erythrocytes resulted in a marked improvement in the rate of clearance in the splenectomized patients. Erythrocytes sensitized with IgG antibody are cleared by the reticuloendothelial system, rather than by intravascular hemolysis; hepatic clearance must occur with a shorter contact time between the particle and the macrophage than is the case in the spleen, and appears to require a higher concentration of surface antibody binding for the hepatic sequestration of bloodborne particles. Splenectomized patients lack the splenic macrophages, which are able to clear bacteria coated with only small amounts of IgG from the blood stream, and they are unable to mount a sufficient antibody response for liver macrophages to overcome the defect (Hosea, 1983).

Pneumococcal polysaccharide encapsulation is antiphagocytic: The bacterium must be phagocytosed to be killed, but the capsule must be neutralized first. Pneumococcal polysaccharide activates the alternative complement pathway, resulting in C3b binding to the bacterial cell surface and clearance of organisms. Coating of the organisms with C3b, however, does not by itself lead to ingestion of the organisms by phagocytes. Consequently, the clearance of these C3b-coated particles is only transient, and the organisms are released back into the blood stream, in splenectomized, nonimmune patients (Hosea, 1983). In patients with pre-existing antibody to specific pneumococcal serotype, antibodies attached to the capsular wall of the pneumococci cause activation of the classical complement pathway, and attachment of C3b molecules to the surface of the bacteria. The presence of antibody on the surface of the bacteria improves Fc-mediated hepatic macrophage clearance of the opsonized pneumococci. Thus, the complement system in splenectomized patients, and in those patients with splenic hypofunction in the absence of sickle cell anemia, seems to be intact, and, in the presence of serotype-specific opsonizing antibody, these patients are better able to defend against challenge with encapsulated organisms.

Other encapsulated organisms have been studied in animal models of hyposplenism. Chen and Moxon (1983) investigated the susceptibility of rats to Hib challenge, in the presence of phenylhydrazine-induced hemolytic anemia. This experimental model of hemolytic anemia results in splenic congestion and a decreased filtering capacity of the spleen, probably because of a decrease in both the open pulp circulation and total splenic blood flow. The phenylhydrazine-treated rats developed levels of bacteremia that were 10× greater than those of control rats, after intranasal inoculation of Hib; the anemic rats also had a higher mortality than control rats after iv bacterial challenge. Moxon et al. (1980) challenged surgically splenectomized rats with Hib, and found the median lethal dose (LD_{50}) after iv administration to be $10^{4.6}$ bacteria, and after intranasal inoculation to be $10^{4.7}$ bacteria. Both doses were significantly lower than in sham-operated rats, which were $10^{8.6}$ and $10^{9.0}$ bacteria, respectively. The phenylhydrazine-treated rats of Chen and Moxon (1983) all died after iv injection of 5×10^7 bacteria at the nadir of their anemia, but an LD_{50} was not determined. As a result, it is difficult to assess the degree of splenic hypofunction induced by splenic congestion during haemolytic anemia as compared to surgical asplenia. These studies support the concept that the spleen is important in the host immune response to H. influenzae infection. The phenylhydrazine-induced hemolytic anemia model shows that splenic congestion, such as that seen during sickle cell sequestration crisis, is a contributing factor to reduced host resistance to encapsulated bacteria. However, when anemia is not associated with splenic congestion, it does not result in similar degrees of splenic hypofunction.

The effect of splenectomy on the host response to challenge with unencapsulated bacteria, such as E. coli, is less well-studied in animal models. Almdahl et al. (1987) found that bacteremia, following intraperitoneal and iv injection of E. coli, was significantly prolonged in splenectomized rats, compared to the effect in sham-operated control animals.

Another important immunological defect noted in patients splenectomized for various underlying diseases is consistently low serum IgM antibody levels. This has been present in many studies reporting mean serum IgM antibody levels, compared to the values in normal subjects, and in those with the same underlying disease, but with an intact spleen (Krivit, 1977). However, the clinical significance of reduced levels of serum IgM is uncertain at this time, since the efficiency of IgM antibody in opsonizing pneumococci is significantly less than that of IgG.

11.7. THE PROTECTION OF THE SPLENECTOMIZED PATIENT FROM ENCAPSULATED BACTERIAL INFECTIONS

Strategies for protection from, and the early treatment of, severe bacterial infections in splenectomized patients have been proposed

Table 11.3
Measures that May Protect
Splenectomized Patient from Overwhelming Sepsis

Vaccination against:
   Streptococcus pneumoniae
   Haemophilus influenzae type b
   Neisseria meningitidis
Oral antibiotic prophylaxis
Preservation of splenic tissue
Provision of medical identification bracelet
Early institution of therapeutic parenteral antibiotics during infection

in the literature (Table 3). Vaccination against encapsulated organisms, such as Hib (at least in children), with *Haemophilus* type b polysaccharide–diphtheria toxoid conjugate vaccine, *N. meningitidis* (meningococcal polysaccharide vaccine, Groups A, C, Y, and W-135 combined), and *S. pneumoniae* (23-valent capsular polysaccharide vaccine) is indicated prior to elective splenectomy, and should also be given to those patients who have already undergone splenectomy, if not already administered. The clearest indication for *Haemophilus* type b conjugate vaccine is in children between the ages of 18 months and 5 years (CDC, 1988). However, the conjugate vaccine (20 μg polyribosephosphate/0.5 mL im dose) has been found to be safe and immunogenic in normal healthy adults (Granoff et al., 1984; Lepow et al., 1984). Administration of conjugate vaccine to hyposplenic adults should be considered.

If chemotherapy is a prospect, vaccination should be given beforehand. Since splenic irradiation with more than 30 Gy results in hyposplenia, vaccination should be accomplished prior to the start of treatment. Chronic oral antibiotic prophylaxis, with agents such as penicillin, amoxicillin, or trimethoprim-sulfamethoxazole, has been advocated during the first 2–3 years after splenectomy, because of the higher number of infections that occur during the early years following splenectomy. However, patients with Hodgkin's disease have developed postsplenectomy sepsis with pneumococcal serotypes contained in the pneumococcal vaccine, while receiving penicillin prophylaxis. Poor compliance with the antibiotic regimen, pneumococcal resistance, and failure to cover other causes of overwhelming infection reduce the effectiveness of chronic antibiotic prophylaxis. Surgical preservation of splenic tissue, whenever possible, would be a desirable goal. An identification bracelet, such as "Medicalert™," advising health care professionals to the presence of the postsplenectomy state, is advisable, because this may help in the institution of appropriately early empirical antibiotic therapy.

Empiric antibiotic therapy should be administered early to the patient who has been splenectomized and is febrile, given the high rate of mortality in these patients due to bacterial septicemia. With rapid treatment, mortality may be reduced. Whether this goal is actually achieved by this form of therapy remains to be proven. Therapeutic regimens chosen empirically at the time of presentation might include a third-generation cephalosporin, such as parenterally administered cefotaxime or ceftriaxone. These agents are effective in the treatment of both bacteremia and meningitis, and use of either of these two antibiotics assures activity against the encapsulated organisms most likely to cause infection in splenectomized patients, including penicillin resistant pneumococci (with minimum inhibitory concentration >1.0 μg/mL) and moderately susceptible *S. pneumoniae* (with minimum inhibitory concentration between

0.1 and 1.0 µg/mL), as well as β-lactamase-producing, ampicillin-resistant *H. influenzae* (Istre et al., 1987). Once the causative organism is isolated and characterized, a narrower-spectrum antimicrobial agent, such as penicillin or ampicillin, can be substituted, when shown to be appropriate. In the patient with significant penicillin allergy, chloramphenicol is empirically the drug of choice.

In subsequent subheadings, evidence supporting strategies for protection against overwhelming bacterial sepsis in the splenectomized patient is described.

11.7.1. IMMUNIZATION AGAINST ENCAPSULATED ORGANISMS The serological response to pneumococcal polysaccharide vaccine has been studied in both animals and humans. In rabbits and mice, the spleen is the primary site of early antibody formation after immunization with pneumococcal polysaccharide antigen. Splenectomy removes most of the lymphocytes that initially respond to antigenic stimulation by polysaccharide antigens. The magnitude of the response to the polysaccharide antigen is possibly affected in these circumstances by normal T-cell suppressor activity and abnormally low T-cell helper activity (Hosea, 1983; Jones et al., 1976). Hosea et al. (1981) investigated serum IgM and IgG antibody responses, measured by ELISA, to pneumococcal vaccine, in nine normal and nine splenectomized human volunteers: Of the latter, four had no disease, three had idiopathic thrombocytopenic purpura, and there were two with idiopathic hemolytic anemia requiring cytotoxic treatment. Significantly higher postvaccination serum IgM antibody titers developed to all nine pneumococcal serotypes tested in the normal volunteers, compared to the splenectomized patients. There were also higher serum IgG antibody titers to 7/9 tested pneumococcal serotypes, in the normal subjects, compared to splenectomized patients.

Ammann et al. (1977) compared the responses to pneumococcal polysaccharide immunization in young subjects aged 2–25 years. 19 patients with congenital or surgical asplenia developed serum antibody responses, measured by indirect hemagglutination, which were not statistically different from those of 38 normal children. A group of 68 patients with homozygous sickle cell disease, seven with sickle-thalassemia and two with hemoglobin SC disease, developed serum antibody responses to the pneumococcal polysaccharide vaccine that were likewise not statistically different from those of 44 healthy African children. In this study, therefore, a humoral response of normal degree developed to the pneumococcal polysaccharide vaccine antigens, in patients with sickle cell disease and in asplenic patients.

The response to pneumococcal polysaccharide vaccine in patients with Hodgkin's disease has also been studied. Siber et al. (1978) evaluated the antibody response of patients with Hodgkin's disease to polysaccharide vaccine after splenectomy and completion of radiation therapy and chemotherapy. The antibody response was impaired, but was relatively normal in those given the polysaccharide vaccine 3 and 4 years after cessation of chemotherapy. Addiego et al. (1980) evaluated the serum antibody response to pneumococcal in 16 normal controls and 27 Hodgkin's disease patients prior to radiation and/or chemotherapy, and either before or after splenectomy. The pneumococcal vaccine was administered 48–72 h before splenectomy, or after staging laparotomy and splenectomy. Serum antibody levels to pneumococcal serotypes were measured using indirect hemagglutination and radioimmunoassay methods. The proportion of fourfold serum antibody responders was not significantly different between the two patient groups. In fact, the mean postimmunization antibody levels to pneumococ-

cal polysaccharide antigen were all >300 ng antibody nitrogen/mL serum, which are levels thought to be protective. No significant difference in serum antibody response was noted when stage I and II Hodgkin's disease patients were compared to stage III and IV Hodgkin's disease patients. Also, there was no significant difference in response when the vaccine was administered 48–72 h prior to splenectomy, compared to administration during the 3–5 d period postsplenectomy.

Sullivan et al. (1978) investigated the route of immunization in patients who had been splenectomized, in comparison to normal controls and patients with Hodgkin's disease. Intravenously administered bacteriophage Φ X174 produced good primary and secondary serum antibody responses in normal controls; however, the primary response was not adequate in the five asplenic patients with Hodgkin's disease. The secondary response was better in these patients, but still abnormal when compared to the normal controls, except in the one Hodgkin's disease patient who had stage IA disease, and had not received chemotherapy. Among patients who were asplenic but did not have Hodgkin's disease, there was significantly decreased serum IgG antibody formation after secondary immunization with bacteriophage, compared to the normal controls, which suggested to Sullivan et al. that switching of the antibody class from IgM to IgG production was not normal in their asplenic patients. These results confirmed previous studies showing deficient antibody response to intravenously administered heterologous red blood cells in anatomically and functionally asplenic individuals (Rowley, 1950; Schwartz and Pearson, 1972).

The geometric mean antibody response (by radioimmunoassay) to subcutaneously injected capsular polysaccharide antigens, in 26 asplenic individuals without Hodgkin's disease was not significantly different from the response of 27 normal control patients with intact spleens. The geometric mean antibody titer in the four Hodgkin's disease patients who had received chemotherapy and radiotherapy did not rise significantly, compared to preimmunization levels; however, the antibody response, in the one Hodgkin's disease patient who had not received chemotherapy was comparable to normal controls and significantly higher than preimmunization antibody level (Sullivan et al., 1978).

These studies support the concept that the spleen is necessary for a normal immune response to bloodborne antigens, but that other parenteral routes of immunization, such as the subcutaneous, circumvent the need for the splenic immune response. They also support the concept that chemotherapy significantly reduces the response to subsequent immunization with parenteral polysaccharide antigen vaccines.

Siber et al. (1986) investigated the serum antibody response to immunization with various capsular polysaccharide antigens, in patients with Hodgkin's disease who received chemotherapy and between 35 and 40 Gy radiation to the spleen, as well as mantle and paraaortic node radiation. The serum antibody response in these patients was compared to that of asplenic controls who did not receive chemotherapy and did not have Hodgkin's disease, and also to healthy controls. All patients received 14-valent pneumococcal polysaccharide vaccine, Hib capsular polysaccharide vaccine, and meningococcal group C vaccine. 3–4 wk after vaccination, serum antibody levels to meningococcal group C polysaccharide antigen were significantly lower in patients with Hodgkin's disease whether they had received radiation, chemotherapy, or both, compared to the asplenic controls and healthy normal controls. The serum antibody response to capsular polysaccharides of

Hib and *S. pneumoniae* were not significantly different in patients with Hodgkin's disease compared to asplenic controls and healthy controls. Those authors found that only the interval between immunization and the beginning of chemotherapy correlated with the antibody response. Those patients who began bimodal therapy or chemotherapy alone, less than 10–14 d after immunization, had a lower mean serum antibody response to pneumococcal antigen.

Molrine et al. (1995) studied 144 patients with Hodgkin disease for at least 2 years prior to enrollment who previously were treated. The group received the Hib-conjugate and 4-valent meningococcal polysaccharide vaccines. Subgroups randomly received either the 23-valent pneumococcal vaccine or a 7-valent pneumococcal-conjugate vaccine (seven pneumococcal serotypes linked to the outer membrane protein complex of *N. meningitidis*). Antigen-specific antibody concentrations were determined at baseline and 3–6 wk after vaccination. Immunization with a single Hib-conjugate dose produced levels of antibody believed to be protective (62% protective at baseline to 99% after vaccination). Protective response was found for both the 4-valent meningococcal polysaccharide and the 23-valent pneumococcal vaccine. The subgroup that received the 7-valent pneumococcal vaccine had a significantly lower response, compared to the standard 23-valent pneumococcal vaccination.

Timing of immunization relative to splenectomy had no apparent effect on serum antibody levels (Siber et al., 1986). In Hodgkin's disease patients, those immunized 2 d prior to splenectomy had similar antibody levels, compared to those immunized on the day of surgery and those receiving pneumococcal vaccine within 2 d of splenectomy. During subsequent follow-up, serum antibody levels declined more significantly in those patients treated with both chemotherapy and radiation, compared to the asplenic and healthy controls. A booster immunization, given 3 mo after the completion of chemotherapy in Hodgkin's disease patients, resulted in no significant change in serum antibody levels.

Ruben et al. (1984) investigated the serum IgM and IgG antibody responses to bivalent meningococcal groups A and C polysaccharide vaccine, given intramuscularly to healthy control subjects and patients who had been splenectomized for trauma, lymphoid tumor, or nonlymphoid tumor. The only antibody responses that were significantly lower, in terms of the number of responding subjects, were the IgM responses to group A and group C meningococcal antigens in the patients with underlying lymphoid tumor. They also had significantly lower mean levels of both IgM and IgG anti-bodies in the postvaccination serum specimens, compared to normal controls. Those who had undergone splenectomy for trauma had a serum antibody response that was nearly the same as that of controls. The authors recommended routine administration of meningococcal vaccine to patients without a spleen or with splenic hypofunction.

The humoral antibody response to pneumococcal polysaccharide vaccine is encouraging; however, whether this humoral immunity prevents subsequent pneumococcal septicemia is not clear (Brivet et al., 1984; Evans, 1984; Giebink et al., 1979; Sumaya et al., 1981). Vaccine efficacy was evident in the study of Ammann et al. (1977). Two year follow-up of their patients revealed the occurrence of eight *S. pneumoniae* infections (all septicemias) in unimmunized sickle cell disease patients, but no pneumococcal infection in the sickle cell disease group immunized with pneumococcal vaccine ($p < 0.025$). Efficacy of vaccination in anatomic asplenia was 77%, in a large study comprised of immunized patients with subsequent pneumococcal infection isolated from blood and cerebrospinal fluid; overall, efficacy was 57% (Butler et al., 1993).

Herbert et al. (1983) compared the cumulative mortality after challenge with aerosolized pneumococci, in three groups of CD-1 mice. The first group of mice was first splenectomized, then vaccinated intraperitoneally with type 3 pneumococcal vaccine. The second group received the same pneumococcal vaccine, then 7 d later, was splenectomized; the third group received the vaccine followed by sham operation. When challenged with aerosolized pneumococci of the same serotype 7 d later, the mice subjected to early splenectomy had a significantly higher mortality. Those authors concluded that asplenic individuals may have impaired immunological responses and increased susceptibility to infection, and that pneumococcal vaccine should be given before elective splenectomy, since the group of mice given the vaccine 7 d before splenectomy had a cumulative mortality that was not significantly different from the group of vaccinated normal mice.

Vaccination with polysaccharide antigen preparations should be accomplished as early as possible, at the latest 1–2 wk prior to elective splenectomy. However, if vaccination is not achieved before splenectomy, there will still be a humoral response with later administration. The serum antibody response will be poor, if the vaccine is administered earlier than the age of 2 years whether or not a normal spleen is present, and if administered after chemotherapy and splenic irradiation. Lower antibody levels, compared to controls, were also found in children who had undergone bone marrow transplantation at least 1 year previously, prior to immunization with the 23-valent pneumococcal vaccine (Lortan et al., 1992). Splenectomy and the presence of chronic graft-vs-host disease did not make a significant difference. Although it is apparent from the literature that type specific serum antibody should improve hepatic macrophage clearance of bacteremia, the literature does contain reports of cases in which pneumococcal vaccine has been unsuccessful in preventing serious infection with vaccine serotypes (Brivet et al., 1984; Evans, 1984; Giebink et al., 1979; Sumaya et al., 1981; Forrester et al., 1987; Fine et al., 1994). Butler et al. (1994) note reduced pneumococcal vaccine efficacy in patients with lymphoma and leukemia, but the number of test subjects in the study was admittedly low. Fedson et al. (1994) suggest that analysis of the effectiveness of the pneumococcal vaccine should not be limited to its ability to limit invasive disease, but also in terms of health care dollars saved and the potential reduction of cases of invasive disease in the general population comparable to the effect of the Hib vaccine. Gable et al. (1990) calculate that $141 (U.S. dollars) would be saved per person vaccinated. Further research is needed in this area.

Recently, a specific defect in the antipneumococcal polysaccharide antibody response has been described, related to immunoglobulin isotype deficiency (Ohga et al., 1995; Sanders et al., 1993; Sanders et al., 1995). In view of the role of the spleen in immunoglobulin production, the relationship of this defect to hyposplenism and diseases of the spleen, such as lymphoma, deserves detailed evaluation.

11.7.2. ANTIBIOTIC PROPHYLAXIS   As yet, no large series or controlled study has effectively demonstrated penicillin prophylaxis to be effective in the prevention of overwhelming postsplenectomy infections. However, there are several recommendations in the literature to the effect that oral penicillin should be given, at least during the first 2 years after splenectomy, and particularly in children. Whether amoxicillin or trimethoprim-sulfamethoxazole should be used, instead, for their activity against *H. influenzae*, particularly in children under the age of 5 years, has likewise not been definitively studied. An alternative to oral penicillin prophylaxis is depot-penicillin injection on a monthly basis (Case records, 1983; Dickerman, 1979; Francke and Neu, 1981; Sherman, 1981). Trimethoprim-sulfamethoxazole or erythromycin prophylaxis have been recommended as a substitute for patients allergic to penicillin. However, there are a number of disadvantages to prophylactic penicillin administration, including noncompliance by patients, uncertainty with respect to dosage, failure to achieve activity against all the organisms commonly responsible for overwhelming postsplenectomy infections, and induction of penicillin-resistant pneumococcal strains in patients taking this antibiotic. Cases of overwhelming pneumococcal infection have been reported in asplenic patients taking penicillin, and these have led to further uncertainty regarding the efficacy of chronic penicillin prophylaxis (Brivet et al., 1984; Evans, 1984). Zarrabi and Rosner (1986) reviewed 14 reported cases of postsplenectomy sepsis in patients who regularly took penicillin prophylaxis. All but one were less than 17-years old, and splenectomy had been performed for various indications, including Hodgkin's disease in nine patients. In six patients, the sepsis was caused by bacteria other than the pneumococcus. However, those authors concluded that failure of penicillin prophylaxis is, in fact, rare.

Nevertheless, there are additional reasons for questioning the usefulness of prolonged oral penicillin prophylaxis, of which the principal one is the potential for poor compliance. Buchanan et al. (1982) studied compliance with an oral penicillin prophylactic regimen in patients splenectomized for miscellaneous conditions, and in a group with homozygous sickle cell anemia. Compliance was monitored by testing for the presence of penicillin in urine; in these two groups, 72 and 64%, respectively, of the urine samples collected showed the presence of penicillin. Those authors felt that compliance tended to improve after reinforcement of the recommendations during follow-up clinic visits. Borgna-Pignatti et al. (1984) found a similar rate of compliance with penicillin prophylaxis in splenectomized thalassemics (79%).

Scher et al. (1983) investigated the effect of penicillin administered to splenectomized rats 1 h prior to intraperitoneal injection of *S. pneumoniae* type 3. Sham-operated control rats, and animals that were splenectomized and given pneumococcal vaccine 2 wk after splenectomy, were both protected significantly better than other groups of rats in the study. The resolution of bacteremia was significantly better in these two groups than in rats in which the only intervention was splenectomy, splenectomized rats given 5000 U of penicillin, and splenectomized rats given 300,000 U penicillin, 1 h prior to the challenge with pneumococci. This suggests that the effectiveness of penicillin prophylaxis may be significantly less than has previously been suggested.

The value of oral penicillin prophylaxis in the splenectomized patient remains controversial. Prophylaxis may be most efficacious in childhood and during the first 2 years following splenectomy. An alternative approach to the use of prolonged oral antibiotic prophylaxis is the institution of therapeutic antibiotics, parenterally, at the first sign of febrile illness. Sherman (1981) has recommended that all splenectomized patients should have penicillin available for oral administration at the time of onset of febrile illness, and that these patients should be promptly evaluated by a physician for any illness accompanied by a temperature greater than 102°F.

11.7.3. PROTECTING THE HYPOSPLENIC PATIENT The patient whose splenic function is not intact requires the implementation of protective strategies. The Working Party of the British Committee for Standards in Hematology Clinical Haematology Task Force have developed the most comprehensive guidelines (1996). Their position paper categorizes patients into those with operative splenectomy, functional hyposplenism, and bone marrow transplant recipients. They emphasize that asplenic children under the age of 5 yr have an infection rate 10×that of adults (10%).

Pneumococcal and Hib immunizations should be routinely administered. When the spleen is removed secondarily to trauma, pneumococcal vaccination should be given after surgery and before discharge to home. If elective splenectomy is scheduled, the pneumococcal vaccine should be administered at least 2 wk prior to the surgery. The meningococcal immunization is provided to those who are at risk of exposure to A, C, Y, or W-135 serogroups, usually encountered when traveling. Because serogroup B is still the more common type of meningococcal infection in both Britain and the United States, the vaccine is of limited utility for routine use. The influenza vaccine may be of value, if, by its administration, a postviral bacterial infection might be prevented. Finally, the patient should be offered lifelong antibiotic prophylaxis with penicillin or amoxicillin, with emphasis on coverage for patients in the first 2 years after splenectomy, for children up to age 16 yr, and for those who have other underlying immunosuppression. Travelers should take chemopropylaxis against malaria, and receive instruction on minimizing contact with mosquitoes. Patients should carry a card or wear a bracelet indicating their hyposplenic state.

If infection is suspected, medical attention should be sought immediately, and antibiotic therapy instituted, with appropriate coverage for pneumococcal, meningococcal, and *H. influenzae* bacteria. The choice of antibiotic should be based on the likelihood of encountering resistance, especially with *S. pneumoniae*.

The Advisory Committee on Immunization Practices (1993) recommends the polyvalent pneumococcal vaccine, if ≥2 years of age, with revaccination at 3–5 years if aged ≤10 yr at the time of reimmunization. There is a similar recommendation for the quadrivalent polysaccharide meningococcal vaccine, but revaccination is not required. Immunization with the Hib vaccine should be given in infancy, as for the schedule for healthy children. It can be considered for use in asplenic adults.

The American College of Physicians' *Guide for Adult Immunization* (1994) advises reimmunization with the 23 polyvalent pneumococcal vaccine for subjects previously immunized with the 14 polyvalent vaccine, and readministering the vaccine every 6 years. The Hib and meningococcal vaccines may be considered. The *Guide* also emphasizes the importance of antimalarial prophylaxis for travelers to endemic areas. The formulations of vaccines and indications for immunization change, because of developments in vaccine technology, change in epidemiology of an infection, and new data in long-term efficacy. There are several resources that are updated frequently; Thompson (1997) revises a practical guide to immunizations annually.

Williams and Kaur (1996) have reviewed postsplenectomy care briefly. There are two excellent reviews by Styrt (1996) and Brozovic (1994) on this subject, which emphasize the importance of antibiotic prophylaxis in children. Lane (1995) reviews the controversies of immunization and antibiotic prophylaxis in asplenic children. Often, the meningococcal vaccine is not administered, although the American Academy of Pediatrics does recommend this immunization. Although many pediatricians prescribe prophylactic antibiotics, others have their patients keep a supply of an antibiotic on hand, to be administered at the first sign of febrile illness.

Prophylaxis in the bone marrow transplant recipient with sple-nectomy includes not only the polyvalent pneumococcal, Hib, and quadrivalent meningococcal immunizations, preferably adminis-tered prior to splenectomy, but also prophylaxis against *Pneumo-cystis carinii* pneumonia and CMV infection (if seropositive for CMV) (Fielding, 1994). A subpopulation at greater risk, given the decreased ability to regain full immune function, are those recipi-ents who develop chronic graft-vs-host disease.

At the present time, asplenic and hyposplenic patients fre-quently do not receive prophylaxis. A survey of medical microbi-ologists in Britain yielded 42 cases of patients with splenectomy over a 2-year period, with a mortality of 45%, caused by OPSI, and only a 20% rate of administration of chemoprophylaxis (Waghorn and Mayon-White, 1997). In a series of 184 patients splenectomized over a 12-year period, only 36% had received the pneumococcal vaccine, and only 42% received prophylaxis or advice regarding infection (Deodhar et al., 1993). In a questionnaire sent to 160 hospital doctors (HDs) and 200 general practitioners (GPs), of which 118 were completed and returned (43% HDs and 25% GPs), 98% were aware of the risk of pneumococcal infection, but only 49% of HDs and 33% of GPs appreciated the increased likelihood of infection secondary to *N. meningitidis* or malaria in splenecto-mized patients (Palejwala et al., 1996). Almost three-fourths of HDs and a little over half of GPs recognized the threat of *H. influ-enzae* in this population. There was knowledge about antibiotic prophylaxis, but only 14% of GPs and 49% of HDs knew of the recommendation for lifelong antibiotic prophylaxis.

Physicians seem to have difficulty in their performance of rel-evant preventive health measures. Although physicians suggest that paucity of time is the problem, Kottke et al. (1993) have ob-served the following effectively limiting implementation of such strategies:

1. Although the ability of physicians to make apparently arbi-trary decisions conveys a sense of independence, the health care system limits their flexibility of behavior.
2. Issues of public health do not compel action in the clinical setting.
3. The health care system prioritizes urgency over severity.
4. Time constraints and patient demand encourage physicians in clinical settings to be respondents, not initiators.
5. Preventive services do not correspond to physicians' images of their work and themselves.
6. The feedback naturally generated from prescribing preven-tive services is primarily negative.
7. Clinicians cannot provide preventive services without ad-equate resources.

Therefore, there is the logical suggestion of developing compu-ter-accessible guidelines and lists of patients subrogated in a public health district (Sarangi et al., 1997). Further analysis is required to determine the effectiveness of this approach.

11.7.4. PRESERVATION OF SPLENIC TISSUE Preservation of splenic tissue by partial (instead of total) splenectomy, splenic autotransplants, or by ectopic splenic tissue may also preserve some aspects of splenic function (*see also* Chapters 10 and 17). Traub et al. (1987) reported that reticuloendothelial function (measured as the mean percentage of pocked erythrocytes and the clearance of antibody-coated autologous erythrocytes) was better preserved after partial splenectomy and splenic repair, than after splenic auto-transplantation, but that autotransplantation was superior to total

splenectomy in a series of 51 patients who had initially presented with abdominal trauma and suspected splenic rupture. However, there is evidence that the presence of splenic tissue is not in itself a guarantee of efficient splenic function (Sass et al., 1983). Preser-vation of the splenic artery and normal splenic architecture appear to be of great importance to the maintenance of effective splenic function; this is shown by cases of fatal pneumococcal septicemia occurring after splenectomy for trauma, in patients found at autopsy to have numerous nodules of splenic tissue present in the perito-neal cavity (Rice and James, 1980).

Animal studies have been used to test various methods of pre-serving splenic function. Livingston et al. (1983) challenged rats with a transtracheal inoculation of *S. pneumoniae* type 3, after one of the following procedures: sham operation, splenectomy with splenic implants within the mesentery or portal vein splenic auto-transplantation, and splenectomy without transplantation of splenic tissue to other sites. Pneumococcal challenge was administered 12 wk after the splenectomy: It was found that rats submitted to sham operation had a significantly lower mortality rate than did rats that were splenectomized, with or without subsequent portal vein splenic autotransplants. The rats with mesenteric splenic autotrans-plants, however, had a mortality rate similar to that of sham-oper-ated rats, showing that this type of splenic implant may have been protective. It was therefore suggested that peritoneal implants after trauma in humans may result in a lower rate of post-splenectomy sepsis for this particular group. However, Schwartz et al. (1978) found that autotransplantation of macerated splenic tissue into the peritoneal cavity of splenectomized rats did not significantly pro-tect these animals from iv challenge with *S. pneumoniae* type 25. The LD_{50} for the autotransplanted rats and for asplenic rats was less than 4×10^3 colony-forming units of bacteria, and all the animals in these two groups died. The LD_{50} for the control sham-operated rats was 8×10^6 colony-forming units, and none of the rats receiving 4×10^5 colony-forming units in this group of controls died as a result of the iv pneumococcal challenge. Thus, there remains some controversy regarding the effectiveness of the re-sidual function of small peritoneal splenic implants.

Alwark et al. (1983) found that rats with a partial (67%) splenic resection had a lower mortality rate, when challenged with *S. pne-umoniae* type 1 intravenously, than did rats that were splenecto-mized, and subsequently had splenic tissue implanted either subcu-taneously or into the omentum, or had dispersed splenic tissue injected subcutaneously, intramuscularly, or retroperitoneally. They found that there was a lesser degree of splenic tissue regeneration in those animals that were injected with dispersed splenic tissue than in those in which pieces of splenic tissue were implanted. This suggested that preservation of the splenic microarchitecture is im-portant for tissue regeneration. In addition, they found that rats with pieces of splenic tissue reimplanted had a significantly longer median survival than rats with reimplantation of dispersed splenic tissue. Steely et al. (1987) reported a decrease in the incidence of septic death following pneumococcal iv challenge, in rats that underwent splenectomy and omental splenic autotransplantation, partial splenectomy, or sham operation, compared with those ani-mals that underwent total splenectomy. Diminished mortality was inversely proportional to, and the incidence of *S. pneumoniae* bac-teremia was parallel to, the amount of splenic remnant present in the respective groups of rats. Van Wyck et al. (1986) found that subtotal splenic resection, with preservation of blood flow and the segmental anatomy of the spleen, resulted in better survival in the face of pneumococcal challenge, than occurred in rats subjected to total splenectomy and splenic autografting.

From this work with animal models, preservation of a portion of the spleen, preferably with arterial structures and splenic architecture intact, appears to be desirable, whenever practicable, in the treatment of patients requiring splenic resection. Indeed, Boles et al. (1978) have reported encouraging results with respect to partial splenectomy during staging laparotomy of patients with Hodgkin's disease and found no evidence that evaluation of splenic involvement was compromised. There is still a pressing need for further data, to assess the indications for partial splenectomy in this and other hematological diseases, and to partial splenectomy and repair of the spleen (splenorrhaphy) in other situations, such as splenic rupture and lacerations, commonly treated by total splenectomy (Werbin and Lodha, 1982). There is an increasing trend toward both nonoperative management and splenorrhaphy in surgical centers around the world (Jalovec et al., 1993; Mustafa, 1994; Van Etten et al., 1995; Garber, 1996). Regional trends are not known, and clinical pathways in use recognize both operative and observational management, initially. A statewide trauma center review found that 1255 patients sustained identifiable splenic injury (Clancy et al., 1997). There was a decline in splenectomies, and greater than half of the patients either were managed nonoperatively (40%) or surgically with splenorrhaphy (12%). The geriatric population (aged ≥65 yr) required greater resources and experienced a greater rate of mortality than younger patients; there was no correlation to the mechanism of injury, or by chosen management. The overall mortality rate was 13%.

The overall trend in splenic preservation is encouraging, and lends optimism that the occurrence of OPSI might be diminished or prevented. Research should be directed to determine the optimal course of treatment for specific presentations of splenic injury. Noninvasive diagnostic modalities, such as computerized tomography, may play an important adjunctive role (Gavant et al., 1997). Further discussion of the surgical approach is given in Chapter 17.

ACKNOWLEDGMENTS

The authors thank Susan Zawodniak for her help in research, and also thank Sherry Puckett for her secretarial services.

REFERENCES

Addiego, J. E. Jr., Ammann, A. J., Schiffman, G., Baehner, R., Higgins, G., and Hammond, D. (1980) Response to pneumococcal polysaccharide vaccine in patients with untreated Hodgkin's disease. *Lancet* ii, 450–453.
Alder, S. P. (1983) Transfusion-associated cytomegalovirus infections. *Rev. Infect. Dis.* **5**, 977–993.
Alwmark, A, Bengmark, S., Gullstrand, P., Idvall, I., and Schalen, C. (1983) Splenic resection or heterotopic transplantation of splenic tissue as alternatives to splenectomy. Regeneration and protective effect against pneumococcal septicemia. *Eur. Surg. Res.* **15**, 217–222.
American College of Physicians' Task Force on Adult Immunization and Infectious Diseases Society of America (1994) *Guide for Adult Immunization*. American College of Physicians, Philadelphia.
Ammann, A. J., Addiego, J., Wara, D. W., Lubin, B., Smith, W. B., and Mentzer, W. C. (1977) Polyvalent pneumococcal-polysaccharide immunization of patients with sickle-cell anemia and patients with splenectomy. *N. Engl. J. Med.* **297**, 897–900.
Askergren, J. and Björkholm, M. (1980) Post-splenectomy septicaemia in Hodgkin's disease and other disorders. *Acta Chir. Scand.* **146**, 569–575.

Athanasios, G., Kaditis, M., O'Marciagh, A., Hable Rhodes, K., Weaver, A., and Henry, N. (1996) Yield of positive blood cultures in pediatric oncology patients by a new method of blood culture collection. *Pediatr. Infect. Dis. J.* **15**, 615–620.
Austin, T. W., Sargeant, H. L., and Warwick, O. H. (1980) Fulminant gonococcaemia after splenectomy. *Can. Med. Assoc. J.* **123**, 195–196.
Barbour, A. G., Krueger, G. G., Feorino, P. M., and Smith, C. B. (1979) Kawasaki-like disease in a young adult: association with primary Epstein-Barr virus infection. *JAMA* **241**, 397–398.
Barbour, M. L. (1996) Conjugate vaccines and the carriage of haemophilus influenzae type b. *Emerg. Infect. Dis.* **2**, 176–182.
Barrett-Connor, E. (1971) Bacterial infection and sickle cell anemia. An analysis of 250 infections in 166 patients and review of the literature. *Medicine* **50**, 97–112.
Baumgartner, J. D., Glauser, M. P., Burgo-Black, A. L., Black, R. D., Pyndiah, N., and Chiolero, R. (1982) Severe cytomegalovirus infection in multiple transfused, splenectomised, trauma patients. *Lancet* **ii**, 63–66.
Bisno, A. L. and Freeman, J. C. (1970) The syndrome of asplenia, pneumococcal sepsis, and disseminated intravascular coagulation. *Ann. Intern. Med.* **72**, 389–393.
Bobo, R. A. and Newton, E. J. (1976) A previously undescribed gram-negative bacillus causing septicemia and meningitis. *Am. J. Clin. Pathol.* **65**, 564–569.
Boles, E. T. Jr., Haase, G. M., and Hamoudi, A. B. (1978) Partial splenectomy in staging laparotomy for Hodgkin's disease: An alternative approach. *J. Pediatr. Surg.* **13**, 581–586.
Boone, K. E. and Watter, D. A. K. (1995) The incidence of malaria after splenectomy in Papua New Guinea. *Br. Med. J.* **311**, 1273.
Borgna-Pignatti, C., De Stefano, P., Barone, F., and Concia, E. (1984) Penicillin compliance in splenectomised thalassemics. *Eur. J. Pediatr.* **142**, 83–85.
Bourgault, A. M., Van Scoy, R. E., Wilkowske, C. J., and Sterioff, S. (1979) Severe infection due to *Streptococcus pneumoniae* in asplenic renal transplant patients. *Mayo Clin. Proc.* **54**, 123–126.
Boustani, M. A. and Gelfand, J. A. (1996) Babesiosis. *Clin. Infect. Dis.* **22**, 611–615.
Brivet, F., Herer, B., Fremaux, A., Dormont, J., and Tchernia, G. (1984) Fatal post-splenectomy pneumococcal sepsis despite pneumococcal vaccine and penicillin prophylaxis. *Lancet* **ii**, 356–357.
Brown, E. J., Hosea, S. W., and Frank. M. M. (1983) The role of antibody and complement in the reticuloendothelial clearance of pneumococci from the bloodstream. *Rev. Infect. Dis.* **5(Suppl.)**, S797–S805.
Brozovic, M. (1994) Infection in non-malignant haematological disease and splenic dysfunction. *Curr. Opin. Infect. Dis.* **7**, 450–455.
Buchanan, G. R., Siegel, J. D., Smith, S. J., and DePasse, B. M. (1982) Oral penicillin prophylaxis in children with impaired splenic function: a study of compliance. *Pediatrics* **9**, 926–930.
Butler, J. C., Breiman, R. F., Campbel, J. F., Lipman, H. B., Broome, C. V., and Facklam, R. R. (1993) Pneumococcal polysaccharide vaccine efficacy, an evaluation of current recommendations. *JAMA* **270**, 1826–1831.
Buchanan, G. R., Smith, S. J., Holtkamp, C. A., and Fuseler, J. P. (1983) Bacterial infection and splenic reticuloendothelial function in children with hemoglobin SC disease. *Pediatrics* **72**, 93–98.
Cartwright, K. A. (1992) Vaccination against haemophilus influenzae b disease. *Br. Med. J.* **205**, 485,486.
Case Records of the Massachusetts General Hospital, Case 20-1983. (1983) *N. Engl. J. Med.* **308**, 1212–1218.
Centers for Disease Control (1996) Serogroup Y meningococcal disease: Illinois, Connecticut, and selected areas, United States. *MMWR* **45**, 1010–1013.
Centers for Disease Control (1996) H. influenzae type b disease: U.S. *MMWR* **45**, 901–906.
Centers for Disease Control (1993) Recommendations of the Advisory Committee on Immunization Practices (ACIP): Use of vaccines and immune globulins in persons with altered immunocompetence. *MMWR* **42**, 4,8.
Centers for Disease Control (1988) Recommendations of the Immunization Practices Advisory Committee (ACIP). Update: prevention of *Haemophilus influenzae* type b disease. *MMWR* **37**, 13–16.

Chaikof, E. L. and McCabe, C. J. (1985) Fatal overwhelming postsplenectomy infection. *Am. J. Surg.* **149**, 534–539.

Chen, T. and Moxon, E. R. (1983) Effect of splenic congestion associated with hemolytic anemia on mortality of rats challenged with *Haemophilus influenzae* b. *Am. J. Hematol.* **15**, 117–121.

Chilcote, R. R., Baehner, R. L., and Hammond, D. (1976) Septicemia and meningitis in children splenectomized for Hodgkin's disease. *N. Engl. J. Med.* **295**, 798–800.

Children's Hospital and the University of Colorado School of Medicine. (1995) The spleen in children. *Curr. Opin. Pediatr.* **7**, 36–41.

Clancy, T. V., Ramshaw, D. G., Maxwell, J. G., Covington, D. L., Churchill, M. P, Rutledge, R. et al. (1997) Management outcomes in splenic injury: a statewide trauma center review. *Ann. Surg.* **226**, 17–24.

Coleman, C. N., McDougall, I. R., Dailey, M. O., Ager, P., Bush, S., and Kaplan, H. S. (1982) Functional hyposplenia after splenic irradiation for Hodgkin's disease. *Ann. Intern. Med.* **96**, 44–47.

Coleman, R. M., Rencricca, N. J., Stout, J. P., Brissette, W. H., and Smith, D. M. (1975) Spenic mediated erythrocyte cytotoxicity in malaria. *Immunology* **29**, 49–54.

Curti, A. J., Lin, J. H., and Szabo, K. (1985) Over-whelming post-splenectomy infection with *Plesiomonas shigelloides* in a patient cured of Hodgkin's disease. *Am. J. Clin. Pathol.* **83**, 522–524.

Cuthbert, R. J., Iqbal, A., Gates, A., Toghill, P. J., and Russell, N. H. (1995) Functional hyposplenism following allogeneic bone marrow transplantation. *J. Clin. Pathol.* **48**, 257–259.

Daily, M. O., Coleman, C. N., and Kaplan, H. S. (1980) Radiation-induced splenic atrophy in patients with Hodgkin's lymphomas. *N. Engl. J. Med.* **302**, 215–217.

Dammin, G. J., Spielman, A., Benach, J. L., and Piesman, J. (1981) The rising incidence of clinical *Babesia microti* infection. *Hum. Pathol.* **12**, 398–400.

Deodhar, H. A., Marshall, R. J., and Barnes, J. N. (1993) Increased risk of sepsis after splenectomy. *Br. Med. J.* **307**, 1408–1409.

Dickerman, J. D. (1979) Splenectomy and sepsis: a warning. *Pediatrics* **63**, 938–941.

Dwyer, D. E. and Kesson, A. M. (1997) Advances in antiviral therapy. *Curr. Opin. Pediatr.* **1**, 24–30.

Ehrbar, H., Gubler, J., Harbarth, S., and Hirschel, B., (1996) Caphocytophaga canimorsus sepsis complicated by myocardial infarction in two patients with normal coronary arteries. *Clin. Infect. Dis.* **23**, 335,336.

Eichner, E. R. (1979) Splenic function: normal, too much and too little. *Am. J. Med.* **66**, 311–320.

Eraklis, A. J., Kevy, S. V., Diamond, L. K., and Gross, R. E. (1967) Hazard of overwhelming infection after splenectomy in childhood. *N. Engl. J. Med.* **276**, 1225–1229.

Evans, D. I. K. (1984) Fatal post-splenectomy sepsis despite prophylaxis with penicillin and pneumococcal vaccine. *Lancet* **i**, 1124.

Farhi, D. C. and Ashfaq, R. (1995) Splenic pathology after traumatic injury. *Am. J. Clin. Pathol.* **105**, 474–477.

Fedson, D. S., Shapiro, E. D., Laforce, F. M., et al. (1994) Pneumococcal vaccine after fifteen years of use. *Arch. Intern. Med.* **154** 2531–2535.

Fielding, A. K. (1994) Prophylaxis against late infection following splenectomy and bone marrow transplant. *Blood Rev.* **3**, 179–191.

Fine, M. J., Smith, M. A., Carson, C. A., Meffe, F., Sankey, S. S., Weissfeld, L. A., Detsky, A. S., Kapoor, W. N. (1994) Efficacy of pneumococcal vaccination in adults; a meta-analysis of randomized controlled trials. *Arch. Intern. Med.* **154**, 2666–2677.

Forrester, H. L., Jahnigen, D. W., and Laforce, F. M. (1987) Inefficacy of pneumococcal vaccine in a high-risk population. *Am. J. Med.* **83**, 425–430.

Foss Abrahamsen, A., Hoiby, E. A., Hannisdal, E., et al. (1997) Systemic pneumococcal disease after staging splenectomy for Hodgkin's disease in 1969-1980 without pneumococcal vaccine protection: a follow-up study *1994. Eur. J. Haematol.* **58**, 73–77.

Foster, K. J., Devitt, N., Gallagher, P. J., and Abbott, R. M. (1982) Overwhelming pneumococcal septicaemia in a patient with ulcerative colitis and splenic atrophy. *Gut* **23**, 630–632.

Foster P. N., Hardy, G. J., and Losowsky, M. S. (1984) Fatal salmonella septicaemia in a patient with systemic lupus erythematosus and splenic atrophy. *Br. J. Clin. Pract.* **38**, 434–435.

Francke, E. L. and Neu, H. C. (1981) Post-splenectomy infection. *Surg. Clin. North Am.* **61**, 135–155.

Freeman, H. J. (1996) Functional asplenia and microscopic (collagenous) colitis. *Can. J. Gastroenterol.* **19**, 443–436.

Gable, C. B., Holzer, S. S., Engelhart, L., Friedman, R. B., Smeltz, F., Schroeder, D., and Baum, K. (1990) Pneumococcal vaccine: efficacy and associated cost savings. *JAMA* **264**, 2910–2915.

Garber, B. G., Yelle, J. D., Fairfull-Smith, R., Lorimer, J. W., and Carson, C. (1996) Management of splenic injuries in a Canadian trauma centre. *Can. J. Surg.* **39**, 474–480.

Gavant, M. L., Schurr, M., Flick, P. A., Croce, M. A., Fabian, T. C., and Gold, R. E. (1997) Predicting clinical outcome of non-surgical management of blunt splenic injury: using CT to reveal abnormalities of splenic vasculature. *Am. J. Roentgenol.* **168**, 207–212.

Giebink, G. S., Schiffman, G., Krivit, W., and Quie, P. G. (1979) Vaccine-type pneumococcal pneumonia. Occurrence after vaccination in an asplenic patient. *JAMA* **241**, 2736,2737.

Gershon, A. A., LaRussa, P., Steinber, S., Mervish, N., Lo, S. H., and Meier, P. (1996) The protective effect of immunologic boosting against zoster: an analysis in leukemic children who were vaccinated against chickenpox. *J. Infect. Dis.* **173**, 450–453.

Giraud, T., Dhainaut, J. F., Schremmer, B., Regnier, B., Desjars, P., Loirat, P., Journois, D., and Lanore, J. J. (1991) Adult overwhelming meningococcal purpura. A study of 35 cases, 1977–1989. *Arch. Intern. Med.* **151**, 310–316.

Giraud, T., Jean-Francois, D., Schremmer, B., Regnier, B., Desjars, P., Loirat, P., Didier-Journois, and Lanore, J. (1991) Adult overwhelming meningococcal purpura; a study of 35 cases, 1977-1989. *Arch. Intern. Med.* **151**, 310–316.

Goffinet, D. R., Glatstein, E. J., and Merigan, T. C. (1972) Herpes zoster-varicella infections and lymphoma. *Ann. Intern. Med.* **76**, 256–240.

Granoff, D. M. Boies, E. G., and Munson, R. S. Jr. (1984) Immunogenicity of *Haemophilus influenzae* type b polysaccharide-diphtheria toxoid conjugate vaccine in adults. *J. Pediatr.* **105**, 22–27.

Green, D. M., Stutzman, L., Blumenson, L. E., Brecher, M. L., Thomas, P. R., Allen, J. E., Jewett, T. C., and Freeman, A. I. (1979) The incidence of post-splenectomy sepsis and herpes zoster in children and adolescents with Hodgkin disease. *Med. Pediatr. Oncol.* **7**, 285–297.

Green, J. B., Shackford, S. R., Sise, M. J., and Fridlund, P. (1986) Late septic complications in adults following splenectomy for trauma: a prospective analysis in 144 patients. *J. Trauma* **26**, 999–1003.

Guertler, A. T. and Carter, C. T. (1996) Fatal pneumococcal septicemia in a patient with a connective tissue disease. *J. Emerg. Med.* **14**, 33–38.

Guinee, V. F., Guido, J. J., Pfalzgraf, K. A., Giacco, G. G., Lagarde, C., Durand, M., et al. (1985) The incidence of herpes zoster in patients with Hodgkin's disease. An analysis of prognostic factors. *Cancer* **56**, 642–648.

Hamilton, D. R. and Pikacha, D. (1982) Ruptured spleen in a malarious area: with emphasis on conservative management in both adults and children. *Aust. NZ J. Surg.* **52**, 310–313.

Heath, T. C., Hewitt, M. C., Jalaludin, B., Roberts, C., Capon, A. G., Jelfs, P., and Gilbert, G., (1997) Invasive haemophilus influenzae type b disease in elderly nursing home residents: two related cases. *Emerg. Infect. Dis.* **3**, 179–182.

Herbert J. C., et al. (1983) Lack of protection by pneumococcal vaccine after splenectomy in mice challenged with aerosolized pneumococci. *J. Trauma* **23**, 1–6.

Herwaldt, B. L., Persing, D. H., Precigout, E. A., et al. (1996) A fatal case of babesiosis in Missouri: identification of another piroplasm that infects humans. *Ann. Intern. Med.* **124**, 643–650.

Heier, H. E. (1980) Splenectomy and serious infections. *Scand. J. Haematol.* **24**, 5–12.

Hicklin, H., Verghese, A., and Alvarez, S. (1987) Dysgonic fermenter 2 septicemia. *Rev. Infect. Dis.* **9**, 884–890.

Hitzig, W. H. (1985) Immunological and hematological consequences of deficient function of the spleen. *Prog. Pediatr. Surg.* **18**, 132–138.

Holmes, B., Pickett, M. J., and Hollis, D. (1995) Unusual gram-negative bacteria, including capnocytophaga, eikenella, pasteurella, and streptobacillus. *Manual Clin. Microbiol.* 499–508.

Holmes, F. F., Weyandt, T., Glazier, J., Cuppage, F. E., Moral, L. A., and Lindsey, N. J. (1981) Fulminant meningococcemia after splenectomy. *JAMA* **246,** 1119,1120.

Horan, M. and Colebatch, F. H. (1962) Relation between splenectomy and subsequent infection. A clinical study. *Arch. Dis. Child.* **37,** 398–414.

Hosea, S. W. (1983) Role of the spleen in pneumococcal infection. *Lymphology* **16,** 115–120.

Hosea, S. W., Brown, E. J., Hamburger, M. I., and Frank, M. M. (1981a) Opsonic requirements for intravascular clearance after splenectomy. *N. Engl. J. Med.* **304,** 245–250.

Hosea, S. W., Burch, C. G., Brown, E. J., Berg, R. A., and Frank, M. M. (1981b) Impaired immune response of splenectomised patients to polyvalent pneumococcal vaccine. *Lancet* **i,** 804–807.

Israeli, A., Shapiro, M., and Ephros, M. A. (1987) *Plasmodium falciparum* malaria in an aplenic man. *Trans. R. Soc. Trop. Med. Hyg.* **81,** 233–234.

Istre, G. R., Tarpay, M., Anderson, M., Pryor, A., and Welch, D. (1987) Invasive disease due to *Streptococcus pneumoniae* in an area with a high rate of relative penicillin resistance. *J. Infect. Dis.* **156,** 732–735.

Jackson, N., Zaki, M., Rahman, A. R., Nazime, M., Win, M. N., and Osman, S. (1997) Fatal campylobacter jejuni infection in a patient splenectomised for thalassaemia. *J. Clin. Pathol.* **50,** 436–437.

Johnston, R. B. Jr., Newman, S., and Struth, A. G. (1973) An abnormality of the alternative pathway of complement activation in sickle-cell disease. *N. Engl. J. Med.* **288,** 803–808.

Jones, J. F., Stutz, F. H., Manuele, V. J., and Allen, R. G. (1975) Atypical rubeola infection after splenectomy. *N. Engl. J. Med.* **292,** 111,112.

Jones, J. M., Amsbaugh, D. F., and Prescott, B. (1976) Kinetics of the antibody response to type III pneumococcal polysaccharide. II. Factors influencing the serum antibody levels after immunization with an optimally immunogenic dose of antigen. *J. Immunol.* **116,** 52–64.

Jalovec, L. M., Boe, B. S., and Wyffels, P. L. (1993) The advantages of early operation with splenorrhaphy versus non-operative management for the blunt splenic trauma patient. *Am. Surg.* **59,** 698–704.

Kalb, R., Kaplan, M. H., Tenenbaum, M. J., Joachim, G. R., and Samuels, S. (1985) Cutaneous infection of dog bite wounds associated with fulminant DF-2 septicemia. *Am. J. Med.* **78,** 697–690.

Katzenstein, D. A., Yu, G. S. M., and Jordan, M. C. (1983) Lethal infection with murine cytomegalovirus after early viral replication in the spleen. *J. Infect. Dis.* **148,** 406–411.

Kim, J. O., Ginsberg, J., and McGowan, K. L. (1996) Capnocytophaga meningitis in a cancer patient. *Ped. Infect. Dis. J.* **15,** 636,637.

King, H. and Shumacker, H. B. Jr. (1952) Splenic studies I. Susceptibility to infection after splenectomy performed in infancy. *Ann. Surg.* **136,** 239–242.

Kingston, M. E. and MacKenzie, C. R. (1979) The syndrome of pneumococcaemia, disseminated intravascular coagulation and asplenia. *Can. Med. Assoc. J.* **121,** 57–61.

Kinnunen, U., Syrjala, H., Koskela, M., Kujala, P., and Koistinen, P. (1996) Continuous monitoring blood culture screening system improves the detection of bacteraemia in neutropenic patients. *Scand. J. Infect. Dis.* **28,** 287–292.

Klein, P., McMeeking, A. A., and Goldenberg, A. (1997) Babesiosis in a patient with sickle cell anemia. *Am. J. Med.* **102,** 416.

Kottke, T. E., Brekke, M. L., and Solberg, L. I. (1993) Making "time" for preventive services. *Mayo Clin. Proc.* **68,** 785–791.

Krivit, W. (1977) Overwhelming postsplenectomy infection. *Am. J. Hematol.* **2,** 193–201.

Kullberg, B. J., Westendorp, R. G., van't Wout, J. W., and Meinders, A. E. (1991) Purpura fulminans and symmetrical peripheral gangrene caused by Capnocytophaga canimorsus (formerly DF-2) septicemia: a complication of dog bite. *Medicine* **70,** 287–292.

Langenhuijsen, M. M. A. C. and van Toorn, D. W. (1982) Splenectomy and the severity of cytomegalovirus infection. *Lancet* **ii,** 820.

Leggiadro, R. J. (1997) The clinical impact of resistance in the management of pneumococcal disease. *Antimicrob. Resistance* **11,** 867–874.

Leopow, M. L., Samuelson, J. S., and Gordon, L. K. (1984) Safety and immunogenicity of *Haemophilus influenzae* type b polysaccharide-diphtheria toxoid conjugate vaccine in adults. *J. Infect. Dis.* **150,** 402–406.

Levin, M. J. and Hayward, A. R. (1996) The varicella vaccine. Prevention of herpes zoster. *Infect. Dis. Clin. North Am.* **10,** 657–675.

Lindquist, S. W., Weber, D. J., Mangum, M. E., Hollis, D. G., and Jordan, J. (1995) *Bordetella holmesii* sepsis in an asplenic adolescent. *Pediatr. Infect. Dis. J.* **14,** 813–815.

Liote, F, Angle, J., Gilmore, N., and Osterland, C. K. (1995) Asplenism and systemic lupus erythematosus. *Clin. Rheumatol.* **2,** 220–223.

Littman, E. (1974) Splenectomy in hereditary spherocytosis: effect on course of relapsing vivax malaria. *Am. J. Med. Sci.* **267,** 53–56.

Livingston, C. D., Levine, B. A., and Sirinek, K. R. (1983) Improved survival rate for intraperitoneal autotransplantation of the spleen following pneumococcal pneumonia. *Surg. Gynecol. Obstet.* **156,** 761–766.

Llende, M., Santiago-Delpín, E. A., and Lavergne, J. (1986) Immunobiological consequences of splenectomy: a review. *J. Surg. Res.* **40,** 85–94.

Loggie, B. W. and Hinchey, J. (1986) Does splenectomy predispose to meningococcal sepsis? an experimental study and clinical review. *J. Pediatr. Surg.* **21,** 326–330.

Looareesuwan, S., Ho, M., and Wattanagoon, Y., White, N. J., Warrell, D. A., Bunnag, D., Harinasuta, T., and Wyler, D. J. (1987) Dynamic alteration in splenic function during acute falciparum malaria. *N. Engl. J. Med.* **317,** 675–679.

Looareesuwan, S., Suntharasamai, P., Webster, H. K., and Ho, M. (1993) Malaria in splenectomised patients: report of four cases and review. *Clin. Infect. Dis.* **16,** 361–366.

Lortan, J. E., Vellodi, A., Jurges, E. S., and Hugh-Jones, K. (1992) Class-and subclass- specific pneumococcal antibody levels and response to immunization after bone marrow transplantation. *Clin. Exp. Immunol.* **88,** 512–519.

Maehlen, J., Heger, B., and Rostrup, M. (1997) Splenic atrophy and fatal pneumococcal infection in inflammatory bowel disease. *Tidsskr. Nor. Laegeforen.* **117,** 1900–1901.

Martone, W. J., Zuehl, R. W., Minson, G. E., and Scheld, W. M. (1980) Post-splenectomy sepsis with DF-2: Report of a case with isolation of the organism from the patient's dog. *Ann. Intern. Med.* **93,** 457–458.

Meier, F. P., Waldvogel, F. A., and Zwahlen, A. (1985) Role of splenectomy in the pathogenesis of *Haemophilus influenzae* type f meningitis. *Eur. J. Clin. Microbiol.* **4,** 598–600.

Mermel, L. A. and Maki, D. G. (1993) Detection of bacteremia in adults: consequences of culturing an inadequate volume of blood. *Ann. Intern. Med.* **119,** 270–272.

Miller, L. H., Usami, S., and Chien, S. (1971) Alteration in the rheologic properties of *Plasmodium knowlesi*-infected red cells: a possible mechanism for capillary obstruction. *J. Clin. Invest.* **50,** 1451–1455.

Molrine, D. C., George, S., Tarbell, N., Mauch, P., Diller, L., Neuberg, D., et al. (1995) Antibody responses to polysaccharide and polysaccharide-conjugate vaccines after treatment of Hodgkin disease. *Ann. Intern. Med.* **123,** 828–834.

Monfardini, S., Bajetta, E., Arnold, C. A., Kenda, R., and Bonadonna, G. (1975) Herpes zoster-varicella infection in malignant lymphomas. Influence of splenectomy and intensive treatment. *Eur. J. Cancer.* **11,** 51–57.

Mossad, S. B., Lichtin, A. E., Hall, G. S., and Gordon, S. M. (1997) Photo quiz: *Capnocytophaga canimorsus* septicemia. *Clin. Infect. Dis.* **24,** 123 and 267.

Moxon, E. R., Goldthorn, J. F., and Schwartz, A. D. (1980) *Haemophilus influenzae* b infection in rats: effect of splenectomy on blood stream and meningeal invasion after intravenous and intranasal innoculations. *Infect. Immun.* **27,** 872–875.

Mufson, M. A. (1981) Pneumococcal infections. *JAMA* **246,** 1942–1948.

Musher, D. M. (1992) Infections caused by *Streptococcus pneumoniae*: clinical spectrum, pathogenesis, immunity, and treatment. *Clin. Infec. Dis.* **14,** 801–809.

Mustafa, N. A. (1994) Splenorrhaphy versus splenectomy. *Acta Chir. Hung.* **34,** 171–176.

Naraqi, S., Jackson, G. G., Jonasson, O., and Yamashiroya, H. M. (1977) Prospective study of prevalence, incidence and source of herpes virus infections in patients with renal allografts. *J. Infect. Dis.* **136,** 531–540.

Nooruddin, H. S. S. (1967) The effects of splenectomy on parasitic infections, and the role of the spleen in filariasis: a brief appraisal of our present knowledge. *J. Trop. Med. Hyg.* **70,** 229–232.

Norris, R. P., Vergis, E. N., and Yu, V. L. (1996) Overwhelming post-splenectomy infection: a critical review of etiologic pathogens and management. *Infect. Med.* **13,** 779–783.

Ohga, S., Okada, K., Asahi, T., Ueda, K., Sakiyama, Y., and Matsumoto, S. (1995) Recurrent pneumococcal meningitis in a patient with transient IgG subclass deficiency. *Acta Pediatr. Jpn.* **37,** 196–200.

Okun, D. B. and Tanaka, K. H. (1978) Profound leukemoid reaction in cytomegalovirus mononucleosis. *JAMA* **240,** 1888–1889.

Otsuji, E., Yamaguchi, T., Sawai, K., Okamoto, K., and Takahashi, T. (1997) End results of simultaneous pancreatectomy, splenectomy and total gastrectomy for patients with gastric carcinoma. *Br. J. Can.* **75,** 1219–1223.

Overturf, G. D., Powars, D., and Baroff, L. J. (1977) Bacterial meningitis and septicemia in sickle cell disease. *Am. J. Dis. Child.* **131,** 784–787.

Palejwala, A. A., Hong, L. Y., and King, D. (1996) Managing patients with an absent or dysfunctional spleen. Under half of doctors know that antibiotic prophylaxis should be life long. *Br. Med. J.* **312,** 1360.

Pearson, H. A., Johnston, D., Smith, K. A., and Touloukian, R. J. (1978) The born-again spleen. Return of splenic function after splenectomy for trauma. *N. Engl. J. Med.* **293,** 1890–1892.

Pers, C., Gahrn-Hansen, B., and Frederiksen, W. (1996) *Capnocytophaga canimorsus* septicemia in Denmark, 1982–1995: review of 39 cases. *Clin. Infect. Dis.* **23,** 71–75.

Peterson, P., Kur, H. H., Marker, S. C., Fryd, D. S., Howard, R. J., and Simmons, R. L. (1980) Cytomegalovirus disease in renal allograft recipients: a prospective study of the clinical features, risk factors and impact on renal transplantation. *Medicine* **59,** 283–300.

Purtilo, D. T., Paquin, L. A., Sakamoto, K., et al. (1980) Persistent transfusion-associated infectious mononucleosis with transient acquired immunodeficiency. *Am. J. Med.* **68,** 437–440.

Quick, R. E., Herwaldt, B. L., Thomford, J. W., Garnett, M. E., Eberhard, M. L., Wilson, M., et al. (1993) Babesiosis in Washington state: a new species of babesia. *Ann. Intern. Med.* **119,** 284–290.

Rebentish, A. and Bernstein, J. (1993) Postsplenectomy sepsis. *Postgrad. Gen. Surg.* **5,** 166–168.

Reboul, F., Donaldson, S. S., and Kaplan, H. S. (1978) Herpes zoster and varicella infections in children with Hodgkin's disease. *Cancer* **41,** 95–99.

Rice, H. M. and James, P. D. (1980) Ectopic splenic tissue failed to prevent fatal pneumococcal septicaemia after splenectomy for trauma. *Lancet* **i,** 565–566.

Rosner, F. and Zarrabi, M. H. (1983) Late infections following splenectomy in Hodgkin's disease. *Cancer Invest.* **1,** 57–65.

Rosner, F., Zarrabi, M. H., Benach, J. L., and Habicht, G. S. (1984) Babesiosis in splenectomized adults. Review of 22 reported cases. *Am. J. Med.* **76,** 696–701.

Rowley, D. A. (1950) The formation of circulating antibody in the splenectomized human being following intravenous injection of heterologous erythrocytes. *J. Immunol.* **65,** 515–521.

Ruben, F. L., Hankins, W. A., Zeigler, Z., et al. (1984) Antibody responses to meningococcal polysaccharide vaccine in adults without a spleen. *Am. J. Med.* **76,** 115–121.

Sanders, L. A., Rijkers, G. T., Kuis, W., Tenbergen-Meekes, A. J., and Graeff-Meeder, B. R. (1993) Defective anti-pneumococcal polysaccharide antibody response in children with recurrent respiratory tract infections. *J. Allergy Clin. Immunol.* **91,** 110–119.

Sanders, L. A., Rijkers, G. T., Tenbergen-Meekes, A. M., Voorhorst-Ogink, M. M., and Zeger, B. J. (1995) Immunoglobulin isotype specific antibody response to pneumococcal polysaccharide vaccine in patients with recurrent bacterial respiratory tract infection. *Ped. Res.* **37,** 812–819.

Salzman, M. B. and Rubin, L. G. (1996) Meningococcemia. *Infect. Dis. Clin. North Am.* **10,** 709–725.

Sarangi, J., Coleby, M., Trivella, M., and Reilly, S. (1997) Prevention of post splenectomy sepsis: a population based approach. *J. Public Health Med.* **19,** 208–212.

Sass, W., Bergolz, M., Kehl, A., Seifert, J., and Hamelmann, H. (1983) Overwhelming infection after splenectomy in spite of some spleen remaining and splenosis. A case report. *Klin. Wochenschr.* **61,** 1975–1979.

Scher, K. S., Wroczynski, A. F., and Jones, C. W. (1983) Protection from post-splenectomy sepsis: effect of prophylactic penicillin and pneumococcal vaccine on clearance of type 3 pneumococcus. *Surgery* **93,** 792–797.

Schilling, R. F. (1995) Estimating the risk for sepsis after splenectomy in hereditary spherocytosis. *Ann. Intern. Med.* **122,** 187–188.

Schimpff, S. C., Serpick, A., Stoler, B., et al. (1972) Varicella-zoster infection in patients with cancer. *Ann. Intern. Med.* **76,** 241–254.

Schoolnik, G. K., Buchanan, T. M., and Holmes, K. (1976) Gonococci causing disseminated gonococcal infection are resistant to the bacterial action of normal human sera. *J. Clin. Invest.* **58,** 1163–1173.

Schwartz, A. D. and Pearson, H. A. (1972) Impaired antibody response to intravenous immunization in sickle cell anemia. *Pediatr. Res.* **6,** 145–149.

Schwartz, P. E., Sterioff, S., Mucha, P., Melton, L. J. III, and Offord, K. P. (1982) Postsplenectomy sepsis and mortality in adults. *JAMA* **248,** 2279–2283.

Seo, I. S. and Chin-Yang, L. (1995) Hyposplenic blood picture in systemic amyloidosis; its absence is not a predictable sign for absence of splenic involvement. *Arch. Pathol. Lab. Med.* **119,** 252–254.

Sherman, R. (1981) Rationale for and methods of splenic preservation following trauma. *Surg. Clin. North Am.* **61,** 127–134.

Shute, P. G. (1975) Splenectomy and susceptibility to malaria and babesia infection. *Br. Med. J.* **1,** 516.

Siber, G. R., Gorham, C., Martin, P., Corkery, J. C., and Schiffman, G. (1978) Impaired antibody response to pre-treatment immunization and post-treatment boosting with bacterial polysaccharide vaccines in patients with Hodgkin's disease. *Ann. Intern. Med.* **104,** 467–475.

Singer, D. B. (1973) Postsplenectomy sepsis. *Perspect. Pediatr. Pathol.* **1,** 285–311.

Siplovich, L. and Kawar, B. (1997) Changes in the management of pediatric blunt splenic and hepatic injuries. *J. Pediatr. Surg.* **32,** 1464, 1465.

Steely, W. M., Satava, R. M., Harris, R. W., and Quispe, G. (1987) Comparison of omental splenic autotransplant to partial splenectomy. Protective effect against septic death. *Am. Surg.* **53,** 702–705.

Styrt, B. A., Piazza-Hepp, T. D., and Chikami, G. K. (1996) Clinical toxicity of antiretroviral nucleoside analogs. *PMID* **3,** 121–135.

Styrt, B. A. (1996) Risks of infection and protective strategies for the asplenic patient. *Infect. Dis. Clin. Pract.* **5,** 94–100.

Sumaya, C. V., Harbison, R. W., and Britton, H. A. (1981) Pneumococcal vaccine failures, two case reports and review. *Am. J. Dis. Child.* **135,** 155–158.

Tapper, M. L. and Armstrong, D. (1976) Malaria complicating neoplastic disease. *Arch. Intern. Med.* **136,** 807–810.

Thompson, R. F. (1997) Travel and routine immunization: a practical guide for the medical office. Shoreland, Inc., Milwaukee, WI.

Traub, A., Giebink, G. S., Smith, C., et al. (1987) Splenic reticuloendothelial function after splenectomy, spleen repair and spleen autotransplantation. *N. Engl. J. Med.* **317,** 1559–1564.

Travel & Routine Immunizations, 1997.

van der Meer, J. T., Drew, W. L., Bowden, R. A., Galasso, G. J., Griffiths, P. D., Jabs, D. A., et al. (1996) Summary of the international consensus symposium on advances in the diagnosis, treatment and prophylaxis and cytomegalovirus infection. *Antiviral Res.* **32,** 119–140.

Van Etten, E. P., Van Popta, T., Van Luyt, P. A., Bode, P. J., and Van Vugt, A. B. (1995) Changes in the diagnosis and treatment of traumatic splenic rupture: a retrospective analysis of 99 consecutive cases. *Eur. J. Emerg. Med.* **2,** 196–200.

Van Wyck, D. B., Witte, M. H., and Witte, C. L. (1986) Compensatory spleen growth and protective function in rats. *Clin. Sci.* **71,** 573–579.

Waghorn, D. J. and Mayon-White, R. T. (1997) A study of 42 episodes of overwhelming post-splenectomy infection: is current guidance for asplenic individuals being followed. *J. Infect.* **35,** 289–294.

Wåhlby, L. and Domellöf, L. (1981) Splenectomy after blunt abdominal trauma. A retrospective study of 413 children. *Acta Chir. Scand.* **147,** 131–135.

Wallace, M. R., Chamberlin, C. J., Sawyer, M. H., Arvin, A. M., Harkins, J., LaRocco, A., et al. (1996) Treatment of adult varicella with sorivudine: a randomized, placebo-controlled trial. *J. Infect. Dis.* **174,** 249–255.

Walzer, P. D., Gibson, J. J., and Schultz, M. G. (1974) Malaria fatalities in the United States. *Am. J. Trop. Med. Hyg.* **23,** 328–333.

Wara, D. W. (1981) Host defense against Streptococcus pneumoniae: the role of the spleen. *Rev. Infect. Dis.* **3,** 299–309.

Ware, R. E. (1997) Salmonella infection in sickle cell disease: a clear and present danger [editorial; comment]. *J. Pediatr.* **130,** 350–351.

Werbin, N. and Lodha, K. (1982) Malign effects of splenectomy: the place of conservative treatment. *Postgrad. Med. J.* **58,** 65–69.

Williams, D. N. and Kaur, B. (1996) Postsplenectomy care. Strategies to decrease the risk of infection. *Postgrad. Med.* **1,** 195–198.

Winkelstein, J. A. and Lambert, G. H. (1975) Pneumococcal serum opsonizing activity in splenectomized children. *J. Pediatr.* **87,** 430–433.

Working Party of the British Committee for Standards in Haematology Clinical Haematology Task Force (1996) *Br. Med. J.* **312,** 430–434.

Wright, J., Thomas, P., and Serjeant, G. R. (1997) Septicemia caused by salmonella infection: an overlooked complication of sickle cell disease. *J. Pediatr.* **130,** 394–399.

Wyler, D. J., Miller, L. H., and Schmidt, L. H. (1977) Spleen function in quartan malaria (due to *Plasmodium inui*): evidence for both protective and suppressive roles in host defense. *J. Infect. Dis,* **135,** 86–93.

Wyler, D. J., Oster, C. N., and Quinn, T. C. (1978) The role of the spleen in malaria infections. *Trop. Dis. Res. Series* **1,** 183–204.

Wyler, D. J., Quinn, T. C., and Chen, L.-T. (1981) Relationship of alterations in splenic clearance function and microciruclation to host defense in acute rodent malaria. *J. Clin. Invest.* **67,** 1400–1404.

Zarrabi, M. H. and Rosner, F. (1984) Serious infections in adults following splenectomy for trauma. *Arch. Intern. Med.* **144,** 1421–1424.

Zarrabi, M. H. and Rosner, F. (1986) Rarity of failure of penicillin prophylaxis to prevent post-splenectomy sepsis. *Arch. Intern. Med.* **146,** 1207–1208.

12 Hemolysis and Thrombocytopenia

DAVID R. ANDERSON, MD AND JOHN G. KELTON, MD

12.1. INTRODUCTION

Some organs of the body are uniquely associated with specific diseases resulting from disturbance or failure of their own structure or function. For example, renal failure is the consequence of disorders of the kidneys, and myocardial infarction results from structural damage to the heart. But the spleen is in many respects unique, and the disorders that are most closely associated with the spleen have their etiological origins elsewhere. For example, hereditary disorders of the red blood cell membrane lead to red blood cell destruction by the spleen. Likewise, in autoantibody-mediated blood cell damage, the spleen may play both a causal and a consequential role. In these conditions, the spleen produces the autoantibodies that initiate cell damage, and also provides the filtration mechanism that destroys the antibody-sensitized cells.

The recognition of the predominant role of the spleen in many autoimmune disorders is recent. This chapter focuses on the clinical and experimental observations that have clarified the role of the spleen in both autoimmune and nonimmune hemolytic and thrombocytopenic disorders, and particularly on two common and important diseases, idiopathic thrombocytopenic purpura (ITP) and autoimmune hemolytic anemia (AIHA). The comparable and contrasting mechanisms of clearance of the red blood cells and platelets in these two autoimmune disorders are addressed.

Once a cell becomes sensitized by immunoglobulin G (IgG) antibody or complement, the fate of this cell is identical, irrespective of whether its removal is useful for the body. Removal of an infecting microorganism, or an antigenically transformed cell, such as a malignant cell, may be regarded, teleologically, as "serving a useful purpose." However, the same mechanism may place the subject at hazard, when removing an otherwise autoantibody-sensitized red blood cell or platelet. Consequently, there is an important relationship between the physiological and pathological aspects of particle clearance.

There is a unique anatomy to the spleen that allows it to function both as a generator of autoantibodies and as a clearance organ of the autoantibody-sensitized cells.

12.2. ANATOMY OF THE SPLEEN

The anatomy of the spleen has been described in detail in Chapters 1–3, and this description is confined to aspects especially relevant to blood cell destruction. Within the spleen are large numbers of lymphocytes, monocytes, and macrophages, so that there is a unique opportunity for communication between blood in the vas-

From: *The Complete Spleen: A Handbook of Structure, Function, and Clinical Disorders* Edited by: A. J. Bowdler © Humana Press Inc., Totowa, NJ

culature and the lymphatic and reticuloendothelial (RE) systems. The white pulp consists of periarterial lymphatic sheaths and lymphatic nodules. The red pulp contains complex vascular pathways identified as splenic cords and sinuses, and there is an abundance of RE cells (monocytes and macrophages). Between the white pulp and the red pulp is the marginal zone (Fig. 1), which is a fine reticular area containing lymphocytes and RE cells.

The spleen receives about 5% of the total cardiac output: Blood passes from the splenic artery to the trabecular arteries, and in turn to the central arteries, which enter the white pulp (Bishop and Lansing, 1982). The central arteries give off lateral branches, which leave at right angles, to penetrate the periarterial lymphatic sheaths (Eichner, 1979). Teleologically, the peculiar anatomy of these arteries, and their orientation at right angles to the parent arteries, can be understood as providing for plasma skimming:Rapidly flowing blood in small vessels assumes a characteristic flow pattern, with the red blood cells in the center of the vessel and the plasma at the periphery. The right-angled arteries of the spleen skim the peripherally situated plasma from the flowing blood, so that the plasma carries soluble antigens to the white pulp, where they are captured by specialized macrophages, termed "dendritic" or "antigen-presenting cells." Second, the monomeric IgG in the plasma, which can inhibit RE cell function, is separated from the cellular elements: This increases the likelihood that IgG-sensitized cells will bind to the Fc-receptor bearing RE cells.

Concentrated blood leaves the white pulp and enters the red pulp via the terminal arterioles. These vessels end in the splenic cords, which form a nonendothelialized reticular meshwork consisting of fibrils and interstitial cells, with a large population of monocytes and macrophages (Chen and Weiss, 1972). Blood cells must traverse these tortuous cords in order to enter the splenic sinuses, which form the first vessels of the venous microcirculation of the red pulp. There are few direct connections between the cords and the sinuses. The cords are actually spaces lying between the sinuses within the red pulp (Weiss and Tavassoli, 1972). In order for a cell to enter the sinus lumen, it must pass through the three-layered wall of the sinus, which is comprised of an inner endothelial layer, a middle basement membrane, and an outer lining of adventitial cells. The endothelial cells contain filaments, which may be contractile, and consequently there is the potential for these cells to regulate the size of the interendothelial cell slits (Bishop and Lansing, 1982). Scanning and transmission electron microscopic pictures of the splenic sinus demonstrate that there are no fixed apertures in the sinus endothelium (Chen and Weiss, 1972; Weiss, 1974). However, potential spaces exist between the endothelial cells, which allow the passage of blood cells into the sinuses.

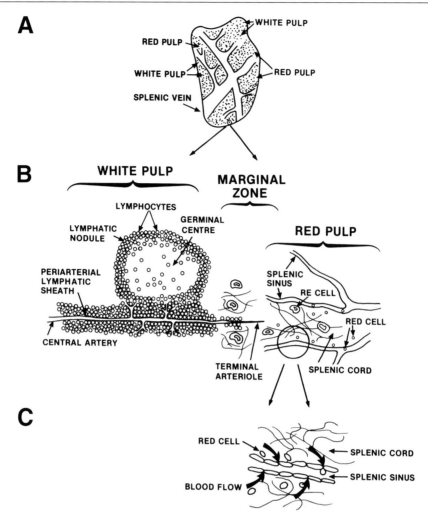

Fig. 12.1. Sequentially magnified diagrams that schematically represent the splenic anatomy as it pertains to blood cell clearance. (**A**) Cross-section of the spleen, its venous tributaries, and the red and white pulp. (**B**) Schematic representation of the white and red pulp. The white pulp is composed of periarterial lymphatic sheaths and lymphatic nodules. The red pulp consists of splenic cords and sinuses. Interspersed between is the marginal zone. Blood enters the white pulp through the central artery, which is enveloped by the periarterial lymphatic sheath. Arteriolar vessels leave the central artery at right angles, and this results in the skimming of the plasma from the parent vessel. The remaining concentrated blood passes through the marginal zone and enters the splenic cords of the red pulp via the terminal arterioles. The splenic cords are a nonendothelialized reticular meshwork rich in RE cells. Blood cells pass through the cords, before entering the splenic sinuses. (**C**) Demonstrates the route blood cells must follow to enter a splenic sinus. There are few direct connections between the cords and sinuses, and most blood cells enter the splenic sinuses by passing through the narrow interendothelial spaces.

Functionally, the direct pathways between the terminal arterioles and the splenic sinuses are unimportant, so that most blood cells must pass through the monocyte and macrophage-rich cordal circulation during each passage through the spleen.

The red pulp plays a dual role in the removal of cells from the circulation: First, antibody-sensitized cells may be removed by the splenic RE cells. Second, cells with reduced deformability are unable to transverse the interendothelial slits of the sinus endothelium, and are retained by the spleen. By these two mechanisms, the red pulp plays a pivotal role in the clearance from the circulation of normal and pathologically altered blood cells.

12.3. THE RETICULOENDOTHELIAL FUNCTION OF THE SPLEEN

The monocytes and macrophages of the spleen effect the removal of infectious agents, foreign antigens, tumor antigens, and antibody-sensitized cells. By the removal of IgG-sensitized platelets

and red blood cells that splenic phagocytes are involved in the pathogenesis of autoimmune thrombocytopenia and hemolysis. This subheading outlines factors influencing splenic RE cell function, the measurement of Fc-dependent RE function, the mechanism of RE-cell-mediated cell destruction, and the importance of the splenic RE cells in the clearance of cells from the circulation.

12.3.1. FACTORS INFLUENCING MACROPHAGE FUNCTION

12.3.1.1. IgG Subclass   The monocytes and macrophages of the spleen have specific binding sites (termed Fc receptors) for the γ-2 region of the heavy chain of IgG (Lobuglio et al., 1967; Huber and Fudenberg, 1968). There are differences in affinity for the different subclasses of IgG, with IgG subclasses 1 and 3 having the highest binding affinity, and IgG subclasses 2 and 4 having a low binding affinity (van der Meulen et al., 1978). The IgG on sensitized cells binds to the unoccupied Fc receptors of the RE cells. There are several different types of Fc receptors on the RE cells: Some have a very high binding affinity for the IgG, and others have

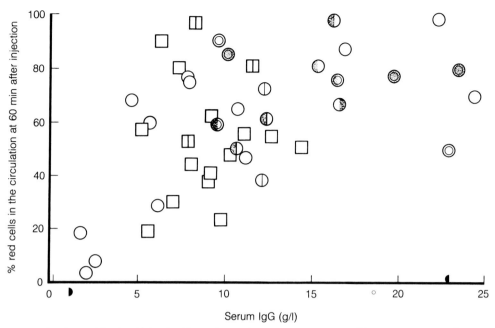

Fig. 12.2.   The clearance of IgG-sensitized red blood cells (ordinate) for 17 control subjects (□) and 27 patients (○), in relation to the serum concentration of IgG (g/L); (▣) indicates that the patient or control subject has the HLA-B8/DR3 haplotype; (◖) indicates a positive PEG assay for immune complexes; (◖) indicates a positive Raji cell assay for immune complexes; (◎) indicates a positive assay for antinuclear antibodies. (Reprinted with permission from Kelton et al., 1985).

a low binding affinity. There are three classes of Fc receptors on the RE cells (Fc-γR), distinguishable by size, gene origin, and reactivity with Fc-γR monoclonal antibodies. Fc-γRI receptors have a very high binding affinity for IgG; Fc-γRIIs and Fc-γRIII receptors have lesser affinity (McKenzie and Schreiber, 1998). All three subclasses can individually mediate phagocytosis of IgG-coated red blood cells, leukocytes, platelets, bacteria, and tumor cells, and other RE cell functions, regardless of the presence of complement and simultaneous activity of complement receptors.

Increasing evidence suggests that the low-affinity Fc receptors are the most important for antibody-mediated cell clearance, because the high-affinity receptors tend to be occupied by the monomeric IgG.

12.3.1.2. Plasma Concentration of Monomeric IgG   The monomeric IgG in the plasma can bind to the Fc receptors. When this occurs, the receptors are unavailable for interacting with IgG-sensitized cells. Indeed, it is likely that, when the plasma concentration of IgG is sufficiently high, even the low-affinity Fc receptors are occupied. This observation has been exploited therapeutically. Intravenous (iv) IgG can dramatically raise the concentration of IgG in the plasma, and this maneuver can prevent the clearance of IgG-sensitized platelets or red blood cells (Fig. 2; Kelton et al., 1985). As noted previously, the anatomy of the spleen counteracts this. As plasma is skimmed from the cellular elements of the blood, the monomeric IgG moves with the plasma. Consequently, as the cellular elements percolate through the splenic cords, there is a significant reduction in the local concentration of monomeric IgG, which might otherwise occupy the Fc receptors of the RE cells. In vitro studies confirm that the decrease in the concentration of IgG, to levels found in the red pulp of the spleen, improves the efficiency of phagocytosis of sensitized red blood cells (Lobuglio et al., 1967). In addition, the slow flow in the splenic cords increases the likelihood that IgG-sensitized cells will have the opportunity of interacting with the Fc receptors on the RE cells within the spleen.

12.3.1.3. Amount of IgG and Complement on Sensitized Cells
IgG-sensitized cells can be cleared by splenic macrophages by two mechanisms. Macrophages and monocytes can bind to the Fc portion of the IgG, and subsequently initiate the phagocytosis of the cell. Surface immunoglobulins on sensitized cells can also induce clearance, by activating the complement system on the cell membrane. Several IgG molecules in close proximity can initiate the complement cascade by activating C1 (Frank, 1987). This event triggers the classical complement cascade, and leads to the cleavage of C4 and C2, and to the formation of the C4b2b complex, also known as the C3 cleaving enzyme. C3 is subsequently proteolyzed to C3a, which is released from the cell surface, and C3b, which remains surface-bound. C3b is the main opsonin of the complement cascade, and RE cells have C3b receptors on their cell membranes (Huber et al., 1968; Lay and Nussenzweig, 1968; Ross et al., 1973). The expression of C3b is under tight control: Two plasma proteins, H and I, can convert C3b to its inactive form, iC3d. As is discussed subsequently, C3b-sensitized cells, both alone and in combination with IgG, play an important role in the antibody-mediated clearance of cells.

12.3.2. MEASUREMENT OF Fc-DEPENDENT RE FUNCTION
Studying the Fc-dependent RE function in humans is accomplished by taking Rh-positive red blood cells from the individual to be tested, labeling the cells with 51-chromate (^{51}Cr), then sensitizing them with a known amount of IgG alloantibody (Kelton, 1987). Anti-D represents an ideal alloantibody, for several reasons. First, its target (the Rh-positive cell) is found with high frequency in the population (85%); second, the Rh antigens are not clustered or mobile, and consequently the anti-D tends not to activate complement; third, anti-D binds with a high affinity, which minimizes in vivo elution of the IgG from the red blood cells.

After injection of the ^{51}Cr-labeled, IgG-sensitized autologous red blood cells, samples of whole blood are collected at various times, and the rate of clearance of these radiolabeled cells is measured. Because the amount of sensitizing alloantibody is controlled, the only variable affecting the rate of clearance of the radiolabeled red blood cells is the functional activity of the RE system. Studies using this technique have established the following:

1. The spleen is the dominant organ for clearance of IgG-sensitized red blood cells. When the red blood cells are moderately sensitized (2000 molecules of IgG/cell), they are rapidly cleared within hours of injection. Following splenectomy, the cells are cleared at a very reduced rate (Kelton et al., 1985; Hosea et al., 1981; *see also* Chapter 7, Subheading 2.6.).

2. The plasma concentration of IgG is an important determinant of the rate of clearance of the IgG-sensitized cells (Kelton et al., 1985). Patients with agammaglobulinemia have an enhanced rate of clearance, and patients with either a naturally occurring or a pharmacologically induced hypergammaglobulinemia have a reduced rate of clearance.

3. Splenic Fc-dependent RE clearance is governed by other, as-yet poorly understood factors, including certain genes, such as those for the HLA B8/DR3 alloantigens (Frank et al., 1983; Lawley et al., 1981), certain disease states, such as systemic lupus erythematosus and HIV infections (Bender et al., 1985; Frank et al., 1979; Van Wyk et al., 1999), and certain medications, especially methyldopa (Kelton, 1985). All of these factors impair splenic Fc-dependent RE cell clearance.

12.4. THE MECHANISM OF DESTRUCTION OF SENSITIZED CELLS

12.4.1. RED BLOOD CELLS Electron and microscopic studies in vitro have shown that the interaction of RE cells and sensitized red blood cells depends on whether IgG or complement coats the red blood cell surface. IgG-sensitized red blood cells form rosettes with monocytes and macrophages (Lobuglio et al., 1967; Rosse et al., 1975) and the red blood cells are either ingested completely or a portion of the red blood cell membrane is removed. Sensitized red blood cells with abnormal shapes, such as spherocytes, are engulfed completely. Light microscopic studies showed that, following monocyte rosette formation, sensitized red blood cells become spherocytic. Sensitized red blood cells which are not rosetted, show no such transformation.

Unlike IgG-sensitized red blood cells which initiate phagocytosis, complement-coated red blood cells adhere efficiently to RE cells, but are rarely ingested (Rosse et al., 1975; Ehlenberger and Nussenzweig, 1977; Bianco et al., 1975). If the cell is ingested by the monocyte or macrophage, it often escapes from the phagocytic vacuole, and is released from the cell. However, when sensitized red blood cells are coated with both IgG and complement, significantly fewer IgG molecules are required for ingestion to occur. The mechanism of this synergism is now apparent. Monocyte and macrophage C3b-receptor binding leads to strong adherence of the red blood cell to the phagocytic cell surface. The Fc receptors for IgG on the RE cells then mediate the ingestion of the already tightly bound red blood cell and this results in phagocytosis.

These observations offer a probable explanation for the clinical observation that spherocytes are commonly found in the circulation in warm autoimmune hemolytic anemia and are usually absent in cold agglutinin disease. Warm autoimmune hemolytic anemia is

mediated by IgG-sensitization of red blood cells. Microscopic studies demonstrate that RE cells are capable of removing portions of the red blood cell membrane from the IgG-sensitized cell, resulting in spherocyte formation. Cold agglutinin disease is mediated solely by IgM-induced complement activation. Because complement-sensitized red blood cells are poorly ingested by RE cells, spherocyte formation is uncommon. Studies in rats have demonstrated that IgG-mediated hemolysis leads to a loss of about 25% of the lipid-rich components of the red blood cell membrane within 24 h of sensitization (Cooper, 1972).

12.4.2. PLATELETS Histological examination of spleens from patients with ITP demonstrates that platelets are phagocytosed as whole cells, usually in the splenic cords (Tavassoli and McMillan, 1975; Luk et al., 1980). Whether IgG and complement-sensitized platelets are processed differently, by the splenic RE cells, is not known.

12.5. THE ROLE OF SPLENIC PHAGOCYTES IN CELL CLEARANCE

Splenic monocytes and macrophages are important in cell clearance under both physiological and pathological circumstances. This subheading outlines their role in the clearance of senescent cell populations and antibody-mediated cell destruction.

12.5.1. THE PHYSIOLOGICAL CLEARANCE OF SENESCENT CELLS

12.5.1.1. Red Blood Cells There is increasing evidence that the clearance of senescent red blood cells is triggered by the binding of autoantibodies to the red blood cell membrane. Kay (1975) first demonstrated that, when red blood cells aged in vitro were incubated with autologous or allogeneic IgG, the cells were phagocytosed by macrophages. They also found that less than 5% of young red blood cells were phagocytosed by macrophages but over 30% of the older cells were destroyed. Kay concluded that an IgG autoantibody attached to the older red blood cells in vivo, and this sensitization initiated the removal of the cells by the RE system. Kay's hypothesis has been confirmed by other groups (Khansari and Fudenberg, 1983). Old red blood cells have elevated levels of surface IgG, bound by the Fab fragment (Lutz et al., 1984; Freedman, 1987). Eluates of IgG from senescent red blood cells rebind to red blood cells, causing the clearance of senescent, but not young, red blood cells (Khansari and Fudenberg, 1983; Kay et al., 1982).

The target of the IgG has been termed the senescent antigen. Subsequent work has located the antigen to band 3, which is an integral protein of the red blood cell membrane (Lutz et al., 1984; Low et al., 1985; Lutz and Wipf, 1982). Although IgG binds to band 3 in vitro, a conformational alteration of this protein may act as the epitope for the immunoglobulin in vivo. This alteration occurs as a consequence of red blood cell aging. The precise characterization of the senescent antigen is not complete. Several groups have confirmed that it is composed of the extracellular and intramembranous portions of band 3, but not the cytoplasmic component of this protein. What also remains unknown is the mechanism of band 3 alteration that causes autoantibody sensitization. Kay et al. (1982) have reported that the senescent antigen forms as a result of the specific proteolytic cleavage of band 3 protein. Low et al. (1985) suggest that the formation of this antigen is secondary to oligomerization of band 3 molecules in the red blood cell membrane. IgG capable of binding to the senescent antigen has been isolated from pooled plasma (Lutz and Wipf, 1982; Lutz et al., 1984); it can be absorbed by incubating plasma with senescent red blood cells, band 3 protein, or the senescent antigen (Kay et al., 1982; Kay, 1984). Lutz et al. (1987) have shown in vitro that the senescent IgG antibody can induce complement deposition on the red blood cell surface, and that complement may contribute to the clearance of senescent red blood cells. Consistent with this hypothesis is the recognition that the small number of IgG molecules, bound per senescent red blood cell is inadequate to cause clearance of the sensitized cells solely by the Fc receptors of the RE system.

Possibly, IgG sensitization represents a general mechanism of cell clearance, e.g., increased red blood cell IgG has also been found in patients with sickle cell anemia (Green et al., 1985; Galili et al., 1986). This disorder is associated with shortened red blood cell survival caused by other factors, but autoantibody sensitization of the red blood cells may represent an additional mechanism of premature cell clearance.

Senescent red blood cells are cleared by the cells of the macrophage system. The evidence that this clearance is mediated by IgG sensitization to a specific band 3 product suggests that the spleen is responsible for the clearance of at least a portion of senescent red blood cells. However, the life-span of red blood cells is apparently unaltered in asplenic individuals, and it may therefore be assumed that other components of the RE system are capable of phagocytosing senescent red blood cells and compensating for the absence of the spleen.

12.5.1.2. Platelets The mechanism of the clearance of senescent platelets is not understood, but is probably similar to that of red blood cells. For example, in normal individuals, the small, low-density platelets, which are probably the oldest, carry large amounts of IgG on their surface (Kelton and Denomme, 1982).

12.5.2. CLEARANCE OF PATHOLOGICALLY SENSITIZED RED BLOOD CELL POPULATIONS

12.5.2.1. Red Blood Cells Jandl and Kaplan (1960) demonstrated the effect of various levels of IgG-sensitization on red blood cell destruction in vivo. They found that low or moderate levels of IgG on the red blood cells resulted in splenic clearance; however, large amounts of antibody led to hepatic clearance. Subsequently, it was shown that high levels of sensitization by IgG resulted in complement deposition on the red blood cells, which is presumed to shift the predominant clearance of red blood cells from the spleen to the liver. Schreiber and Frank (1972b) demonstrated that 1.4 complement molecules/cell were capable of decreasing the survival of IgG-sensitized cells. Work in both guinea pigs and humans has shown that, with low levels of IgG sensitization, clearance of ^{51}Cr-labeled red blood cells is predominantly by the spleen (Schreiber and Frank, 1972a; Frank et al., 1977). Furthermore, animals and humans with C4 deficiency or C1-esterase deficiency showed a reduced rate of clearance of IgG-sensitized red blood cells. However, the clearance rate does not return to normal, suggesting that IgG alone can accelerate red blood cell clearance, and that the effect of complement is synergistic. With increasing levels of IgG sensitization, more C3b activation occurs, and the survival of the sensitized cells is further shortened (Frank et al., 1977; Mollison et al., 1965).

The clearance of IgM-sensitized red blood cells is quite different from that of IgG-coated cells. There are no specific receptors on macrophages for IgM, and IgM can only mediate cell clearance through the activation of complement. IgM is much more efficient in activating complement than IgG, and only one molecule of IgM is required to initiate the complement cascade (Frank, 1987). With low levels of IgM sensitization, most red blood cells are removed

from the circulation and sequestered in the liver. However, a portion of these cells returns to the circulation, where they have a normal survival (Frank et al., 1977). These cells have iC3d on their surface, which protects them from being subjected to further cell clearance.

If the level of IgM sensitization is increased, the initial sequestration in the liver is increased, and fewer cells are returned to the circulation. Patients with C1-esterase deficiency show no significant clearance of IgM-sensitized red blood cells at levels that would normally lead to hemolysis.

12.5.2.2. Platelets Understanding of the importance of antibody and complement sensitization to the clearance of platelets comes principally from studying patients with idiopathic thrombocytopenic purpura (ITP). Human and animal studies have demonstrated low baseline levels of IgG on normal platelets (Winiarsky and Holm, 1983). Increased levels of IgG result in rapid clearance of the platelets by the spleen. Increased platelet-associated complement has been reported in some, but not all, patients with immune thrombocytopenia, with some patients having marked elevations in platelet-bound complement. Comparisons between the various studies that have been made are difficult, because of the different techniques used for measuring complement, and the use of measurements of different complement components. However, platelet-associated C3b, C3c, C3d, C4, and C9 have all been reported to be elevated on ITP platelets (Winiarski and Holm, 1983; Kurata et al., 1986; Cines and Schreiber, 1979; Panzer et al., 1986; Lehman et al., 1987; Hegde et al., 1988; Myers et al., 1982; Hauch and Rosse, 1977; Kayser et al., 1983).

There has been speculation on how complement is bound to the platelet surface. McMillan and Martin (1981) demonstrated that purified antiplatelet autoantibody, produced in vitro by splenic cells from patients with ITP, causes the binding of C3 to the platelet surface, which suggests that complement can be activated in vivo, with resulting augmentation of the clearance of IgG-sensitized platelets. Complement on the platelet surface has the potential for shifting the primary organ of clearance from the spleen to the liver, and this was found in one study (Panzer et al., 1986). This is of more than theoretical importance, because it may imply that splenectomy would be unsuccessful in such patients.

A recent case report provides evidence that complement-mediated immune platelet destruction can occur (Lehman et al., 1987). A patient with a lymphoreticular disease was shown to have increased levels of platelet-associated IgG (PAIgG), IgM, C3c, and C3d. Serum from this patient was reported to deposit complement on the platelet surface, and result in platelet lysis. This mechanism of platelet destruction may account for the patient's unresponsiveness to therapy.

The relationship between PAIgG, platelet-associated IgM, and platelet-associated complement remains unclear. Some authors have reported correlations between PAIgG and platelet-associated complement (Winiarski and Holm, 1983; Kurata et al., 1986; Myers et al., 1982; Kayser et al., 1983);, others have reported an association between platelet-associated IgM and platelet-associated complement (Lehman et al., 1987; Hegde et al., 1985).

12.6. SPLENIC ANTIBODY FORMATION

The spleen has an important function in forming antibodies against soluble plasma antigens. As arterial blood passes through the spleen, plasma is separated from the cellular elements, and directed to the white pulp. Soluble antigens in the plasma bind to the antigen processing cells. These cells partially digest the antigens, then present them to adjacent T-lymphocytes, where the process of antibody formation begins. Following splenectomy, the levels of serum IgG and IgA do not change, although the level of IgM drops slightly. There is a significant increase in the risk of serious infection following splenectomy, especially infections caused by encapsulated organisms, such as *Streptococcus pneumoniae* and *Haemophilus influenzae* (Eraklis et al., 1967; *see also* Chapters 10 and 11).

The spleen is a major source of antiplatelet autoantibody in patients with ITP. Evidence supporting this statement is both direct and indirect. The indirect evidence comes from measuring PAIgG on platelets from patients with ITP, before and after splenectomy. In most patients, as the platelet count rises to normal levels, the level of PAIgG drops to normal levels (Cines and Schreiber, 1979; Karpatkin et al., 1972; Dixon et al., 1975). However, this fall in PAIgG may also be dilutional: Thus, if the total amount of antiplatelet antibody is constant, the quantity of antiplatelet antibody per platelet will fall, because the PAIgG will be distributed throughout a larger platelet mass. Hence, it is important to examine more direct evidence implicating the spleen as a major site for antiplatelet antibody production. McMillan et al. (1972, 1974) demonstrated that in vitro spleen cultures from patients with ITP have IgG production that is several times higher than that of controls. In most patients, the IgG has specific antiplatelet activity. These observations have been confirmed and extended by others, who have shown that lymphocytes obtained from the spleens of ITP patients produce antiplatelet autoantibody, both spontaneously and following stimulation with B-lymphocyte activators, such as pokeweed mitogen (Karpatkin et al., 1972). The cytokine pattern in the serum of individuals with ITP shows increases in interleukin-2, interleukin-11 and interferon-γ; interleukin-4 is decreased. Thrombopoietin has been found at normal levels. These show a Th1 type of T-helper cytokine response, with Th2 downregulated (Andersson, 1998). The increase in interleukin-11 suggests that the number of platelets produced by each megakaryocyte is increased.

12.7. THE FILTERING FUNCTION OF THE SPLEEN

The anatomy of the spleen provides the means for it to act as a fine filter. In the present context, its most important function is the removal from the circulation of abnormal red blood cells or their inclusions, such as the physiological inclusions of reticulocytes and siderocytes, and also of red blood cells with pathological inclusions such as parasites. Conversely, the filtering function of the spleen appears to have a limited role in platelet pathophysiology.

12.7.1. THE REMOVAL OF INTRACELLULAR INCLUSIONS

Reticulocytes, which are the youngest circulating red blood cells, have the largest surface area:volume ratio of all red blood cells. During the first few passages of reticulocytes through the spleen, some of the cell membrane is lost (Come et al., 1974; Shattil and Cooper, 1972). The membrane lost is mostly lipid in composition, although a specific high-mol-wt protein is also removed (Lux and John, 1977). Simultaneously, nuclear remnants, termed "Howell-Jolly bodies" are also removed (Crosby, 1957).

The spleen removes other red blood cell inclusions, including iron-containing particles from siderocytes, Heinz bodies consisting of hemoglobin denatured by oxidative stress (Chen and Weiss, 1973), and intraerythrocytic parasites (Schnitzer et al., 1972), following which the red blood cells are returned to the circulation.

Electron microscopy studies have demonstrated that inclusion bodies are "pitted" from red blood cells as they pass through the interendothelial slits of the sinus endothelium. Probably, the inclusion is physically trapped and forced to remain within the splenic cords (Fig. 3). Whether there is an additional recognition signal, which optimizes the conformation of splenic structures for the removal of an inclusion, is unknown.

12.7.2. THE REMOVAL OF INDIVIDUAL CELLS

12.7.2.1. Red Blood Cells
For passage through narrow apertures, such as the interendothelial slits of the splenic sinuses, the red blood cells depend on their high surface:volume ratio and the flexibility of the cell membrane. Factors affecting red blood cell deformability include the viscoelastic properties of the membrane, the geometry of the cell, and the viscosity of the intracellular haemoglobin (Mohandas et al., 1979). Congenital and acquired conditions that adversely affect these will lead to decreased red blood cell survival. The major obstacle to survival in most of these disorders is the red blood cells' inability to pass through the splenic microcirculation.

The fate of antibody-sensitized red blood cells depends on both the immune and the filtration functions of the spleen. Once a red blood cell is sensitized by IgG, there are several possible sequelae. First, the surface concentration of the autoantibody may be so low, or the functional activity of the reticuloendothelial system may be sufficiently impaired, that the cell is not cleared from the circulation. Second, IgG-sensitized red blood cells may be removed from the circulation by binding to the Fc or complement receptors on the RE cells. This outcome is most likely for those cells carrying the largest amount of IgG on the cell surface. Third, the IgG-sensitized red blood cells may bind to the RE cells, without being destroyed during this first interaction: The red blood cell escapes complete phagocytosis, but leaves a portion of its membrane behind, which in turn causes it to assume a spherical shape (Fig. 4). The change of shape increases the risk of removal by means of the spleen's filtering function.

The filtering capacity of the spleen can be measured in vivo by determining the clearance of radiolabeled (usually ^{51}Cr), heat-treated autologous red blood cells or by measuring the clearance of radiolabeled aggregates of albumin. Heat treatment denatures spectrin, and causes the red blood cells to become spherocytic (Palek and Lux, 1983).

12.7.2.2. Platelets
The filtration function of the spleen is unimportant in platelet destruction. There is, however, indirect evidence that the spleen retains the youngest and most hemostatically active platelets. Transfusion studies have shown that platelets from asplenic donors have a 2-d-longer survival than those from normal controls (Shulman et al., 1968).

In a few uncommon disorders, the spleen modifies the platelets, and possibly contributes to their subsequent destruction. The Wiskott-Aldrich syndrome is a severe X-linked platelet and immunodeficiency syndrome arising from mutation of the gene *WASP*. It is characterized by frequent infections, eczema, and thrombocytopenia with small platelets. Splenectomy has been shown to partially alleviate the thrombocytopenia and bleeding symptoms in one group of 16 patients (Lum et al., 1980). The morphology of the platelets returned to normal after removal of the spleen; the mechanism of interaction between the platelet and the spleen in this condition has been obscure. Shcherbina et al. (1999) have shown high levels of calcium (Ca^{2+}) in the platelets and enhancement of the Ca^{2+}-dependent processes of surface exposure of phosphatidylserine (PS) and microparticle release. Furthermore fluorescence microscopy of spleen sections showed co-localization of platelet

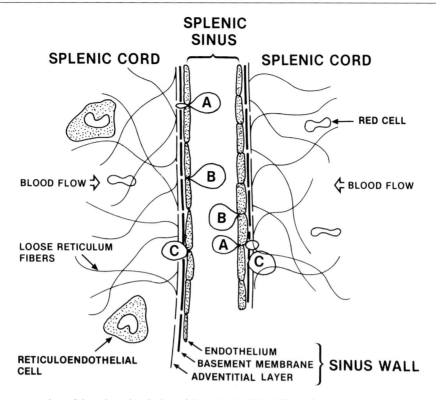

Fig. 12.3. Schematic representation of the microcirculation of the red pulp. Blood flows from the splenic cords to the sinuses. The sinus endothelium is incompletely covered by a basement membrane and an adventitial cell lining. Red blood cells must undergo dramatic changes in shape to pass through the interendothelial cell slits. Alterations in red blood cell deformability may slow or prevent the passage of the cells. In the diagram, the red blood cells labeled "A" contain inclusion bodies. Although the greater part of the cell may pass through the sinus endothelium, the inclusions are pinched off and remain in the splenic cord. Removal of pathological inclusions by the spleen results in the loss of small amounts of the red blood cell membrane. The loss of membrane further reduces the red blood cell deformability, and increases the likelihood of subsequent splenic retention. Red blood cells labeled B are normal red blood cells, which are able to pass through the sinus endothelium unhindered. Red blood cells labeled C are spherocytes, which, because of their reduced deformability, are unable to pass through the interendothelial slits. Red blood cells and inclusions unable to penetrate the sinus endothelium will be removed by the RE cells.

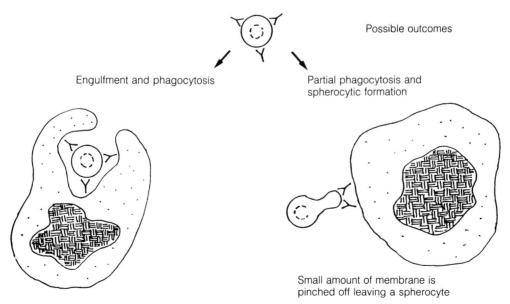

Fig. 12.4. IgG-sensitized red blood cells show three possible outcomes when interacting with splenic RE cells: (1) The red blood cells may be engulfed and phagocytosed by the RE cells; (2) the red blood cells may be partially phagocytosed, resulting in the formation of spherocytes; or (3) the red blood cells may not interact with the RE cells. Phagocytosis is most likely to occur with high levels of IgG sensitization, surface complement activation, and normal RE cell function. This diagram schematically outlines the first two possibilities. (Reproduced with permission from Murphy, W. G. and Kelton, J. G., 1989).

Table 12.1
Conditions Associated with Enhanced or Decreased Splenic RE Cell and Filtration Activity

Splenic RE cell activity
    Increased
        Chronic infection
        Agammaglobulinemia
        ITP
        AIHA
        Collagen-vascular diseases

    Decreased
        Systemic lupus erythematosus
        Acquired immunodeficiency syndrome/
          immunodeficiency virus infection
        Drugs: methyldopa
        Hypergammaglobulinemia
        Certain leukocyte alloantigens (B8/DR3)

Splenic filtering activity
    Increased
        Congenital red blood cell membrane abnormalities
        Hemoglobinopathies and thalassemias
        Essential thrombocythemia
        AIHA
        Splenomegaly with hypersplenism

    Decreased[a]
        Celiac disease
        Sickle cell anemia
        Graves disease

[a]*See also* Chapter 11.

and macrophage markers, suggesting macrophage destruction of platelets in the spleen, possibly induced by PS exposure.

Case reports have also suggested a role for the spleen in the destruction of platelets in patients with the Bernard-Soulier syndrome and the grey platelet syndrome (Najean et al., 1963; Raccuglia, 1971). Whether the thrombocytopenia of these two conditions, associated with large platelets, is related to the filtration system of the spleen is unknown.

12.7.3. CELL POOLING BY THE SPLEEN (*see also* Chapter 7)

12.7.3.1. Red Blood Cells Despite the extensive filtering system, there is little retention of normal red blood cells by the spleen in humans. Following intravenous injection of radiolabeled red blood cells, less than 5% of the cells are retained by the spleen (Hegde et al., 1973). With splenomegaly, the splenic red blood cell pool may increase to more than 20% of the red blood cell mass (Jandl and Aster, 1967) (in some instances, the splenic red blood cell pool may contain more than 40% of the total red blood cells in the circulation [*see also* Chapter 7]—the editor.) Increased red blood cell pooling is found with lymphoproliferative disorders, myeloproliferative disorders, and warm AIHA (Christensen, 1973a; Lewis et al., 1977; Bateman et al., 1978; *see* Chapter 7).

The transit time of a red blood cell through the normal spleen is relatively brief, and usually less than 1 min (Ferrant et al., 1987). The splenic transit time is increased in patients with splenomegaly, and is especially increased in patients with hereditary spherocytosis and AIHA in association with splenomegaly (Bowdler, 1962), which suggests that red blood cell abnormalities and splenic enlargement are additive in delaying the passage of erythrocytes through the spleen.

12.7.3.2. Platelets The relationship of platelets to the spleen differs from the interaction of red blood cells with the organ. First, in healthy individuals, between 25 and 45% of the platelet mass is found in the spleen (Peters and Lavender, 1983; Aster, 1966; Penny et al., 1966). These platelets can be mobilized by stress or the infusion of adrenaline. The mechanism maintaining these platelets within the spleen is unknown, but it could be age-related or antibody-dependent. Also, the average transit time of platelets through the spleen is much longer than that of red blood cells, being approx 10 min, compared to 1 min (Peters et al., 1980). As in the case of red blood cells, splenomegaly leads to an increase in the splenic

platelet mass, but there is no increase in the transit time of platelets through the spleen (Aster, 1966; Penny et al., 1966; Peters, 1983).

12.8. DISEASES ASSOCIATED WITH SPLENIC IMMUNOLOGICAL AND FILTERING ABNORMALITIES

Some diseases are associated with either enhanced or impaired splenic function: These are summarized in Table 1. Important examples of the role of the spleen are provided by two major autoimmune disorders, ITP and AIHA, and by hereditary red blood cell abnormalities associated with decreased cell deformability. These conditions illustrate a complex but dominant role played by the spleen in blood cell destruction.

12.8.1. IDIOPATHIC THROMBOCYTOPENIC PURPURA

ITP is an autoimmune disease of uncertain etiology, despite which much of the mechanism of platelet destruction is well understood. In this condition, platelet destruction is initiated by the binding of IgG antiplatelet autoantibodies to specific platelet glycoproteins and the secondary binding of IgG and other plasma proteins to the platelet membrane. The sensitized platelets are subsequently removed by the RE cells (Kelton and Steeves, 1983; Kelton, 1983; McMillan et al., 1987).

There are two basic patterns of ITP, which depend on the age of the patient at presentation. Acute ITP occurs principally in young children, and usually follows a viral infection, and spontaneously resolves in over 75% of cases (Karpatkin, 1985). In most, the disease lasts for less than 6 mo. By contrast, chronic ITP is a disease that typically occurs in adults, and spontaneous recovery is the exception (Difino et al., 1980; McMillen, 1981). Occasionally, autoimmune thrombocytopenia is associated with a lymphoproliferative disorder such as chronic lymphocytic leukemia. Sometimes, thrombocytopenia complicates a more generalized autoimmune disorder, such as systemic lupus erythematosus or rheumatoid arthritis. However, for most patients, there are no predisposing factors or associated diseases.

Most patients with ITP are asymptomatic, but some have evidence of hemostatic impairment, which parallels the platelet count. When this is above 20×10^9/L, most patients do not bleed, and the disease is often discovered by routine laboratory testing. Once the platelet count falls below $10–20 \times 10^9$/L, petechiae and purpura often occur. Very low platelet counts are associated with evidence of generalized hemostatic impairment, including mucous membrane bleeding, hematuria, melena, and menorrhagia. Life-threatening bleeding, such as intracerebral hemorrhage, is rare, but does occur (Karpatkin, 1985; McMillen, 1981; Komrower and Watson, 1954).

12.8.1.1. Clinical and Laboratory Investigations Physical ex-amination is usually normal in patients with ITP, except for the petechiae and purpura. Patients at especially high risk for serious bleeding are more likely to have "wet purpura," with blood blisters in the mouth and evidence of mucous membrane bleeding (Crosby, 1975). Splenomegaly does not occur in ITP, and its presence should lead one to search for alternative causes of the thrombocytopenia.

Laboratory investigation, in the majority of adults and children with ITP, is characterized by isolated thrombocytopenia. Often, the platelets are increased in size, which may reflect increased platelet turnover and increased megakaryocyte ploidy. White cell and red blood cell changes are nonspecific, and can indicate an associated illness, such as infectious mononucleosis or a chronic bleeding disorder that has resulted in iron deficiency anemia. Bone marrow examination demonstrates normal-to-increased numbers of megakaryocytes. Other exclusionary laboratory tests are often performed in these patients, and include the rheumatoid factor, antinuclear antibody tests, and serological tests for infectious mononucleosis, and, when appropriate, the human immunodeficiency virus. These tests are negative in patients with ITP. Because ITP may be associated with an abnormally functioning thyroid gland, thyroid function studies should be performed in adult ITP patients at presentation, and periodically during the management of the patient.

12.8.1.2. Special Tests Used in the Investigation of ITP; Measurement of PAIgG and Platelet Survival Studies There are two special tests that may be useful in the investigation of ITP patients: platelet antibody tests, and the measurement of platelet survival and sequestration studies, using radiolabeled platelets.

12.8.1.2.1. Measurement of PAIgG Immunoglobulins have been measured on platelets for more than 30 years, and, as yet, an ideal assay remains to be identified. Perhaps the best evidence for this is that there are available more than 100 assay methods for measuring platelet-associated PAIgG. These can be grouped into several categories, and the following briefly summarizes them in relation to the chronological order of their introduction.

12.8.1.2.1.1. PHASE I ASSAYS These were developed following the observation of Harrington et al., that thrombocytopenia develops in healthy individuals after infusion of plasma from patients with ITP. All phase I assays share the same basic principle: Test serum is mixed with normal platelets, and a platelet-dependent end point is measured. End points have included platelet aggregation, platelet release of radioactive tracers, platelet factor 3 availability, and inhibition of specific platelet functions, such as platelet migration or clot retraction. Phase I assays are no longer regarded as satisfactory, because they lack both sensitivity and specificity.

12.8.1.2.1.2. PHASE II ASSAYS These share the general characteristic of directly measuring IgG, or other immunoglobulins, proteins, or complement, on the surface of washed platelets. The test may be performed directly on platelets collected from the patient; alternatively, test serum from the patient is mixed with normal platelets, and the IgG adsorbed onto the platelets is measured. All phase II assays measure IgG, using an antibody or staphylococcal

protein A as the probe. Staphylococcal protein A binds to IgG subclasses 1, 2, and 4, and is a very specific ligand.

Phase II assays may be divided into three general groups: The first includes the direct-binding assays, in which the ligand is labeled directly with fluorescein, an enzyme, or a radioactive marker, then mixed with the test platelets, and, after the reaction has reached equilibrium, unbound ligand is separated by washing. Direct-binding assays are simple to perform, but difficult to quantitate. The second general type of phase II assay is the two-stage assay, in which the ligand is incubated with the washed test platelets, and, after this reaction has achieved equilibrium, residual unbound ligand is measured in a second phase by measuring its interaction with IgG (or another protein of interest) bound to a solid phase. Two-stage assays are more complex than direct-binding assays, but are simpler to quantitate. The final type of phase II assay includes assays for total PAIgG, in which the platelet membrane is dissolved and all platelet IgG, both surface and internal, is measured.

There is now general agreement that all phase II assays have a similar sensitivity and specificity: In ITP, positive reactions are obtained in the majority of thrombocytopenic patients. However, there is a low specificity for ITP, and positive results may occur in many different thrombocytopenic disorders, some of which are usually considered not to be caused by immune mechanisms.

12.8.1.2.1.3. PHASE III ASSAYS These have been introduced in the past several years, and there is still little information on their overall sensitivity and specificity. Phase III assays measure the binding of IgG to individual platelet glycoproteins, in the expectation that this maneuver may overcome the low specificity of phase II assays. There are three general types of phase III assays, including immunoblotting, in which the platelet membrane glycoproteins are separated according to size, and fixed to a solid surface (nitrocellulose); following this the binding of the test serum to the glycoproteins is measured. Radioimmunoprecipitation is performed by radiolabeling the surface platelet glycoproteins, solubilizing the membranes, then reacting the patient's serum with this mixture. Patient IgG binding to the radiolabeled platelet glycoproteins is separated by an immunoprecipitation step, then the radiolabeled glycoproteins are isolated according to size. The final type of phase III assay is the antigen capture assay, in which a monoclonal antibody is attached to a solid phase, such as a bead or a microtiter well. Solubilized platelets are incubated with this, and, after a further wash, the patient's serum is allowed to react. If the patient's serum carries an antibody against the particular glycoprotein, then increased binding of IgG to the monoclonal antibody-platelet glycoprotein will be detected.

12.8.1.2.1.4. THE CLINICAL USEFULNESS OF ANTIPLATELET ANTIBODY ASSAYS IN ITP Phase I assays lack sufficient sensitivity and specificity to be used as diagnostic tests for ITP. The clinical usefulness of phase II assays in ITP remains controversial, but there is little evidence that any particular phase II assay differs significantly in overall sensitivity and specificity for ITP. Major differences among the various assays concerning sensitivity and specificity are probably related principally to differences in assay experience between laboratories, rather than to any intrinsic advantages for a particular assay. Second, there is general agreement that PAIgG is elevated in 80–90% of ITP patients, with the increase being inversely proportional to the platelet count (Panzer et al., 1986; Karpatkin, 1985; McMillan, 1981; Kernoff et al., 1980). Consequently, patients with severe thrombocytopenia almost always have elevated levels of PAIgG; those with mild thrombocytopenia often have normal levels of PAIgG. Finally, there is general agreement that these assays are nonspecific, and positive results are observed in many different thrombocytopenic disorders (Kelton et al., 1982), and in patients who are not thrombocytopenic (Kelton et al., 1984). We believe that increased PAIgG characterizes a variety of thrombocytopenic disorders, including some that traditionally have not been considered to be caused by immune mechanisms.

PAIgG assays are positive in most thrombocytopenic patients with ITP. A positive test is consistent with ITP, but not diagnostic of it. As previously discussed, platelet-associated complement components have been found in elevated quantities in many patients with ITP. The pathological significance of this finding remains unclear.

12.8.1.3. Platelet Survival Studies Using Radionuclides

Platelet survival studies can be performed in patients with ITP, using sodium 51-chromate (^{51}Cr) or 111-Indium Oxine (^{111}In). These studies have provided important information concerning the mechanism of platelet destruction in ITP. Before summarizing these studies, the advantages and disadvantages of each label are described.

Both ^{51}Cr and ^{111}In are taken up by platelets, and both are γ emitters. However, the platelet-labeling efficiency of ^{111}In is far higher (over 80%) than ^{51}Cr (less than 10%), which has a major impact on labeling procedures, especially when using autologous platelets. The low labeling efficiency of ^{51}Cr means that far more platelets are required to provide a sufficiently high level of radioactive emissions to be counted. Consequently, autologous platelet survival studies cannot be accurately performed in severely thrombocytopenic patients, using ^{51}Cr. In contrast, the high labeling efficiency of ^{111}In allows the performance of autologous platelet survival studies, even in thrombocytopenic patients. The pattern of γ emission for ^{111}In is also better than ^{51}Cr, for counting and organ visualization. Finally, there is evidence that ^{51}Cr can be released from platelets by several stimuli, including that of certain antiplatelet autoantibodies (Nagasawa et al., 1977; Baldini, 1978; Joist and Baker, 1981); ^{111}In binds to a large-mol-wt protein within the platelets, and is not released unless the platelets are destroyed. The major disadvantages of ^{111}In are its expense and its much shorter decay half-life (2.8 d), compared with ^{51}Cr.

12.8.1.3.1. Application of Platelet Life-Span Studies in ITP

As with many aspects of ITP, there is still no complete agreement concerning typical platelet survival in an ITP patient, the dominant organ of clearance, and whether platelet survival studies or measurement of organ clearance predict response to therapy. Nevertheless, recent work has developed increased understanding of several aspects.

12.8.1.3.1.1. Platelet Life-Span Measurements in ITP   Virtually all thrombocytopenic ITP patients show shortening of platelet life-span, whether this is measured by ^{51}Cr or ^{111}In (Peters and Lavender, 1983; Peters et al., 1980; Kernoff et al., 1980; Aster, 1972; Branehog et al., 1974). However, the reported degree of shortening of the platelet life-span differs dramatically among the various studies. In some studies, an inverse correlation was found between the level of PAIgG and the platelet survival (Kernoff et al., 1980; Mueller-Eckhardt et al., 1980; Mueller-Eckhardt et al., 1982), but in other patients this relationship was not observed (Ballem et al., 1987).

The results of platelet survival studies have been used to elucidate the pathophysiology of thrombocytopenia in ITP. Two major platelet kinetic studies in the 1970s, using ^{51}Cr-labeled platelets, supported the view that the thrombocytopenia was secondary to a marked increase in platelet destruction (Harker, 1970; Branehog et al., 1975). In those studies, the mean platelet count was 21 and 27 $\times 10^9$/L, respectively, and the average platelet survival was 0.34 and 0.57 d. Both studies showed increases in megakaryocytic size and number, and elevated platelet turnover values, compared to controls. Those results strongly suggested that the major mechanism of the thrombocytopenia was peripheral destruction, and that there was a compensatory increase in platelet production.

Later, those observations were questioned: Ballem et al. (1987) reported that the majority of their patients with chronic ITP had only moderate shortening of platelet survival, and normal rates of platelet turnover. They used ^{111}In-labeled autologous platelets in their study. The platelet life-spans ranged from 1 to 7 d. Those investigators suggested that the discrepancy between their data and previous studies resulted from the use of autologous, rather than homologous, labeled platelets. Ballem et al. also reported a threefold increase in DNA synthetic activity by megakaryocytic stem cells, in nonsplenectomized ITP patients. Despite this finding, most of these patients had normal platelet turnover rates.

These results suggest that, although there is a stimulus for increased platelet production at the level of the stem cells and early megakaryocytic forms, the platelet precursors are not reaching full maturation, or are not releasing platelets into the circulation. An observation consistent with this is the finding that some patients with ITP have cytotoxic antibodies directed against megakaryocytes (Hoffman et al., 1985). Isaka et al. (1990) made similar studies, using ^{111}In-labeled autologous platelets, and found low platelet turnovers in 8/12 patients, the others being within the normal range. They concluded that the platelet destruction in the RE system was the principal pathogenetic mechanism, but impaired thrombopoiesis also contributed to the severity of the condition.

Sequestration studies, using ^{111}In-labeled autologous platelets in ITP, appear to be more useful than similar studies using ^{51}Cr-labeled red blood cells in hemolytic disorders (see and Subheading 8.2.2. Chapter 7). Lamy et al. (1993) showed splenic sequestration of platelets in 81% of ITP patients, and 33/38 such patients normalized the platelet counts after splenectomy. The sequestration site was hepatic in 7% of cases, and mixed in 12%. Of 13 cases without specifically splenic sequestration, only two cases produced normal platelet counts after splenectomy. Other studies have also supported the value of this method in predicting the outcome of splenectomy in ITP (Najean et al., 1991; Najean et al., 1991).

12.8.1.3.1.2. Correlation of the Level of PAIgG with Platelet Survival, Organ Clearance and Response to Therapy   The platelets with the most IgG on their surface might be expected to be destroyed not only in the spleen, but also in the liver. Some investigators have in fact reported just that: Patients with moderately increased levels of PAIgG show principally splenic destruction; those with the largest amount of PAIgG have mostly hepatic destruction (Kernoff et al., 1980). However, other investigators have not confirmed this correlation between the level of PAIgG and the pattern of destruction (Panzer et al., 1986; Mueller-Eckhardt et al., 1982). There is now some evidence that the pattern of platelet clearance evaluated with ^{111}In-labeled platelets assists in predicting the response to splenectomy in individual patients (see Subheading 8.1.2.1.1.).

12.8.1.3.1.3. Splenic Pathology and ITP   The pathology of the spleen in ITP is nonspecific. The organ is normal in size (Tavassoli and McMillan, 1975; Hayes et al., 1985), and an enlarged spleen suggests that the patient does not have ITP. Luk et al. (1980) have reported that the white pulp has increased numbers of germinal centers, and that they contain increased numbers of activated lymphocytes. More recently, others have observed these findings in only about half of all cases of ITP. However, even those who do not report an increase in germinal centers have observed increased numbers of plasma cells within the germinal centers of such spleens (Kristensen and Jensen, 1985). Changes in the microcirculatory pathways have been demonstrated in chronic ITP by Schmidt et al. (1991), who found a striking proliferation of arterioles and capillaries in the white pulp and marginal zone, with extensive vascularization in the majority of lymphatic nodules. Likewise, the marginal sinus was absent in a high portion of nodules. It is suggested that this diverts the distribution of blood flow, causing platelets to be delayed in transit, and leading to greater exposure to macrophages.

The splenic red pulp of ITP patients contains increased numbers of RE cells and neutrophils. Many of the monocytes and macrophages have a lipid-laden cytoplasm, and are termed foamy histiocytes. Some investigators have described partially degraded platelets within these macrophages, which may account for the cytoplasmic lipids (Tavassoli and McMillan, 1975). Although foamy histiocytes are not observed by light microscopy in every ITP patient, they can be observed in most when the histiocytes are examined using electron microscopy (Hayes et al., 1985; Kristensen and Jensen, 1985).

12.8.2. AUTOIMMUNE HEMOLYTIC ANEMIA   Warm-antibody autoimmune hemolytic anemia (AIHA) is an uncommon acquired disorder caused by the development of IgG anti-red blood cell autoantibodies. Additionally, the autoantibody sometimes deposits complement on the red blood cell surface. Hemolysis is almost exclusively extravascular, with RE cells phagocytosing the IgG-sensitized red blood cells. The IgG is referred to as a warm antibody, because it is preferentially active at 37°C. In a majority of patients with warm-antibody AIHA, the disease is idiopathic, although this depends in part on the rigor with which associated disorders are distinguished from "primary" in the various series. However, in about one-third, the anemia is clearly associated with a lymphoproliferative disorder, other autoimmune disease, or a collagen-vascular disorder, most commonly systemic lupus erythematosus (Chaplin and Avioli, 1977). There is a wide range of age at presentation, with three-forths of patients being over the age of 40 yr (Petz and Garratty, 1980). In patients under 50 years of age, the idiopathic form is much more common. The principal symptoms on presentation are highly variable, and are usually related to the severity of the patient's anemia; physical examination is often remarkable only for the patient's pallor, and sometimes slight icterus, and most (57%) have a palpable spleen (Allgood and Chaplin, 1967), which is usually only slightly or moderately enlarged.

Warm-antibody AIHA is usually a chronic disease. Patients have periodic exacerbations, and the response to different therapeutic agents varies appreciably. Prognosis is difficult to estimate on an individual basis, but earlier series suggested an overall mortality of 30–50% (Crosby and Rappaport, 1957; Dacie, 1962; Allgood and Chaplin, 1967). Later studies have suggested a lower mortality, possibly as the result of improved management (Worlledge et al., 1982; Silverstein et al., 1972).

12.8.2.1. Clinical and Laboratory Investigations   Most patients are anemic at presentation, and 40% have an initial hemoglobin of <70 g/L. The red blood cells may show spherocytosis, with

Table 12.2
Participation of the Spleen in Pathogenesis of ITP and AIHA

	ITP	AIHA
Antibody production	++	+
IgG-dependent RE cell clearance	+++	++
Filtration capacity	–	++
Response to splenectomy	+++	++

increased osmotic fragility. The reticulocyte count is usually elevated, but, exceptionally, cases with reticulocytopenia can occur (Liesveld et al., 1987; Conley et al., 1982). The indirect bilirubin and LDH levels are elevated with moderate hemolysis. The direct antiglobulin test for surface immunoglobulin or complement is positive in more than 95% of cases. Bone marrow examination usually shows erythroid hyperplasia.

12.8.2.2. ^{51}Cr-Labeled Red Blood Cell Survival Studies   These demonstrate a shortened survival in patients with warm-antibody AIHA. The site of red blood cell destruction is usually the spleen. ^{51}Cr red blood cell studies have a limited value in predicting the efficacy of splenectomy in patients with this disorder, because this depends critically on the positioning of the external counter, the frequency of observations, and the mathematical analysis of the pattern of spleen-related uptake (see also discussion in Chapter 7).

12.8.2.3. Pathology of the Spleen in Warm-Antibody AIHA   In contrast to its normal size in ITP, the spleen is usually enlarged in patients with warm-antibody AIHA (Jensen and Kristensen, 1986; Schwartz et al., 1970). Histological examination of splenic tissue from patients with AIHA demonstrates that the enlargement is principally within the red pulp, and particularly the cords, where there is a striking increase in the number of trapped red calls and spherocytes. In addition, there are also increased numbers of monocytes and macrophages.

Splenomegaly also characterizes other extravascular hemolytic disorders (Jandl et al., 1965; Molnar and Rappaport, 1972). Histologically, the red pulp in such cases also contains many red blood cells, which emphasizes the lack of specificity of this appearance in hemolytic anemias, and also the importance of the filtration function of the spleen in these disorders. The difficulty with which spherocytic red blood cells pass through the splenic sinus wall leads to obstruction of the passage of red blood cells with slowing of flow through the spleen: This enhances the interaction of RE cells with sensitized red blood cells within the splenic cords as well as causing the cords to enlarge. The combination of macrophage activity and passive filtration by the spleen are additive in producing increased destruction of sensitized red blood cells (Table 2). The interactions of the microvasculature of the spleen and blood cells in passage are discussed in detail in Chapters 2 and 3.

12.8.3. TREATMENT OF ITP AND AIHA   The various approaches to therapy for both ITP and warm-antibody AIHA are discussed together, because of their similarity with respect to the role of the spleen in their pathophysiology, predisposing causes, and response to therapy. The modalities of treatment are summarized according to the probable mechanism of effect. A treatment often acts by more than one mechanism, and, in these instances, the effects are discussed under the response most likely to be predominant.

12.8.3.1. Impairment of RE Function and Suppression of Autoantibody Formation   The spleen is the dominant organ of autoantibody formation in both warm-antibody AIHA and ITP. In addition, the spleen removes the IgG-sensitized red blood cells and platelets from the circulation. However, it is not the only organ that can serve both functions; this poses a problem for the clinician, because the relative importance of the spleen, compared to other lymphocyte-rich macrophage-rich, organs in autoantibody generation and cell clearance, cannot be unequivocally determined in individual patients.

12.8.3.1.1. Corticosteroids
Corticosteriods are the first choice of treatment for both ITP and AIHA. A typical dose is 1–2 mg/kg body wt of prednisone per day, although there have been studies suggesting that much lower doses can be equally efficacious in ITP (Bellucci et al., 1988). A positive response with a rise in the platelet count (ITP) or a rise in the hemoglobin level (AIHA) can be anticipated in at least two-thirds of patients (Karpatkin, 1985; Difino et al., 1980; Allgood and Chaplin, 1967; Bellucci et al., 1988; Christensen, 1973b).

The mechanism of the effect of corticosteroids in these diseases has been studied in detail: The major mechanism is probably the impairment of RE cell function. In vitro studies have shown that corticosteroids inhibit RE receptors for IgG and C3, and cause a dose-dependent decrease in the numbers of RE cell Fc-receptors (Schreiber et al., 1975; Fries et al., 1985). Consequently corticosteroids inhibit the adhesion, ingestion, and subsequent destruction of platelets and red blood cells by mononuclear cells (Verp and Karpatkin, 1975), and also inhibit chemotaxis and the migration of monocytes (Rinehart et al., 1974).

There is indirect evidence to suggest that corticosteroids decrease autoantibody production in patients with AIHA and ITP (Rosse, 1971), based mostly on the observation that the amount of cell-specific antibody is decreased in those patients with AIHA or ITP who respond to corticosteroid therapy. Finally, corticosteroids may have a unique action in ITP, which could account for the rapid reduction of bleeding, even before there is a rise in platelet count. Corticosteroids have been reported to decrease capillary fragility, and thus decrease the local risk of bleeding, by a mechanism that involves the impairment of prostaglandin I2 biosynthesis (Faloon et al., 1952; Stefanini and Martino, 1956; Kitchens, 1977; Blajchman et al., 1979).

Because of the potential for serious long-term side effects with corticosteroids, once a patient has achieved an optimal clinical response, which is usually within 1–2 wk, the dose of corticosteroid should be reduced, with tapering from high to low doses over 1–2 mo. Frequently, the patient shows evidence of relapse during this time, with a fall in the platelet count (ITP), or a fall in hemoglobin level (AIHA). In such patients, it is appropriate to resume high-dosage corticosteroids, and, after a response is achieved, to taper them for a second time. However, in the majority of adult patients, ITP and AIHA are chronic illnesses, and to continue long-term corticosteroid therapy in the hope of ultimate remission may represent an undue hazard for a patient with little chance of long-lasting remission (Difino et al., 1980; Allgood and Chaplin, 1967; Thompson et al., 1972; Doan Wisem et al., 1960).

12.8.3.1.2. Splenectomy
This is the definitive treatment for both ITP and warm-antibody AIHA, because the spleen is both a major site of autoantibody formation and an important site for red blood cell and platelet destruction. Evidence confirming its role in autoantibody formation comes from the in vitro studies discussed previously, in which splenic lymphocytes produce antiplatelet autoantibodies. The levels of antiplatelet autoantibody (Myers et al.,

1982) and anti-red blood cell autoantibody (Allgood and Chaplin, 1967) fall dramatically in the majority of patients following splenectomy. Evidence implicating the role of the spleen in IgG-mediated cell clearance also is strong. IgG-sensitized red blood cells are rapidly removed from the circulation in healthy individuals, but are cleared at a very slow rate in patients following splenectomy (Hosea et al., 1981). A fourfold increase in the IgG sensitization of red blood cells is required for the clearance rate in splenectomized subjects to be comparable to that in nonsplenectomized subjects. Similar results have been found for IgG-mediated platelet clearance. The amount of antiplatelet antibody must be increased at least sixfold, to produce a similar degree of thrombocytopenia in individuals who have undergone splenectomy, by comparison with individuals with a normal spleen (Shulman et al., 1965).

In both ITP and AIHA, attempts have been made to predict which patients are the more likely to respond to splenectomy, but at present it is not possible to state with certainty which prognostic factors are important. Both very high and very low levels of PAIgG have been associated with a poor response to splenectomy (Dixon et al., 1975; Court et al., 1987). Patients with cold agglutinin disease, with only complement on the red blood cells, are unlikely to respond to splenectomy, and this procedure is generally avoided in these patients.

Measurement of platelet life-span, and splenic–hepatic sequestration patterns, have not in general been predictive of response to splenectomy (Nagasawa et al., 1977; Najean and Ardaillou, 1971; Ries and Price, 1974; Gugliotta et al., 1981; Najean et al., 1967). Indeed, potential pitfalls in using the pattern of platelet destruction in deciding on therapy are illustrated by one patient, whose pattern of sequestration varied throughout the illness (Aster and Keene, 1969).

There is better agreement concerning the predictive nature of a previous response to therapy. Patients with ITP, who have had a good response to corticosteroids, defined as a dramatic rise in platelet count, or who respond to a lower-than-expected dose of corticosteroids, are more likely to respond to splenectomy (Brennan et al., 1975; Difino et al., 1980; Karpatkin, 1985). Unfortunately, such correlates do not necessarily hold for the individual patient.

Following splenectomy, about 20% of patients with ITP will show clinical relapse. Unfortunately, the results with AIHA are not as good, and more than one-third of complete responders will relapse within 1 year of therapy. When a late relapse in ITP occurs, the possibility of an accessory spleen should be considered. The presence of Howell-Jolly bodies, siderocytes, and other evidence of hyposplenism in the peripheral blood film does not exclude the possibility of an accessory spleen (Verheyden et al., 1978; Gibson et al., 1986), because the filtering capacity of the spleen differs from its antibody-based, Fc-dependent clearing function. Accessory spleens can be observed using technetium scanning (Gibson et al., 1986), but it appears that more sensitive techniques are radionuclide scanning following ^{111}In-labeled platelet life-span measurements, and CT scans of the abdomen (Verheyden et al., 1978; Hansen and Jarhult, 1986; see also Chapter 17).

The acute mortality of splenectomy in patients with ITP and AIHA is very low. There exists a low but real long-term risk of septicemia, which is, however, not as pronounced as in children under 4 years of age, and in patients with otherwise impaired immunity. Postsplenectomy septicemia can occur in otherwise healthy individuals (Eraklis et al., 1967; Whitaker, 1969); therefore, any patient not previously immunized should receive multivalent pneumococcal vaccine 1–2 wk before elective surgery. Occasionally, pneumococcal vaccine has been found to exacerbate immune thrombocytopenia (Kelton, 1981). The infectious sequelae of splenectomy are also addressed in Chapters 10 and 11.

12.8.3.2. Agents Acting by Reticuloendothelial Cell Blockade Most agents effective in ITP and AIHA have more than one mechanism of action. However, in several instances, the mechanism of action appears to be highly focused, and acts by preventing the clearance of IgG-sensitized cells. The first to be described is still experimental; the second is already widely used.

12.8.3.2.1. RE Blockade Using Monoclonal Antibodies At least one report has described the use of a monoclonal antibody in a patient with refractory ITP (Clarkson et al., 1986). The monoclonal antibody had activity against the low-affinity Fc-receptors on macrophages. The patient was treated with this monoclonal antibody on two separate occasions, and both were followed by an increase in the platelet count. The mechanism was presumed to be one of specific RE blockade, and this was supported by demonstration of impaired clearance of ^{51}Cr-labeled, IgG-sensitized autologous red blood cells. This study appears to be important, not only because it offers the promise of a new approach to clinical management, but also because of its contribution to understanding the pathophysiology of this and related diseases.

12.8.3.2..2. High-Dose Intravenous Immunoglobulin-G (IV-IgG) Several years ago, it was observed that treatment of children with large doses of IV-IgG for agammaglobulinemia might result in resolution of associated autoimmune thrombocytopenia. This observation was soon confirmed, and now IV-IgG provides an important therapy for children with acute immune thrombocytopenia, and for patients of all ages with chronic ITP (Bussel et al., 1983a; Bussel et al., 1983b; Bussel et al., 1985; Mori et al., 1983; Newland et al., 1983; Oral et al., 1984; Imbach et al., 1981). Clinical trials have shown that the administration of IV-IgG in doses of 2 g/kg body wt, to children with acute ITP produces in many patients a significantly more rapid rise in the platelet count than with corticosteroids (Imbach et al., 1985).

In both children and adults with chronic ITP, IV-IgG raises the platelet count in about 75% of patients. Although the rise tends to be less dramatic in chronic than in acute ITP, in most patients, the increase results in the patient achieving safe platelet levels. Unfortunately, for most patients with chronic ITP, the response is short-lived, and the platelets return to their original levels within ~1 mo. Rarely, a patient will have a long-term remission following the administration of high doses of IV-IgG (Mori et al., 1983; Oral et al., 1984).

IV-IgG significantly impairs Fc-dependent macrophage function, while the plasma concentration of IgG remains at high levels. Consequently, it is likely that the mechanism of action of IV-IgG is mediated by preventing the clearance of IgG-sensitized platelets. In patients with acute ITP, the platelet count is kept at safe levels by the RE blockade. Simultaneously, the antiplatelet autoantibody in the plasma slowly declines in amount, and the patient has an apparently spontaneous cure of the illness. In patients with chronic ITP, the platelet count rises because of RE blockade, but, as the plasma concentration of IgG declines, and normal RE function returns, the continued formation of autoantibodies causes the patient to relapse.

Although high-dose IV-IgG has been used in small numbers of patients with AIHA, experience is not sufficiently large to allow one to comment on the efficacy of this therapy. The early pessimistic reports were followed by more hopeful descriptions of IV-IgG in AIHA (Stiehm et al., 1987; Besa, 1988). Consequently, the usefulness of IV-IgG in AIHA still remains to be defined.

The mechanism of action of IV-IgG in ITP and AIHA may be more complex than simple Fc-dependent RE blockade. Some patients have a long-term remission following treatment with IV-IgG. In these patients, it has been postulated that an anti-idiotypic interaction interrupts the formation of autoantibody, and alters the basic pathophysiology of the disease. This possibility implies that, in these patients, a small fraction of the IV-IgG is responsible for the long-term benefit.

12.8.3.2.3. Treatment with Anti-D Salama et al. (1984, 1986) have reported that the administration of 1–2 mg anti-D, to Rh-positive individuals with ITP, resulted in a rise in the platelet count in many of these patients. We have observed similar benefit from anti-D in ITP patients. Presumably, the mechanism of action is by a temporary RE blockade. Anti-D is much less expensive than IV-IgG, and can be given rapidly, subcutaneously or intravenously, depending on the preparation. This may prove useful in the ambulatory management of patients with chronic ITP.

12.8.3.2.4. Danazol This is an attenuated androgen with limited virilizing effects. It was first reported to be effective in ITP by Ahn et al. (1983), using relatively high doses (400–800 mg/d). Subsequent reports by the original investigators have found that danazol may also be used successfully in the treatment of AIHA, and that doses as low as 50 mg/d could be effec-tive in some patients with ITP (Ahn et al., 1985; Ahn et al., 1987). Initially, it was felt that the medication suppressed autoantibody formation, as shown by a fall in the level of antiplatelet autoantibody. A more recent study has suggested that the mechanism of action is principally by RE blockade: In a longitudinal study of six patients with ITP, Schreiber et al. (1987) demonstrated that the level of PAIgG did not change in patients responding to danazol. However, there was a reduction in the number of Fc receptors on monocytes.

Danazol is generally well-tolerated. Side effects include myalgias, headaches, occasional nausea, and weight gain (Ahn et al., 1983); it should not be used during pregnancy, because it may be teratogenic (Wentz, 1982).

12.8.3.3. Agents Acting by Suppression of Autoantibody Formation Azathiaprine and cyclophosphamide have been used successfully in patients with chronic ITP (Finch et al., 1974) and AIHA. These agents act by decreasing the formation of antiplatelet and anti-red blood cell autoantibodies. Evidence for this is given by the reduction in the level of antiplatelet and anti-red blood cell autoantibodies and the delay in response, which often does not occur for several months following the initiation of therapy. Because secondary malignancies have been associated with these medications, their use is limited essentially to cases in which other therapies have failed.

12.8.4. CONDITIONS ASSOCIATED WITH DECREASED RED BLOOD CELL DEFORMABILITY Reduced red blood cell deformability is the consequence of alterations in the red blood cell membrane, an increase in intracellular viscosity, or a decrease in the surface area:volume ratio of the cells. Subtle alterations in deformability can lead to splenic sequestration; when more marked changes in red blood cell properties occur, an increasing proportion of the red blood cell destruction occurs in other RE-rich organs, such as the liver. Intravascular red blood cell destruction may also occur under these circumstances. This pattern of clearance of abnormal red blood cells has been confirmed by experimental, red blood cell survival, and pathological studies.

12.8.4.1. Experimental Studies Much has been learned about the patterns of red blood cell destruction, by using phenylhydrazine as an oxidizing agent to induce Heinz body formation. Rifkind (1965) showed that, when phenylhydrazine is injected into rabbits, about 50% of the circulating blood cells contain Heinz bodies within 24 h. Histological examination of the liver reveals little or no red blood cell ingestion by the Kupffer cells. However, the spleen shows a marked increase in the numbers of red blood cells within the cords: Almost all these red blood cells contain Heinz bodies, and many of the cells are in process of ingestion by monocytes and macrophages. Fewer red blood cells are seen in the splenic sinuses.

When high doses of phenylhydrazine are administered, the red blood cells are ingested by the hepatic Kupffer cells, and there is evidence of intravascular hemolysis. Microscopic examination of the liver shows red blood cell ingestion by the RE cells, but there is no extracellular sequestration, such as occurs in the splenic cords. Rifkind's study (1965) emphasizes the importance of the microcirculation of the spleen in the clearance of red blood cells with mild to moderate impairment in deformability. The interendothelial slits, between the cords and sinusoids, act as an important barrier to the passage of deformed red blood cells. This obstruction promotes increasing contact between abnormal red blood cells and cordal RE cells, and subsequently leads to erythrophagocytosis. However, when damage to the red blood cell is severe, the major site of clearance becomes the liver (see also Chapters 2 and 3).

12.8.4.2. Clinical Data: Thalassemia, Hemoglobinopathies, and Red Blood Cell Membrane Abnormalities

12.8.4.2.1. Thalassemia   The pathogenesis of the anemia of thalassemia is multifactorial. Inclusion bodies are rarely found in the peripheral blood of thalassemic patients with a normally functioning spleen. However, splenectomized patients with thalassemia major show inclusion bodies within their red blood cells indicating that the spleen is important for the clearance of globin chain precipitates (Rigas and Koler, 1961; Slater et al., 1968; Wennberg and Weiss, 1968). ^{51}Cr-labeled red blood cell studies show increased uptake of the thalassemic cells by the spleen.

Light microscopic examination of splenic tissue from patients with thalassemia major shows an accumulation of red blood cells within the splenic cords. The interendothelial slits are the most important barrier to red blood cell passage: electron microscopic studies demonstrate a marked distortion of the thalassemic cells as they pass through these apertures, and red blood cells containing inclusion bodies are disrupted during their passage through them (Fig. 3). The red blood cells become teardrop in shape, and pass into the splenic sinuses; however, the inclusion bodies remain in the splenic cords, where phagocytosis occurs. The formation of teardrop cells (dacryocytes) and red blood cell fragments by the microcirculation of the spleen accounts for the finding of these cells in the peripheral blood of patients with thalassemia major. However, after splenectomy, these abnormal cells are not as commonly seen (Wennberg and Weiss, 1968; Slater et al., 1968; Nathan and Gunn, 1966). Splenomegaly is a common sequela of thalassemia major. This can result in hypersplenism and increased red blood cell transfusion requirements. Hypertransfusion programs, designed to maintain the patient's hemoglobin within the normal range, have decreased the spleen size in some patients (Beard et al., 1969; O'Brien et al., 1977), which may be caused by diminished red blood cell pooling, or possibly a reduction in extramedullary hematopoiesis within the spleen.

Some thalassemia patients benefit from splenectomy performed to alleviate the hypersplenism and decrease red blood cell transfu-

sion requirements. Several studies have attempted to define factors capable of predicting the optimal time for splenectomy in these patients. Some would recommend splenectomy when transfusion requirements progressively rise above their previous baseline (Modell, 1977). In a study analyzing the transfusion requirements and hemoglobin levels of a group of thalassemic patients before and after splenectomy, the mean transfusion requirements were found to be significantly higher in the presplenectomy group (Cohen et al., 1980).

There is some disagreement about the long-term benefit of splenectomy in patients with thalassemia: Opinion is at present divided between those who believe that most patients with increasing transfusion requirements have a long-term benefit from splenectomy (Modell, 1977), and others who feel that the improvement is at best temporary (Engelhard et al., 1975).

12.8.4.2.2. Hemoglobinopathies

12.8.4.2.2.1. SICKLE CELL ANEMIA   In young patients with homozygous sickle cell anemia, splenomegaly is common, although splenic function is usually impaired (Pearson et al., 1979; see also Chapter 15). By the age of 8 years, ~50% of affected children will develop splenic fibrosis and functional asplenia, probably caused by recurrent splenic thromboses. However, patients with splenomegaly, who develop increasing transfusion requirements or thrombocytopenia, may be helped by splenectomy. In these cases, the splenectomy will usually lead to resolution of thrombocytopenia, reduce the transfusion requirements, and increase the red blood cell lifespan (Sprague and Paterson, 1958; Szwed et al., 1980; Emond et al., 1984).

Patients with functioning spleens are also susceptible to the development of acute splenic red blood cell sequestration, characterized by a sudden fall in the hemoglobin concentration, hypovolemia, and evidence of rapid splenic enlargement. This condition usually occurs in children, although it is known to occur in adults (Solanki et al., 1986). In some patients, the splenic sequestration crisis is triggered by acute splenic venous occlusion. Treatment involves red blood cell transfusions, and exchange transfusion may need to be considered. This complication may be fatal, and splenectomy is indicated for recurrent cases (Seelder and Shwiaki, 1972). For further consideration of the significance of the spleen in sickle cell disease, see Chapter 15.

12.8.4.2.2.2. UNSTABLE HEMOGLOBINS   Such hemoglobins result in hemoglobinopathies, in which a structural abnormality of hemoglobin leads to the formation in red blood cells of insoluble hemoglobin inclusions, known as Heinz bodies. The disorder is diagnosed by showing that hemolysates containing these hemoglobins denature when heated in iso-osmotic phosphate buffer to 50°C. The spectrum of clinical disease associated with unstable hemoglobins varies from mild hemolysis to severe, life-threatening red blood cell destruction; splenomegaly may be present. Patients with mild-to-moderate disease principally show spleen-mediated red blood cell destruction, and will respond to splenectomy. More severe, unstable hemoglobinopathies are less likely to benefit from splenectomy (Miller et al., 1971; White and Dacie, 1971).

12.8.4.2.3. Red Blood Cell Membrane Abnormalities

12.8.4.2.3.1. HEREDITARY SPHEROCYTOSIS   This is an inherited hemolytic disorder, with extravascular hemolysis caused by structural red blood cell membrane abnormalities (Weed and Bowdler, 1966; Becker and Lux, 1985). Inheritance is usually as an autosomal dominant. Patients with this disorder have laboratory evidence of chronic but low-grade hemolysis, spherocytic red blood cell morphology, and commonly splenomegaly.

[51]Cr red blood cell survival studies demonstrate that the red blood cells have a shortened life-span, with destruction occurring predominantly in the spleen. Splenectomy cures the expression of the disorder, although it does not alter the abnormality of the red blood cell membrane or the increased osmotic fragility of the red blood cells.

Investigation of the role of the spleen in the pathogenesis of the hemolysis of hereditary spherocytosis has provided a unique insight into the manner in which the spleen is capable of conditioning red blood cells to premature destruction. The filtration system of the splenic microcirculation delays or prevents the passage of the poorly deformable spherocytic cells, and this results in loss of cell membrane (fragmentation) during the slow passage through the red pulp and the interendothelial slits of the sinus wall. This progressively decreases the surface area:volume ratio of the cell. The conditions in the splenic pulp appear to create a metabolic competition, which aggravates the loss of integrity of the membrane. The RE cells of the splenic cords are exceptionally active and phagocytose many of the trapped spherocytic cells; however, it is clear that this accounts for only part of the total cells destroyed. A significant fraction is conditioned by the spleen, and destroyed at other sites (Bowdler, 1962; Ferrant, 1983).

One characteristic abnormality of red blood cells in hereditary spherocytosis is their high sodium flux, which requires a highly active sodium–potassium pump to maintain normal intracellular electrolytes. This is not, however, the cause of the spherocytosis. When the red blood cells are trapped in the splenic cords, cellular adenosine triphosphate levels remain normal, but there is a decrease in intracellular glucose and pH, which could impair activity of the sodium–potassium pump and lead to further cell membrane damage (Becker and Lux, 1985; Emerson et al., 1956; Prankerd, 1963; Murphy, 1967).

12.8.4.2.3.2. HEREDITARY ELLIPTOCYTOSIS This abnormality is also caused by a congenital defect of the red blood cell membrane, and is morphologically characterized by elliptical red blood cells. Inheritance is as an autosomal dominant, and the homozygous form is associated with a severe hemolytic disorder in affected infants. However, in most instances, the heterozygous form is found to be a clinical epiphenomenon, without significant anemia or hemolysis. Occasional cases show severe hemolysis and splenomegaly, and the severity of the anemia is usually improved by splenectomy. As with hereditary spherocytosis, the morphological abnormality of the red blood cells continues after splenectomy (Palek, 1985).

12.8.4.2.3.3. HEREDITARY PYROPOIKILOCYTOSIS This is a rare condition, related to hereditary elliptocytosis, in that both conditions show an inherent instability in the cytoskeleton, in this case, expressed by heat-induced cell fragmentation at temperatures lower than for normal red blood cell membranes. The red blood cell morphology shows microspherocytes and a wide variety of bizarre red shapes. Splenectomy lessens the hemolysis, and the spleen is probably a major site of cell destruction.

12.8.5. HYPERSPLENISM Hypersplenism is essentially a clinical syndrome, rather than a process, and it can be defined as the condition present when there are decreased numbers of cells of one or more blood cell lines in the peripheral blood; there is at least a normal, and sometimes increased, production of that cell line present on bone marrow examination; splenomegaly is present; and splenectomy corrects the cytopenia. Anemia, leucopenia, and thrombocytopenia occur to differing degrees in association with splenomegaly and hypersplenism, and it is difficult to define any predictable relationship between splenomegaly and the degree of cytopenia induced by the wide variety of primary and secondary disorders that can cause splenic enlargement (see also Chapter 9).

12.8.5.1. Anemia Splenomegaly from many causes tends to increase the mass of red blood cells pooled in the spleen (see Chapter 7), and this may lead to a moderate shortening of the red blood cell life-span. In itself, this is seldom sufficient in degree to exceed the compensatory reserve of the bone marrow, but the volume of pooled red blood cells, in the presence of a slight shortening of red blood cell survival, may diminish the sustainable population of red blood cells in the extrasplenic circulation. Of greater importance is the dilutional effect of an expansion of blood volume caused by splenomegaly, in the presence of a limited productive capacity for red blood cells (see Chapter 9).

12.8.5.2. Thrombocytopenia The thrombocytopenia of hypersplenism is principally caused by the increased pooling of platelets in the spleen with a normal (or only slightly shortened) platelet survival. That is, it is predominantly distributional in origin (Najean et al., 1967; Cooney and Smith, 1968; Toghill et al., 1977; Heyns et al., 1985). Karpatkin and Freedman (1978) studied platelet size as a means of differentiating the thrombocytopenia of ITP from that of hypersplenism, and showed that the mean platelet volume was significantly greater in patients with ITP than in those with hypersplenism. Karpatkin (1978, 1983) hypothesized that the spleen is enriched with young and large platelets, termed "megathrombocytes," and speculated that these platelets could be released into the circulation at times of stress. This would explain the low degree of hemostatic impairment in patients with thrombocytopenia secondary to hypersplenism.

REFERENCES

Ahn, Y. S., Harrington, W. J., Simon, S. R., Mylvaganam, R., Pall, L. M., and So, A. G. (1983) Danazol for the treatment of idiopathic thrombocytopenic purpura. *N. Engl. J. Med.* **308,** 1396–1399.

Ahn, Y. S., Harrington, W. J., Mylvaganam, R., Ayub, J., and Pall, L. M. (1985) Danazol therapy for autoimmune hemolytic anemia. *Ann. Int. Med.* **102,** 298–301.

Ahn, Y. S., Mylvaganam, R., Garcia, R. O., Kim, C. I., Palow, D., and Harrington, W. J. (1987) Low dose danazol therapy in idiopathic thrombocytopenic purpura. *Ann. Int. Med.* **107,** 177–181.

Allgood, J. W. and Chaplin, H. Jr. (1967) Idiopathic acquired autoimmune hemolytic anemia: a review of 47 cases treated from 1955 through 1965. *Am. J. Med.* **43,** 254–273.

Andersson, J. (1998) Cytokines in idiopathic thrombocytopenic purpura (ITP). *Acta Pediatr.* **424(Suppl.),** 61–64.

Aster, R. H. (1966) Pooling of platelets in the spleen: role in the pathogenesis of "hypersplenic" thrombocytopenia. *J. Clin. Invest.* **45,** 645–657.

Aster, R. H. (1972) Platelet sequestration studies in man. *Br. J. Haematol.* **22,** 259–263.

Aster, R. H. and Keene, W. R. (1969) Sites of platelet destruction in idiopathic thrombocytopenic purpura. *Br. J. Haematol.* **16,** 61–73.

Baldini, M. G. (1978) Platelet production and destruction in idiopathic thrombocytopenic purpura: a controversial issue. *JAMA* **239,** 2477–2479.

Ballem, P. J., Segal, G. M., Stratton, J. R., Gernsheimer, T., Adamson, J. W., and Slichter, S. J. (1987) Mechanisms of thrombocytopenia in chronic autoimmune thrombocytopenic purpura. Evidence of both impaired platelet production and increased platelet clearance. *J. Clin. Invest.* **80,** 33–40.

Bateman, S., Lewis S. M., Nicholas, A., and Zaafran, A. (1978) Splenic red cell pooling: a diagnostic feature in polycythaemia. *Br. J. Haematol.* **40,** 389–396.

Beard, M. E. J., Necheles, T. F., and Allen, D. M. (1969) Clinical experience with intensive transfusion therapy in Cooley's anemia. *Ann. NY Acad. Sci.* **165,** 415–422.

Becker, P. S. and Lux, S. E. (1985) Hereditary spherocytosis and related disorders. *Clin. Haematol.* **14,** 15–43.

Bellucci, S., Charpak, Y., Chastang, C., and Tobelem, G. (1988) Low doses v conventional doses of corticoids in immune thrombocytopenic purpura (ITP): results of a randomized clinical trial in 160 children, 223 adults. *Blood* **71,** 1165–1169.

Bender, B. S., Frank, M. M., Lawley, T. J., Smith, W. J., Brickman, C. M., and Quinn, T. C. (1985) Defective reticuloendothelial system Fc-receptor function in patients with acquired immunodeficiency syndrome. *J. Infect. Dis.* **152,** 409–412.

Besa, E. C. (1988) Rapid transient reversal of anemia and long-term effects of maintenance intravenous immunoglobulin for autoimmune hemolytic anemia in patients with lymphoproliferative disorders. *Am. J. Med.* **84,** 691–697.

Bianco, C., Griffin, F.M., and Silverstein, S. C. (1975) Studies of the macrophage complement receptor: alteration of receptor function macrophage upon activation. *J. Exper. Med.* **141,** 1278–1290.

Bishop, M. D. and Lansing, L. S. (1982) The spleen: a correlative overview of normal and pathologic anatomy. *Hum. Pathol.* **13,** 334–342.

Blajchman, M. A., Senyi, A. F., Hirsh, J., Surya, Y., Buchanan, M., and Mustard, J. F. (1979) Shortening of the bleeding time in rabbits by hydrocortisone caused by inhibition of prostacyclin generation by the vessel wall. *J. Clin. Invest.* **63,** 1026–1035.

Bowdler, A. J. (1962) Theoretical considerations concerning measurement of the splenic red cell pool. *Clin. Sci.* **23,** 181–195.

Branehog, I., Kutti, J., and Weinfeld, A. (1974) Platelet survival and platelet production in idiopathic thrombocytopenic purpura. *Br. J. Haematol.* **27,** 127–143.

Branehog, I., Kutti, J., Ridell, B., Swolin B., and Weinfeld, A. (1975) The relation of thrombokinetics to bone marrow megakaryocytes in idiopathic thrombocytopenic purpura. *Blood* **45,** 551–562.

Brennan, M. F., Rappeport, J. M., Moloney, W. C., and Wilson, R. E. (1975) Correlation between response to corticosteroids and splenectomy for adult idiopathic thrombocytopenic purpura. *Am. J. Surg.* **129,** 490–492.

Bussel, J. B. Schulman, I., Hilgartner, M. W., and Barandun, S. (1983a) Intravenous use of gammaglobulin in the treatment of chronic immune thrombocytopenic purpura as a means to defer splenectomy. *J. Pediatr.* **103,** 651–654.

Bussel, J. B., Kimberly, R. P., Inman, R. D., Schulman, I., Cunningham-Rundles, C., Cheung, N., et al. (1983b) Intravenous gammaglobulin treatment of chronic idiopathic thrombocytopenic purpura. *Blood* **62,** 480–486.

Bussel, J. B., Goldman, A., Imbach, P., Schulman, I., and Hilgartner, M. W. (1985) Treatment of acute idiopathic thrombocytopenia of childhood with intravenous infusions of gammaglobulin. *J. Pediatr.* **106,** 886–890.

Chaplin, H. and Avioli, L. V. (1977) Autoimmune hemolytic anemia. *AMA Arch. Int. Med.* **137,** 346–351.

Chen, L. and Weiss, L. (1972) Electron microscopy of the red pulp of human spleen. *Am. J. Anat.* **134,** 425–458.

Chen, L. and Weiss, L. (1973) The role of the sinus wall in the passage of erythrocytes through the spleen. *Blood* **41,** 529–537.

Christensen, B. E. (1973a) Erythrocyte pooling and sequestration in enlarged spleens. Estimations of splenic erythrocyte and plasma volume in splenomegalic patients. *Scand. J. Haematol.* **10,** 106–119.

Christensen, B. E. (1973b) The pattern of erythrocyte sequestration in immunohemolysis: effects of prednisone treatment and splenectomy. *Scand. J. Haematol.* **10,** 120–129.

Cines, D. B. and Schreiber, A. D. (1979) Immune thrombocytopenia: use of a Coombs' antiglobulin test to detect IgG and C3 on platelets. *N. Engl. J. Med.* **300,** 106–111.

Clarkson, S. B., Bussel, J. B., Kimberly, R. P., Valinsky, J. E., Nachman, R. L., and Unkeless, J. C. (1986) Treatment of refractory immune thrombocytopenic purpura with an anti-Fc gamma-receptor antibody. *N. Engl. J. Med.* **314,** 1236–1239.

Cohen, A., Markenson, A. L., and Schwartz, E. (1980) Transfusion requirements and splenectomy in thalassemia major. *J. Pediatr.* **97,** 100–102.

Come, S. E., Shohet, S. B., and Robinson, S. H. (1974) Surface remodeling vs whole-cell hemolysis of reticulocytes produced with erythroid stimulation or iron deficiency anemia. *Blood* **44,** 817–829.

Conley, C. L., Lippman, S. M., Ness, P. M., Petz, L. D., Branch, D. R., and Gallagher, M. T. (1982) Autoimmune hemolytic anemia with reticulocytopenia and erythroid marrow. *N. Engl. J. Med.* **306,** 281–286.

Cooney, D. P. and Smith, B. A. (1968) The pathophysiology of hypersplenic thrombocytopenia. *AMA Arch. Int. Med.* **121,** 332–337.

Cooper, R. A. (1972) Loss of membrane components in the pathogenesis of antibody-induced spherocytosis. *J. Clin. Invest.* **51,** 16–21.

Court, W. S., Bozeman, J. M., Soong, S. J., Saleh, M. N., Shaw, D. R., and LoBuglio, A. F. (1987) Platelet surface-bound IgG in patients with immune and nonimmune thrombocytopenia. *Blood* **69,** 278–283.

Crosby, W. H. (1957) Siderocytes and the spleen. *Blood* **12,** 165–170.

Crosby, W. H. (1975) Wet purpura, dry purpura. *JAMA* **232,** 7441–7745.

Crosby, W. H. and Rappaport, H. (1957) Autoimmune hemolytic anemia. I. Analysis of hematologic observations with particular reference to their prognostic value. A survey of 57 cases. *Blood* **12,** 42–49.

Dacie, J. F. (1962) *The Haemolytic Anaemias, Congenital and Acquired,* 2nd ed. Churchill, London.

Difino, S. M., Lachant, N. A., Kirshner, J. J., and Gottlieb, A. J. (1980) Adult idiopathic thrombocytopenic purpura. Clinical findings and response to therapy. *Am. J. Med.* **69,** 430–442.

Dixon, R., Rosse, W., and Ebbert, L. (1975) Quantitative determination of antibody in idiopathic thrombocytopenic purpura: correlation of serum and platelet-bound antibody with clinical response. *N. Engl. J. Med.* **292,** 230–236.

Doan, C. A., Bouroncle, B. A., and Wiseman, B. K. (1960) Idiopathic and secondary thrombocytopenic purpura: clinical study and evaluation of 381 cases over a period of 28 years. *Ann. Int. Med.* **53,** 861–876.

Ehlenberger, A. G. and Nussenzweig, V. (1977) The role of membrane receptors for C3b and C3d in phagocytosis. *J. Exper. Med.* **145,** 357–371.

Eichner, E. R. (1979) Splenic function: normal, too much and too little. *Am. J. Med.* **66,** 311–320.

Emerson, C. P., Shu, C. S., Ham, T. H., Fleming, E. M., and Castle, W. B. (1956) Studies on the destruction of red blood cells. IX. Quantitative methods for determining the osmotic and mechanical fragility of red cells in the peripheral blood and splenic pulp: the mechanism of increased hemolysis in hereditary spherocytosis (congenital hemolytic jaundice) as related to the functions of the spleen. *AMA Arch. Int. Med.* **97,** 1–38.

Emond, A. M., Morais, P., Venugopal, S., Carpenter, R. G., and Serjeant, G. R. (1984) Role of splenectomy in homozygous sickle cell disease in childhood. *Lancet* **1,** 88–91.

Engelhard, D., Cividalli, G., and Rachmilewitz, E. A. (1975) Splenectomy in homozygous beta-thalassaemia: a retrospective study of 30 patients. *Br. J. Haematol.* **31,** 391–403.

Eraklis, A. J., Kevy, S. V., Diamond, L. K., and Gross, R. E. (1967) Hazard of overwhelming infection after splenectomy in childhood. *N. Engl. J. Med.* **276,** 1225–1229.

Faloon, W. W., Green, R. W., and Lozner, E. L. (1952) The hemostatic defect in thrombocytopenia as studied by the use of ACTH and cortisone. *Am. J. Med.* **13,** 12–20.

Ferrant, A. (1983) Role of the spleen in haemolysis. *Clin. Haematol.* **12,** 489–504.

Ferrant, A., Leners, N., Michaux, J. L., Verwilghen, R. L., and Sokal, G. (1987) The spleen and haemolysis: evaluation of the intrasplenic transit time. *Br. J. Haematol.* **65,** 31–34.

Finch, S. C., Castro, O., Cooper, M., Covey, W., Erichson, R., and McPhedran, P. (1974) Immunosuppressive therapy of chronic idiopathic thrombocytopenic purpura. *Am. J. Med.* **56,** 4–12.

Frank, M. M. (1987) Complement in the pathophysiology of human disease. *N. Engl. J. Med.* **316,** 1525–1530.

Frank, M. M., Schreiber, A. D., Atkinson, J. P., and Jaffe, C. J. (1977) Pathophysiology of immune hemolytic anemia. *Ann. Int. Med.* **87,** 210–222.

Frank, M. M., Hamburger, M. I., Lawley, T. J., Kimberly, R. P., and Plotz, P. H. (1979) Defective reticuloendothelial system Fc-receptor function in systemic lupus erythematosis. *N. Engl. J. Med.* **300,** 518–523.

Frank, M. M., Lawley, T. J., Hamburger, M. I., and Brown, E. J. (1983) Immunoglobulin G Fc receptor-mediated clearance in autoimmune diseases. *Ann. Int. Med.* **98,** 206–218.

Freedman, J. (1987) The significance of complement on the red cell surface. *Transfusion Med. Rev.* **1,** 58–70.

Fries, L. F., Brickman, C. M., and Frank, M. M. (1983) Monocyte receptors for the Fc portion of IgG increase in number in autoimmune hemolytic anemia and other hemolytic states and are decreased by corticosteroid therapy. *J. Immunol.* **131,** 1240–1245.

Galili, U., Clark, M. R., and Shohet, S. B. (1986) Excessive binding of natural anti-alpha-galactosyl immunoglobin G to sickle erythrocytes may contribute to extravascular cell destruction. *J. Clin. Invest.* **77,** 27–33.

Gibson, J., Rickard, K. A., Bautovich, G., May, J., and Kronenberg, H. (1986) Management of splenectomy failures in chronic immune thrombocytopenic purpura: role of accessory splenectomy. *Aust. NZ J. Med.* **16,** 695–698.

Green, G. A., Rehn, M. M., and Kalra, V. K. (1985) Cell-bound autologous immunoglobulin in erythrocyte subpopulations from patients with sickle cell disease. *Blood* **65,** 1127–1133.

Gugliotta, L., Isacchi, G., Guarini, A., Ciccone, F., Motta, M. R., Lattarini, C., et al. (1981) Chronic idiopathic thrombocytopenic purpura:site of platelet sequestration and results of splenectomy. A study of 197 patients. *Scand. J. Haematol.* **26,** 407–412.

Hansen, S. and Jarhult, J. (1986) Accessory spleen imaging: radionuclide, ultrasound and CT investigations in a patient with thrombocytopenia 25 years after splenectomy for ITP. *Scand. J. Haematol.* **37,** 74–77.

Harker, L. A. (1970) Thrombokinetics in idiopathic thrombocytopenic purpura. *Br. J. Haematol.* **19,** 95–104.

Hauch, T. W. and Rosse, W. F. (1977) Platelet-bound complement (C3) in immune thrombocytopenia. *Blood* **50,** 1129–1136.

Hayes, M. M., Jacobs, P., Wood, L., and Dent, D. M. (1985) Splenic pathology in immune thrombocytopenia. *J. Clin. Pathol.* **38,** 985–988.

Hegde, U. M., Williams, E. D., Lewis, S. M., Szur, L., Glass, H. I., and Pettit, J. E. (1973) Measurement of splenic red cell volume and visualization of the spleen with ^{99m}Tc. *J. Nucl. Med.* **14,** 769–771.

Hegde, U. M., Bowes, A., and Roter, B. L. T. (1985) Platelet associated complement components (PAC_{3c} and PAC_{3d}) in patients with autoimmune thrombocytopenia. *Br. J. Haematol.* **60,** 49–55.

Heyns, A. duP., Badenhorst, P. N., Lotter, M. G., Pieters, H., and Wessels, P. (1985) Kinetics and mobilization from the spleen of indium-111-labeled platelets during platelet apheresis. *Transfusion* **25,** 215–218.

Hoffman, R., Zaknoen, S., Yang, H. H., Bruno, E., LoBuglio, A. F., Arrowsmith, J. B., and Prchal, J. T. (1985) An antibody cytotoxic to megakaryocyte progenitor cells in a patient with immune thrombocytopenic purpura. *N. Engl. J. Med.* **312,** 1170–1174.

Hosea, S. W., Brown, E. J., Hamburger, M. I., and Frank, M. M. (1981) Opsonic requirements for intravascular clearance after splenectomy. *N. Engl. J. Med.* **304,** 245–250.

Huber, H., Polley, M. J., Linscott, W. D., Fudenberg, H. H., and Muller-Eberhard, H. J. (1968) Human monocytes: distinct receptor sites for the third component of complement and for immunoglobulin G. *Science* **162,** 1281–1283.

Huber, H. and Fudenberg, H. H. (1968) Receptor sites of human monocytes for IgG. *Int. Arch. Allergy* **34,** 18–31.

Imbach, P., Barandun, S., d'Apuzzo, V., Baumgartner, C., Hirt, A., Morell, A., et al. (1981) High-dose intravenous gammaglobulin for idiopathic thrombocytopenic purpura in childhood. *Lancet* **1,** 1228–1231.

Imbach, P., Wagner, H. P., Berchtold, W., Gaedicke, G., Hirt, A., Joller, P., et al. (1985) Intravenous immunoglobulin versus oral corticosteroids in acute immune thrombocytopenic purpura in childhood. *Lancet* **2,** 464–468.

Isaka, Y., Kambayashi, J., Kimura, K., Matsumoto, M., Uehara, A., Hashikawa, K., et al. (1990) Platelet production, clearance and distribution in patients with idiopathic thrombocytopenic purpura. *Thromb. Res.* **60,** 121–131.

Jandl, J. H., Files, N. M., Barnett, S. B., and Macdonald, R. A. (1965) Proliferative response of the spleen and liver to hemolysis. *J. Exp. Med.* **122,** 299–325.

Jandl, J. H. and Aster, R. H. (1967) Increased splenic pooling and the pathogenesis of hypersplenism. *Am. J. Med. Sci.* **253,** 383–398.

Jandl, J. H. and Kaplan, M. E. (1960) The destruction of red cells by antibodies in man. III. Qualitative factors influencing the patterns of hemolysis in vivo. *J. Clin. Invest.* **39,** 1145–1156.

Jensen, O. M. and Kristensen, J. (1986) Red pulp of the spleen in autoimmune haemolytic anemia and hereditary spherocytosis: morphometric light and electron microscopic studies. *Scand. J. Haematol.* **36,** 263–266.

Joist, J. H. and Baker, R. K. (1981) Loss of 111Indium as indicator of platelet injury. *Blood* **58,** 350–353.

Karpatkin, S. (1978) Heterogeneity of human platelets. VI. Correlation of platelet function with platelet volume. *Blood* **51,** 307–316.

Karpatkin, S. (1983) The spleen and thrombocytopenia. *Clin. Haematol.* **12,** 591–604.

Karpatkin, S. (1985) Autoimmune thrombocytopenic purpura. *Semin. Hematol.* **22,** 260–288.

Karpatkin, S. and Freedman, M. L. (1978) Hypersplenic thrombocytopenia differentiated from increased peripheral destruction by platelet volume. *Ann. Int. Med.* **89,** 200–203.

Karpatkin, S., Strick, N., and Siskind, G. W. (1972) Detection of splenic anti-platelet antibody synthesis in autoimmune thrombocytopenic purpura. *Br. J. Haematol.* **23,** 167–176.

Kay, M. M. B. (1975) Mechanism of removal of senescent cells by human macrophages *in situ. Proc. Natl. Acad. Sci. USA* **72.** 3521–3525.

Kay, M. M. B. (1984) Localization of senescent cell antigen on band 3. *Proc. Natl. Acad. Sci. USA* **81,** 5753–5757.

Kay, M. M. B., Sorensen, K., Wong, P., and Bolton, P. (1982) Antigenicity, storage, and aging: physiologic autoantibodies to cell membrane and serum proteins and the senescent cell antigen. *Mol. Cell. Biochem.* **49,** 65–85.

Kayser, W., Mueller-Eckhardt, C., Bhakdi, S., and Ebert, K. (1983) Platelet associated complement C3 in thrombocytopenic states. *Br. J. Haematol.* **54,** 353–363.

Kelton, J. G. (1981) Vaccination-associated relapse of immune thrombocytopenia. *JAMA* **245,** 369–371.

Kelton, J. G. (1983) The measurement of platelet-bound immunoglobulins: an overview of the methods and the biological relevance of platelet-associated IgG. In: *Progress in Hematology,* vol. XIII (Brown, E. B., ed.), Grune & Stratton, New York, pp. 163–199.

Kelton, J. G. (1985) Impaired reticuloendothelial function in patients treated with methyldopa. *N. Engl. J. Med.* **313,** 596–600.

Kelton, J. G. (1987) Platelet and red cell clearance is determined by the interaction of the IgG and complement on the cells and the activity of the reticuloendothelial system. *Transfusion Med. Rev.* **1,** 75–84.

Kelton, J. G. and Denomme, G. (1982) The quantitation of platelet-associated IgG on cohorts of platelets separated from healthy individuals by buoyant density centrifugation. *Blood* **60,** 136–139.

Kelton, J. G. and Steeves, K. (1983) The amount of platelet-bound albumin parallels the amount of IgG on washed platelets from patients with immune thrombocytopenia. *Blood* **62,** 924–927.

Kelton, J. G., Powers, P. J., and Carter, C. J. (1982) A prospective study of the usefulness of the measurement of platelet-associated IgG for the diagnosis of idiopathic thrombocytopenic purpura. *Blood* **60,** 1050–1053.

Kelton, J. G., Carter, C. J., Rodger, C., Bebenek, G., Gauldie, J., Sheridan, D., et al. (1984) The relationship among platelet-associated IgG, platelet lifespan, and reticuloendothelial cell function. *Blood* **63,** 1434–1438.

Kelton, J. G., Singer, J., Rodger, C., Gauldie, J., Horsewood, P., and Dent, P. (1985) The concentration of IgG in the serum is a major determinant of Fc-dependent reticuloendothelial function. *Blood* **66,** 490–495.

Kernoff, L. M., Blake, K. C. H., and Shackleton, D. (1980) Influence of the amount of platelet-bound IgG on platelet survival and site of sequestration in autoimmune thrombocytopenia. *Blood* **55,** 730–733.

Khansari, N. and Fudenberg, H. H. (1983) Phagocytosis of senescent erythrocytes by autologous monocytes: requirement of membrane-specific autologous IgG for immune elimination of aging red blood cells. *Cell. Immunol.* **78**, 114–121.

Kitchens, C. S. (1977) Amelioration of endothelial abnormalities by prednisone in experimental thrombocytopenia in the rabbit. *J. Clin. Invest.* **60**, 1129–1134.

Komrower, G. M. and Watson, G. H. (1954) Prognosis of idiopathic thrombocytopenic purpura of childhood. *AMA Arch. Dis. Child.* **29**, 502–506.

Kristensen, J. and Jensen, O. M. (1985) Splenic pulp, plasma cells and foamy histiocytes in immune thrombocytopenia: combined morphometric, immunohistochemical and ultrastructural studies. *Scand. J. Haematol.* **34**, 340–344.

Kurata, Y., Curd, J. G., Tamerius, J. D., and McMillan, R. (1985) Platelet-associated complement in chronic ITP. *Br. J. Haematol.* **60**, 723–733.

Lamy, T., Moisan, A., Dauriac, C., Ghandour, C., Morice, P., and Le Prise, P. Y. (1993) Splenectomy in idiopathic thrombocytopenic purpura: its correlation with the sequestration of autologous indium-111-labeled platelets. *J. Nucl. Med.* **34**, 182–186.

Lawley, T. J., Hall, R. P., Fauci, A. S., Katz, S. I., Hamburger, M. I., and Frank, M. M. (1981) Defective Fc-receptor functions associated with the HLA-B8/DRw3 haplotype: studies in patients with dermatitis herpetiformis and normal subjects. *N. Engl. J. Med.* **304**, 185–192.

Lay, W. H. and Nussenzweig, V. (1968) Receptors for complement on leukocytes. *J. Exper. Med.* **128**, 991–1009.

Lehman, H. A., Lehman, L. O., Rustagi, P. K., Rustagi, R. N., Plunkett, R. W., Farolino, D. L., Conway, J. and Logue, G. L. (1987) Complement-mediated autoimmune thrombocytopenia. Monoclonal IgM antiplatelet antibody associated with lymphoreticular malignant disease. *N. Engl. J. Med.* **316**, 194–198.

Lewis, S. M., Catovsky, D., Hows, J. M., and Ardalan, B. (1977) Splenic red cell pooling in hairy cell leukaemia. *Br. J. Haematol.* **35**, 351–357.

Liesveld, J. L., Rowe, J. M., and Lichtman, M. A. (1987) Variability of the erythropoietic response in autoimmune hemolytic anemia: analysis of 109 cases. *Blood* **69**, 820–826.

Lobuglio, A. F., Cotran, R. S., and Jandl, J. H. (1967) Red cells coated with immunoglobulin G: binding and sphering by mononuclear cells in man. *Science* **158**, 1582–1585.

Low, P. S., Waugh, S. M., Zinke, K., and Drenckhahn, D. (1985) The role of hemoglobin denaturation and band 3 clustering in red blood cell aging. *Science* **227**, 531–533.

Luk, S. C., Musclow, E., and Simon, G. T. (1980) Platelet phagocytosis in the spleen of patients with idiopathic thrombocytopenic purpura. *Histopathology* **4**, 127–136.

Lum, L. G., Tubergen, D. G., Corash, L., and Blaese, R. M. (1980) Splenectomy in the management of the thrombocytopenia of the Wiskott-Aldrich syndrome. *N. Engl. J. Med.* **302**, 892–896.

Lutz, H. U. and Wipf, G. (1982) Naturally occurring autoantibodies to skeletal proteins from human red blood cells. *J. Immunol.* **128**, 1695–1699.

Lutz, H. U., Flepp, R., and Stringaro-Wipf, G. (1984) Naturally occurring autoantibodies to exoplasmic and cryptic regions of band 3 protein, the major integral membrane protein of human red blood cells. *J. Immunol.* **133**, 2610–2618.

Lutz, H. U., Bussolino, F., Flepp, R., Fasler, S., Stammler, P., Kazatchkine M. D., and Arese, P. (1987) Naturally occurring anti-band-3 antibodies and complement together mediate phagocytosis of oxidatively stressed human erythrocytes. *Proc. Natl. Acad. Sci. USA* **84**, 7368–7372.

Lux, S. E. and John, K. M. (1977) Isolation and partial characterization of a high molecular weight red cell membrane protein complex normally removed by the spleen. *Blood* **50**, 625–641.

McKenzie, S. E. and Schreiber, A. D. (1998) Fc gamma receptors in phagocytes. *Curr. Opin. Hematol.* **5**, 16–21.

McMillan, R. (1981) Chronic idiopathic thrombocytopenic purpura. *N. Engl. J. Med.* **304**, 1135–1147.

McMillan, R, Tani, P., Millard, F., Berchtold, P., Renshaw, L., and Woods, V. L. Jr. (1987) Platelet-associated and plasma anti-glycoprotein autoantibodies in chronic ITP. *Blood* **70**, 1040–1045.

McMillan, R. and Martin, M. (1981) Fixation of C3 to platelets *in vitro* by antiplatelet antibody from patients with immune thrombocytopenic purpura. *Br. J. Haematol.* **47**, 251–256.

McMillan, R., Longmire, R. L., Yelenosky, R., Smith, R. S., and Craddock, C. G. (1972) Immunoglobulin synthesis in vitro by splenic tissue in idiopathic thrombocytopenic purpura. *N. Engl. J. Med.* **286**, 681–684.

McMillan, R., Longmire, R. L., Yelenosky, R., Donnell, R. L., and Armstrong, S. (1974) Quantitation of platelet-binding IgG produced in vitro by spleens from patients with idiopathic thrombocytopenic purpura. *N. Engl. J. Med.* **291**, 812–817.

van der Meulen, F. W., van der Hart, M., Fleer, A., von dem Borne, A. E., Engelfriet, C. P., and van Loghem, J. J. (1978) The role of adherence to human mononuclear phagocytes in the destruction of red cells sensitized with non-complement binding IgG antibodies. *Br. J. Haematol.* **38**, 541–549.

Miller, D. R., Weed, R. I., Stamatoyannopoulos, G., and Yoshida, A. (1971) Hemoglobin Köln disease occurring as a fresh mutation: erythrocyte metabolism and survival. *Blood* **38**, 715–729.

Modell, B. (1977) Total management of thalassemia major. *AMA Arch. Dis. Child.* **52**, 489–500.

Mohandas, N., Phillips, W. M., and Bessis, M. (1979) Red blood cell deformability and hemolytic anemias. *Semin. Hematol.* **16**, 95–114.

Mollison, P. L., Crome, P., Hughes-Jones, N. C., and Rochna, E. (1965) Rate of removal from the circulation of red cells sensitized with different amounts of antibody. *Br. J. Haematol.* **11**, 461–470.

Molnar, Z. and Rappaport, H. (1972) Fine structure of the red pulp of the spleen in hereditary spherocytosis. *Blood* **39**, 81–98.

Mori, P. G., Mancuso, G., del Principe, D., Duse, M., Miniero, R., Tovo, R., et al. (1983) Chronic idiopathic thrombocytopenia treated with immunoglobulin. *AMA Arch. Dis. Child.* **58**, 851–855.

Mueller-Eckhardt, C., Kayser, W., Mersch-Baumert, K., Mueller-Eckhardt, G., Breidenbach, M., Kugel, H. G., and Graubner, M. (1980) The clinical significance of platelet- associated IgG: a study on 298 patients with various disorders. *Br. J. Haematol.* **46**, 123–131.

Mueller-Eckhardt, C., Mueller-Eckhardt, G., Kayser, W., Voss, R. M., Wegner, J., and Kuenzlen, E. (1982) Platelet associated IgG, platelet survival, and platelet sequestration in thrombocytopenic states. *Br. J. Haematol.* **52**, 49–58.

Murphy, J. R. (1967) The influence of pH and temperature on some physical properties of normal erythrocytes and erythrocytes from patients with hereditary spherocytosis. *J. Lab. Clin. Med.* **69**, 758–775.

Myers, T. J., Kim, B. K., Steiner, M., and Baldini, M. G. (1982) Platelet-associated complement C3 in immune thrombocytopenic purpura. *Blood* **59**, 1023–1028.

Nagasawa, T., Kim, B. K., and Baldini, M. G. (1977) In vivo elution of ^{51}Cr from labeled platelets induced by antibody. *Fed. Proc.* **36**, 380.

Najean, Y. and Ardaillou, N. (1971) The sequestration site of platelets in idiopathic thrombocytopenic purpura: its correlation with the results of splenectomy. *Br. J. Haematol.* **21**, 153–164.

Najean, Y., Ardaillou, N., Caen, J., Larrieu, M.-J., and Bernard, J. (1963) Survival of radiochromium-labeled platelets in thrombocytopenias. *Blood* **22**, 718–732.

Najean, Y., Ardaillou, N., Dresch, C., and Bernard, J. (1967) The platelet destruction site in thrombocytopenic purpuras. *Br. J. Haematol.* **13**, 409–426.

Najean, Y., Dufour, V., Rain, J. D., and Toubert M. E. (1991) The site of platelet destruction in thrombocytopenic purpura as a predictive index of the efficacy of splenectomy. *Br. J. Haematol.* **79**, 271–276.

Najean, Y., Rain, J. D., and Dufour, V. (1991) The sequestration of 111-In-labelled autologous platelets and the efficiency of splenectomy. *Nouv. Rev. Fr. Hematol.* **33**, 449,450.

Nathan, D. G. and Gunn, R. B. (1966) Thalassemia: the consequences of unbalanced hemoglobin synthesis. *Am. J. Med.* **41**, 815–830.

Newland, A. C., Treleaven, J. G., Minchinton, R. M., and Waters, A. H. (1983) High-dose intravenous IgG in adults with autoimmune thrombocytopenia. *Lancet* **1**, 84–87.

O'Brien, R. T., Pearson, H. A., and Spencer, R. P. (1977) Transfusion induced decrease in spleen size in thalassemia major: documentation by radioisotopic scan. *J. Pediatr.* **81**, 105–107.

Oral, A., Nusbacher, J., Hill, J. B., and Lewis, J. H. (1984) Intravenous gamma globulin in the treatment of chronic idiopathic thrombocytopenic purpura in adults. *Am. J. Med.* **76**, 187–192.

Palek, J. (1985) Hereditary elliptocytosis and related disorders. *Clin. Haematol.* **14**, 45–87.

Palek, J. and Lux, S. E. (1983) Red cell membrane skeletal defects in hereditary and acquired hemolytic anemias. *Semin. Hematol.* **20**, 189–224.

Panzer, S., Niessner, H., Lechner, K., Dudczak, R., Jager, U., and Mayr, W. R. (1986) Platelet-associated immunoglobulins IgG, IgM, IgA and complement C3c in chronic idiopathic autoimmune thrombocytopenia: relation to the sequestration pattern of 111Indium labelled platelets. *Scand. J. Haematol.* **37**, 97–102.

Pearson, H. A., McIntosh, S., Ritchey, A. K., Lobel, J. S., Rooks, Y., and Johnston, D. (1979) Developmental aspects of splenic function in sickle cell diseases. *Blood* **53**, 358–365.

Penny, R., Rozenberg, M. C., and Firkin, B. G. (1966) The splenic platelet pool. *Blood* **27**, 1–16.

Peters, A. M. (1983) Splenic blood flow and blood cell kinetics. *Clin. Haematol.* **12**, 421–447.

Peters, A. M., Klonizakis, I., Lavender, J. P., and Lewis, S. M. (1980) Use of 111Indium-labelled platelets to measure splenic function. *Br. J. Haematol.* **46**, 587–593.

Peters, A. M. and Lavender, J. P. (1983) Platelet kinetics with indium-111 platelets: comparison with chromium-51 platelets. *Semin. Thromb. Hemostasis* **9**, 100–114.

Petz, L. D. and Garratty, G. (1980) *Acquired Immune Hemolytic Anemias.* Churchill Livingstone, New York.

Prankerd, T. A. J. (1963) The spleen and anaemia. *Br. Med. J.* **2**, 517–524.

Raccuglia, G. (1971) Gray platelet syndrome: a variety of qualitative platelet disorder. *Am. J. Med.* **51**, 818–828.

Ries, C. A. and Price, D. C. (1974) [51Cr]Platelet kinetics in thrombocytopenia: correlation between splenic sequestration of platelets and response to splenectomy. *Ann. Int. Med.* **80**, 702–707.

Rifkind, R. A. (1965) Heinz body anemia: an ultrastructural study. II. Red cell sequestration and destruction. *Blood* **26**, 433–448.

Rigas, D. A. and Koler, R. D. (1961) Decreased erythrocyte survival in hemoglobin H disease as a result of the abnormal properties of hemoglobin H: the benefit of splenectomy. *Blood* **18**, 1–17.

Rinehart, J. J., Balcerzak, S. P., Sagone, A. L., and LoBuglio, A. F. (1974) Effect of corticosteroids on human monocyte function. *J. Clin Invest.* **54**, 1337–1343.

Ross, G. D., Polley, M. J., Rabellino, E. M., and Grey, H. M. (1973) Two different complement receptors on human lymphocytes. One specific for C3b and one specific for C3b inactivator-cleaved C3b. *J. Exper. Med.* **138**, 798–811.

Rosse, W. F. (1971) Quantitative immunology of immune hemolytic anemia. II. The relationship of cell-bound antibody to hemolysis and the effect of treatment. *J. Clin. Invest.* **50**, 734–743.

Rosse, W. F., de Boisfleury, A., and Bessis, M. (1975) The interaction of phagocytic cells and red cells modified by immune reactions. Comparison of antibody and complement coated red cells. *Blood Cells* **1**, 345–358.

Salama, A., Kiefel, V., Amberg, R., and Mueller-Eckhardt, C. (1984) Treatment of autoimmune thrombocytopenic purpura with rhesus antibodies [anti-RhoD)]. *Blut* **49**, 29–35.

Salama, A., Kiefel, V., and Mueller-Eckhardt, C. (1986) Effect of IgG anti-Rho(D) in adult patients with chronic autoimmune thrombocytopenia. *Am. J. Hematol.* **22**, 241–250.

Schmidt, E. E., MacDonald, I. C., and Groom, A. C. (1991) Changes in splenic microcirculatory pathways in chronic thrombocytopenic purpura. *Blood* **78**, 1485–1489.

Schnitzer, B., Sodeman, T., Mead, M. I., and Contacos, P. G. (1972) Pitting function of the spleen in malaria: ultrastructural observations. *Science* **177**, 175–177.

Schreiber, A. D. and Frank, M. M. (1972a) Role of antibody and complement in the immune clearance and destruction of erythrocytes. I. *In vivo* effects of IgG and IgM complement-fixing sites. *J. Clin. Invest.* **51**, 575–582.

Schreiber, A. D. and Frank, M. M. (1972b) Role of antibody and complement in the immune clearance and destruction of erythrocytes. II.

Molecular nature of IgG and IgM complement-fixing sites and effects of their interactions with serum. *J. Clin. Invest.* **51**, 583–589.

Schreiber, A. D., Parsons, J., McDermott, P., and Cooper, R. A. (1975) Effect of corticosteroids on the human monocyte IgG and complement receptors. *J. Clin. Invest.* **56**, 1189–1197.

Schreiber, A. D., Chien, P., Tomaski, A., and Cines, D. B. (1987) Effect of danazol in immune thrombocytopenic purpura. *N. Engl. J. Med.* **316**, 503–508.

Schwartz, S. I., Bernard, R. P., and Adams, J. T. (1970) Splenectomy for hematologic disorders. *Arch. Surg.* **101**, 338–347.

Seelder, R. A. and Shwiaki, M. Z. (1972) Acute splenic sequestration crisis (ASSC) in young children with sickle cell anemia: clinical observations in 20 episodes in 14 children. *Clin. Pediatr.* **11**, 701–704.

Shattil, S. J. and Cooper, R. A. (1972) Maturation of macroreticulocyte membrane in vivo. *J. Lab. Clin. Med.* **79**, 215–227.

Shcherbina, A., Rosen, F. S., and Remold-O'Donnell, E. (1999) Pathological events in platelets of Wiscott-Aldrich syndrome patients. *Br. J. Haematol.* **106**, 875–883.

Shulman, N. R., Marder, V. J., and Weinrach, R. S. (1965) Similarities between known antiplatelet antibodies and the factor responsible for thrombocytopenia in idiopathic purpura. Physiologic, serologic, and isotopic studies. *Ann. NY Acad. Sci.* **124**, 499–542.

Shulman, N. R., Watkins, S. P. Jr., Itscoitz, S. B., and Students, A. B. (1968) Evidence that the spleen retains the youngest and hemostatically most effective platelets. *Trans. Assoc. Am. Physiol.* **81**, 302–313.

Silverstein, M. N., Gomes, M. R., Elveback, L. R., ReMine, W. H., and Linman, J. W. (1972) Idiopathic acquired hemolytic anemia. Survival in 117 cases. *AMA Arch. Int. Med.* **129**, 85–87.

Slater, L. M., Muir, W. A., and Weed, R. I. (1968) Influence of splenectomy on insoluble hemoglobin inclusion bodies in β-thalassemic erythrocytes. *Blood* **31**, 766–777.

Solanki, D. L., Kletter, G. G., and Castro, O. (1986) Acute splenic sequestration crisis in adults with sickle cell disease. *Am. J. Med.* **80**, 985–990.

Sprague, C. C. and Paterson, J. C. S. (1958) Role of the spleen and effect of splenectomy in sickle cell disease. *Blood* **13**, 569–581.

Stefanini, M. and Martino, N. B. (1956) Use of prednisone in the management of some hemorrhagic states. *N. Engl. J. Med.* **254**, 313–317.

Stiehm, E. R., Ashida, E., Kim, K. S., Winston, D. J., Haas, A., and Gale, R. P. (1987) Intravenous immunoglobulins as therapeutic agents. *Ann. Int. Med.* **107**, 367–382.

Szwed, J. J., Yum, M., and Hogan, R. (1980) A beneficial effect of splenectomy in sickle cell anemia and chronic renal failure. *Am. J. Med. Sci.* **279**, 169–172.

Tavassoli, M. and McMillan, R. (1975) Structure of the spleen in idiopathic thrombocytopenic purpura. *Am. J. Clin. Pathol.* **64**, 180–191.

Thompson, R. L., Moore, R. A., Hess, C. E., Wheby, M. S., and Leavell, B. S. (1972) Idiopathic thrombocytopenic purpura. Long-term results of treatment and the prognostic significance of response to corticosteroids. *AMA Arch. Int. Med.* **130**, 730–734.

Toghill, P. J., Green, S., and Ferguson, R. (1977) Platelet dynamics in chronic liver disease with special reference to the role of the spleen. *J. Clin. Pathol.* **30**, 367–371.

Verheyden, C. N., Beart, R. W. Jr., Clifton, M. D., and Phyliky, R. L. (1978) Accessory splenectomy in management of recurrent idiopathic thrombocytopenic purpura. *Mayo Clin. Proc.* **53**, 442–446.

Verp, M. and Karpatkin, S. (1975) Effect of plasma, steroids or steroid products on the adhesion of human opsonized thrombocytes to human leukocytes. *J. Lab. Clin. Med.* **85**, 478–486.

Weed, R. I. and Bowdler, A. J. (1966) Metabolic dependence of the critical hemolytic volume of human erythrocytes: relationship to osmotic fragility and autohemolysis in hereditary spherocytosis and normal red cells. *J. Clin. Invest.* **45**, 1137–1149.

Weiss, L. (1974) A scanning electron microscopic study of the spleen. *Blood* **43**, 665–91.

Weiss, L. (1983) The red pulp of the spleen: structural basis of blood flow. *Clin. Haematol.* **12**, 375–393.

Weiss, L. and Tavassoli, M. (1972) Anatomic hazards to the passage of erythrocytes through the spleen. *Semin. Hematol.* **7**, 372–380.

Wennberg, E. and Weiss, L. (1968) Splenic erythroclasia: an electron microscopic study of hemoglobin H disease. *Blood* **31,** 778–790.

Wentz, A. C. (1982) Adverse effects of danazol in pregnancy. *Ann. Int. Med.* **96,** 672–673.

Whitaker, A. N. (1969) Infection and the spleen: association between hyposplenism, pneumococcal sepsis and disseminated intravascular coagulation. *Med. J. Aust.* **1,** 1213–1219.

White, J. M. and Dacie, J. V. (1971) The unstable hemoglobins: molecular and clinical features. *Progr. Hematol.* **7,** 69–109.

Winiarski, J. and Holm, G. (1983) Platelet associated immunoglobulins and complement in idiopathic thrombocytopenic purpura. *Clin. Exp. Immunol.* **53,** 201–207.

Worlledge, S., Hughes Jones, N. C., and Bain, B. (1982) *Blood and Its Disorders* (Hardisty, R. M. and Weatherall, D. J., eds.), Blackwell, Oxford, pp. 485–493.

13 Myeloproliferative Disorders

Michael T. Shaw, MD, FRCP, FACP, DCH

13.1. INTRODUCTION

"Myeloproliferative syndrome" was a term coined by Dameshek (1960). Most hematologists today regard the myeloproliferative disorders (MPDs) as pathological entities that include polycythemia vera, essential thrombocythemia, agnogenic (primary) myeloid metaplasia and chronic myeloid leukemia. With the possible exception of essential thrombocythemia, they are considered to be panmyeloses, and are clonal hemopathies arising from the pluripotent stem cell (Adamson and Fialkow, 1978). In each disease, there is an emphasis on the proliferation of one cell line. Thus, in polycythemia vera, erythropoiesis predominates; in essential thrombocythemia and chronic myeloid leukemia, thrombopoiesis and granulopoiesis are the predominant events, respectively. In agnogenic myeloid metaplasia fibrosis, which is found in the bone marrow, does not seem to be part of the myeloproliferation, and is probably a reactive process produced as a result of abnormal myeloid cell development. The most consistent abnormality in this group of diseases is the Philadelphia chromosome (Ph^1) found in all the hematopoietic cell precursors of patients with chronic myeloid leukemia. The Ph^1 represents reciprocal translation of sections of the long arms of chromosomes 9 and 22. The principal molecular event involves translocation of the Abelson proto-oncogene (c-*abl*) from chromosome 9 to the breakpoint cluster region (bcr) of chromosome 22, resulting in the formation of a chimeric *bcr*/c-*abl* gene (Champlin et al., 1986).

The spleen is an organ that is intimately associated with the hematopoietic system. Physiologically, it is responsible for trapping effete circulating blood cells, as part of the reticuloendothelial system. Pathologically, this removal of cells may become excessive, as in patients with immune thrombocytopenic purpura, various hemolytic anemias, and certain MPDs. In many mammals, the spleen plays a prominent role in the development of hematopoiesis during embryonic life, and therefore, is involved in the hematopathology of the MPDs. This chapter reviews the pathophysiological processes that occur in the spleen in these diseases, the clinical implications of splenomegaly, and the indications and results of splenectomy and splenic radiation therapy.

From: *The Complete Spleen: A Handbook of Structure, Function, and Clinical Disorders* Edited by: A. J. Bowdler © Humana Press Inc., Totowa, NJ

13.2. SPLENIC HEMATOPOIESIS AND MYELOID METAPLASIA

Extramedullary hematopoiesis has been said to occur in the spleen, to some extent, during embryonic life, from the twelfth week of gestation to birth (Wintrobe et al., 1976; Lewis, 1983). Embryologically, the spleen originates as a thickening of the mesenchyme of the gastric mesentery. Large basophilic stem cells differentiate into erythroblasts and megakaryocytes within the sinusoids, and to granulocytes in the adjacent arterioles. In mice, stromal cells have been found to proliferate in the embryonic spleen, prior to the appearance of splenic hematopoiesis, and to decrease when splenic hematopoiesis becomes established (Van den Heuvel et al., 1987). The hematopoietic tissue completely fills the spleen, prior to the development of lymphatic tissue(Thiel and Downey, 1921; Block, 1964; Ward and Block, 1971). In most mammals, myeloid tissue persists in the red pulp after embryonic life, but, in humans, only a few erythroblasts, granulocytes, and megakaryocytes are found here at birth, and these totally disappear soon after, according to Ward and Block (1971), who observe that, as far as embryonic hematopoiesis is concerned, ontogeny recapitulates phylogeny, in that mature fishes, amphibia, and reptiles show splenic hematopoiesis. Because extramedullary hematopoiesis in man occurs in sites of normal hematopoiesis in lower vertebrates, these areas, such as the spleen, must either retain mesenchymal cells capable of differentiating into hematopoietic stem cells, or, alternatively, the microenvironment is suitable for recolonization by such cells. The potential for splenic hematopoiesis remains after birth, and, when there is hematological stress, such as megaloblastic or hemolytic anemia, extramedullary erythropoiesis and megakaryopoiesis, may be found in the spleen. It is further postulated that, in these conditions, there is injury to the endothelial cells of the bone marrow sinuses, allowing immature cells to escape into the blood and become trapped in the splenic red pulp. Further mitotic divisions result in the formation of "nests" of erythroid and megakaryocytic cells (Lewis, 1983).

By contrast, some investigators believe that hematopoietic cells found in embryonic spleens merely reflect splenic trapping of these cells from the peripheral blood. Their evidence is persuasive: Keleman et al. (1979) claim that the spleen is not a significant organ of hematopoiesis in the human fetus, most observations from previous studies having been made in nonhuman mammals. Wolf et al. (1983) studied the spleens from 65 aborted human fetuses and stillborn infants, the gestational age varying from 12 to 40 weeks. They used immunohistological and cytochemical methods to study hematopoiesis, and found surprisingly few blood precursor cells. Those few erythroid precursors seen were scattered in the red pulp, and were not in clusters. Furthermore, most of them were late normoblasts. There were even fewer granulocytic precursors and very few megakaryocytes. These findings were confirmed by Wilkins et al. (1994), using similar techniques. Similar conclusions have been drawn from observations made using monoclonal antibodies prepared against transferrin receptors, to demonstrate erythroid and myeloid precursors.

Pluripotential stem cells (colony-forming units [CFUs]) are considered by many to occur normally in the spleen, as well as in the bone marrow of mature humans (Schofield, 1979). In fact, Murphy (1983) suggested that erythroid-committed stem cells (burst-forming unit, erythrocytes [BFU-E] and CFU-E) migrated from the bone marrow into the spleen. This is also supported by the work of Lutton and Levere (1979), who demonstrated that the peripheral blood mononuclear cell fraction, obtained by density-gradient centrifugation from patients with polycythemia vera and myelofibrosis with myeloid metaplasia, contained erythroid precursor cells of high proliferative capacity. The erythroid precursor cells formed colonies, which appeared in culture within 5–7 d, in the absence of exogenous erythropoietin, in contrast to normal peripheral blood cells, in which erythroid colonies appeared later (in 10–14 days), and only in the presence of exogenous erythropoietin. Spleen cells from a patient with myelofibrosis behaved like spleen cells in patients with polycythemia vera. In addition, patients with agnogenic myeloid metaplasia and chronic myeloid leukemia have increased numbers of circulating myeloid precursors capable of producing colony forming units (CFU-C) in vitro. Splenic irradiation in patients with agnogenic myeloid metaplasia and chronic myeloid leukemia produces a marked fall in circulating CFU-C, which remain depressed for several weeks (Fig. 1; Barret et al., 1977; Koeffler et al., 1979), suggesting that radiation therapy destroys splenic proliferating precursor cells. One patient with probable chronic myeloid leukemia was found to have higher numbers of granulocyte-monocyte committed stem cells (CFU-GM) in the splenic vein blood than in the peripheral blood (Bagby, 1978). CFU-GM numbers fell rapidly after splenectomy. Greenberg and Steed (1981) found a 100-fold increase of CFU-GM in spleens removed from chronic myeloid leukemia patients, compared to normal spleens. In patients with agnogenic myeloid metaplasia the splenic vein blood has also been found to have more CFU-GM than peripheral venous blood. The numbers of CFU-GMs in the splenic vein blood of two patients with agnogenic myeloid metaplasia were shown to be much higher than in blood from other peripheral veins, suggesting granulocyte production by the spleen (Kirschner et al., 1980).

In patients with MPDs, especially chronic myeloid leukemia and agnogenic myeloid metaplasia, a great proportion of hematopoietic stem cell proliferation may be shifted from the bone marrow to the spleen (Adler, 1976). In a few cases, there is evidence that virtually the entire hematopoietic stem cell population may have shifted to the spleen. An analogous situation may be demonstrated experimentally in mice in which a few CFUs are always present in the spleen. When the bone marrow has been ablated with ^{89}Sr, there is a marked increase in the number of splenic CFUs. If such mice are splenectomized 2–3 weeks after ^{89}Sr has been administered, they die from complications of pancytopenia (Adler, 1976).

It is postulated that, in agnogenic myeloid metaplasia and chronic myeloid leukemia, the site in which the hematopoietic cells proliferate depends, first, on the character of the hematopoietic population itself (Moore, 1975), and, second, on the characteristics of the environment of the supporting organs (Wolf and Trentin, 1968). Possibly, the cells acquire "fetal characteristics," resulting in a predilection for growth in fetal hematopoietic tissue. In agnogenic myeloid leukemia metaplasia, alteration of the microenvironment may be caused by myeloid fibrosis. In chronic myeloid infiltration of the microenvironment with myeloid elements could result in suppression of local stem cell proliferation.

Extramedullary hematopoiesis in the spleen occurs in those conditions that result in stressed bone marrow producing normal or megaloblastic myeloid elements. Myeloid metaplasia, on the other hand, is a specific form of extramedullary hematopoiesis in which the myeloid cells, found in both bone marrow and spleen, are dysplastic and/or neoplastic. In the latter situation, the spleen is participating in this pathological process.

12.3. THE PATHOLOGY OF THE SPLEEN IN MYELOPROLIFERATIVE SYNDROMES

Similarities and differences in the pathological processes, which occur in the spleen in the MPDs are summarized in Table 1.

12.3.1. POLYCYTHEMIA VERA   Slight to moderate splenomegaly is the rule in this disease (Westin et al., 1972). The spleen often reveals vascular thromboses and infarcts. Histologically, the sinuses are engorged with blood, the splenic cords may show histiocytic hyperplasia, and hemosiderin is scant or absent. Extramedullary hematopoiesis is usually absent, but when present is limited to a few foci of erythropoiesis. If extramedullary hematopoiesis is more than scanty, it usually signifies conversion to myelofibrosis (Rappaport, 1966; Pettit et al., 1979).

13.3.2. ESSENTIAL THROMBOCYTHEMIA   The spleen in this disorder is either enlarged (weighing from 400 to more than 2000 g) or is found to be atrophic (weighing less than 15 g) (Rappaport, 1966). The most prominent microscopic feature is the large number of clumped platelets in the sinuses. Very few megakaryocytes are seen, but, when found, are occasionally atypical. No extramedullary hematopoiesis is present. It has been suggested that the spleen traps some of the excess of platelets, and that patients with splenic atrophy reveal the hematological and clinical manifestations of thrombocythemia before those with splenomegaly (Rappaport, 1966; Pettit et al., 1979). The spleen often also shows widening of the pulp cords, probably caused by reticulin fibrosis.

13.3.3. AGNOGENIC MYELOID METAPLASIA   The spleen is almost always enlarged in this disease, and weighs between 700 and 4000 g. However, increasing spleen weight was not found to correlate with disease duration or progression, by Wolf and Neiman (1985), although this does not appear to correlate with clinical observations of individual patients. The splenic capsule tends to be thickened by the scars of previous infarcts, which have been said to occur less frequently than in chronic myeloid leukemia (Rappaport, 1966; Jackson et al., 1940), although this has been challenged (Ward and Block, 1971).

Microscopically, extramedullary hematopoiesis is always found in the red pulp (Fig. 2). The trabeculae and malpighian corpuscles are widely separated. Hematopoietic islands are found in the cords and sinuses, together with nucleated red blood cells and granulocytes in varying proportions. Megakaryocytes are prominent, and sometimes they predominate and may be dysplastic (Wolf and

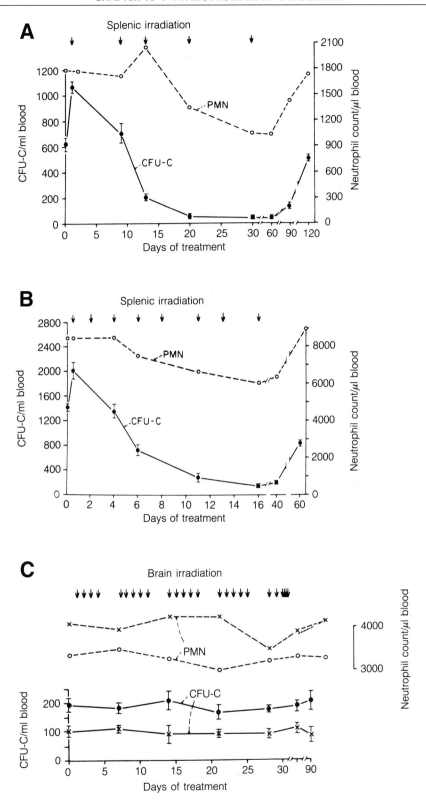

Fig. 13.1. Number of granulocyte colonies (CFU-C)/mL blood and neutrophil count/μL blood assayed 1 h after irradiation. Solid line represents mean CFU-C ± SE/mL of blood. The mean represents triplicate cultures plated at 0.5, 1.0, and 2.0×10^5 peripheral blood cells/dish. Dotted line shows neutrophil concentration/μL, and arrows indicate time of irradiation. Patients 1 and 2 had myelofibrosis, and received splenic irradiation. Patients 3 and 4 had malignant gliomas, and received brain irradiation. (**A**) Patient 1. (**B**) Patient 2. (**C**) Astrocytoma control patients 3(x) and 4(.). (Reproduced with permission from Koeffler et al., 1979).

Neiman, 1985). Splenic cords show increased cellularity or fibrosis, or both; increased reticulin can be seen when specimens are examined with silver stains (Rappaport, 1966). However, Ward and Block (1971) claimed that fibrosis occurred in mild to moderate amounts in only a few progressive cases. Many histiocytes have been observed in the splenic cords, and, in some cases, hemosiderin

Table 13.1
Splenic Pathology in MPDs

	PCV	E. Thromb.	AMM	CML
Splenomegaly	+	±	++	++
Splenic infarcts	+	?	++	++
Myeloid metaplasia	–	–	+	+
Reticulin fibrosis of cords	–	+	+	±

MPD, myeloproliferative disorder; PCV, polycythemia vera; E. Thromb, essential thrombocythemia; AMM, Agnogenic myeloid metaplasia; CML, Chronic myeloid leukemia.

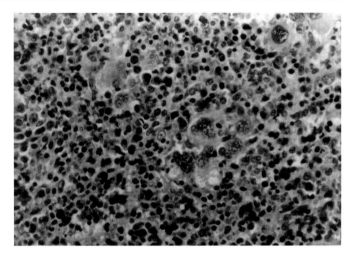

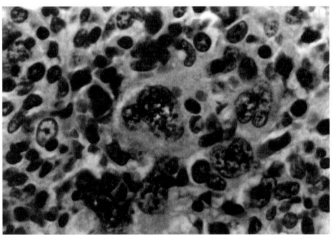

abounds in macrophages. On electron microscopy, the hematopoietic cells demonstrate loops and blebs in the nucleus. There is also cytoplasmic degeneration, suggesting that that hematopoiesis may, to a great extent, be ineffective (Tavassoli and Weiss, 1973). In the white pulp, the malpighian corpuscles are atrophic. Tavassoli (1973), in describing the ultrastructure, found focal cytoplasmic degeneration, involving mitochondria and elements of endoplasmic reticulum, in lymphocytes and reticulum cells.

13.3.4. CHRONIC MYELOID LEUKEMIA
The spleen is often very large in this condition, with weight varying from 1500 to 4000 g. The capsule reveals adhesions. Obliteration of the normal architecture can be seen on cut sections, and ischemic and hemorrhagic infarcts may be observed. Histologically, myeloid metaplasia, predominantly granulocytic, is the most notable feature. The pulp cords are infiltrated with granulocytes at all stages of maturation. Neutrophil and eosinophil myelocytes predominate, and basophils may be conspicuous. Myeloid foci are seen in the splenic sinuses, together with nucleated red blood cells, granulocytes, and megakaryocytes (Fig. 3). In long-standing cases, or after splenic radiation therapy, fibrosis of the splenic cords may be noticeable. In the white pulp, the malpighian corpuscles become atrophic and widely separated, as the disease progresses (Rappaport, 1966).

13.4. CLINICAL IMPLICATIONS OF SPLENOMEGALY IN MPDS

13.4.1. POLYCYTHEMIA VERA
Splenomegaly is present in about 40% of patients with polycythemia vera, on physical examination. When the spleen is scanned by means of radioisotopic techniques, splenomegaly is found in 90% of patients, although one recent study (Carnesog et al., 1996) found this in no more than 60% of patients. The spleen size is variable, but usually modest. Increasing size of the spleen or massive splenomegaly in a patient with polycythemia vera usually signifies progression to myelofibrosis. In some cases, the spleen remains impalpable during the whole course of the disease. Splenic vein thrombosis is a rare complication leading to portal hypertension and bleeding from esophageal varices.

Splenic pain may occasionally occur, and is more likely to result from splenic enlargement than from splenic infarcts (Wetherley-Mein and Pearson, 1982). There is evidently no change in the size of the spleen, after phlebotomy, sufficient to produce a normal packed cell volume, but it does shrink after treatment with myelosuppressive agents (Westin et al., 1972). Splenic rupture occurs rarely (Fernandez et al., 1983).

Ferrokinetic studies indicate minimal, if any, extramedullary erythropoiesis; however, a few patients present with features of both polycythemia and myelofibrosis. In these patients [52]Fe uptake in the spleen resembles that seen in myelofibrosis, rather than polycythemia vera. Clinically and hematologically, patients may

Fig. 13.2. (A) Section of spleen from a patient with agnogenic myeloid metaplasia showing complete replacement of normal architecture with myeloid metaplasia. (H&E ×200). (B) Same, showing megakaryocytic hyperplasia with atypical features (H&E ×500).

remain in a steady state for several years; so that this syndrome has been called "transitional myeloproliferative disorder" (Pettit et al., 1979).

A "spent" phase of polycythemia vera has been described by Najean et al. (1984), in which there is persistent splenomegaly, despite treatment, frequent cytopenia of one or more cell lines, persistent red blood cell hypervolemia, persistence of myeloid hyperplasia without collagen fibrosis, and no hepatosplenic erythroblastic metaplasia, as measured by radioiron studies or [111]Indium transferrin scintigraphy. This phase is significantly more common in patients treated by phlebotomy than by myelosuppressive therapy.

13.4.2. ESSENTIAL THROMBOCYTHEMIA
As stated earlier, patients with this condition may have either splenomegaly or splenic atrophy, and, in some the spleen size may be normal. In one series of 94 patients, splenomegaly occurred in 48% (Belucci et al., 1986). Splenomegaly was always moderate, not exceeding palpability beyond 4 cm below the costal margin. In another series, 30% of the patients had splenomegaly (Murphy et al., 1982). Revesz et al. (1993), using γ camera scintigraphy, concluded that 39% had splenic enlargement. Carneskog et al. (1996), using a similar method, put the number at no less than 50%. Splenic scintigraphy may be

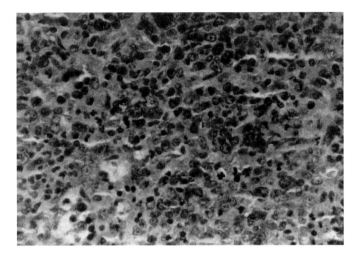

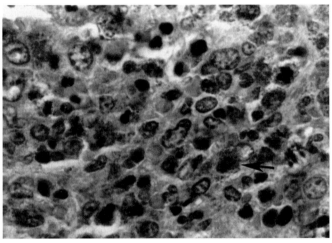

Fig. 3. (A) Section of spleen from a patient with chronic myeloid leukemia showing myeloid infiltration (H&E ×500). **(B)** Same. Note eosinophil myelocyte, shown with arrow (H&E ×500).

a useful tool in differentiating the disease from other causes of unexplained thrombocytosis.

The spleen does enlarge when complications, such as portal vein thrombosis or hepatic vein thrombosis, occur, and also in those few cases progressing to myelofibrosis (Waweru and Lewis, 1985). Marsh et al. (1966), using ^{51}Cr-labeled, heat-damaged red blood cells to study splenic function, described splenic atrophy in a subset of patients with essential thrombocythemia. It is not known whether the etiology of splenic atrophy is splenic infarction caused by multiple splenic arterial thrombi, comparable to the autosplenectomy that occurs in adults with sickle cell disease, or whether it has unrelated causes. Patients with splenic atrophy tend to have higher platelet counts, presumably because of the absence of platelet pooling by the spleen. Ferrokinetic studies with [52]Fe have also been used to demonstrate the absence of extramedullary hematopoiesis (Waweru and Lewis, 1985).

13.4.3. AGNOGENIC MYELOID METAPLASIA Moderate-to-massive splenomegaly is found in this disease, and is progressive. The duration of the disease can be roughly correlated with the degree of splenomegaly (Hickling, 1937; Ward and Block, 1971). Patients in whom the spleen extends into the iliac fossa probably have had the disease for 13–27 years. Rarely, rapid enlargement of

the spleen occurs over 1–2 years (Chevalier, 1949; Skinner and Sophean, 1951). In a few cases, the spleen is not palpable, but, in all cases, enlargement later develops and becomes apparent (Silverstein et al., 1973).

Portal hypertension is a well-documented complication of agnogenic myeloid metaplasia and may compound the degree of splenomegaly. The cause is obscure, but it has been suggested to arise from cirrhosis caused by hepatitis following blood transfusion, hemosiderosis from Fe storage and accumulation, while portal and splenic vein thromboses may be contributary factors (Ward and Block, 1971). In addition, liver biopsies, performed in patients with agnogenic myeloid metaplasia demonstrate myeloid metaplasia (Silverstein et al., 1973; Ligumski et al., 1978), the presence of which may result in atrophy or necrosis of the liver parenchyma, followed by reparative fibrosis. Increased portal blood flow has also been shown to be important in the pathogenesis of portal hypertension.

As the spleen enlarges, other effects on the blood elements may be seen. Anemia may be caused by various factors, including splenic pooling of the red blood cells, hemolysis, and the apparent effects on the hemoglobin level of the increased plasma volume (Bowdler, 1983). The theoretical proposal, that ineffective erythropoiesis in the bone marrow results from a humoral substance produced by the large spleen, has not been convincingly supported by experimental studies (Goldman and Nolasco, 1983). The hypersplenic effect often involves platelets, and, in patients with markedly enlarged spleens, more than 90% of the circulating platelets may be intrasplenic (Bowdler, 1983). This can result in profound thrombocytopenia. Neutropenia may be caused by increased margination of the polymorphonuclear leukocytes in the splenic blood vessels, thus depleting the counts of circulating cells (Fieschi and Sacchetti, 1964; Scott et al., 1971).

Laboratory evidence, that splenic erythropoiesis makes a useful contribution to red blood cell production, is inconclusive. [52]Fe and ^{59}Fe studies often show uptake and release of the isotope similar to that seen in normal marrow, confirming the presence of splenic erythropoiesis, but not the effective production of functional circulating red blood cells (Wetherley-Mein and Pearson, 1982).

13.4.4. CHRONIC MYELOID LEUKEMIA In this condition, the spleen size tends to correlate with the duration of the disease; the spleen is nearly always palpably enlarged at presentation. In six cases in which the spleen was not palpably enlarged, the peripheral blood leukocyte count was less than 100×10^9/L (Thompson and Stainsby, 1982). It is generally agreed that splenic size at the time of diagnosis of the chronic phase of the disease is an important prognostic indicator, a small spleen being associated with a longer survival, and, conversely, a large spleen being indicative of a short survival (Medical Research Council, 1983). During treatment of the chronic phase, rapid shrinkage occurs when adequate control is achieved. Often, a previously easily palpable or massively enlarged spleen becomes impalpable. In others, however, a palpable spleen remains the only clinical hint of the continued presence of the disease.

The spleen is not usually tender to palpation during the chronic phase of chronic myeloid leukemia. Abdominal discomfort or vague digestive complaints, such as early satiety, may be noticed by the patient. During the accelerated phase, the spleen enlarges rapidly, and splenic pain, either felt locally or referred to the tip of the shoulder, is common. This symptom is often associated with splenic infarcts. The pain is exacerbated by breathing or movement, and a splenic rub may be evident on auscultation. Portal hypertension, as previously noted in agnogenic myeloid metaplasia, has occasionally been described, and the cause may be similar (Thompson and Stainsby, 1982). Increased plasma volume and red blood cell pooling play a part in the production of anemia. Splenic rupture has been described (Bauer et al., 1981), but is uncommon. The spleen is certainly important as an organ of pathological hematopoiesis in this disease, being secondary only to the bone marrow, and considerable traffic of granulocytes takes place between the marrow and the spleen (Pederson, 1979). Sometimes, however, a falling myeloid and rising splenic contribution to granulopoiesis occurs, coincident with the development of relapse. Indeed, it has been suggested that the spleen may be the initial site of evolution of the cytogenetic changes leading to the terminal phase of the disease, because aneuploidy has been seen in cells of the spleen, before the bone marrow has shown any chromosomal changes. However, one case has been described, in which chromosomal changes, associated with the accelerated phase, occurred in the bone marrow and not in the spleen (Brandt, 1975). Furthermore, splenectomy has not been successful in delaying the terminal phase, so evidence for the splenic origin of the accellerated phase is lacking.

13.5. SPLEEN-RELATED THERAPY IN MPDS

13.5.1. SPLENECTOMY
The two MPDs in which splenectomy has been performed most appropriately are agnogenic myeloid metaplasia and chronic myeloid leukemia. Historically, Hickling (1953) reviewed 27 patients with agnogenic myeloid metaplasia who underwent splenectomy, and noted that 15 died in the immediate postoperative period, and 6 others died within the first year. He therefore concluded that this operation is contraindicated in patients with this disease, probably because the patient has become dependant on the hematopoiesis of the removed spleen. Green et al. (1953), reviewing a series of splenectomized patients with agnogenic myeloid metaplasia, pointed out that only 6/29 had died within 6 months of the operation. They concluded that deaths following splenectomy had previously been related to frequent postoperative complications, rather than to anemia caused by erythropoietic deprivation. The pendulum of thought about the advisability of this procedure then swung in the opposite direction, until Crosby (1972) recommended splenectomy for all cases of agnogenic myeloid metaplasia as soon as the diagnosis of the condition had been made.

In agnogenic myeloid metaplasia the indications for which splenectomy is now considered appropriate are hypersplenism, especially with increasing anemia and thrombocytopenia, resulting in increasing transfusion requirements, and symptomatic splenomegaly (Garrison et al., 1984). Lafaye et al. (1994) believed that the operation should be limited to patients with splenic pain and increasing transfusion requirements. Certainly, the most pressing indication is thrombocytopenia. Studies in some patients have shown increased splenic accumulation of autologous ^{51}Cr-labeled red blood cells (Cabot et al., 1978). Ideally, prior demonstration of adequate bone marrow function, by such means as ferrokinetic studies with ^{59}Fe, ^{52}Fe sacral uptake, or ^{111}Indium scanning, should be shown. Results have been far from conclusive in predicting outcome, however, and are now performed much less frequently than formerly (Wilson et al., 1985). Of interest are ferrokinetic studies made before and after splenectomy, in two series of patients with agnogenic myeloid metaplasia which showed increased myeloid erythropoiesis, as measured by the ^{59}Fe sacral uptake, following splenectomy (Wetherley-Mein and Pearson, 1982; Barosi et al.,

1984). This has suggested that, after splenectomy, there is reorganization of erythropoiesis. A theory formerly current was that a humoral agent produced by the spleen acts as an inhibitor of erythropoiesis in the marrow, and these studies appear to offer support to this concept.*

Other less common indications for splenectomy in patients with agnogenic myeloid metaplasia are ruptured spleen and portal hypertension, provided that adequate liver function is maintained (Sullivan et al., 1974; Silverstein and ReMime, 1974). A contraindication to splenectomy is the presence of thrombocytosis, because of the hazard of postsplenectomy thromboses (Ward and Block, 1971) and consumption soagulopathy.

The operative details of splenectomy vary, but the operation is usually performed through a midline or left paramedian incision (Cabot et al., 1978; Goldstone, 1978). To decrease the risk of hemorrhage, the spleen is mobilized and the short gastric vessels, the lienogastric, and lienocolic ligaments are divided, before approach is made to the markedly enlarged splenic artery and vein (Goldstone, 1978; Coon and Liepman, 1982). In a review of the literature, Benbasset et al. (1990) reported an average operative mortality of 13.4%. Postoperative complications include subphrenic abscess and other intra-abdominal infections, postoperative bleeding, pleural effusion, pneumonia, thrombosis and pulmonary embolism, hepatic failure, and, occasionally, pericardial effusion (Nagler et al., 1986). The later complication is reported of an unexpectedly high rate of blastic transformation (Barosi et al., 1984). Postoperative survival is said to be shorter in males than in females (Silverstein and ReMime, 1974), and it is also shortened in patients with anemia, massive splenomegaly, and elevated serum alkaline phosphatase levels (Barosi et al., 1993).

Splenectomy in agnogenic myeloid metaplasia results in hematological and clinical changes. The most profound hematological effect is the often dramatic rise in the platelet count (Garrison et al., 1984; Cabot et al., 1978; Heaton et al., 1976; Mulder et al., 1977). The hemoglobin and hematocrit values often rise, and, in one study, polycythemia occurred following splenectomy in three cases (Barosi et al., 1984). The peripheral white blood count also tends to rise (Garrison et al., 1984; Mulder et al., 1977). In another study, the number of teardrop poikilocytes in the peripheral blood fell (DiBella et al., 1977). An interesting observation was made by Aviram et al. (1986) observed that the spleen plays an important role in cholesterol and lipoprotein metabolism: They showed that, after splenectomy in patients with MPDs, cholesterol, apolipoprotein B, and low density lipoproteins were significantly increased. In general, the quality of life may be considerably improved in those patients who have needed frequent red blood cell and/or platelet transfusions. However, the natural history of the disease is not significantly altered, and there is little evidence of a survival benefit to be obtained from the operation.

Longer-term complications include thromboses, including mesenteric venous and arterial thrombosis, portal vein thrombosis, deep vein thrombosis and pulmonary embolism, related to the rapid rise of platelet count (Garrison et al., 1984; Cabot et al., 1978; Goldstone, 1978; Heaton et al., 1976; Wobbes et al., 1984). There is

---

*It may simply be that the distribution of Fe is modified by increased accumulation in the bone marrow, when competition from a splenic "sink" is removed, and a higher proportion of the standard dose of radionucleide can be taken up by the marrow erythroid component, when this is a greater fraction of the total active erythropoiesis of the body.   –Editor

always a long-term risk of bacterial infection as with other splenectomized patients. Slow enlargement of the liver is an invariable consequence following splenectomy, but, although explosive hepatomegaly has been described, this has not been confirmed (Ward and Block, 1971). Massive liver enlargement has, however, been described by Barosi et al. (1993).

Splenectomy in patients with chronic myeloid leukemia was for many years, not regarded as a useful form of treatment. However, Baikie (1968) suggested that elective splenectomy, early in the course of the disease, might prolong survival by delaying metamorphosis. This proposition was made because of the cytogenetic evidence, referred to previously in this chapter, that, in some cases, the spleen may be the initial site of evolution of the terminal phase. Spiers et al. (1975) reviewed 26 patients in whom splenectomy had been performed. They found that the number who entered the terminal phase was significantly fewer than those in a comparable retrospective group of nonsplenectomized patients. Two further retrospective studies showed no evidence of prolongation of survival in splenectomized patients (Ihde et al., 1976; McBride and Hester, 1977). A controlled trial from Italy, of early splenectomy in patients in the chronic phase, revealed no benefit in the splenectomized group (Baccarini et al., 1981). A similar British Medical Research Council trial (1983) also reported negative findings.

One benefit of splenectomy in the chronic phase of the illness is the reduction of morbidity during the terminal phase, symptoms from a rapidly enlarging spleen being prevented (Coon, 1985). However, an uncomplicated chronic phase is not now generally regarded as a sufficient indication for splenectomy. Nevertheless, there are circumstances in symptomatic patients with chronic myeloid leukemia and those in the terminal phase, in which splenectomy may produce some beneficial effects. Canellos et al. (1982) reported benefit in patients made thrombocytopenic by treatment with busulfan. In the terminal phase, some patients have had short-term improvement after splenectomy for severe splenic pain from splenomegaly with or without infarction, and, when thrombocytopenia or anemia required frequent transfusions (Gomez et al., 1976).

In patients with polycythemia vera and essential thrombocythemia, a high portion of the total body platelet population is pooled in the spleen (Aster, 1966). If splenectomy is performed, the resulting severe thrombocytosis is very likely to result in thrombotic or hemorrhagic complications (Murphy, 1983). Bensinger et al. (1970) described the effectiveness of melphalan in four such patients with postsplenectomy thrombosis. Therefore splenectomy is strongly contraindicated in patients with polycythemia or essential thrombocythemia.

13.5.2. SPLENIC RADIATION THERAPY
In MPDs the use of radiation therapy to the spleen as a modality has been recognized as an option for the treatment of chronic myeloid leukemia in the chronic phase, since the beginning of the twentieth century (Pusey, 1902; Senn, 1903). This form of therapy remained standard for several years. It was found to alleviate the symptoms, shrink the spleen, and produce a marked improvement of the blood counts, in total doses of 6–10 Gy (Hotchkiss and Block, 1962; Schoen and Bauer, 1968).

In 1968, the British Medical Research Council (1968) published the results of a randomized trial of busulfan vs radiation therapy in the treatment of chronic myeloid leukemia. Those patients who received radiation therapy had a median survival time of 2.5 years, compared to 3.5 years in those treated with busulfan. This trial has been criticized because of the lack of standardization of radiation

therapy. However, the results were supported by others (Gollerkeri and Shah, 1971; Conrad, 1973), since then, radiation therapy as a definitive form of treatment has been superseded by chemotherapy and bone marrow tranplantation. Splenic radiation therapy is now reserved for symptomatic splenomegaly unresponsive to chemotherapy. It is also used for patients unable to tolerate chemotherapy, and for women in pregnancy (Richards and Spiers, 1975).

In patients with agnogenic myeloid metaplasia radiation therapy has not been used to the same extent. Hickling (1953) described the use of radiation therapy as an effective method of reducing the white cell count in this disease, but Ward and Block (1971) concluded that radiation therapy was seldom indicated, and suggested that only an occasional patient might obtain transient relief of abdominal symptoms. In general, it is now held that the use of low-dose radiation therapy to the spleen is an acceptable means of alleviating splenic pain and of reducing the size of a massively enlarged spleen (Szur et al., 1973; Parmentier et al., 1977; Greenberger et al., 1977; Canellos et al., 1979). Doses delivered vary from 1 to 15 gy, given over 9–15 days. Radiation therapy may also be indicated for patients in whom splenectomy is contraindicated. The treatment results in a moderate-to-marked fall in the peripheral granulocyte count. The mechanism seems to be destruction of proliferating precursor cells in the splenic tissue and sinuses (Koeffler et al., 1979). The effects on bone marrow erythropoiesis, as shown by ferrokinetic studies, are variable (Szur et al., 1973; Parmentier et al., 1977).

13.5.3. OTHER METHODS OF TREATING SPLENOMEGALY
Canellos et al. (1979) treated five patients in the blastic phase of chronic myeloid leukemia with symptomatic splenomegaly, by splenic artery infusions of cytosine arabinoside. All patients showed reduction in the size of the spleen, and achieved symptomatic relief. In another study, Hocking et al. (1980) advocated splenic embolization with inert materials, prior to splenectomy, to alleviate the complications of removing a massively enlarged spleen. Neither of these procedures has gained universal acceptance, although splenic embolization is still employed.

REFERENCES

Adamson, J. W. and Fialkow, P. J. (1978) The pathogenesis of myeloproliferative syndromes. *Br. J. Haematol.* **38**, 299–303.

Adler, S. S. (1976) The pathogenesis of spleen mediated phenomena in chronic myeloid leukemia and agnogenic myeloid metaplasia: a non-abscopal mechanism. *Scand. J. Haematol.* **17**, 153–159.

Aster, R. H. (1966) Pooling of platelets in the spleen: role in the pathogenesis of "hypersplenic" thrombocytopenia. *J. Clin. Invest.* **45**, 645–657.

Aviram, M., Brook, J. G., Tatarski, I., Levy, Y., and Carter, A. (1986) Increased low-density lipoprotein levels after splenectomy: role for the spleen in cholesterol metabolism in myeloproliferative disorders. *Am. J. Med. Sci.* **291**, 25–28.

Baccarini, M., Corbelli, G., Tura, S., and the Italian Group on Chronic Myeloid Leukemia (1981) Early splenectomy and polychemotherapy versus polychemotherapy alone in chronic myeloid leukemia. *Leukemia Res.* **5**, 149–157.

Bagby, G. C. (1978) Stem cell (CFU-C) proliferation and emergence in a case of chronic granulocytic leukaemia. *Scand. J. Haematol.* **20**, 193–199.

Baikie, A. G. (1968) The place of splenectomy in the treatment of chronic granulocytic leukaemia: some random observations, a review of the earlier literature and a plea for its proper study in a co-operative therapeutic trial. *Aust. Ann. Med.* **71**, 175,176.

Barosi, G., Ambrosetti, A., Buratti, A., Finelli, C., Liberato, N. L., Quaglini, S., et al. (1993) Splenectomy for patients with myelofibrosis with myeloid metaplasia: pretreatment variables and outcome prediction. *Leukemia* **7**, 200–206.

Barosi, G., Baraldi, A., Cazzola, M., Fortunato, A., Palestra, P., Polino, G., Ramella, S., and Spriano, P. (1984) Polycythaemia following splenectomy in myelofibrosis with myeloid metaplasia. A reorganization of erythropoiesis. *Scand. J. Haematol.* **32**, 12–18.

Barret, A. J., Longhurst, P., Humble, J. G., and Newton, A. K. (1977) Effect of splenic irradiation on colony-forming cells in chronic granulocytic leukaemia. *Br. Med. J.* i, 1259.

Bauer, T. W., Haskins, G. E., and Armitage, J. O. (1981) Splenic rupture in patients with hematological malignancies. *Cancer* **48**, 2729–2733.

Belucci, S., Janvier, M., Tobelem, X., Flandrin, G., Charpak, Y., Berger, R., and Boiron, M. (1986) Essential thrombocythemia. Clinical, evolutionary and biological data. *Cancer* **58**, 2440–2447.

Benbassat, J., Gilon, D., and Penchas, S. (1990) The choice between splenectomy and medical treatment in patients with advanced agnogenic myeloid metaplasia. *Am. J. Hematol.* **33**, 128–135.

Bensinger, T. A., Logue, G. L., and Rundles, R. W. (1970) Hemorrhagic thrombocythemia: control of postsplenectomy thrombocytosis with melphalan. *Blood* **36**, 61–68.

Block, M. (1964) Studies on the blood and blood-forming tissues of the newborn opossum. I. Normal development. *Ergeb. Anat. Entwick. Gesch.* **37**, 237.

Bowdler, A. J. (1983) Splenomegaly and hypersplenism. *Clin. Haematol.* **12**, 467–488.

Brandt, L. (1975) Comparative study of bone marrow and extramedullary haemopoietic tissue in chronic myeloid leukaemia. *Ser. Haematol.* **8**, 75–80.

Cabot, E. B., Brennan, M. F., Rosenthal, D. S., and Wilson, R. E. (1978). Splenectomy in myeloid metaplasia. *Ann. Surg.* **187**, 24–30.

Canellos, G. P., Nordland, J., and Carbone, P. P. (1972) Splenectomy for thrombocytopenia in chronic granulocytic leukemia. *Cancer* **29**, 660–665.

Canellos, G. P., Sutcliffe, S. B., DeVita, V. T., and Lister, T. A. (1979) Treatment of refractory splenomegaly in myeloproliferative disease by splenic artery infusion. *Blood* **53**, 1014–1017.

Carnesog, J., Wadenvik, H., Fjalling, M., and Kutti, J. (1996) Assessment of spleen size using gamma camera scintigraphy in newly diagnosed patients with essential thrombocythaemia and polycythaemia vera. *Eur. J. Haematol.* **56**, 158–162.

Champlin, R. E., Gale, R. P., Foon, K. A., and Golde, D. W. (1986) Chronic leukemias: oncogenes, chromosomes and advances in therapy. *Ann. Int. Med.* **104**, 671–688.

Chevalier, P. (1949) Les splenomegalies myeloides et leurs formes complexes. *Sang* **29**, 112.

Conrad, R. G. (1973) Survival in chronic granulocytic leukemia. *Arch. Intern. Med,* **131**, 684,685.

Coon, W. W. (1985) The limited role of splenectomy in leukemia. *Surg. Gynecol. Obstet.* **160**, 291–294.

Coon, W. W. and Liepman, M. K. (1982) Splenectomy for agnogenic myeloid metaplasia. *Surg. Gynecol. Obstet.* **154**, 561–563.

Crosby, W. H. (1972) Splenectomy in hematologic disorders. *N. Engl. J. Med.* **286**, 1252–1254.

Dameshek, W. (1960) Some speculations on the myeloproliferative syndromes. *Blood* **6**, 372–375.

DiBella, N. J., Silverstein, M. N., and Hoagland, H. (1977) Effect of splenectomy on teardrop-shaped erythrocytes in agnogenic myeloid metaplasia. *Arch. Intern. Med.* **137**, 380,381.

Fernandez, S. F., Y Benitez de Lugo, A. S., Reimers, E. G., et al. (1983) Rotura patologica del bazo secundaria a policitema vera. *Rev. Clin. Esp.* **168**, 139–141.

Fieschi, A. and Sacchetti, C. (1964). Clinical assessment of granulopoiesis. *Acta Haematol.* **31**, 150–162.

Garrison, R. N., McCoy, M., Winkler, C., Yam, L., and Fry, D. E. (1984) Splenectomy in hematologic malignancy. *Am. Surg.* **50**, 428–432.

Goldman, J. M. and Nolasco, I. (1983) The spleen in myeloproliferative disorders. *Clin. Haematol.* **12**, 505–516.

Goldstone, J. (1978) Splenectomy for massive splenomegaly. *Am. J. Surg.* **135**, 385–388.

Gollerkeri, M. P. and Shah, G. B. (1971) Management of chronic myeloid leukemia: a five-year survey with a comparison of busulfan and splenic irradiation. *Cancer* **21**, 596– 601.

Gomez, G. A., Sokal, J. E., Mittleman, A., and Aungst, C. W. (1976) Splenectomy for palliation of chronic myelocytic leukemia. *Am. J. Med.* **16**, 14–22.

Green, T. W., Conley, C. L., Ashburn, L. L., and Peters, H. R. (1953) Splenectomy for myeloid metaplasia of the spleen. *N. Engl. J Med.* **248**, 211–219.

Greenberg, P. L. and Steed, S. M. (1981) Splenic granulocytopoiesis and production of colony-stimulating activity in lymphoma and leukemia. *Blood* **57**, 119–121.

Greenberger, J. S., Chaffery, J. T., Rosenthal, D. S., and Moloney, W. C. (1977) Irradiaton for control of hypersplenism and painful splenomegaly in myeloid metaplasia. *Int. J. Radiat. Oncol. Biol. Phys.* **2**, 1083–1090.

Heaton, A., Jacobs, P., Dent, D. M., and Louw, J. H. (1976) Experience with splenectomy in auto-immune thrombocytopenia and agnogenic myeloid metaplasia. *S. Afr. Med. J.* **50**, 1506–1512.

Hickling, R. A. (1937) Chronic non-leukaemic myelosis. *Q. J. Med.* **6**, 253–275.

Hickling, R. A. (1953) Treatment of patients with myelosclerosis. *Br. Med. J.* ii, 411–413.

Hocking, W. G., Machleder, H. I., and Golde, D. W. (1980) Splenic artery embolism prior to splenectomy in end-stage polycythemia vera. *Am. J. Hematol* **8**, 123–127.

Hotchkiss, D. R. and Block, M. A. (1962) Effect of spenic irradiation on systemic hematopoiesis. *Ann. Intern. Med.* **109**, 697–711.

Ihde, D. C., Canellos, G. P., Schwartz, J. H., and DeVita, V. T. (1976) Splenectomy in the chronic phase of chronic granulocytic leukemia. *Ann. Intern. Med.,* **84**, 17–21.

Jackson, H. Jr., Parker, F. Jr., and Lemon, H. M. (1940) Agnogenic myeloid metaplasia of the spleen. *N. Engl. J. Med.* **222**, 985.

Keleman, E., Calvo, W., and Fliedner, T. M. (1979) *Atlas of Hematopoietic Development,* Springer-Verlag, New York, pp. 156–171.

Kirschner, J. J., Goldberg, J., and Landaw, S. A. (1980) The spleen as a site of colony-forming cell production in myelofibrosis. *Proc. Exp. Biol. Med.* **165**, 279–282.

Koeffler, H. P., Cline, M. J., and Golde, D. W. (1979) Splenic irradiation in myelofibrosis: effect on circulating myeloid progenitor cells. *Br. J. Haematol.* **43**, 69–77.

Lafaye, F., Rain, J. D., Clot, P., and Najean, Y. (1994) Risks and benefits of splenectomy in myelofibrosis: an analysis of 39 cases. *Nouv. Rev. Fr. Hematol.* **36**, 359–362.

Lancet editorial (1985) Splenectomy-risk of infection, long-term. *Lancet* ii, 928,929.

Lewis, S. M. (1983) The spleen: mysteries solved and unresolved. *Clin. Haematol.* **12**, 363–373.

Ligumski, M., Polliack, A., and Benbasset, J. (1978) Nature and incidence of liver involvement in agnogenic myeloid metaplasia. *Scand. J. Haematol.* **21**, 81–93.

Lutton, J. D. and Levere, R. D. (1979) Endogenous erythroid colony formation by peripheral blood mononuclear cells from patients with myelofibrosis and polycythaemia vera. *Acta Haematol.* **62**, 94–99.

Marsh, G. W., Lewis, S. M., and Szur, L. (1966) The use of ^{51}Cr-labelled heat-damaged red cells to study splenic function. *Br. J. Haematol.* **12**, 167–171.

McBride, C. M. and Hester, J. P. (1977) Chronic myelogenous leukemia: management of splenectomy in a high risk population. *Cancer* **39**, 653–658.

Medical Research Council (1983) Randomised trial of splenectomy in Ph^1-positive chronic granulocytic leukaemia including an analysis of prognostic features. *Br. J. Haematol.* **54**, 415–430.

Moore, M. A. S. (1975) Embryologic and phylogenetic development of the hematopoietic systems. In: *Advances in the Biosciences* 16, Pergamon, Vieweg, Germany, pp. 87–101.

Mulder, H., Steenbergen, J., and Haanen, C. (1977) Clinical course and survival after elective splenectomy in 19 patients with primary myelofibrosis. *Br. J. Haematol.* **35**, 419–427.

Murphy, S. (1983) Thrombocytosis and thrombocythaemia. *Clin. Haematol.* **12**, 89–106.

Murphy, S., Rosenthal, D. S., Weinfeld, A., Briere, J., Faguet, G. B., Knospe, W. H., et al. (1982) Essential thrombocythemia: response during first year of therapy with melphalan and radioactive phosphorus: a Polycythemia Vera Study Group report. *Cancer Treat. Rep.* **66**, 35–40.

Nagler, A., Brenner, B., Argov, S., and Tatarsky, I. (1986) Postsplenectomy pericardial effusion in two patients with myeloid metaplasia. *Arch. Intern. Med.* **146**, 600,601.

Najean, Y., Arrago, J. P., Rain, J. D., and Desch, C. (1984) The "spent" phase of polycythaemia vera: hypersplenism in the absence of myelofibrosis. *Br. J. Haematol.* **56**, 1163–1170.

Parmentier, C., Charbord, P., Tibi, M., and Tubiana, M. (1977) Splenic irradiation in myelofibrosis. Clinical findings and ferrokinetics. *Int. J. Radiat. Oncol. Biol. Phys.* **2**, 1075–1081.

Pederson, B. (1979) Spleen and relapse in chronic myeloid leukaemia. *Scand. J. Haematol.* **22**, 369–374.

Pettit, J. E., Lewis, S. M., and Nicholas, A. W. (1979) Transitional myeloproliferative disorder. *Br. J. Haematol.* **43**, 167–184.

Pusey, W. A. (1902) Report of cases treated with Roentgen rays. *JAMA* **38**, 911–919.

Rappaport, H. (1966) Tumors of the hemopoietic system. In: *An Atlas of Tumor Pathology.* Armed Forces Institute of Pathology, Washington, DC, pp. 237–336.

Revesz, P., Carneskog, J., Wadenvik, H., Jarneborn, L., and Kutti, J. (1993) Measurement of spleen size using gamma camera scintigraphy in essential thrombocythaemia. *Eur. J. Haematol.* **51**, 141–143.

Richards, H. G. H. and Spiers, A. S. D. (1975) Chronic granulocytic leukaemia in pregnancy. *Br. J. Radiol.* **48**, 261–264.

Schoen, D. and Bauer, R. (1968) Ergebnisse mit der Milzbestralung bei 175 fallen mit chronischer myelischer Leukamie. *Strahlentherapie* **135**, 1–10.

Schofield, R. (1979) The pluripotent stem cell. *Clin. Haematol.* **8**, 221–237.

Scott, J. L., McMillan, R., Davidson, J. G., and Marino, J. V. (1971) Leukocyte labelling with ⁵¹chromium. II. Leukocyte kinetics in chronic myelocytic leukemia. *Blood* **38**, 162–173.

Senn, N. (1903) Case of splenomedullary leukemia successfully treated by the use of Roentgen ray. *Med. Rec.* **64**, 281,282.

Shaw, M. T. (1982) Clinical and haematological manifestations in the terminal phase, in *Chronic Granulocytic Leukaemia* (Shaw, M. T., ed.), Praeger, Eastbourne, UK, pp. 169–188.

Silverstein, M. N. and ReMime, W. H. (1974) Sex, splenectomy, and myeloid metaplasia. *Blood* **53**, 515–518.

Silverstein, M. N., Wollaeger, E. E., and Baggentoss, A. H. (1973) Gastrointestinal and abdominal manifestations of agnogenic myeloid metaplasia. *Arch. Intern. Med.* **131**, 532–537.

Skinner, H. C. and Sophean, L. S. (1951) Agnogenic myeloid metaplasia of the spleen: follow-up after splenectomy. *J. Int. Coll. Surg.* **15**, 343–346.

Spiers, A. S. D., Baikie, A. G., Galton, D. A. G., et al. (1975) Chronic granulocytic leukaemia: effect of elective splenectomy on the course of the disease. *Br. Med. J.* **i**, 175–179.

Sullivan, A. Rheinlander, H., and Weintraub, L. R. (1974) Esophageal varices in myeloid metaplasia. *Gastroenterology* **66**, 429–432.

Szur, L., Pettit, J. E., Lewis, S. M., Bruce-Tagoe, A. A., and Short, M. D. (1973) The effect of radiation on splenic function in myelosclerosis: studies with ⁵²Fe and ⁹⁹Tc. *Br. J. Radiol.* **46**, 295–301.

Tavassoli, M. (1973) Splenic white pulp in myeloid metaplasia. *Arch. Pathol.* **95**, 419–421.

Tavassoli, M. and Weiss, L. (1973) An electron microscopic study of spleen in myelofibrosis with myeloid metaplasia. *Blood* **42**, 267–279.

Thiel, G. and Downey, H. (1921) The development of the mammalian spleen, with special reference to its hemopoietic activity. *Am. J. Anat.* **28**, 279.

Thompson, R. B. and Stainsby, D. (1982) The clinical and haematological features of chronic granulocytic leukaemia in the chronic phase. In: *Chronic Granulocytic Leukaemia* (Shaw, M. T., ed.), Praeger, Eastbourne, UK, pp. 137–168.

Van Den Heuvel, R. L., Versele, S. R. M., Schoeters, G. E. R., and Vanderborght, O. L. J. (1987) Stromal stem cells (CFU-f) in yolk sac, liver, spleen and bone marrow of pre- and postnatal mice. *Br. J. Haematol.* **66**, 15–20.

Wagner, H., McKeogh, P. G., Desforges, J., and Madoc-Jones, H. (1986) Splenic irradiation in the treatment of patients with chronic myelogenous leukemia or myelofibrosis with myeloid metaplasia. *Cancer* **58**, 1204–1207.

Ward, H. P. and Block, M. H. (1971) The natural history of agnogenic myeloid metaplasia (AMM) and a critical evaluation of its relationship with the myeloproliferative syndrome. *Medicine* **50**, 357–421.

Waweru, F. and Lewis, S. M. (1985) Blood volume, erythrokinetics and spleen function in thrombocythaemia. *Acta Haematol.* **73**, 219–223.

Westin, J., Lanner, L., Larsson, A, and Weinfeld, A. (1972) Spleen size in polycythaemia. *Acta Med. Scand.* **191**, 431–436.

Wetherley-Mein, G. and Pearson, T. C. (1982) The myeloproliferative disorders. In: *Blood and its Disorders* (Hardisty, R. M. and Weatherall, D. J., eds.), Blackwell, Oxford.

Wilkins, B. S., Green, A., Wild, A. E., and Jones, D. B. (1994) Extramedullary hemopoiesis in fetal and adult human spleen: a quantitative immunohistological study. *Histopathology* **24**, 241–247.

Wilson, R. E., Rosenthal, D. S., Moloney, W. C., and Osteen, R. T. (1985) Splenectomy for, myeloproliferative disorders. *World J. Surg.* **9**, 431–436.

Wintrobe, M., M., Lee, G. R., and Boggs, D. R., eds. (1976) *Clinical Hematology,* 7th ed. Lee and Febiger, Philadelphia.

Wobbes, T., van der Sluis, R. F., and Lubbers, E. C. (1984) Removal of the massive spleen: a surgical risk? *Am. J. Surg.* **147**, 800–802.

Wolf, B. and Neiman, R. S. (1985) Myelofibrosis with myeloid metaplasia: pathophysiologic implications of the correlation between bone marrow changes and progression of splenomegaly. *Blood* **65**, 803–809.

Wolf, B. C., Luevano, E., and Neiman, R. S. (1983) Evidence to suggest that the human fetal spleen is not a hematopoietic organ. *Am. J. Clin. Pathol.* **80**, 140–144.

Wolf, N. S. and Trentin, J. J. (1968) Hemopoietic colony studies, V. Effect of hemopoietic stroma on differentiation of pluripotent stem cells. *J. Exp. Med.* **127**, 205–214.

14 The Spleen in Lymphoproliferative Disease

Peter C. Raich, MD

14.1. INTRODUCTION

Because the spleen is the largest lymphoid organ in the body, it is frequently involved in the lymphoproliferative disorders (Table 1). In the malignant lymphomas, splenic involvement, manifested by splenomegaly and at times the associated features of hypersplenism, may be a presenting feature, together with lymph node enlargement, or it may appear later in the course of the disease, on relapse, or with disease resistant to therapy. Occasionally, lymphomas present with involvement limited to the spleen. In chronic lymphocytic leukemia, splenomegaly may be one of the earliest findings, but this appears to have little influence on the outcome of the disease. The presence of splenomegaly may be the major physical finding in hairy cell leukemia (HCL), alerting the physician to the possibility of that diagnosis, and subsequent removal of the spleen will frequently be associated with lasting remission.

In this chapter, the extent of splenic involvement observed in the malignant lymphoproliferative disorders (MLPDs) is discussed, as well as how this involvement pertains to the diagnosis, staging, prognosis, and treatment of each disorder.

14.2. CLASSIFICATION OF LYMPHOID NEOPLASMS

The MLPDs initially and primarily involve the lymphoid system. The malignant cells represent a monoclonal population of cells characterized by surface markers having predominantly B- or T-lymphocyte features (Greaves, 1975; Seligmann et al., 1973). The marked pleomorphism observed in Hodgkin's disease has been attributed to the host's reaction to the malignant cells; the cells in non-Hodgkin's lymphomas (NHLs) have been shown to be expanded clones of specific lymphocyte precursors and functional cell types. The increased availability and application of specific monoclonal antibodies directed against cell surface antigens (Uckun, 1990) has led to the identification of malignant lymphoma cells corresponding to various stages of differentiation of B- and T-cells, as well as of antigenically stimulated, activated cell types (Table 2).

More recently, chromosomal and molecular biologic defects have been defined in various NHLs. These frequently involve genes controlling cell growth. Chromosome translocations have been identified, involving sites of immunoglobulin heavy- and light-chain genes, especially chromosomes 2, 14, and 22, as summarized in Table 3.

Since these immunoproliferative cells retain many of the characteristics of normal B- and T-cells, they probably will retain other traits, such as recirculation through the lymphatic (immune) system, as well as the predilection to accumulate and proliferate in certain compartments of the immune system. Malignancies arising from cells corresponding to the primary differentiation pathway, such as acute lymphocytic leukemia (ALL), involve the bone marrow, but less often the spleen; those linked to the secondary differentiation pathway, including most of the lymphomas, frequently involve the lymph nodes and spleen.

The presence of certain adhesion molecules may explain unusual organ involvement and peculiar infiltrative patterns of some of the MLPDs. For example, neoplastic cells in HCL characteristically express large amounts of the CD11c molecule on their surface. This and other surface molecules have a high affinity for postcapillary (high endothelial) venules, possibly explaining the prominent red pulp infiltration and vascular plugging (Vincent et al., 1996), as well as the good response to immune modulation therapy characteristic for this disease. Another example is the interaction of the β-1 integrin very late antigen 4 (VLA-4) on B-lymphocytes, with the vascular cell adhesion molecule-1 (VCAM-1) expressed on follicular dendritic cells, which leads to the homing of malignant cells preferentially to the lymphatic germinal centers in follicle center cell lymphoma (Freedman et al., 1992).

The adhesion molecule, ICAM-1 (CD54-IOL54), has been linked to tumor dissemination, especially with the growth pattern and organ distribution of indolent and aggressive lymphomas (Terol et al., 1998). Additional adhesion molecules, including CD44 and Mel-14, have been described, which are also involved in lymphocyte–high endothelial venule interactions (Picker et al., 1989; Berg et al., 1989; Haynes et al., 1989). The degree of expression of these and other adhesion molecules may determine the unique dissemination and infiltration patterns characteristic of the MLPD family (Stamenkovic et al., 1989).

Several classification systems of these immunoproliferative diseases, based on functional and immunological studies, have been proposed and used over the past four decades, including those by Lukes et al. (1966), Lennert (1967), Lukes and Collins (1974), the Kiel Classification (Lennert, 1978; Meugè et al., 1978), the Working Formulation (WF) (Non-Hodgkin's Lymphoma Classification Project, 1982), and, most recently, the Revised European American Lymphoma (REAL) Classification (Harris et al., 1994).

Table 4 compares the major entities included within each of the three most frequently used systems for classification of lymphoid neoplasms: the WF, the REAL Classification, and the Kiel

From: *The Complete Spleen: A Handbook of Structure, Function, and Clinical Disorders* Edited by: A. J. Bowdler © Humana Press Inc., Totowa, NJ

Table 14.1
Splenic Involvement in Lymphoproliferative Malignancies

Disease	Splenomegaly	White pulp	Red pulp
CLL	Common	Early	Late
Waldenstroem's	Common	Early	Late
HCL	Common	Late	Early
NHL			
Marginal zone	Common	Early	Late
Mantle cell	Common	Early	Late
T-cell MLPDs	Variable	Early	Early
ALL	In children	Early	Late
Hodgkin's disease	Late	Early	Late

Table 14.2
B-Lymphocyte Differentiation and Origins of B-Cell Lymphoproliferative Disorders

B-cell differentiation	Lymphoid malignancy equivalent (REAL Classification)
Primary Differentiation	
Antigen-independent	
(Bone marrow and thymus)	
Multipotential stem cell	ALL (Null-cell type)
↓	
Pre-B-cell	ALL (Pre-B-cell type)
↓	
B-cell with SIgM	Burkitt-like lymphoma
↓	
B-cell with SIg, CR, FcR	
↓	
Immunocompetent lymphocyte	B-cell CLL/lymphoma
Secondary Differentiation	
Antigen-dependent	
(Spleen and lymph nodes)	
Centrocyte	Follicle center cell lymphoma (grade I, II, and III)
↓	
Centroblast	Mantle cell lymphoma
↓	
Immunoblast	Immunoblastic lymphoma
↘	
Memory lymphocyte	B-cell lymphocytic lymphoma/ CLL
↓	
Plasmablast	Lymphoplasmacytoid lymphoma
↓	
Plasma cell	Multiple myeloma

SIg, Surface immunoglobulin-bearing cells; CR, complement receptors; FcR, receptors for Fc portion of Ig; ALL, acute lymphocytic leukemia; CLL, chronic lymphocytic leukemia.

Classification. The WF is presently the most widely used classification system in the United States; the modified Kiel Classification (Stansfeld et al., 1988) is popular in Europe.

Both of the latter classifications have significant problems, although each has its staunch defenders. For example, neither provides a logical place for the recently described entities of marginal zone and mantle cell lympomas. In order to develop more encompassing consensus criteria for distinct pathologic and clinical entities, a large group of pathologists from throughout the world met during the early 1990s, to develop a new classification schema. This group, the International Lymphoma Study Group, published its proposed classification, the REAL Classification, in 1994 (Harris et al., 1994). A thorough discussion of the advantages and disadvantages of the REAL Classification, compared to the other two commonly used classification systems, has been provided by Longo (1995) and others (Armitage, 1997; Skarin and Dorfman, 1997).

The concept of the REAL Classification was tested in 1400 lymphoma patients from around the world (The Non-Hodgkin's Lymphoma Classification Project, 1997). This analysis confirmed that diagnoses could be made more accurately than with previous systems, and led to the delineation of clinically relevant subgroups. A wealth of information is available from this data. For example, an analysis of the effect of age on the characteristics and clinical behavior of NHL patients showed that splenic involvement was observed less frequently in young and old patients, 13 and 14%, respectively, compared to 17–24% for intermediate age patients.

Although the REAL Classification is not perfect regarding its clinical applicability (Hiddemann et al., 1996; Engelhard et al., 1997; Melnyk et al., 1997), this chapter follows this classification in discussing splenic involvement by the major MLPDs. Accordingly, under the REAL Classification, one can divide the various diagnoses into five clinical disease syndromes:

1. Chronic leukemia/lymphoma
2. Nodal or extranodal lymphoma
   a. Indolent
   b. Aggressive
3. Acute leukemia/lymphoma
4. Plasma cell disorders
5. Hodgkin's disease

14.2.1. CHRONIC LYMOPHOCYTIC LEUKEMIA AND ITS VARIANTS

Chronic lymphocytic leukemia (CLL) is a generalized lymphoproliferative disease affecting the small lymphocyte (Dame-shek and Gunz, 1964). A variety of cell markers and clinical features delineate several subtypes (Cheson et al., 1996).

14.2.1.1. B-Cell Chronic Lymphocytic Leukemia (B-Cell CLL) In approx 95% of cases, cell surface membrane immunoglobulin markers will identify the small abnormal lymphocytes of CLL as B-cells (Foucar, 1992). They proliferate slowly, and circulate through the blood, the spleen, bone marrow and lymph nodes. The spleen is often involved, and may occasionally present as an isolated initial manifestation (Dighiero et al., 1979; see Subheading 2.2.1.4.). The spleen is palpably enlarged in 50% of patients at diagnosis (Hansen, 1973), and splenomegaly progresses with advancing disease (Videbaek et al., 1982). Total body tumor mass, as reflected by areas of involvement and symptoms, is related to prognosis. To assist in making treatment decisions in CLL patients, a clinical staging system was proposed in the 1970s by Rai et al. (1975), as shown in Table 5. This system is still commonly in use, although, subsequently, a simpler staging scheme has been adopted by an international study group (Binet et al., 1981).

The most common pattern of splenic involvement in CLL is expansion of the white pulp and infiltration of the red pulp (Lampert et al., 1980a). The white pulp may be infiltrated in either a nodular or diffuse fashion. The degree of red pulp infiltration will usually parallel the degree of peripheral blood lymphocytosis. T-cells are displaced from their usual periarterial location, and appear more often in the red pulp (Lampert, 1983). Praz et al. (1984) have demon-

Table 14.3
Summary of Immunophenotypic and Genetic Findings in NHLs

Lymphoma subtype	Pan-B	SIg	CD5	CD10	CD23	Pan-T	TdT	Cytogenetic findings
Small lymphocytic	+	+	+	−	+	−	−	+12; 13q14; 14q+
Follicular center cell	+	+	−	+	+/−	−	−	t(14:18) (*bcl-2*)
Marginal zone	+	+	−	−	−	−	−	+3
Diffuse large B-cell	+/−	+/−	−	−/+	+/−	−	−	t(14;18) *bcl-2*; 3q27 (*bcl-6*)
Mantle cell	+	+	+	−	−	−/+	−	t(11;14) (cyclin D1)
Small noncleaved cell	+	+	−	+	−	−	−	t(2;8); t(8;14); t(8;22) (c-*myc*)
Peripheral T-cell	−	−	+	−	−/+	+	−	t(2;5)
Lymphoblastic	−/+	−	+/−	−/+	−/+	+/−	+	Multiple

Pan-B, pan B-cell markers such as CD19, CD20; Pan-T, pan T-cell markers such as CD2, CD3, CD7; SIg, surface immunoglobuin staining; TdT, terminal deoxynucleotidyl transferase. +, positive; −, negative; +/ −, often positive, but may be negative; −/+, often negative, but may be positive. (Adapted with permission from Skarin and Dorfman, 1997.)

Table 14.4
Comparison of Revised European American Lymphoma (REAL) Classification,
Working Formulation (WF), and Kiel Classification for MLPDs

REAL Classification	Working Formulation	Kiel Classification
Chronic leukemia/lymphoma		
Chronic leukemia/lymphoma, B- and T-cell type	Small lymphocytic lymphoma/CLL	Lymphocytic, B- and T-cell type
Lymphoplasmacytoid lymphoma/WM	Small lymphocytic, plasma-cytoid	Lymphoplasmacytic immunocytoma
Prolymphocytic leukemia, B-and T-cell type	Small lymphocytic, plasma-cytoid	Prolymphocytic leukemia
Large granular lymphocytic leukemia	Small lymphocytic leukemia	T-lymphocytic, CLL type
HCL	HCL	HCL
Indolent lymphomas		
Follicle center cell lymphoma, follicular, small-cell type (grade I)	Follicular, predominantly small cleaved cell	Centroblastic-centrocytic, follicular

Marginal zone lymphoma, B-cell:
    Extranodal (MALT)
    Nodal (monocytoid)
    Splenic
	Small lymphocytic, diffuse, small cleaved cell, or mixed small- and large-cell	Monocytoid, including marginal zone

Aggressive lymphomas		
Diffuse, large B-cell, including immunoblastic and diffuse mixed-cell	Diffuse, large-cell Immunoblastic, large-cell Diffuse mixed-cell	Centroblastic Immunoblastic
Follicle center cell, follicular (grade II and III)	Follicular, mixed small- and large-cell Follicular, large-cell	Centroblastic-centrocytic, follicular
Follicle center cell, diffuse	Diffuse, small cleaved cell, or mixed small and large	Centroblastic-centrocytic, diffuse
Mantle cell	Diffuse, small cleaved cell, or mixed small and large	Centrocytic Centroblastic
High grade B-cell, Burkitt-like	Small noncleaved cell, non-Burkitt's	Centroblastic Immunoblastic
Peripheral T-cell	Diffuse, mixed Large-cell immunoblastic	Pleomorphic
Angioimmunoblastic, T-cell	Diffuse, mixed Large-cell immunoblastic	Angioimmunoblastic
Anaplastic large-cell	Large-cell immunoblastic	Large-cell anaplastic
Acute leukemia/lymphoma		
Lymphoblastic, T- and B-cell	Lymphoblastic	Lymphoblastic, T- and B-cell
Burkitt's lymphoma	Small noncleaved cell, Burkitt's	Burkitt's lymphoma
Adult T-cell	Lymphoblastic	T-lymphoblastic
Plasma cell disorders		
Solitary plasmacytoma	Extramedullary plasmacytoma	Plasmacytic
Multiple myeloma	Myeloma	Plasmacytic

WM, Waldenstroem's macroglobulinemia; MALT, Mucosal-associated lymphatic tissue; HCL, hairy cell leukemia.

Table 14.5
Rai Clinical Staging System for CLL

Stage	Findings at diagnosis
0	Lymphocytes in blood 15,000/μL or higher, and 40% marrow lymphocytosis.
I	Above, plus enlarged lymph nodes.
II	Above, plus splenomegaly, hepatomegaly, or both.
III	Above, plus anemia (hemoglobin less than 11 g/dL).
IV	Above, plus thrombocytopenia (platelets less than 100,000/μL).

(Adapted with permission from Rai et al., 1975.)

strated that CLL cells can activate the alternative complement pathway in vitro, and that C3 molecules are detectable on CLL cells in vivo. Those authors postulate that these CLL cells could interact with splenic and hepatic macrophages, thereby sequestering preferentially in these organs.

14.2.1.2. T-Cell Chronic Lymphocytic Leukemia (T-Cell CLL)
T-cell CLL is rare in the Western world, but is the most common type of CLL in Japan (Hanaoka et al., 1979). It is frequently associated with splenomegaly, skin infiltration, and early neurologic manifestations (Brouet et al., 1975). The involved spleen shows enlargement of both the red and white pulp, with, however, prominent residual germinal centers (Lampert, 1983). Cell typing has shown these cells, phenotypically and functionally, to be suppressor T-cells, which may explain the hypogammaglobulinemia observed in many cases.

More recently, several publications have provided additional information about natural killer (NK) cell and NK-like T-cell malignancies (Emile et al., 1996; Macon et al., 1996). Jaffe (1996), in an editorial accompanying the previous reports, provides a schema for the differential diagnosis of these T-cell malignancies. Included is the entity called "aggressive NK-cell leukemia," which usually presents with widespread disease, including peripheral blood and skin involvement, and prominent hepatosplenomegaly (Imamura et al., 1990; Wong et al., 1992; Sun et al., 1993). The presence of azurophilic granules in the T-cells suggests a derivation from NK cells.

A second more recently described entity is aggressive, T-cell, large granular lymphocyte (NK-like) leukemia (Gentile et al., 1994; Macon et al., 1996). This entity is characterized by peripheral blood, bone marrow and gastrointestinal tract involvement, along with prominent hepatosplenomegaly. The malignant cells subserve many of the functions of NK cells, but are phenotypically and genotypically true T-cells (MacDonald, 1995). Like the aggressive NK-cell leukemia described above, it is also clinically aggressive, more common in Asia, and has a variable association with Epstein-Barr virus (Jaffe, 1996). These two entities need to be distinguished from the more common, indolent, large granular lymphocyte lymphoproliferative disorder described below.

14.2.1.3. Lymphoproliferative Disease of Granular Lymphocytes (LDGL) The lymphoproliferative disease of large granular lymphocytes is now felt to be a distinct, though heterogeneous disorder, resulting from a clonal proliferation of granular lymphocytes with $CD3^+$ or $CD3^-$ phenotype. Both types of T-cells from patients with this syndrome have been shown to express NK-related antigens (Loughran, 1993; Newland et al., 1984; Pandolfi et al., 1984; Loughran et al., 1985; McKenna et al., 1985; Grillot-

Courvalin et al., 1986). LDGL does not generally present with features of an invasive malignancy, but rather as a chronic lymphocytosis with complications of neutropenia, thrombocytopenia, anemia, and autoimmune disorders, such as rheumatoid arthritis (Pandolfi et al., 1990; Semenzato et al., 1997). Organ enlargement is generally limited to the spleen (20–50%), and lymph node enlargement is rare. The pathology includes distinctive sinusoidal infiltration of spleen, liver, and, less consistently, the bone marrow. Polyclonal plasma cell infiltration can also often be found in the bone marrow and spleen. Despite these clinical and pathologic signs of low-grade malignancy, the clinical course of these patients may be distinctly unfavorable, because of the profound pancytopenia. This pancytopenia is felt to be not related to the splenomegaly, but rather on an autoimmune or marrow-suppressive basis (Lamy and Loughran, 1998). It is best addressed by elucidating a possible autoimmune mechanism, or by the use of growth factors, such as granulocyte- or granulocyte-macrophage colony-stimulating factors, rather than antineoplastic therapy (Lamy and Loughran, 1998).

14.2.1.4. Prolymphocytic Leukemia Prolymphocytic leukemia is a much less common, but more aggressive disease than CLL, with a poor response to alkylating chemotherapy (Melo et al., 1985). It typically presents with massive splenomegaly and marked leukocytosis, but no lymphadenopathy (Galton et al., 1974). Prolymphocytes are of intermediate size, with a characteristic nucleus showing well-condensed chromatin and a prominent nucleolus (Catovsky, 1977). The majority of spleens in this condition have shown enlargement of the white pulp and infiltration of the red pulp (Lampert, 1983). A nodular pattern is often seen, with the larger, abnormal cells at the periphery of the nodules (Lampert et al., 1980b). Splenectomy and leukapheresis have led to temporary therapeutic responses (Buskard et al., 1976), but, more successful, definitive treatment includes the purine analog, 2-deoxycoformin, pentostatin, or fludarabine (El'Agnaf et al., 1986; Mercieca et al., 1994).

With the advent of broader availability of immunophenotyping of the lymphoproliferative disorders, some patients will present with findings common to several of the MLPDs. For example, there are three reports of patients with $CD5^+$, $CD11c^+$, TRAP-positive B-cell CLL/prolymphocytic leukemia, with splenomegaly, but little lymph node enlargement, and with peripheral blood prolymphocytes (Prince et al., 1992; Hanson et al., 1990; Wormsley et al., 1990).

14.2.1.5. Heavy Chain Disease 6/7 patients with μ heavy-chain disease, reported by Franklin (1975), presented clinically as CLL, often with marked splenomegaly, but infrequently with peripheral lymphadenopathy (Jonsson et al., 1976). Associated findings are κ light chains in the urine and vacuolated plasma cells in the marrow (Franklin, 1975). γ heavy-chain disease frequently presents as a lymphoma, with lymphadenopathy, hepatosplenomegaly, and systemic symptoms (Franklin et al., 1964). α heavy-chain disease may present with enteric manifestations and abdominal masses (Mediterranean lymphoma), or with respiratory tract infiltration (Seligmann et al., 1968). Spleen and liver are usually not involved, but such involvement has been described (Plesnicar et al., 1975).

14.2.1.6. Waldenstroem's Macroglobulinemia Clinically, this condition mimics aleukemic CLL, with manifestations of hyperviscosity caused by the immunoglobulin M monoclonal gammopathy (Kyle and Garton, 1987). Moderate hepatosplenomegaly and lymph node enlargement are also part of the clinical presentation. Splenomegaly was reported in 37% of patients described by McCallister et al. (1967) and MacKenzie and Fudenberg (1972), and in

Table 14.6
Hepatosplenomegaly in HCL

Authors	Splenomegaly (%)	Hepatomegaly (%)
Catovsky (1977)	85	35
Golomb et al. (1978)	82	19
Bouroncle (1979)	93	40
Cawley et al. (1980)	84	40
Flandrin et al. (1984)	72	20

23% of those described by Andriko et al. (1997). Immunoblastic transformation of Waldenstroem's macroglobulinemia limited to the spleen, and treated successfully by splenectomy, has been described (Winter et al., 1995).

14.2.1.7. Hairy Cell Leukemia Hairy cell leukemia (HCL), or leukemic reticuloendotheliosis, accounts for 2–5% of all leukemias (Bouroncle, 1979; Katayama and Finkel, 1974; Golomb et al., 1978). Evidence points to a B-lymphocyte as the malignant cell, which, however, possesses certain monocyte characteristics (Catovsky, 1977; Meijer et al., 1984). The hairy cell can be shown to have numerous cytoplasmic filamentous projections, when observed by phase microscopy of the peripheral blood, the bone marrow, and the spleen. The malignant cells usually demonstrate typical acid phosphatase positivity resistant to tartrate, or TRAP (Yam et al., 1972); however, cases with negative TRAP reactivity have been described (Schaefer et al., 1975). The typical appearance of the marrow, infiltrated with a loose network of mononuclear cells, is diagnostic, especially when associated with prominent splenomegaly and pancytopenia (Catovsky, 1977).

Splenomegaly is present in 80–90% of cases (Table 6). In a review by Maurer (1985) of three reported series (Katayama and Finkel, 1974; Mintz and Golomb, 1979; Burke et al., 1974), the average spleen weight was 1500 g, with a range of 250 to 4650 g. At surgery, involved spleens typically have a homogeneous, red, fleshy appearance, without nodularity (Maurer, 1985; Breitfeld and Lee, 1975). It is one of few lymphoproliferative that primarily involves the red pulp of the spleen (Table 1). The microscopic picture is distinctive and diagnostic: the white pulp is atrophic, and may be partially obliterated in massively enlarged spleens (Burke, 1981). The hairy cells diffusely infiltrate the cords of the red (but not the white) pulp, and the sinusoids are filled with similar cells. This obliteration of red pulp architecture differs from other MLPDs, and is considered pathognomic for HCL. Subendothelial infiltration of the trabecular veins by hairy cells has also been described as characteristic (Burke and Rappaport, 1984). This finding, and a monoclonal antibody phenotype characteristic of HCL, led to the confirmation of splenic involvement in a 140-g spleen (Burke et al., 1987).

Pseudosinuses and red blood cell pools are located within the splenic cords of patients with HCL (Nanba et al., 1977). The hairy cells tend to attach to endothelial cells, via specific receptors (Vincent et al., 1996), and to each other, as well as to red blood cells, leading to plugging of sinus pores, increased intrasinusal pressure, and dilatation of the cord structures to form blood lakes (Burke et al., 1976; Pilon et al., 1981, 1982). These structural abnormalities of the spleen would explain the prominent functional hypersplenism

and the cases of splenic rupture observed in patients with HCL (*see* Subheadings 4.1. and 4.2.). The splenic blood pool is especially prominent in HCL (Maurer, 1985). The increased splenic blood pool, and the congestion and decreased blood flow of the cords, leads to increased exposure of blood cells to the cordal macrophages, and results in removal of these cells from the circulation, contributing to the peripheral cytopenias.

14.2.2. NODAL AND EXTRANODAL LYMPHOMAS The malignant cells in the great majority of these disorders are B-lymphocytes in varying degrees of differentiation (Tables 2 and 3). In contrast to Hodgkin's disease, the NHLs more often present in disseminated fashion. Malignant lymphoma presenting in the spleen as the only site of involvement, is rare (*see* Subheading 2.2.1.4.), but involvement of the spleen during the course of lymphoma is common (Ahmann et al., 1966). In an extensive review by Rosenberg et al. (1961) of 1269 patients with NHL, 0.8% of patients presented with a palpable spleen, 35.9% developed a palpable spleen during the course of the disease, and 53.7% showed splenic involvement at autopsy, which is comparable to previously reported series, which observed palpable spleens during the patients' lifetime in 21–56% of cases (Sugarbaker and Craver, 1940; Gall and Mallory, 1942; Wetherley-Mein et al., 1952). Nodular lymphomas involve the spleen in 50–60% of cases; the diffuse types show this in about 30% (Heifetz et al., 1980). Since the classification of lymphomas has changed drastically over the latter half of the twentieth century, it is very difficult to extrapolate these earlier reports to present classification systems.

Initial splenic involvement in NHL typically involves the white pulp, and therefore presents in nodular fashion in both the nodular and diffuse types of lymphomas. Small-cell lymphomas usually form small uniform nodules, representing infiltration and enlargement of the malpighian corpuscles evenly distributed throughout the spleen; the large-cell lymphomas form bulky and irregular nodules (Maurer, 1985; Kim and Dorfman, 1974; Galton et al., 1978). In the follicular lymphomas, it is not unusual to observe lymphoma cells in the red pulp. This would seem to correspond to the relatively high percentage of lymphosarcoma cell leukemia presentations in patients with follicular lymphomas (Spiro et al., 1975).

Splenic size in NHL is not a reliable indicator of lymphoma involvement. Although large spleens are commonly involved, splenic lymphoma may also be found in spleens of normal weight (Kim and Dorfman, 1974). Involved spleens weighed from 75 to 4500 g in NHL patients (Skarin et al., 1971); uninvolved spleens weighed less than 270 g (Lotz et al., 1976). Rosenberg et al. (1961) showed that 59% of spleens involved with lymphoma at autopsy were palpable premortem; 29% of palpable spleens showed no lymphoma in the spleen postmortem. Although it is difficult to assess splenic involvement by noninvasive methods, definite documentation of disease in the spleen is much less important than in Hodgkin's disease: Because of the more generalized presentation of NHL, the question of splenic involvement seldom influences treatment.

14.2.2.1. Indolent Lymphomas The indolent, or low-grade, lymphomas have a natural history that is measured in years, although they are seldom truly cured. Even when in complete remission, clonal excess has been found in the lymphocyte population of approximately one-third of such patients (Ault, 1979; Ligler et al., 1980; Berliner et al., 1986). The indolent lymphomas include grade I follicle cell lymphoma, mycosis fungoides, and marginal zone lymphomas (MZL).

14.2.2.1.1. Follicle Center Cell Lymphoma, Small-cell Type (Grade I) This is the most common of the indolent lymphomas, presenting primarily with widespread lymphadenopathy. Grade I, and the more aggressive grades II and III follicle cell lymphomas, grow in a nodular pattern. The cell population ranges from predominantly small cleaved cells (grade I; WF: follicular small cleaved-cell lymphoma), a mixture of small and large cells (grade II; WF: follicular mixed cell), to almost entirely large cells (grade III; WF: follicular large cell).

Grade I follicle center cell lymphoma is a node-based disease that is disseminated, at diagnosis, in approx 85% of cases. The spleen is enlarged in about 40% of these patients at diagnosis. The spread and the histologic pattern of the disease may result from retained cell-adhesion characteristics of these lymphoma cells. Normal B-cells bind to lymphatic germinal centers (Freedman et al., 1992). This interaction is mediated by a receptor–ligand pair consisting of the β-1 integrin very late antigen 4 (VLA-4) on B-cells, and the vascular cell adhesion molecule-1 (VCAM-1) expressed on follicular dendritic cells. Cells from involved lymph node tissues, from patients with grades I and II follicle cell lymphomas, also were shown to bind to normal germinal centers and to neoplastic follicles, by the same mechanism (Freedman et al., 1992). This adhesion was inhibited by monoclonal antibodies directed against VLA-4 and VCAM-1.

14.2.2.1.2. Mycosis Fungoides/Sezary Syndrome Mycosis fungoides and the Sezary syndrome are closely related, and are commonly grouped as part of the spectrum of postthymic, T-cell-origin lymphomas with a predilection for skin infiltration (Crossen et al., 1971; Edelson et al., 1974). The malignant cells in both disorders are mature T-lymphocytes, often with helper-inducer phenotypes (Brouet et al., 1973; Braylan et al., 1975; Broder et al., 1979; Broder et al., 1976; Kung et al., 1981), and express CD3 and CD4 on their surface. These cells also demonstrate a striking convoluted and cerebriform nuclear contour (Zucker-Franklin, 1974), and frequently have nonspecific chromosomal abnormalities (Whang-Peng et al., 1979). These cutaneous T-cell lymphoma cells have been shown to have active T-cell growth factor (TCGF) receptors on their surface (Gootenberg et al., 1981).

Individuals with these disorders usually progress through stages from the initial premycotic, to infiltrating plaque, to cutaneous tumor, and finally to generalized erythrodermia associated with the presence of abnormal T-lymphocytes in the blood (Lutzner et al., 1975). In the leukemic phase, lymphadenopathy and hepatosplenomegaly are common. The clinical features heralding the onset of extracutaneous dissemination of mycosis fungoides include fever, weight loss, widespread lymphadenopathy, and often hepatosplenomegaly. In the series by Long and Mihm (1974), 6/15 patients presented with splenomegaly at the time of dissemination. At autopsy, 12/15 had splenic involvement, with a mean spleen weight of 310 g, and a range of 110 to 2050 g.

Staging laparotomy may be of some value in assessing extracutaneous spread, and for the definition of treatment options (Variakojis et al., 1974). Staging evaluation employing noninvasive methods, including cytological and chromosomal evaluation of blood and lymph node cells, shows a high percentage of cases with extracutaneous dissemination (Bunn et al., 1980). Several clinical and histological staging systems have been employed in the past (Bunn and Lamberg, 1979; Griem et al., 1975), and have been proposed (Willemze et al., 1997; *see* Table 7).

14.2.2.1.3. Marginal Zone B-Cell Lymphomas Marginal zone lymphoma (MZL) is a recently identified entity, previously classi-

Table 14.7
EORTC Classification for Primary Cutaneous Lymphomas

Primary CTCL	Primary CBCL
Indolent	Indolent
Mycosis fungoides (MF)	Follicle center cell lymphoma
MF + follicular mucinosis	Immunocytoma (marginal zone B-cell lymphoma)
Pagetoid reticulosis	
Large-cell CTCL, CD30+	
Anaplastic	
Immunoblastic	
Pleomorphic	
Lymphomatoid papulosis	
Aggressive	Intermediate
Sezary syndrome	Large B-cell lymphoma of the leg
Large-cell, CTCL, CD30−	
Immunoblastic	
Pleomorphic	
Provisional	Provisional
Granulomatous slack skin	Intravascular large B-cell lymphoma
CTCL, pleomorphic small or medium-sized	Plasmacytoma
Subcutaneous panniculitis-like T-cell lymphoma	

CTCL, cutaneous T-cell lymphoma; CBCL, cutaneous B-cell lymphoma. (Adapted with permission from Willemze et al., 1997.)

fied as small lymphocytic lymphoma (Fisher et al., 1995; Pittaluga et al., 1996). The marginal zone of the lymph node is an area at the margin of the follicle, adjacent to the follicular mantle. A characteristic finding in involved lymph nodes is the so-called inverted follicular appearance, caused by expansion of neoplastic monocytoid B-cells. These lighter-staining cells surround the darker staining normal germinal centers. This picture is the inverse of that found in normal lymph node follicles.

When MZLs involve the lymph nodes, they are called "monocytoid B-cell lymphomas" (Ngan et al., 1991; Nizze et al., 1991); when they involve extranodal sites, they are called "mucosal-associated lymphatic tissue" (MALT) lymphomas (Isaacson and Wright, 1983; Ferry et al., 1996; Thieblemont et al., 1997). A study by the Southwest Oncology Group showed a better prognosis for the node-based MZLs, compared with the MALT lymphomas (Fisher et al., 1995). Recent studies, however, have shown an association between gastric low-grade MALT lymphomas and *Heliobacter pylori* infection. In a number of these cases, regression of the lymphoma was associated with treatment of the *H. Pylori* infection (Roggero et al., 1997; Wotherspoon et al., 1993; Neubauer et al., 1997).

14.2.2.1.4. Splenic MZL (With or Without Villous Lymphocytes) This proposed provisional entity in the REAL classification is thought to be related to MZL. This entity was previously described as splenic lymphoma with villous lymphocytes (SLVL) (Melo et al., 1987; Mulligan et al., 1991). Most patients are older than 60 years of age, present with a markedly enlarged spleen without lymph node involvement, a diffusely involved bone marrow, circulating lymphocytes with villous cytoplasmic projections, and a low level of paraproteinemia. The diagnosis is made from the characteristic involvement of the splenic white pulp, although moderate or extensive red pulp involvement has been reported (Melo et al., 1987; Palutke et al., 1988; Salgado et al., 1993). Immuno-phenotyping and cytogenetic studies have established a distinct profile for this entity (Zhu et al., 1995; Wu et al., 1996; Oscier et al., 1993; Baldini et al., 1994; Matutes et al., 1994). Kettle et al. (1990) described four patients presenting with splenic B-cell lymphoma, whose malignant cells were TRAP-positive.

Spleen weights ranged from 525 to 2850 g in a series of nine splenic MZL patients (Pittaluga et al., 1996). The clinical course of patients with splenic MZL is usually indolent, and splenectomy alone may be curative in some patients (Vandenberghe, 1994; De Wolf-Peeters and Pittaluga, 1994; Schmid et al., 1992; Fisher et al., 1995; Mollejo et al., 1995; Rosso et al., 1995; Pittaluga et al., 1996).

Primary malignant lymphoma of the spleen (PMLS) is rare, accounting for less than 2% of all NHLs (Long and Aisenberg, 1974). Whether the cases of primary lymphoma of the spleen reported in the earlier literature represent this entity is unclear, but most probably did. In a series from the Memorial Sloan Kettering Institute, 2.6% of stage I cases showed localization to the spleen only (Straus et al., 1983). Primary lymphoma of the spleen was known to develop after chronic immune stimulation, including infection and idiopathic splenomegaly (Stahel et al., 1982; Dacie et al., 1969), and possibly hepatitis C infection and chronic hepatitis (Satoh et al., 1997).

Skarin et al. (1971) described 11 patients with primary lymphosarcoma of the spleen confirmed by splenectomy. All presented with palpably enlarged spleens, and eight with features of hypersplenism and mild lymphocytosis in the bone marrow. A blood picture of CLL subsequently developed in six of the 11 patients. The latter cases are similar to the so-called "splenomegalic aleukemic CLL" as identified by Videbaek et al. (1982). Although, in most cases, unexplained splenomegaly is the major presenting feature of PMLS (Kehoe and Strauss, 1988; Falk and Stutte, 1990), one case presented with chronic hemorrhagic ascites (Hacker, Richter, Pyatt et al., 1982), another with autoimmune hemolytic anemia (Sawamura et al., 1994), and a third with leukemic meningitis (Yamazaki et al., 1994). Immunophenotyping usually correlates with the histological and cytological features of the malignant population (Hollema et al., 1991; Stroup et al., 1992).

14.2.2.2. The Aggressive Lymphomas The aggressive lymphomas include a large number of entities, such as all variants of diffuse large-cell lymphoma, grades II and III follicle center cell lymphoma, mantle cell lymphoma (MCL), Burkitt-like lymphoma, peripheral T-cell lymphoma, angiocentric lymphoma, angioimmunoblastic T-cell lymphoma, intestinal T-cell lymphoma, and anaplastic large cell lymphoma. The aggressive lymphomas have a natural history measured in months, although a portion can be cured with intensive chemotherapy.

14.2.2.2.1. Diffuse Large B-Cell Lymphoma This is the most common of the aggressive lymphomas and of all NHLs. Included in this category are immunoblastic lymphoma and Burkitt-like lymphoma of the WF. A subset of patients with diffuse large-cell lymphoma present with predominantly mediastinal disease (Yousem et al., 1985). These patients are usually younger, male, with tumor tissue showing significant fibrosis, reminiscent of nodular sclerosing Hodgkin's disease. Splenic involvement is usually a late event.

14.2.2.2.2. Follicle Center Cell Lymphoma (Grades II and III) Follicle center cell lymphoma accounts for ~35% of NHLs in adults. Histologically, they consist of a variable mixture of small cleaved and large cells. Grades II and III have the propensity to pro-

gressively increase the proportion of their large cells over time, and to accumulate genetic damage that can lead to histologic transformation to a more aggressive diffuse large-cell lymphoma (Hubbard et al., 1982; Sander et al., 1993). As with grade I follicle center cell lymphoma, these patients usually present with advanced nodal disease. Bone marrow involvement (usually with small cleaved cells) is uncommon; abdominal masses, including splenomegaly, are common.

14.2.2.2.3. Mantle Cell Lymphoma Patients presenting with NHL with prominent splenomegaly, but little lymphadenopathy, usually fall into one of two categories; splenic MZL described previously, or MCL (Fisher et al., 1995; Pittaluga et al., 1996). The latter entity is also known as MZL, as intermediate lymphocytic lymphoma, and as mixed-cell lymphoma, in the WF. MCL is considerably more aggressive, clinically, than the other small-cell lymphomas, including MZL (Fisher et al., 1995). MCL is diagnosed in 5–10% of NHL patients. They tend to be older males, present in advanced stage, and respond poorly to chemotherapy, with a median survival of 2–3 years (Banks et al., 1992; Fisher et al., 1995, 1996; Norton et al., 1995; Argatoff et al., 1997).

Extranodal disease is common. The spleen is often involved, particularly in the mantle zone (nodular) type (Weisenburger et al., 1982; Duggan et al., 1990; Majlis et al., 1997). In a series of eight patients with MCL, spleen weights ranged from 1050 to 2600 g (Pittaluga et al., 1996). Microscopically, the white pulp is markedly expanded by the abnormal cell proliferation, and reactive-appearing germinal centers may be present in these areas (Weisenburger and Armitage, 1996).

MCLs have a characteristic morphologic appearance, with distinctive microanatomic and cytologic features (Weisenburger et al., 1981; Weisenburger et al., 1982; Swerdlow et al., 1983; Banks et al., 1992). The malignant tissue is comprised of small lymphoid cells with slightly irregular nuclear outlines, without admixed large transformed cells. Initially, MCL grows around residual normal germinal centers, giving an expanded mantle zone pattern. The MCL phenotype is characterized by expression of pan-B antigens, monotypic immunoglobulin, co-expression of the pan-T antigen CD5 (Weisenburger, 1984; Lardelli et al., 1990; Bookman et al., 1990), and a characteristic chromosomal translocation, t(11;14) (Weisenburger et al., 1987; Leroux et al., 1991; Pittaluga et al., 1995; *see* Table 3).

14.2.2.2.4. Peripheral T-Cell Lymphomas The term "peripheral" refers to the cell surface phenotype of the T-cell, namely, that it is postthymic or peripheral, and expresses either CD4 or CD8. These lymphomas have an aggressive natural history, with poor response to therapy (Coiffier et al., 1988). Recently, a distinct clinicopathologic entity of cytotoxic γδ T-cell origin was described in predominantly young male patients, who presented with marked hepatosplenomegaly, but without lymphadenopathy or significant peripheral blood lymphocytosis, and with a median survival of less than 1 year (Cooke et al., 1996). Those authors called this entity "hepatosplenic T-cell lymphoma." Histologically, it was characterized by a monomorphic population of medium-sized lymphocytes, with clumped chromatin and a rim of pale cytoplasm infiltrating the sinusoids of the spleen, liver, and bone marrow.

14.2.2.2.5. Anaplastic Large-Cell Lymphoma Anaplastic large-cell lymphoma has recently been recognized as a subtype of aggressive lymphomas. The neoplastic cells of this disorder have no obvious normal cellular counterpart, and resemble cells of non-lymphoid anaplastic malignancies, such as carcinomas and melanoma (Zinzani et al., 1996). The tumor cells express CD30 antigen, contain a characteristic chromosomal abnormality [t(2;5)], and express a unique chimeric NPM-ALK protein (Benharroch et al., 1998). Clinically, skin involvement is common, and lymphadenopathy and extranodal disease, including spleen involvement, may be present (Mason et al., 1990).

14.2.2.2.6. AIDS-Associated Lymphomas Although of B-cell lineage, the NHLs, associated with HIV infection and AIDS demonstrate several striking differences from the other aggressive B-cell lymphomas. The majority are of high-grade histological type, either small noncleaved lymphoma (undifferentiated, Burkitt's, or Burkitt-like), or immunoblastic lymphoma (Ziegler, 1981; Levine and Gill, 1987; Ioachim et al., 1985; Levine et al., 1984; Ziegler et al., 1984; Kalter et al., 1985; Knowles et al., 1988). Most patients present with "B" symptoms, and with a high proportion of extranodal involvement, especially of the gastrointestinal tract, central nervous system, bone marrow, and myocardium. In this respect, they are very similar to the malignant lymphomas associated with other immunosuppressive states, such as accompany cardiac and renal allotransplantation (Penn, 1990; Weintraub and Warnke, 1982; Matas et al., 1976; Swinnen et al., 1990), and primary immunodeficiency syndromes. Splenomegaly was present in 2/21 patients with AIDS-associated lymphoma (Ioachim et al., 1985). T-cell leukemia/lymphoma, which has been linked to infection with human T-cell leukemia/lymphoma virus I (HTLV-I), and has been described in some AIDS patients, is discussed in more detail in Subheading 2.3.3. below.

14.2.3. ACUTE LYMPHOCYTIC LEUKEMIA (ALL)

14.2.3.1. Lymphoblastic Leukemia/Lymphoma Lymphoblastic leukemia may be of either T-cell or B-cell phenotype, with B-cell phenotype more common in ALL of children. Splenomegaly, lymphadenopathy, and hepatomegaly are common in childhood ALL. However, such organomegaly is seldom prominent, and may be absent. In adults with ALL, which is more often of T-cell type, extramedullary manifestations, such as splenomegaly and adenopathy are rare. Splenomegaly appearing in children who have achieved hematological remission does not necessarily indicate a relapse. Manoharan et al. (1980) described five children in whom an isolated finding of splenomegaly was evaluated. Splenectomy was performed in three: None of the spleens was involved with leukemia. However, all three died in leukemic recurrence within 28 months, while the two nonsplenectomized children remained in complete remission, 2 and 6 years after the appearance of splenomegaly.

14.2.3.2. Burkitt's Lymphoma/Leukemia Burkitt's lymphoma typically presents with disease outside the lymphatic system (Burkitt and O'Connor, 1961). Splenomegaly may be found, occasionally; however, other tumor masses usually predominate in the abdomen (Wright, 1970).

14.2.3.3. Adult T-Cell Leukemia/Lymphoma Uchiyama et al. (1977) first reported a distinct T-cell lymphoproliferative disorder affecting adults in the southwestern part of Japan, especially in Kyushu. Subsequently, clusters of an aggressive T-cell malignancy were described in Caribbean black immigrants in London (Catovsky et al., 1982), and in blacks from the southeastern part of the United States (Blayney et al., 1983). The clinical features of this adult T-cell leukemia/lymphoma (ATL) have been described in several hundred cases from Japan, but in only a few from other endemic areas, including the Caribbean basin and the southeastern United States (Urba and Longo, 1985; Bunn et al., 1983; Swerdlow et al., 1984; Takatsuki et al., 1985; Gibbs et al., 1987). The syn-

drome presents with nearly identical features in these different geographic areas, with an aggressive clinical course, peripheral lymph node enlargement (86%), hepatomegaly (72%), splenomegaly (51%), lytic bone lesions (50%), often with hypercalcemia, and skin lesions (49%). In other series, splenomegaly was present in 63% of Japanese cases (Uchiyama et al., 1977), in 25% of Jamaican cases (Gibbs et al., 1987), but in none of the U.S. patients with ATL (Blayney et al., 1983). The bone marrow and peripheral blood was involved in all cases, and a high incidence of CNS involvement and of opportunistic infections has been noted (Cappell and Chow, 1987).

The pleomorphic neoplastic cells show irregular nuclear contours and characteristic lobulation, and are difficult to distinguish from Sezary cells. Cell surface marker analysis has identified the malignant cells in ATL as mature T-lymphocytes, often of helper-inducer phenotype, with T1, T3, T4, and T11 positivity and T8 negativity (Hattori et al., 1981; Catovsky et al., 1982; Takatsuki et al., 1982). However, in approx 50% of cases, the leukemic T-cells appeared to act as suppressor cells (Uchiyama et al., 1978). These cells have been shown to display IL-2 receptors, and to release biologically active IL-1 (Wano et al., 1987), which possibly explains the osteoclast activation and fever observed in such patients. In 1980, Poiesz et al. isolated a retrovirus, termed HTLV-I, from a cell line from a black patient with what was thought to be mycosis fungoides. This virus could be definitely linked to ATL, when seroepidemiological studies showed that more than 90% of cases from the endemic areas were HTLV-I antibody positive (Gallo, 1981, 1984; Gallo and Wong-Staal, 1982; Wong-Staal and Gallo, 1985; Gallo et al., 1983; Essex et al., 1984). Although some patients who present with typical ATL do not show the presence of HTLV-I infection (Shimoyama et al., 1983), they still demonstrate the typical chromosomal changes of HTLV-I-associated ATL (Shimoyama et al., 1987). The presence of TCGF receptors (Tac) on ATL cells, as measured by reactivity with anti-Tac antibody, can help to distinguish HTLV-I-associated ATL from other T-cell malignancies (Broder et al., 1984).

A second transforming retrovirus (HTLV-II) has been found to be associated with a T-cell HCL (Kalyanaraman et al., 1982), but has been isolated only rarely worldwide.

14.2.4. PLASMA CELL DISORDERS Only rarely has splenomegaly been observed in multiple myeloma. In a review of plasma cell leukemia by Kosmo and Gale (1987), a 5% incidence of splenomegaly was derived from a combined analysis of 1045 cases of multiple myeloma. By contrast, a 60% frequency of splenomegaly was noted in 30 patients with primary (*de novo*) plasma cell leukemia, and, in 3/8 patients with the secondary form, the late leukemic phase of multiple myeloma.

14.2.5. HODGKIN'S DISEASE In the 1960s, in contrast to most of the other MLPDs, Hodgkin's disease was thought to begin locally in one lymphoid organ, then to spread, in an orderly, centripetal fashion, to adjacent lymphoid structures and, at times, adjacent non-lymphoid structures. This concept of spread by contiguity was favored by Rosenberg and Kaplan (1966), after careful assessment of a large number of patients with Hodgkin's disease. This approach, when applied to the design of radiation therapy to include the adjacent uninvolved lymphoid areas (extended field), resulted in high cure rates in early stage Hodgkin's disease (Kaplan, 1980).

However, it is difficult to accept that spread into the abdomen occurs frequently in retrograde fashion via the thoracic duct, or that it spreads from one side of the neck to the other or from the neck to the axillae. Staging laparotomy studies in Hodgkin's disease patients have shown that the spleen is the most frequently involved intra-abdominal site. Rates of 36–44% for splenic involvement, compared to 6–28% for para-aortic lymph node involvement, have been reported (Aisenberg and Qazi, 1974; Glees et al., 1982). Splenic involvement as the only site of intra-abdominal disease has been reported in 3–14% (Mann et al., 1986); intra-abdominal lymph disease without splenic involvement occurs in less than 10% (Krikorian et al., 1986; Mauch et al., 1983). In a review by Leibenhaut et al. (1987), patients with CS (clinical stage) I-A subdiaphragmatic disease, with negative lymphoangiograms, had only a 10% probability of splenic involvement, contrasting with a 30% probability in patients with supradiaphragmatic disease and negative lymphoangiograms.

The susceptibility theory developed by Smithers (Smithers, 1970; Smithers et al., 1974) presents a more plausible concept to explain intra-abdominal spread. According to this concept, malignant cells migrate via the lymph to the blood stream, then localize preferentially at certain sites. Initial spread to the spleen is thought to be by hematogenous routes, independent of other intra-abdominal disease. From there, Hodgkin's disease can spread to other intra-abdominal sites, such as lymph nodes and liver, as well as to the bone marrow. That Hodgkin's disease can spread through the blood is supported by the finding of characteristic Reed-Sternberg cells circulating in peripheral blood in some Hodgkin's disease patients (Bouroncle, 1966; Schiffer et al., 1975).

In an evaluation of staging laparotomy data for 76 patients, Stein et al. (1982) showed a correlation between anatomical substaging and splenic involvement in patients with pathological stage III Hodgkin's disease. Patients with substage III-1 more often had minimal involvement of the spleen (1–4 nodules), compared to extensive involvement (>4 nodules), the proportions being 56 and 44%, respectively. Extensive involvement of the spleen was seen in 76% of patients with substage III-2. Thus, involvement of the spleen *per se* does not necessarily imply a bad prognosis or a high probability of hematogenous spread to liver, bone marrow and other extralymphatic organs. Patients with substage III-1 disease have experienced generally good results with a treatment program of total nodal irradiation only (Stein et al., 1982). Splenic vascular invasion, however, has been associated with systemic involvement and a poor prognosis (Haskell, 1981; Strum et al., 1971; Kirschner et al., 1974).

Splenomegaly is rarely present at the initial presentation of Hodgkin's disease. In late stages of the disease, however, it may become massive. In a series reported by Glatstein et al. (1969), spleen weights ranged from 100 to 1300 g, with those weighing more than 400 g invariably containing Hodgkin's disease. The difficulty of establishing splenic involvement by means short of splenectomy is borne out by data presented by Kaplan (1970). In a series of 340 consecutive untreated patients with biopsy-proven Hodgkin's disease, evaluated principally by thorough clinical staging, 44 (13%) were felt to have splenic involvement. In a second series of untreated patients, evaluated by clinical staging and laparotomy with splenectomy, 58/160 (36%) patients had documented splenic disease. Spleen involvement becomes progressively greater with advancing disease. In three large series of autopsy evaluation in 335 Hodgkin's disease patients, 59–69% had documented splenic involvement (Uddstroemer, 1934; Westling, 1965; Jackson and Parker, 1947). Liver involvement is usually associated with massive splenomegaly, although it may occur without splenic disease (Sextro et al., 1997).

Hodgkin's disease nodules in the spleen range from a few millimeters in diameter to multiple large masses almost completely replacing the normal parenchyma. It is, therefore, crucial that the spleen be carefully examined following staging laparotomy. This includes slicing the entire spleen at less than 5-mm intervals, and sampling all suspicious areas for microscopic examination (Farrer-Brown et al., 1972). Since small nodules of Hodgkin's disease may be scattered randomly throughout the spleen, it would appear that partial splenectomy, at times recommended in children with Hodgkin's disease, would not be as accurate for staging (Boles et al., 1978).

Early lesions of Hodgkin's disease in the spleen are usually found near the central artery in the periarterial lymphatic sheaths of the white pulp or in adjacent lymphoid follicles (Butler, 1983; Yam and Li, 1976; Halie et al., 1978). As these initially small nodules grow and expand, they tend to compress the red pulp rather than invade it, perhaps because of characteristics of the special splenic environment. Such small Hodgkin's disease nodules frequently show a halo or corona of small lymphocytes surrounding the nodule. The prominence of this lymphocyte layer tends to decrease in larger nodules and in spleens involved by lymphocyte-depletion Hodgkin's disease. This finding, and the observation that the splenic follicles nearest to the Hodgkin's disease nodule are larger, with centers nearly devoid of small lymphocytes, but with prominent large cells, implies an immune reaction to the malignant nodule (Halie et al., 1978).

The histological criteria applied to foci of Hodgkin's disease in the spleen are the same as those for involved lymph nodes (Lukes, 1971). The presence of typical Reed-Sternberg and Hodgkin's cells, in a background of a mixed-cell population of lymphocytes, plasma cells, and eosinophils, leads to the diagnosis of involvement by Hodgkin's disease. It is, however, important not to over-interpret such findings, since multinucleated giant cells, closely resembling Reed-Sternberg cells, have been found in other malignant and nonmalignant disorders (Lukes et al., 1969; Strum et al., 1970). Furthermore, epithelioid granulomas are commonly seen in the spleens of Hodgkin's disease patients; they are observed in 9% of otherwise uninvolved spleens. The presence of these granulomas without splenic involvement is considered a favorable prognostic sign (O'Connell et al., 1975; Sacks et al., 1978).

Recent work indicates that the Reed-Sternberg cells, as well as the lymphocytic and histiocytic cells from lymphocyte-predominant Hodgkin's disease, are clones of neoplastic B-cells that originate from the germinal centers of antigenically stimulated lymphoid tissue (Kuppers et al., 1994; Kanzler et al., 1996) or from "Hodgkin's transformation" of B-cell CLL (Ohno et al., 1998). Furthermore, there is evidence that these neoplastic clones secrete potent cytokines, leading to the B symptoms of Hodgkin's disease, promoting their own growth, and evading immune surveillance (Gruss et al., 1997).

14.3. DIAGNOSIS OF SPLENIC INVOLVEMENT

14.3.1. PHYSICAL EXAMINATION The frequent finding of Hodgkin's disease in spleens of normal size and weight, at routine staging laparotomy became apparent early on (Enright et al., 1970; Glatstein et al., 1969, 1970). Between one-third and one-half of spleens, removed from patients without clinically or radiographically detectable splenomegaly, were found to have gross or microscopic involvement. In addition to this false-negative error, false-positive findings of splenomegaly prior to laparotomy could not be attributed to splenic Hodgkin's disease in 35–40% of cases (Rosenberg and Kaplan, 1970; Glatsteing et al., 1969, 1970). In a series reported by Askergren et al. (1981), 17/48 nonpalpable spleens showed tumor involvement; palpable spleens, all of which weighed over 600 g, were all involved. In one patient with Hodgkin's disease, cyclical splenomegaly was associated with cyclical fever and hemolysis (McKenna et al., 1979).

The spleen must to be enlarged from 1.5 to 3× its normal size for it to become palpable (Barkun et al., 1991). In addition, a palpable spleen is not necessarily enlarged, but a moderately enlarged spleen may not be palpable by the most skilled examiner. Radiographical methods, especially CT scanning, are considerably more reliable as indicators of splenic enlargement (*see* Subheading 3.5.; *see also* Chapters 9 and 16).

In contrast to Hodgkin's disease, clinically detectable splenomegaly in the NHLs, CLL, and HCL usually does reflect splenic involvement. At autopsy, 40–50% of patients with NHL have documented splenic disease (Risdall et al., 1979; Rosenberg et al., 1961). Patients with early-stage NHL, who underwent staging laparotomy and splenectomy, showed involvement in 30–40% of cases (Goffinet et al., 1973; Moran et al., 1975).

14.3.2. LABORATORY EVALUATION   Hematological abnormalities may be pronounced in the lymphoproliferative diseases. Often, these can be directly attributed to the enlarged or involved spleen. In such cases, the hematological changes are part of the wider array of symptoms and signs ascribed to hypersplenism (Dameshek and Estren, 1947), big spleen disease (Hamilton et al., 1967) or splenomegaly syndrome (Videbaek et al., 1982). The pathophysiological mechanisms observed in the hypersplenism associated with MLPDs are discussed in more detail in Subheading 4.1.

The presence of pancytopenia, with a normocellular or hyperplastic bone marrow is usually attributed to hypersplenism, no matter what its cause. Anemia has been attributed to erythrocyte pooling in the spleen, hemodilution anemia (Bowdler, 1967), and excessive destruction of red blood cells caused by the increased time spent in the unfavorable splenic environment (Videbaek et al., 1982). In HCL, the splenic erythrocyte pool is especially large, possibly because of the prominent red pulp involvement (Lewis et al., 1977).

Autoimmune hemolytic anemia (AIHA) is common in the MLPDs, especially in CLL and the NHLs. In CLL, approx 30% of patients will develop a positive Coombs' test at some stage of their disease (Hansen, 1973). The onset of this hemolytic anemia may precede the diagnosis of CLL or lymphoma, by several years (Bowdler and Glick, 1966). In a series of 234 patients with AIHA reported by Pirofsky (1969), 48% were found to result from an associated MLPD. In 190 cases of secondary AIHA, 60% were seen in patients with MLPDs. Especially in those patients with warm-reacting antibody type AIHA, the spleen plays a major role in red blood cell destruction, and splenectomy or corticosteroids often improve the anemia (Christensen, 1973b).

At times, despite the absence of a positive Coombs' test, immune hemolysis may still exist. These cases have a small number of antibody molecules per red blood cell (Gilliland et al., 1971; Videbaek et al., 1982), but, because of the high number of Fc receptors on splenic phagocytes, even sensitized red blood cells with few surface antibody molecules attach to monocytes, and are partially or entirely phagocytosed (LoBuglio et al., 1967).

Thrombocytopenia in lymphoproliferative splenomegaly has been ascribed to intensified pooling of platelets in the enlarged spleen (Aster, 1966); platelet survival is usually normal. Neutropenia has been ascribed to both splenic sequestration and increased destruction.

Wedelin et al. (1981) correlated the results of a number of routine laboratory tests, in 39 untreated patients with Hodgkin's disease, with the size and degree of splenic involvement. They found that large spleens, irrespective of tumor involvement, were correlated with lower hemoglobin, decreased lymphocyte counts, elevated reticulocyte counts, and lower IgG and IgM levels. No such correlations were found when involved spleens weighed less than 500 g. Other laboratory tests showed no differences, and those authors concluded that other routine laboratory tests yield no specific information with respect to spleen size or involvement in Hodgkin's disease.

The erythrocyte sedimentation rate (ESR) is elevated in approximately half of Hodgkin's disease patients at presentation, and is increased in almost all patients with large body tumor burden, B symptoms and extensive prior treatment (Le Bourgeois and Tubiana, 1977; Jaffe et al., 1970). An increase in ESR is strongly suggestive of relapse (Henry-Amar et al., 1991). There appears to be no specific correlation between splenic involvement or enlargement and elevation of the ESR. This also seems true for other nonspecific laboratory abnormalities, including the levels of serum copper, zinc, uric acid, lactic dehydrogenase, alkaline phosphatase, haptoglobin, and acute-phase reactants (Ray et al., 1973). Serum iron and iron-binding capacity are decreased in Hodgkin's disease, presenting a picture of anemia of chronic disease. This does not represent an iron deficiency state, since tissue iron stores, including those in the spleen, are frequently increased (Britten et al., 1986). This increase is reflected in elevated serum ferritin levels, which may be up to 10× normal, especially in extensive and advanced disease (Bieber and Bieber, 1973; Jaffe et al., 1970; Jones et al., 1972).

Anemia, neutropenia, and thrombocytopenia are commonly observed in patients with HCL. In a series of 211 patients reported by Flandrin et al. (1984), the mean hemoglobin was 10.2 g/dL, the mean platelet count 92,000/mm^3, the mean white blood count 5000/mm^3, and the mean neutrophil count 949/mm^3. Pancytopenia was present in 59% of patients. They found no significant correlation between hemoglobin or white blood count and spleen size. A weak inverse relationship was found between spleen size and platelet counts, and between spleen size and neutrophil counts. In a comparison of patients presenting with and without splenomegaly, those authors found no statistically significant difference between the two groups, regarding to clinical features and survival, or with laboratory findings, such as anemia, thrombocytopenia and neutropenia. Jansen and Hermans (1981), in a series of 391 patients with HCL, did demonstrate a negative prognostic effect of decreased hemoglobin, neutrophils, and platelets on presentation. They concluded that the larger the spleen and the lower the hemoglobin level, the poorer the prognosis. Catovsky (1977) also linked low levels of hemoglobin, neutropenia, and thrombocytopenia with survival.

Reed-Sternberg cells are only occasionally encountered in the peripheral blood of patients with Hodgkin's disease (Bouroncle, 1966); in the NHLs, morphologically abnormal, and presumably malignant, lymphocytes are observed in approx 10%. Such abnormal cells are especially common in patients with the follicular small cleaved cell and the diffuse large-cell types of NHL (Come et al., 1980). By using cytofluorometric methods, with monoclonal surface immunoglobulins, to identify such abnormal lymphocyte clones, clonal excess has been detected in 30–40% of NHL patients, without morphological blood involvement (Ault, 1979; Ligler et al., 1980; Berliner et al., 1986).

14.3.3. RADIONUCLIDE SCANNING Because physical examination and customary X-rays of the abdomen have been unreliable in assessing splenic involvement in malignancy, a number of special, noninvasive techniques have been applied to the spleen, in an effort to provide such information prior to, or instead of, splenectomy (*see also* Chapter 16). This is especially important in Hodgkin's disease, in which the extent of disease and specific organ involvement frequently determines the best treatment for individual patients.

In the early days of organ scanning with radionuclides, 51-chromate (^{51}Cr), attached to heat-damaged red blood cells was employed to measure microvascular function of the spleen. In a series of 68 patients with Hodgkin's disease reported by Ell et al. (1975), this method was found to be an unreliable technique for staging. Splenic contraction, in response to adrenalin following the administration of ^{51}Cr-labeled red blood cells, was found, by spleen scanning, to be less in those patients with Hodgkin's disease involving the spleen (Osadchaya et al., 1980). This has been confirmed with ^{99m}Tc-labeled heat-treated red blood cells (Rosen et al., 1982). ^{67}Ga-labeled citrate scanning is also unreliable in detecting splenic disease (Kay and McCready, 1972; Horn et al., 1976; Johnston et al., 1974; Levi et al., 1975; Seabold et al., 1976), but it has been found to be more useful in detecting disease above the diaphragm than abdominal involvement (Ben-Haim et al., 1996; Salloum et al., 1997), and may have prognostic significance (Janicek et al., 1997).

The splenic scintigram with [^{99m}Tc]-sulfur colloid has been the most commonly employed radionuclide scanning method for the spleen. When the results of such scanning are compared to the findings at laparotomy and splenectomy, however, this method is found to lack sensitivity with respect to borderline splenic enlargement, especially for Hodgkin's disease involvement (Askergren et al., 1981). In a study from the Walter Reed Army Hospital, 15/66 spleens judged normal by spleen scan were found to be positive for tumor, whereas 13/23 spleens considered to be enlarged on scan contained no disease (Harris et al., 1978). Similar results have been reported by others (Hermreck et al., 1975; Silverman et al., 1972; Milder et al., 1973; *see* Table 8). In Table 8, "Sensitivity" refers to the percentage of patients with histologically proven disease in the spleen, whose imaging studies were correctly interpreted as positive. "Specificity" refers to the percentage of patients with no histological disease in the spleen, whose imaging studies were correctly interpreted as negative. Overall "Accuracy" is the percentage of patients whose imaging studies were correctly interpreted as either positive or negative.

Even the finding of definite large filling defects on the scan of an enlarged spleen is not always evidence for active or persistent disease. A patient with stage IV-A nodular sclerosing Hodgkin's disease, with a large filling defect seen on spleen scan prior to treatment, showed a persistent defect following 6 months of MOPP chemotherapy. Subsequent laparotomy showed the spleen to be disease-free and histologically normal (Dickerman and Clements, 1975). With the advent of CT and MRI technology, splenic scintiscans may remain useful as a secondary method to assess splenic function and blood flow, and to differentiate between splenic hilar nodes and accessory spleens (Frick et al., 1981). The presence of an ectopic, or wandering, spleen may be suspected, when no splenic

Table 14.8
Comparison of Noninvasive Imaging Methods of the Spleen

	No. Patients	Sensitivity	Specificity	Accuracy
Computed tomography				
Alcorn et al. (1977)	16	–	–	0.78
Redman et al. (1977)	22	0.50	–	0.80
Breiman et al. (1978)	16	0.90	1.00	0.94
Frick et al. (1981)	18	0.75	1.00	0.89
Castellino et al. (1984)	121	0.33	0.76	0.58
Strijk et al. (1985)	35	0.57	1.00	0.77
Ultrasound				
Glees et al. (1977)	20	0.77	0.72	0.75
Frick et al. (1981)	22	0.35	0.82	0.68
King et al. (1985)	22	0.60	0.88	0.82
Radionuclide scan (^{99m}Tc-sulfur colloid)				
Alcorn et al. (1977)	15	–	–	0.66
Glees et al. (1977)	19	0.61	0.66	0.55
Frick et al. (1981)	39	0.75	0.88	0.86
Hermreck et al. (1975)	28	0.36	0.65	0.53
Milder et al. (1973)	50	0.74	0.63	0.70
Silverman et al. (1972)	42	0.40	0.82	0.62
Harris et al. (1978)	87	0.40	0.79	0.67

image is seen in its usual location, and definite uptake is noted elsewhere in the abdomen or pelvis (Waldman and Suissa, 1978).

In the NHLs, the finding of focal splenic defects usually correlates with splenic disease (Lindfors et al., 1984). Large-cell lymphomas with splenic involvement are especially prone to show this pattern, which usually improves or disappears with effective chemotherapy (Sagar et al., 1979). In CLL, the increase in spleen size was found to be primarily caused by increased cellularity; in HCL, it was caused by both increased splenic vascularity and cellularity (Zhang and Lewis, 1989). Immunoscintography utilizing radionuclide-labeled monoclonal antibodies may offer increased specificity in scanning for areas of lymphomatous involvement in the future (Carde et al., 1988).

14.3.4. ULTRASONIC SCANNING The usefulness of ultrasound examination lies primarily in detecting borderline enlargement of the spleen, which may not be palpable on physical examination, but which, because of its size, has a greater likelihood of being diseased (Hofmann, 1985; Koga and Morikawa, 1975; Frick et al., 1981; King et al., 1985; Glees et al., 1977). Both decreased and increased splenic echogenicity have been associated with malignant involvement (Siler et al., 1980). The calculated sensitivity, specificity, and accuracy of ultrasound in detecting splenic lymphoma from three series of patients are listed in Table 8, and are compared to other imaging methods. Sonography has also been employed as an adjunct to splenic aspiration and biopsy (Solbiati et al., 1983; Lindgren et al., 1985).

14.3.5. COMPUTED TOMOGRAPHY Computed tomography (CT) has revolutionized the noninvasive staging of patients with malignancies, especially the assessment of the intra-abdominal extent of the malignant lymphomas. Lymphoma nodules of 1 cm or greater can usually be well identified in the spleen as single or multiple low-density lesions (Earl et al., 1980; Piekarski et al., 1980). Early studies indicated that this would prove to be a much more sensitive noninvasive method than others in assessing spleen size and tumor involvement (Jones et al., 1978; Redman et al., 1977). However, small miliary deposits of lymphoma remain elusive, even with this methodology.

Many reports have appeared in the literature, assessing the usefulness and accuracy of CT scanning of the spleen, in detecting lymphoma involvement. Several are summarized in Table 8, and are compared to a similar assessment for ultrasound and radionuclide scanning (Frick et al., 1981; Alcorn et al., 1977; Redman et al., 1977; Breiman et al., 1978; Castellino et al., 1984; Strijk et al., 1985).

Although CT has been shown to be the most useful and reliable noninvasive method to detect splenic disease, a number of problems remain. In approximately two-thirds of cases of splenic involvement with Hodgkin's disease, the tumor nodules measure less than 1 cm in diameter (Castellino et al., 1984), a size usually not detectable by CT. Although it is excellent for assessing spleen size, not all large spleens are involved by lymphoma, and many normal-sized spleens have been shown to contain lymphoma nodules. Calculation of total splenic volume, by deriving a splenic index from the CT, has been proposed as a means for improving diagnostic accuracy (Strijk et al., 1985). Splenic hilar nodes and accessory spleens are well detected by CT (Frick et al., 1981), although, at times, ^{99m}Tc-sulfur colloid scanning may provide additional useful information. Use of dynamic CT scans, following bolus administration of iodinated contrast material, does not add to the accuracy of detecting splenic disease, but will distinguish accessory spleens from enlarged lymph nodes or splenic varices (Glazer et al., 1981).

Magnetic resonance imaging (MRI) has two major applications to the monitoring of malignancy: It can produce high-resolution images without the use of ionizing radiation, and it can chemically characterize the tumor and tissues in vivo, and yield biochemical information on metabolic differences (Smith, 1984; Smith et al., 1989). It remains to be seen if and when MRI will replace CT as the definitive noninvasive procedure of choice for the imaging of splenic disease.

14.3.6. SPLENIC ASPIRATION AND BIOPSY Splenic aspiration or biopsy is seldom performed in the United States or Britain, primarily because of its perceived limited usefulness and the possibility of hemorrhage. However, in the earlier hematological literature, there is considerable evidence that this is a safe procedure. During the 1950s and 1960s, splenic puncture results were described in over 1600 patients, with very few minor complications (Moeschlin, 1957; Soederstroem, 1970, 1979; Dameshek and Gunz, 1964). In other parts of the world, splenic aspiration and biopsy continue to be used in the diagnosis of infectious and malignant diseases involving the spleen (Pinto et al., 1995; Kager et al., 1983; Zeppa et al., 1994). In a report from Sweden, TrueCut needle biopsies were performed in 32 patients with a variety of malignant and nonmalignant disorders (Lindgren et al., 1985). Of eight patients with focally abnormal ultrasound evaluation, seven had lymphoma documented on splenic biopsy. Four of the 32 patients experienced bleeding requiring transfusions: Two of these occurred in patients with HCL, and splenectomy had to be performed in one of the HCL patients.

In one of very few more recent reports on this subject from the United States, Moriarty et al. (1993) performed 11 fine-needle aspirate biopsies over a 3-year period, in cases in which the spleen was the only, or the most accessible, organ for biopsy. No significant complications occurred, and all specimens were sufficiently cellular to establish the diagnosis. A specific MLPD was diagnosed in four, with the help of ancillary techniques, including surface markers, immunocytochemistry, and enzyme-histochemical methods.

Splenic aspiration or biopsy has been recommended as an alternative to diagnostic splenectomy in children with Hodgkin's disease who appear most susceptible to serious postsplenectomy sepsis. However, the incomplete information obtained from such a procedure seriously limits its usefulness for this purpose (Lampert, 1983).

14.3.7. DIAGNOSTIC AND STAGING LAPAROTOMY AND SPLENECTOMY From the discussion so far, it is apparent that none of the noninvasive methods of evaluating splenic disease is sufficiently accurate to replace direct examination of the spleen. This is especially crucial in those patients in whom the presence of splenic disease would modify the treatment. Aside from diagnostic laparotomy and splenectomy in previously undiagnosed patients, this situation exists today principally in the pretreatment evaluation of patients with an early stage of Hodgkin's disease.

14.3.7.1. Diagnostic Splenectomy The removal of an enlarged spleen for histological examination is often required when noninvasive investigations fail to elicit a definite diagnosis. This may include a small number of patients with protracted fever of undetermined origin (Greenall et al., 1983). The spleen, however, should not be removed simply because it is enlarged: The diagnostic and therapeutic benefits should be carefully weighed against the potential morbidity and mortality. Exploratory laparotomy has been associated with a mortality rate of 0.5–1.0%, and a surgical complication rate of 9–15%, even in experienced hands (Larson and Ultmann, 1982; Mitchell and Morris, 1983; Klaue et al., 1979; Traetow et al., 1980; Kawarada et al., 1976; Goffinet et al., 1977).

Where diagnostic and staging laparotomies are performed frequently, about 12% are for undiagnosed splenomegaly (Long and Aisenberg, 1974; Mitchell and Morris, 1983; Goonewardene et al., 1979; Letoquart et al., 1993; Cronin et al., 1994). Of these, 90% have yielded a definite diagnosis, usually of one of the lymphoproliferative disorders. One group of patients, with splenomegaly that remains undiagnosed following splenectomy, are those with nontropical splenomegaly (Dacie et al., 1969). In up to 20% of these patients, malignant lymphoma has occurred after several years (Dacie et al., 1978).

14.3.7.2. Staging Laparotomy and Splenectomy Laparotomy with splenectomy and biopsy of the liver and para-aortic lymph nodes was initially performed on selected patients with Hodgkin's disease presenting special diagnostic problems (Glatstein et al., 1969). Because of an unexpectedly high frequency of Hodgkin's disease involvement of the resected spleens (61%), the value of routine laparotomy and splenectomy in unselected, previously untreated patients was evaluated (Rosenberg and Kaplan, 1970; Kadin et al., 1971; Glatstein et al., 1970). In 100 consecutive untreated patients reported by Rosenberg and Kaplan (1970), 50% of the clinically enlarged spleens, and 24% of the clinically negative spleens, contained histologically documented disease. A later review of 160 cases gave an overall frequency of splenic involvement of 36% (Kaplan, 1980).

The primary purpose of the staging laparotomy is to determine as accurately as possible the extent of intra-abdominal disease. It is not considered a therapeutic procedure, although it does preclude the development of hypersplenism, which may decrease tolerance to subsequent chemotherapy (Salzman and Kaplan, 1971). Absence of the spleen also avoids the need for irradiation of the splenic region, which overlaps with the left kidney and the base of the left lung (Greenberger et al., 1979). The noninvasive methods of CT and radionuclide scanning cannot replace splenectomy as a staging procedure (Aisenberg, 1978).

Table 14.9
Potential Role for Staging Laparotomy in Lymphoma Patients

Hodgkin's disease:
    Clinical stage IA and IIA, except:
        (a) isolated high cervical nodes only
        (b) bulky mediastinal disease
    Clinical stage IIIA (without involvement of lower abdominal nodes)
    Presence of splenomegaly when radiation therapy main therapy
    Equivocal lymphangiogram/abdominal CT
    Preservation of ovarian function prior to radiation therapy
NHLs:
    Clinical stage I (diffuse large-cell lymphomas)

Staging laparotomy and splenectomy for Hodgkin's disease and the NHLs is indicated only if the findings may lead to a change in treatment from that planned from clinical staging (Table 9). In several series assessing changes in stage, pre- and postoperatively, the findings at laparotomy led to changes in stage in 30–43% of Hodgkin's disease patients (Kaplan, 1972; Sterchi and Myers, 1980; Gill et al., 1980; Glees et al., 1982). Hodgkin's disease patients with stage III disease, who had splenic involvement, were found to have a shorter disease-free interval than those who did not (Worthy, 1981; Levi and Wiernik, 1977; Shipley et al., 1974). Several authors have suggested that patients with stage IIIA disease, whose abdominal disease is limited to the spleen and the upper abdominal nodes (anatomical substage III-1), respond well to radiotherapy alone; those with lower abdominal disease (anatomical substage III-2) respond poorly, and require primary treatment with chemotherapy (Desser et al., 1973; Stein et al., 1978; Stein et al., 1982). Assessment of data from Stanford University, however, found no prognostic advantage to such substaging, and identified a group of pathologic stage (PS) patients with extensive splenic disease (defined as >4 nodules), who benefited from chemotherapy in addition to radiation therapy (Hoppe et al., 1982). Data from the University of Chicago did show a correlation between anatomical substaging and splenic involvement, in 76 patients with PS IIIA Hodgkin's disease (Larson and Ultmann, 1982). Patients with stage III-2 disease tended to have extensive involvement, with >4 splenic nodules; stage III-1 patients more often had minimal splenic disease, and were therefore felt to be at lower risk for occult liver involvement.

The likelihood of splenic involvement has been shown to be strongly dependent on the histological subtype of Hodgkin's disease (Kaplan, 1972). The spleen was found to be involved in 16% of lymphocyte-predominant (LP), in 35% of nodular-sclerosing (NS), in 59% of mixed-cellularity (MC), and in 83% of lymphocyte-depletion Hodgkin's disease cases. The probability of change in stage following laparotomy could also be correlated with histological subtype: A change in stage was seen in 13% of LP, in 19% of NS, and in 37% of MC types.

With the development of more effective combination chemotherapy regimens and the judicious combination of radiation and chemotherapy, laparotomy has become less important as a routine staging procedure (Rosenberg, 1988). Its present indications are outlined in Table 9. For Hodgkin's disease, staging laparotomy is recommended for clinical stage (CS) IA and IIA disease, except for those with nodal disease limited to one high cervical area, who carry an excellent prognosis with local treatment only, and those with bulky mediastinal adenopathy, who should receive chemo-

therapy with or without irradiation. Patients presenting with subdiaphragmatic CS IIB disease generally do not require laparotomy, because of a high probability of splenic involvement (89%), which is best treated with combination chemotherapy (Leibenhaut et al., 1987). Laparotomy may also be useful in CS IIIA, in which evidence for lower abdominal disease is absent or equivocal, in whom chemotherapy is not the treatment of choice, and in those with splenomegaly, in whom radiation therapy is planned as the initial treatment. Women who wish to preserve ovarian function may benefit from the surgical relocation of the ovaries at laparotomy.

The role of staging laparotomy with splenectomy in NHL is much less clearly defined. The great majority of these patients present with advanced, stage III and IV disease, and in only few will surgical staging affect treatment decisions (Come and Chabner, 1979). Although splenic involvement was noted in 32% of a series of unselected and untreated lymphoma patients who underwent staging laparotomy (Goffinet et al., 1973), 60–75% of NHL patients are stage IV by virtue of bone marrow, liver, or other extranodal involvement (Come and Chabner, 1979). Splenic evaluation in such cases is superfluous. On the other hand, splenic involvement is uncommon in diffuse large cell lymphoma (Goffinet et al., 1973; Heifetz et al., 1980). This type of NHL also presents more often as stage I and II, compared with the nodular lymphomas (Rosenberg et al., 1978). Therefore, in patients presenting as CS I diffuse large B-cell lymphoma, staging laparotomy may be an important aspect of their overall evaluation, to exclude intra-abdominal and splenic disease, unless chemotherapy is already planned.

14.3.7.3. Restaging Laparotomy Restaging, or "second-look," laparotomy for Hodgkin's disease patients, in clinical complete remission following treatment, has been studied by several groups (Sutcliffe et al., 1978; Goodman et al., 1982; Sutcliffe et al., 1982), in order to document a pathologic complete remission. These studies showed that residual disease is only rarely found in patients with normal clinical restaging following completion of therapy. Of 46 Hodgkin's disease patients who underwent posttreatment laparotomy, four patients with a normal clinical evaluation showed splenic involvement only; of 14 patients with clinically suspicious findings, only two had evidence of active disease on laparotomy (Sutcliffe et al., 1982). Restaging laparotomy is not recommended as a routine procedure, especially in patients who have undergone pretreatment laparotomy with removal of the spleen.

14.3.7.4. Partial Splenectomy Because of the high risk of post-splenectomy sepsis in children with Hodgkin's disease (Singer, 1973; Dickerman, 1979; Chilcote et al., 1976; Lanzkowsky et al., 1976), which has been estimated at about 10% incidence, with a 30–50% mortality rate, partial splenectomy has been recommended and performed at a number of institutions (Pearson, 1980; Katz and Schiller, 1980; Boles et al., 1978). The use of an ultrasonic scalpel has been proposed for this procedure for better hemostasis (Hodgson and McElhinney, 1982). Boles et al. (1978) estimated only a 2–3% understaging of patients with Hodgkin's disease, when partial splenectomy was performed. However, data from other authors point to a larger error: Dearth et al. (1978) reported that 11.6% of splenic disease would have been missed with partial splenectomy; Sterchi et al. (1984) found a 6.2% understaging of splenic involvement.

A plea has been made to preserve accessory spleens at the time of initial staging laparotomy and splenectomy, in patients with Hodgkin's disease (Strauch, 1979), although accessory spleens do not always protect from postsplenectomy sepsis, and a critical mass of functioning splenic tissue may be required to provide adequate protection (Goldthorn and Schwartz, 1978; Moore et al., 1983). Splenic autotransplantation has also been proposed to provide some degree of splenic function after splenectomy (Traub et al., 1987).

14.3.7.5. Laparoscopy Laparoscopy has been proposed as an alternative to staging laparotomy and splenectomy, because of the decreased risk of postsplenectomy infections, the avoidance of operative risk and the fact that chemotherapy is being employed more frequently, with or without radiation therapy, whether the spleen is involved or not (DeVita et al., 1971; Bagley et al., 1973; Beretta et al., 1976). In a series of 121 unselected and previously untreated patients with Hodgkin's disease reported by Beretta et al. (1976), findings on laparoscopy were compared with subsequent laparotomy and splenectomy. Needle biopsy of the liver during laparoscopy was helpful in detecting extranodal disease. Although needle biopsies of the spleen were positive in 13%, subsequent laparotomy and splenectomy demonstrated disease in an additional 26 spleens. Those authors concluded that, although laparoscopy appears to be a useful staging procedure in Hodgkin's disease patients, especially for the detection of liver involvement, it is not recommended in patients in whom splenic evaluation is an important part of staging prior to therapy.

In NHL, laparoscopy may be useful in clinically localized disease, in which combined radiotherapy and chemotherapy is indicated, to detect stage IV disease by virtue of hepatic involvement. This procedure has also been employed to re-evaluate NHL patients for completeness of response, and to detect sites of relapse (Anderson et al., 1976)

14.4. COMPLICATIONS OF SPLENIC INVOLVEMENT AND SPLENECTOMY

14.4.1. HYPERSPLENISM The problems encountered in patients with enlarged spleens, designated as the "splenomegaly syndrome" by Videbaek et al. (1982), center principally on the pancytopenia of hypersplenism, although other complications, such as hypermetabolic symptoms, including fever (McKenna et al., 1979) and mechanical problems of pain and rupture, should also be included. This subheading addresses those complications specifically encountered in patients with splenomegaly associated with the MLPDs, as well as problems that follow splenectomy (*see also* Chapters 9 and 17).

Anemia, thrombocytopenia, and leukopenia, in the presence of a normocellular or hypercellular bone marrow are the presenting features of hypersplenism (Dameshek and Estren, 1947; Hamilton et al., 1967). Anemia is especially common in the MLPDs, which, however, may not reflect a true reduction in total red blood cell volume. In patients with enlarged spleens, no matter what the cause, expansion of plasma volume leads to a hemodilutional anemia (Bowdler, 1970), which is sometimes exaggerated by the diversion of red blood cells into a large splenic pool. As discussed in Subheading 2.2., splenic involvement by the MLPDs leads to expansion of the extrasinusal space by lymphocytes (Harris et al., 1958), but the red pulp remains relatively intact, allowing for increased blood flow and for accumulation of red blood cells (Videbaek et al., 1982). In patients with CLL, Christensen (1973a) has shown a direct correlation between the degree of splenomegaly and size of the splenic erythrocyte pool. For spleens weighing ~1000 g, the erythrocyte pool was 10% of the total red blood cell mass, increasing to 40% for spleens weighing 4000 g (*see also* Chapter 9).

In HCL, because of the especially prominent parenchymal changes described in Subheading 2.1.7., the splenic erythrocyte pool is unusually large (Lewis et al., 1977), and contributes to the prominent anemia of this disorder (Flandrin et al., 1984). In this disease also, expansion of plasma volume and dilutional anemia are related to the degree of splenomegaly, and contribute to the reduced hemoglobin levels (Castro-Malaspina et al., 1979).

There appears to be a relationship, between spleen size and splenic pooling of platelets, similar to red blood cell pooling. Normally, about 30% of the circulating platelet mass is pooled in the spleen (Aster, 1966). As the size of the spleen increases, the platelet pool expands, reaching values up to 90% of the total circulating platelet mass. On the other hand, despite significant splenic enlargement, platelet survival usually remains normal (Aster and Jandl, 1964). There is some evidence for splenic pooling of granulocytes, which increases with splenomegaly (Vincent, 1977). There also appears to be increased margination of granulocytes in the splenic vessels, thereby reducing the peripheral neutrophil count (Fieschi and Sacchetti, 1964; Scott et al., 1971).

Hypermetabolic manifestations are at times a prominent feature of the hypersplenism observed in MLPDs, including weight loss, fever, hyperhydrosis, and increased basal metabolic rate, and are often reversed by splenectomy (Christensen et al., 1977; McKenna et al., 1979).

14.4.2. SPLENIC PAIN AND RUPTURE The discomfort experienced by MLPD patients with splenomegaly is usually vague and nondramatic, except when caused by splenic infarction. In general, splenic infarction is more common in the chronic leukemias than in acute leukemia or the lymphomas, and is often associated with the sudden onset of left flank, back, or shoulder pain, at times pleuritic in nature, or sometimes mimicking an acute abdomen.

Splenic infarction may predispose to splenic rupture, although acute rupture of the spleen occurs more often in the acute than the chronic MLPDs. Bauer et al. (1981) have reviewed the diagnoses in 53 cases of splenic rupture. The following number of cases were observed; 11 AML, 10 ALL, 9 unclassified acute leukemia, 9 NHL, 6 CML, 5 Hodgkin's disease, and 3 CLL. A report by Johnson, Rosen and Sheehan (1979) noted that 1% of patients with acute leukemia experience splenic rupture. In 34% of ruptured spleens in cases of acute leukemia, this was the presenting event for the leukemia (Bauer et al., 1981). Possibly, the leukemic infiltration of the spleen contributes to spontaneous rupture, either by causing capsular invasion or ischemic infarction.

Splenic rupture has also been observed in HCL (Rosier and Lefer, 1977; Yam and Crosby, 1979; Schmitt et al., 1981). Again, a major correlation appears to be with the frequency of splenic infarction (Yam and Crosby, 1979), which in turn is most likely related to the vascular changes observed in such spleens (*see* Subheading 2.1.7.). Two cases of splenic rupture in plasma cell leukemia have been described (Stephens and Hudson, 1969; Rogers and Shah, 1980). Infarction, followed by subcapsular hematoma, was postulated as the possible mechanism for the splenic rupture. Spontaneous rupture of the spleen as an initial manifestation of splenic lymphoma is rare (Fausel et al., 1990; Berrebi et al., 1984).

14.4.3. IMMUNE DEFICIENCIES The immune function of the spleen, and the consequences of hyposplenism, including infectious complications, are discussed in detail in Chapters 9 and 16.

14.4.4. SECOND MALIGNANCIES The greater-than-expected incidence of second malignancies, especially acute leukemia, in patients treated for Hodgkin's disease, has been known for some time (Cadman et al., 1977; Arseneau et al., 1972; Raich et al., 1975). Those patients treated with sequential radiation and intensive chemotherapy, including alkylating agents, were felt to be especially at risk. There is some evidence that splenectomy may be associated with the subsequent appearance of acute nonlymphocytic leukemia in Hodgkin's disease patients who have received chemotherapy with alkylating agents, such as MOPP combination chemotherapy (Rosenberg, 1988; van Leeuwen et al., 1987). The data from Stanford (Rosenberg, 1988) implies that this is an especially high risk in patients over the age of 40 years. It will be of interest to see if other chemotherapy combinations containing nonalkylating agents will show a lesser risk of leukemia, even in the face of splenectomy (Hoppe et al., 1985).

14.5. TREATMENT OF SPLENIC INVOLVEMENT

14.5.1. SPLENECTOMY

"Splenectomy should be done when the patient does not need it. If one waits until the patient needs the operation he may not be able to tolerate it."

William H. Crosby (1972)

During the past 75 years, splenectomy has become a common procedure in the treatment of hypersplenism. This generalization includes the lymphoproliferative disorders which are often complicated by symptomatic splenomegaly. The first successful splenectomies employed in the treatment of MLPDs were reported by Giffin (1921). A number of more recent studies have confirmed the therapeutic value of splenectomy in this setting (Crosby, 1972; Strumia et al., 1966; Christensen et al., 1970; Neal et al., 1992; Seymour et al., 1997).

As defined by Dameshek and Estren (1947), hypersplenism is characterized by the tetralogy of peripheral blood cytopenias, bone marrow hyperplasia, splenomegaly, and correction of these cytopenias following splenectomy. In the MLPDs, blood cytopenias most often reflect the combined effects of splenic sequestration, splenic pooling, increased plasma volume, bone marrow infiltration and replacement, and possibly marrow suppression caused by therapy. Correction of the hematological abnormalities following splenectomy is commonly observed in hypersplenism associated with malignant lymphomas and CLL. Morris et al. (1975) and, later, Gill et al. (1981), reported nearly identical results following splenectomy in such patients. Of the patients with Hodgkin's disease, 53% obtained a hematological remission of the hypersplenism, as did 55% of NHL patients (Mitchell and Morris, 1983). Approximately 50% of the patients were able to return to full chemotherapy doses. Clinically significant hypersplenism develops in 5–10% of patients with Hodgkin's disease (Crosby, 1972), and splenectomy may allow more effective therapy and a reduction of complications (Cooper et al., 1974). The great majority of splenectomies performed in Hodgkin's disease patients are for the purpose of accurate surgical staging early in the course of the disease, as discussed in Subheading 3.6.2.

14.5.1.1. Chronic Lymphocytic Leukemia In the past, splenectomy had a limited role in CLL, and was associated with a high operative mortality (Christensen et al., 1970), because the fact that the standard approach to treatment of CLL usually consists of chemotherapy and possibly radiotherapy, and only late in the course of the disease, when the patient is refractory and presents with massive splenomegaly, is splenectomy considered. An 8% perioperative mortality and a 20% complication rate were reported by MacRae et al. (1992) in 34 patients with MLPDs following therapeutic splenectomy.

Yam and Crosby (1974) showed that early splenectomy for hypersplenism was well-tolerated in patients with CLL, well-differentiated lymphomas, and HCL, in contrast to the poor results observed in large cell lymphomas. In a series reported by Christensen et al. (1977), a group of CLL patients was splenectomized electively at a early stage of their disease, and compared with a nonsplenectomized control group. Generally, splenectomy was performed for progressive splenomegaly and hypersplenism. The mean survival for the splenectomized group was 54 months, compared to 30 months for the control group. The median hemoglobin values rose from 100 to 130 g/L within 3 months of operation, and platelet counts rose from a median of 90,000 to 270,000/mm^3. The need for transfusion was considerably reduced, and hypermetabolic symptoms associated with hypersplenism were frequently improved. No cases of fulminant postsplenectomy septicemia were observed. Dramatic improvements in platelet counts in CLL patients with refractory thrombocytopenia have also been reported following splenectomy (Merl et al., 1983).

Neal et al. (1992) concluded that splenectomy remains a reasonable and effective treatment option for cytopenic CLL patients who have failed after chemotherapy, or whose peripheral blood counts may not permit additional cytotoxic therapy. Almost all of the 50 patients studied had Rai stage III or IV disease and a palpable spleen. Significant improvement was observed in 77% of patients with anemia, in 70% of patients with thrombocytopenia, and in 64% with both. Transfusion requirements were reduced, and responses usually lasted for at least 1 year. The operative mortality was 4% and the morbidity 26%.

A recent report by Seymour et al. (1997) compared the results of splenectomy in 55 CLL patients with 55 patients treated with fludarabine, matched for major prognostic factors. Among Rai stage IV patients, a trend for improved survival was seen in the splenectomized patients ($p = .15$). The 2-year survival rate for stage IV patients was 51% in the splenectomy group and 28% in the fludarabine group. The only predictor for blood count improvement was spleen weight ($p < .05$). Perioperative mortality was 9% and morbidity 43%, both caused primarily by infection.

14.5.1.2. Hairy Cell Leukemia Hairy cell leukemia (HCL) is known to have a variable natural history. There is a subset of approx 10% of patients who remain clinically stable, without treatment for several years (Champlin et al., 1986). However, for patients who present with an enlarged spleen and peripheral blood cytopenias, splenectomy remains an effective initial treatment. The usual indications for such treatment include progressive cytopenias, massive splenomegaly, and recurrent infections. Although most patients with enlarged spleens will present more frequently with significant pancytopenia, it is not possible to predict, by spleen size, which patient will respond to splenectomy (Golomb, 1987; Flandrin et al., 1984), although the degree of response tends to be greater in patients with massive splenomegaly (Mintz and Golomb, 1979). Golomb and Vardiman (1983) reported that patients with pancytopenia, but without a palpable spleen, may respond to splenectomy; Jansen and Hermans (1981) found such treatment unsuccessful. It should be borne in mind that, in patients with HCL, the spleen may be found to be enlarged to 2–3× normal at surgery, but escape detection by clinical examination (Golomb, 1987).

In most series, a good hematological response is observed in more than 50% of HCL patients undergoing splenectomy (Golde, 1982; Schrek and Donnelly, 1966; Naeim and Smith, 1974; Bouroncle et al., 1958; Yam et al., 1972; Burke et al., 1974; Golomb et al., 1986; Rubin et al., 1969; Flandrin et al., 1973, 1984; Catovsky et al., 1974). In 28 splenectomized patients with HCL followed by Catovsky (1977), 61% achieved complete remission and 39% partial remission within 2 weeks of splenectomy. Complete remission was defined as a rise in hemoglobin above 110 g/L, neutrophils above 1000/mm^3, and platelets >100,000/mm^3. In 85 splenectomized patients reported by Flandrin et al. (1984), 61% achieved a complete remission of HCL, as defined by Catovsky (1977). In 170 patients reviewed by Golomb et al. (1986), the mean pre- and post-splenectomy values changed as follows, hemoglobin rising from 104 to 115 g/L, granulocytes from 552 to 1754/mm^3, and platelets from 87,000 to 211,000/mm^3.

In the series reported by Catovsky (1977) and Flandrin et al. (1984), the survival for splenectomized patients was better than for nonsplenectomized patients. Although both were nonrandomized studies, a clear advantage is evident for the splenectomized patients. The median survival time was more than 5× that of the nonsplenectomized patients in Catovsky's series; Flandrin et al. (1984) reported a median survival time of more than 200 months in splenectomized patients and 37 months in nonsplenectomized patients. There was no significant difference in survival in those patients whose spleens were palpable at 4 cm or less below the costal margin: Their survival rate was, in fact, similar to those with larger spleens, who underwent splenectomy.

Golomb et al. (1986) reported that approximately one-third of their patients required further therapy after splenectomy, with a median interval to additional treatment of 8.3 months. In the Catovsky (1977) series, relapse of pancytopenia occurred in all patients who achieved partial responses, and in one-half of those who showed a complete response. However, the median time to relapse was 16 months in the complete responders, compared to 2.5 months in the remaining patients.

Most reported cases of HCL, with prolonged remissions and survival, have been in splenectomized patients. Catovsky (1977) describes three long-term complete responders, continuing between 37 and 180 months following splenectomy, and Myers et al. (1981) describe a case continuing in complete remission 21 years after removal of the spleen. Flink (1988) observed a similar survival in a patient with HCL, diagnosed initially as lymphosarcoma of the spleen, who remained in peripheral remission 22 years following splenectomy.

The precise mechanism by which such excellent responses occur following splenectomy is not clear. The spleen is a preferred area of infiltration and growth for the neoplastic hairy cells. As discussed in Subheading 2.1.7., hypersplenism is the major mechanism for the paneytopenia in these patients. In addition to improvement in absolute blood counts, improvement in platelet function has also been observed following splenectomy (Champlin et al., 1986). Rosove et al. (1980) describe degranulation of platelets circulating through the HCL spleen, leading to an acquired storage pool functional defect.

Because of the strong susceptibility of the pancytopenic HCL patient to infections, including those caused by opportunistic organisms, care must be taken before and after surgery, to investigate and treat all sources of infection. Among the splenectomized patients reported by Catovsky (1977), one patient died of bronchopneumonia 2½ weeks following surgery, and six other patients died during the first 6 months, all from infections. Four of these patients had received chemotherapy just prior to the infections, and Catovsky warns that cytotoxic drugs are contraindicated in the pre- and immediately postoperative periods. The usefulness of protective measures, such as prophylactic antibiotics, remains to be evaluated in such patients.

14.5.2. RADIATION THERAPY Although a splenic irradiation port is included in patients with Hodgkin's disease receiving total nodal radiation therapy, this is associated with radiation damage to the left kidney and the base of the left lung (Greenberger et al., 1979; Le Bourgeois et al., 1979). Staging laparotomy with splenectomy removes the need to irradiate the spleen. Furthermore, the increased effectiveness of combination chemotherapy programs in achieving prolonged complete remissions, in patients with more advanced stages of Hodgkin's disease, has also decreased the need to add radiation therapy to the spleen.

In early-stage Hodgkin's disease, patients with a supradiaphragmatic presentation may be considered for radiation to the upper abdomen, in place of staging laparotomy and splenectomy. In a controlled clinical trial by the European Organization for the Research and Treatment of Cancer (EORTC), reported by Tubiana et al. (1981), 300 patients with clinical stages I and II Hodgkin's disease were randomized to receive either splenic irradiation or splenectomy. All patients received mantle-field irradiation, as well as para-aortic lymph node irradiation. Both the survival rates and relapse-free survival rates were almost identical in the two groups. However, the authors state that the prognostic significance of the finding of splenic involvement is valuable in selecting patients who benefit from prophylactic para-aortic node irradiation, even in those patients with otherwise good prognostic indicators, such as young age, absence of symptoms, and favorable histology.

In the NHLs, radiation of the spleen may be included as part of abdominal radiation fields, or as part of total abdominal irradiation (Goffinet et al., 1976). Radiation to an enlarged spleen may also be beneficial later in the course of the disease, to relieve pain not responding to chemotherapy, or for hypersplenism in patients who are not candidates for surgery or chemotherapy (Newell, 1963; Comas et al., 1968). Transient decreases in blood counts may be encountered during and following such radiation.

Patients with Hodgkin's disease and NHL, who have undergone radiation therapy to the spleen, have experienced atrophy and functional hyposplenism, occasionally leading to fatal pneumococcal sepsis (Dailey et al., 1980). When irradiated spleens, obtained at autopsy from patients with Hodgkin's disease and other lymphomas, are compared to nonirradiated spleens, major differences are observed (Dailey et al., 1981). After an interval of 1–8 years, and following an average radiation dose of 3900 cGy, most of the irradiated spleens, were found to be small, with an average weight of 75 g, with a thickened capsule and diffuse fibrosis of the red pulp. Intimal thickening of the arteries, and, at times, of the veins, was also observed. In one study, ^{99m}Tc-sulfur colloid scans did not reflect splenic atrophy or decrease in reticuloendothelial function following radiation (Spencer and Knowlton, 1975).

Splenic irradiation in CLL dates back to the early therapeutic use of radiation (Senn, 1903). More extensive lymphoid irradiation, including total body irradiation (Del Regato, 1974), has been explored during the past quarter-century. These techniques do not appear to be consistently superior to chemotherapy, and are often associated with excessive marrow suppression. In a review of the role of radiotherapy in CLL by Paule et al. (1985), only fractional low-dose splenic irradiation was found to lead to a long-lasting decrease in the lymphocyte count, and improvement in anemia and thrombocytopenia. Most patients treated show relief of painful splenomegaly, as well as improvement in blood counts (Byhardt et al., 1975; Singh et al., 1986; Parmentier et al., 1974). These studies have shown a reduction of lymphocytic bone marrow infiltration by 20–50% with total doses of 600–800 cGy to the spleen.

Splenic irradiation in CLL leads to the destruction of a large portion of the malignant B-cell clone, with low doses, and, potentially, the more-resistant subset of T-suppressor cells present in the spleen is affected by higher doses of radiation (Paule et al., 1985). T-suppressor cells have been shown to contribute to bone marrow stem cell inhibition, resulting in anemia and thrombocytopenia in some patients with CLL (Nagasawa et al., 1981; Mangan et al., 1982). Normalization of helper:suppressor T-cell ratios have been observed following splenic irradiation (Paule and Cosset, 1985; McCann et al., 1982). An additional mechanism for improvement of anemia in these patients is suggested by Awwad et al. (1967), who showed decreased red blood cell destruction and increased red blood cell survival after splenic irradiation.

Splenic irradiation in patients with CLL is generally well-tolerated, with little hematological toxicity. A transient decrease in neutrophils and platelets occurs, but is seldom severe (Singh et al., 1986). Occasionally, hyperkalemia (Kurlander et al., 1975) and a transient increase in liver size have been described following splenic irradiation. Apart from these occasional problems, splenic irradiation is a useful mode of treatment in CLL, especially in patients refractory to chemotherapy, and a safer alternative than total body irradiation.

Prolymphocytic leukemia appears more resistant to splenic radiation: Only 1/3 patients reported by Singh et al. (1986) responded.

Several reports have demonstrated complete and partial remissions of HCL with splenic irradiation (Plenderleith, 1970; Bouroncle, 1979; Schrek and Donelly, 1966; Jansen and Hermans, 1981; Sharp and MacWalter, 1983; Gosselin et al., 1956). Yam et al. (1972), however, found splenic irradiation ineffective. In those patients with HCL, in whom splenectomy is inadvisable, or is refused, and other modalities, such as interferon or chemotherapeutic agents, are not available, splenic irradiation may be considered as an alternative treatment.

14.5.3. CHEMOTHERAPY AND BIOLOGIC RESPONSE MODIFIERS The initial management of patients with CLL and the indolent lymphomas include watchful waiting, if asymptomatic, or chemotherapy with single agents or combinations of chemotherapeutic agents and corticosteroids. The newer agents, fludarabine or cladribine (2-chlorodeoxyadenosine [2-CdA]), are often the initial treatment of choice (Tallman and Hakimian, 1995; Saven et al., 1995; Juliusson et al., 1996; Solal-Celigny et al., 1996). Biologic therapy of the malignant lymphomas has been limited to the use of α-interferon to prolong chemotherapeutic responses in the low-grade lymphomas (Andersen and Smalley, 1993; Cole et al., 1995), and, more recently, the demonstration that chimeric anti-CD20 monoclonal antibody led to a 46% partial and complete response rate in patients with relapsed or refractory, low-grade NHL (Maloney et al., 1997). Work with anti-idiotype immunization in follicular low-grade lymphomas is promising, but not yet of practical applicability (Kobrin and Kwak, 1997).

In patients with Hodgkin's disease and the aggressive NHLs, combination chemotherapy has been effective in advanced stages,

including those with splenic involvement (Gaynor and Fisher, 1998; Canellos et al., 1992; Fisher et al., 1993). Long-term disease-free remissions are common. Splenic involvement and enlargement may be associated with lower blood counts and a decreased ability to tolerate full chemotherapy doses. Splenectomy has been proposed as a means for improving tolerance to chemotherapy in such patients.

For many years, splenectomy and α interferon (Golomb, 1987; Spiegel, 1987; Thompson and Fefer, 1987; Fahey et al., 1987) were the standard treatment approaches to HCL. The majority of patients on α interferon are known to relapse after stopping therapy (Jaiyesimi et al. 1993). A more promising agent for the treatment of HCL was initially reported by Spiers et al. (1984): pentostatin (2-deoxycoformycin) acts as an inhibitor of adenosine deaminase, an enzyme of purine metabolism. Since then, a number of additional reports have attested to the effectiveness of pentostatin (Kraut et al., 1986; Spiers et al., 1985; Johnston et al., 1986; Grever et al., 1995). Prolonged, unmaintained remissions were achieved in 50–90% of patients, including regression of splenomegaly, clearing of bone marrow infiltration, and normalization of blood counts.

More recently, cladribine (2-CdA) has been shown to have considerable activity in HCL, initially described by Piro et al. (1990). This agent is a deoxyadenosine analog that is resistant to deamination by adenosine deaminase. Since the initial report, additional investigators have reported high rates of complete remissions with a single course of 2-CdA therapy (Juliusson and Lilliemark, 1992; Lauria et al., 1991; Estey et al., 1992; Tallman et al., 1992; Saven et al., 1993). Hoffman et al. (1997) reported on the long-term follow-up of 49 patients with HCL treated with one 7-day course of intravenous 2-CdA. 76% achieved complete remission, and the remainder were partial remissions. At a median follow-up of 55 months, the relapse-free survival was 80%, and the overall survival 95%. Oral 2-CdA has been found to be equally effective to intravenous administration (Juliusson et al., 1996).

14.6. CONCLUSION

The spleen has been implicated in diseases afflicting mankind for the duration of recorded medical history. Because it represents the largest concentration of lymphocytes in the body, and is continuously perfused by blood, the spleen is involved in many diseases initiated by the immune system, and in the majority of malignancies involving the immune system. Although the spleen is seldom the only organ involved in such disorders, they do afford a window to observe the disease mechanisms operative in the spleen.

The onset and extension of splenic involvement by the MLPDs are determined by cell kinetics and circulation patterns, cell surface markers and stromal cell receptors, as by well as local factors within the spleen. For many disorders, reasons are beginning to be learned for the degree and timing of splenic involvement.

In addition to exploring these specific pathogenic factors, we have made extensive use of a wealth of clinical observations regarding the role of the spleen in these disorders. Staging laparotomy and splenectomy, for example, have added much information about the natural history of Hodgkin's disease, and have allowed for the development of more rational and effective treatment. Splenectomy remains an effective treatment for HCL, although, in other disorders, altered or absent splenic function is associated with immediate and long-term problems, which may need clinical attention.

In continuing to provide new knowledge concerning the MLPDs, the spleen deserves continued interest and inquiry.

ACKNOWLEDGMENTS

P. R. acknowledges the assistance of Jennifer Sheaffer in the preparation of this chapter.

REFERENCES

Ahmann, D. L., Kiely, J. M., Harrison, E. G., and Payne, W. S. (1966) Malignant lymphoma of the spleen. A review of 49 cases in which the diagnosis was made at splenectomy. *Cancer* **19**, 461–469.

Aisenberg, A. C. (1978) The staging and treatment of Hodgkin's disease. *N. Engl. J. Med.* **299**, 1228–1232.

Aisenberg, A. C. and Qazi, R. (1974) Abdominal involvement at the onset of Hodgkin's disease. *Am. J. Med.* **57**, 870–874.

Alcorn, F. S., Mategrano, V. C., Petasnick, J. P., and Clark, J. W. (1977) Contributions of computed tomography in the staging and management of malignant lymphomas. *Radiology* **125**, 717–723.

Andersen, J. W. and Smalley, R. V. (1993) Interferon alfa plus chemotherapy for non-Hodgkin's lymphoma: five-year follow-up. *N. Engl. J. Med.* **329**, 1821.

Anderson, T., Rosenoff, S., Bender, R., et al. (1976) Peritoneoscopy: a useful tool in restaging lymphoma patients. *Proc. AACR ASCO,* **17,** 268.

Andriko, J. W., Ives Aguilera, N. S., Chu, W. S., Nandedkar, M. A., and Cotelingam, J. D. (1997) Waldenström's macroglobulinemia. *Cancer* **80**, 1926–1935.

Argatoff, L. H., Connors, J. M., Klasa, R. J., Horsman, D. E., and Gascoyne, R. D. (1997) Mantle cell lymphoma: a clinicopathologic study of 80 cases. *Blood* **89**, 2067–2078.

Armitage, J. O. (1997) The changing classification of non-Hodgkin's lymphomas. *CA. Cancer J. Clin.* **47**, 323–325.

Arseneau, J. C., Sponzo, R. W., Levin, D. L., Schnipper, L. E., Bonner, H., Young, R. C., et al. (1972) Non-lymphomatous malignant tumors complicating Hodgkin's disease. Possible association with intensive therapy. *N. Engl. J. Med.* **287**, 1119–1122.

Askergren, J., Björkholm, M., Holm, G., Johansson, B., and Sundblad, R. (1981) On the size and tumour involvement of the spleen in Hodgkin's disease. *Acta Med. Scand.* **209**, 217–220.

Aster, R. H. (1966) Pooling of platelets in the spleen: role in the pathogenesis of 'hypersplenic' thrombocytopenia. *J. Clin. Invest.* **45**, 645–657.

Aster, R. H. and Jandl, J. H. (1964) Platelet sequestration in man. II. Immunological and clinical studies. *J. Clin. Invest.* **43**, 856–869.

Ault, K. A. (1979) Detection of small numbers of monoclonal B lymphocytes in the blood of patients with lymphoma. *N. Engl. J. Med.* **300**, 1401–1405.

Awwad, H. K., Badeeb, A. O., Massoud, G. E., and Salah, M. (1967) The effect of splenic irradiation on the ferrokinetics of chronic leukemia with a clinical study. *Blood* **29**, 242–256.

Bagley, C. M. Jr., Thomas, L. B., Johnson, R. E., Chretien, P. B., and DeVita, V. T. (1973) Diagnosis of liver involvement by lymphoma: results in 96 consecutive peritoneoscopies. *Cancer* **31**, 840–847.

Baldini, L., Fracchiolla, N. S., Cro, L. M., et al. (1994) Frequent p53 gene involvement in splenic B-cell leukemia/lymphomas of possible marginal zone origin. *Blood* **84**, 270–278.

Banks, P. M., Chan, J., Cleary, M. L., Delson, G., De Wolf-Peeters, C., Gatter, K., et al. (1992) Mantle cell lymphoma: a proposal for unification of morphologic, immunologic, and molecular data. *Am. J. Surg. Pathol.* **16**, 637–640.

Barkun, A. N., Camus, M., Green, L., Meagher, T., Coupal, L., De Stempel, J., and Grover, S. A. (1991) Bedside assessment of splenic enlargement. *Am. J. Med.* **91**, 512–518.

Bauer, T. W., Haskins, G. E., and Armitage, J. O. (1981) Splenic rupture in patients with hematologic malignancies. *Cancer* **48**, 2729–2733.

Ben-Haim, S., Bar-Shalom, R., Israel, O., Haim, N., Epelbaum, R., Ben-Shachar, M., et al. (1996) Utility of gallium-67 scintigraphy in low-grade non-Hodgkin's lymphoma. *J. Clin. Oncol.* **14**, 1936–1942.

Benharroch, D., Meguerian-Bedoyan, Z., Lamant, L., Amin, C., Brugières, L., Terrier-Lacombe, M.J., et al. (1998) ALK-positive lymphoma: a single disease with a broad spectrum of morphology. *Blood* **91**, 2076–2084.

Beretta, G., Spinelli, P., Rilke, F., et al. (1976) Sequential laparoscopy and laparotomy combined with bone marrow biopsy in staging Hodgkin's disease. *Cancer Treat. Rep.* **60**, 1231–1237.

Berg, E. L., Goldstein, L. A., Jutila, M. A., Nakache, M., Picker, L. J., Streeter, P. R., et al.. (1989) Homing receptors and vascular addressins: cell adhesion molecules that direct lymphocyte traffic. *Immunol. Rev.* **108**, 5–18.

Berliner, N., Ault, K. A., Martin, P., and Weinberg, D. S. (1986) Detection of clonal excess in lymphoproliferative disease by kappa/lambda analysis: correlation with immunoglobulin gene DNA rearrangement. *Blood* **67**, 80–85.

Berrebi, B. A., Bustan, A., Mashiah, A., and Hurwitz, N. (1984) Splenic rupture as a presenting sign of lymphoma of the spleen. *Isr. J. Med. Sci.* **20**, 66–67.

Bieber, C. P. and Bieber, M. M. (1973) Detection of ferritin as a circulating tumor associated antigen in Hodgkin's disease. *Natl. Cancer Inst. Monogr.* **36**, 147–153.

Binet, J. L., Auquier, A., Dighiero, G., Chastang, C., Piquet, H., Goasguen, J., et al. (1981) A new prognostic classification of chronic lymphocytic leukemia derived from multivariate survival analysis. *Cancer* **48**, 198–206.

Blayney, D. W., Jaffe, E. S., Blattner, W. A., et al. (1983) The human T-cell leukemia/lymphoma virus associated with American adult T-cell leukemia/lymphoma. *Blood* **62**, 401–405.

Boles, E. T. Jr., Haase, G. M., and Hamoudi, A. B. (1978) Partial splenectomy in staging laparotomy for Hodgkin's disease: an alternative approach. *J. Pediatr. Surg.* **13**, 581–586.

Bookman, M. A., Lardelli, P., Jaffe, E. S., Duffey, P. L., and Longo, D. L. (1990) Lymphocytic lymphoma of intermediate differentiation: morphologic, immunophenotypic, and prognostic factors. *J. Natl. Cancer Inst.* **82**, 742.

Bouroncle, B. A. (1966) Sternberg-Reed cells in the peripheral blood of patients with Hodgkin's disease. *Blood* **27**, 544–556.

Bouroncle, B. A. (1979) Leukemic reticuloendotheliosis (hairy cell leukemia). *Blood* **53**, 412–436.

Bouroncle, B. A., Wiseman, B. K., and Doan, C. A. (1958) Leukemic reticuloendotheliosis. *Blood* **13**, 609–630.

Bowdler, A. J. (1967) Dilution anaemia associated with enlargement of the spleen. *Proc. R. Soc. Med.* **60**, 44–47.

Bowdler, A. J. (1970) Blood volume studies in patients with splenomegaly. *Transfusion* **10**, 171–181.

Bowdler, A. J. and Glick, I. W. (1966) Autoimmune hemolytic anemia as the herald state of Hodgkin's disease. *Ann. Intern. Med.* **65**, 761–767.

Braylan, R., Variakojis, D., and Yachnin, S. (1975) The Sezary syndrome lymphoid cell: abnormal surface properties and mitogen responsiveness. *Br. J. Haematol.* **31**, 553–564.

Breiman, R. S., Castellino, R. A., Harell, G. S., Marshall, W. H., Glatstein, E., and Kaplan, H. S. (1978) CT-pathologic correlations in Hodgkin's disease and non-Hodgkin's lymphoma. *Radiology* **126**, 159–166.

Breitfeld, V. and Lee, R. E. (1975) Pathology of the spleen in hematologic disease. *Surg. Clin. North Am.* **55**, 233–251.

Britten, K. J. M., Jones, D. B., De Sousa, M., and Wright, D. H. (1986) The distribution of iron and iron binding proteins in spleen with reference to Hodgkin's disease. *Br. J. Cancer* **54**, 277–286.

Broder, S., Uchiyama, T., and Waldmann, T. A. (1979) Current concepts in immunoregulatory T-cell neoplasms. *Cancer Treat. Rep.* **63**, 607–612.

Broder, S., Edelson, R. L., Lutzner, M. A., Nelson, D. L., MacDermott, R. P., Durm, M. E., et al. (1976) The Sezary syndrome: a malignant proliferation of helper T-cells. *J. Clin. Invest.* **58**, 1297–1306.

Broder, S., Bunn, P. A., Jaffe, E. S., Blattner, W., Gallo, R. C., Wong-Staal, F., et al. (1984) T-cell lymphoproliferative syndrome associated with human T-cell leukemia/lymphoma virus. *Ann. Intern. Med.* **100**, 543–557.

Brouet, J. C., Flandrin, G., and Seligmann, M. (1973) Indications of the thymus-derived nature of the proliferating cells in six patients with Sezary's syndrome. *N. Engl. J. Med.* **289**, 341–344.

Brouet, J. C., Flandrin, G., Sasportes, M., Preud'Homme, J. L., and Seligmann, M. (1975) Chronic lymphocytic leukaemia of T-cell origin. Immunological and clinical evaluation in eleven patients. *Lancet* **ii**, 890–893.

Bunn, P. A. and Lamberg, S. I. (1979) Report of the Committee on Staging and Classification of Cutaneous T-cell Lymphomas. *Cancer Treat. Rep.* **63**, 725–736.

Bunn, P. A. Jr., Huberman, M. S., Whang-Peng, J., Schechter, G. P., Guccion, J. G., Matthews, M. J., et al. (1980) Prospective staging evaluation of patients with cutaneous T-cell lymphomas. Demonstration of a high frequency of extracutaneous dissemination. *Ann. Intern. Med.* **93**, 223–230.

Bunn, P. A. Jr., Schechter, G. P., Jaffe, E., Blayney, D., Young, R. C., Matthews, M. J., et al. (1983) Clinical course of retrovirus-associated adult T-cell lymphoma in the United States. *N. Engl. J. Med.* **309**, 257–264.

Burke, J. S. (1981) Surgical pathology of the spleen: an approach to the differential diagnosis of splenic lymphomas and leukemias. Diseases of the white pulp. Diseases of the red pulp. *Am. J. Surg. Pathol.* **5**, 681–694.

Burke, J. S. and Rappaport, H. (1984) The diagnosis and differential diagnosis of hairy cell leukemia in bone marrow and spleen. *Semin. Oncol.* **11**, 334–346.

Burke, J. S., Byrne, G. E., and Rappaport, H. (1974) Hairy cell leukemia (leukemic reticuloendotheliosis). A clinical pathologic study of 21 patients. *Cancer* **33**, 1399–1410.

Burke, J. S., Mackay, B., and Rappaport, H. (1976) Hairy cell leukemia (leukemic reticuloendotheliosis). Ultrastructure of the spleen. *Cancer* **37**, 2267–2274.

Burke, J. S., Sheibani, K., Winberg, C. D., and Rappaport, H. (1987) Recognition of hairy cell leukemia in a spleen of normal weight. *J. Clin. Pathol.* **87**, 276–281.

Burkitt, D. and O'Connor, G. T. (1961) Malignant lymphoma in African children. I. A clinical syndrome. *Cancer* **14**, 258–269.

Buskard, N. A., Catovsky, D., Okos, A., Goldman, J. M., and Galton, D. A. G. (1976) Prolymphocytic leukemia. *Hämatol. Bluttransfus.* **18**, 237–253.

Butler, J. J. (1983) Pathology of the spleen in benign and malignant conditions. *Histopathology* **7**, 453–474.

Byhardt, R. W., Brace, K. C., and Wiernik, P. H. (1975) The role of splenic irradiation in chronic lymphocytic leukemia. *Cancer* **35**, 1621–1625.

Cadman, E. C., Capizzi, R. L., and Bertino, J. R. (1977) Acute non-lymphocytic leukemia. A delayed complication of Hodgkin's disease therapy: analysis of 109 cases. *Cancer* **40**, 1280–1296.

Canellos, G., Anderson, J., Propert, K., Nissen, N., Cooper, M., Henderson, E., et al. (1992) Chemotherapy of advanced Hodgkin's disease with MOPP, ABVD, or MOPP alternating with ABVD. *N. Engl. J. Med.* **327**, 1478–1484.

Cappell, M. S. and Chow, J. (1987) HTLV-I-associated lymphoma involving the entire alimentary tract and presenting with an acquired immune deficiency. *Am. J. Med.* **82**, 649–654.

Carde, P., Manil, L., Da Costa, L., Pfreundschuh, M., Lumbroso, J., Saccavini, J.C., et al. (1988) Hodgkin's disease (Hodgkin's disease) and immunoscintigraphy (IS): use of anti-Reed-Sternberg cells H-RS-1 monoclonal antibody (Mab) in 9 patients (pts). *Proc. ASCO* **7**, 227.

Castellino, R. A., Hoppe, R. T., Blank, N., et al. (1984) Computed tomography, lymphography, and staging laparotomy: correlations in initial staging of Hodgkin's disease. *Am. J. Roentgenology* **143**, 37–41.

Castro-Malaspina, H., Najean, Y. and Flandrin, G. (1979) Erythrokinetic studies in hairy-cell leukaemia. *Br. J. Haematol.* **42**, 189–197.

Catovsky, D. (1977) Hairy-cell leukaemia and prolymphocytic leukaemia. *Clin. Haematol.* **6**, 245–268.

Catovsky, D., Pettit, J. E., Galton, D. A. G., Spiers, A. S. D., and Harrison, C. V. (1974) Leukaemic reticuloendotheliosis (hairy-cell leukaemia), a distinct clinico-pathological entity. *Br. J. Haematol.* **26**, 9–27.

Catovsky, D., Rose, M., Goolden, A. W. G., White, J. M., Bourikas, G., Brownell, A. I., et al. (1982) Adult T-cell lymphoma-leukaemia in blacks from the West Indies. *Lancet* **i**, 639–642.

Cawley, J. C., Burns, G. F., and Hayhoe, F. G. J. (1980) *Hairy Cell Leukaemia*, Springer-Verlag, Berlin.

Champlin, R., Gale, R. P., Foon, K. A., and Golde, D. W. (1986) Chronic leukemias: oncogenes, chromosomes, and advances in therapy. *Ann. Intern. Med.* **104**, 671–688.

Cheson, B. D., Bennett, J., Grever, M., Kay, N., Keating, M. J., O'Brien, S., and Rai, K. R. (1996) National Cancer Institute-sponsored working group guidelines for chronic lymphocytic leukemia: revised guidelines for diagnosis and treatment. *Blood* **87**, 4990–4997.

Chilcote, R. R., Baehner, R. L., and Hammond, D., Investigators and Special Studies Committee of the Children's Cancer Study Group (1976) Septicemia and meningitis in children splenectomized for Hodgkin's disease. *N. Engl. J. Med.* **295**, 798–800.

Christensen, B. E. (1973a) Erythrocyte pooling and sequestration in enlarged spleens. Estimations of splenic erythrocyte and plasma volume in splenomegalic patients. *Scand. J. Haematol.* **10**, 106–119.

Christensen, B. E. (1973b) The pattern of erythrocyte sequestration in immunohaemolysis. Effects of prednisone treatment and splenectomy. *Scand. J. Haematol.* **10**, 120–129.

Christensen, B. E., Hansen, M. M., and Videbaek, A. A. (1977) Splenectomy in chronic lymphocytic leukaemia. *Scand. J. Haematol.* **18**, 279–287.

Christensen, B. E., Kuld Hansen, L., Kvist Kristensen, J., and Videbaek, A. A. (1970) Splenectomy in haematology. Indications, results and complications in 41 cases. *Scand. J. Haematol.* **7**, 247–260.

Coiffier, B., Berger, F., Bryon, P. A., and Magaud, J. P. (1988) T cell lymphomas: immunologic, histologic, clinical and therapeutic analysis of 63 cases. *J. Clin. Pathol.* **6**, 1584–1589.

Cole, B., Solal-Celigny, P., and LePage, E. (1995) Interferon alpha for the treatment of advanced follicular lymphoma: an analysis of quality-of-life-adjusted survival. *Blood* **86**, 440a.

Comas, F. V., Andrews, G. A., and Nelson, B. (1968) Spleen irradiation in secondary hypersplenism. *Am. J. Roentgenol. Rad. Ther. Nucl. Med.* **104**, 668–673.

Come, S. E. and Chabner, B. A. (1979) Staging in non-Hodgkin's lymphoma: approach, results and relationship to histopathology. *Clin. Haematol.* **8**, 645–656.

Come, S. E., Jaffe, E. S., Andersen, J. C., Mann, R. B., Johnson, B. L., DeVita, V. T., and Young, R. C. (1980) Non-Hodgkin's lymphomas in leukemic phase: clinicopathologic correlations. *Am. J. Med.* **69**, 667–674.

Cooke, C.B., Krenacs, L., Stetler-Stevenson, M., Greiner, T.C., Raffeld, M., Kingma, D.W., et al. (1996) Hepatosplenic T-cell lymphoma: a distinct clinicopathologic entity of cytotoxic γδ T-cell origin. *Blood* **88**, 4265–4274.

Cooper, I. A., Ironside, P. N. J., Madigan, J. P., Morris, P. J., and Ewing, M. R. (1974) The role of splenectomy in the management of advanced Hodgkin's disease. *Cancer* **34**, 408–417.

Crosby, W. H. (1972) Splenectomy in hematologic disorders. *N. Engl. J. Med.* **286**, 1252–1254.

Cronin, C. C., Brady, M. P., Murphy, C., Kenny, E., Whelton, M. J. and Hardiman, C. (1994) Splenectomy in patients with undiagnosed splenomegaly. *Postgrad. Med. J.* **70**, 288–291.

Crossen, P. E., Mellor, J. E. L., Finley, A. G., Ravich, R. B. M., Vincent, P. C., and Gunz, F. W. (1971) The Sezary syndrome. *Am. J. Med.* **50**, 24–34.

Dacie, J. V., Brain, M. C., Harrison, C. V., Lewis, S. M., and Worlledge, S. M. (1969) Non-tropical idiopathic splenomegaly (primary hypersplenism): a review of ten cases and their relationship to malignant lymphomas. *Br. J. Haematol.* **17**, 317–333.

Dacie, J. V., Galton, D. A. G., Gordon-Smith, E. C., and Harrison, C. V. (1978) Non-tropical idiopathic splenomegaly: a follow-up study of ten patients described in 1969. *Br. J. Haematol.* **38**, 185–193.

Dailey, M. O., Coleman, C. N., and Kaplan, H. S. (1980) Radiation-induced splenic atrophy in patients with Hodgkin's disease and non-Hodgkin's lymphomas. *N. Engl. J. Med.* **302**, 215–217.

Dailey, M. O., Coleman, C. N., and Fajardo, L. F. (1981) Splenic injury caused by therapeutic irradiation. *Am. J. Surg. Pathol.* **5**, 325–331.

Dameshek, W. S. and Estren, S. (1947) *The Spleen and Hypersplenism.* Grune and Stratton, New York.

Dameshek, W. and Gunz, I. (1964) *Leukemia*, 2nd ed. Grune and Stratton, New York.

Dearth, J. C., Gilchrist, G. S., Telander, R. L., O'Connell, M. J., and Weiland, L. H. (1978) Partial splenectomy for staging Hodgkin's disease: risk of false-negative results. *N. Engl. J. Med.* **299**, 345–346.

Del Regato, J. A. (1974) Total body irradiation in the treatment of chronic lymphogenous leukemia. *Am. J. Roentgenol. Rad. Ther. Nucl. Med.* **120**, 504–520.

Desser, R. K., Moran, E. M., and Ultmann, J. E. (1973) Staging of Hodgkin's disease and lymphoma. *Med. Clin. North Am.* **57**, 479–498.

DeVita, V. T. Jr., Bagley, C. M., Goodell, B., O'Kieffe, D. A., and Trujillo, N. P. (1971) Peritoneoscopy in the staging of Hodgkin's disease. *Cancer Res.* **31**, 1746–1750.

De Wolf-Peeters, C. and Pittaluga, S. (1994) Mantle-cell lymphoma. *Ann. Oncol.* **5(Suppl. 1)**, S35–S37.

Dickerman, J. D. (1979) Splenectomy and sepsis: a warning. *Pediatrics* **63**, 938–941.

Dickerman, J. D. and Clements, J. P. (1975) Abnormal spleen scan following MOPP therapy in a patient with Hodgkin's disease: case report. *J. Nucl. Med.* **16**, 457–458.

Dighiero, G., Charron, D., Debre, P., Le Porrier, M., Vaugier, G., Follezou, J. Y., et al. (1979) Identification of a pure splenic form of chronic lymphocytic leukaemia. *Br. J. Haematol.* **41**, 169–176.

Duggan, M. J., Weisenburger, D. D., Ye, Y. L., Bast, M. A., Pierson, J. L., Linder, J., and Armitage, J. O. (1990) Mantle zone lymphoma. A clinicopathologic study of 22 cases. *Cancer* **66**, 522.

Earl, H. M., Sutcliffe, S. B. J., Fry, I. K., Tucker, A. K., Young, J., Husband, T., Wrigley, P. F. M., and Malpas, J. S. (1980) Computerized tomographic (CT) abdominal scanning in Hodgkin's disease. *Clin. Radiol.* **31**, 149–153.

Edelson, R. L., Kirkpatrick, C. H., Shevach, E. M., Schein, P. S., Smith, R. W., Green, I., and Lutzner, M. (1974) Preferential cutaneous infiltration by neoplastic thymus-derived lymphocytes. *Ann. Intern. Med.* **80**, 685–692.

El'Agnaf, M. R., Ennis, K. E., Morris, T. C., Robertson, J. H., Markey, G., and Alexander, H. D. (1986) Successful remission induction with deoxycoformycin in elderly patients with T-helper prolymphocytic leukaemia. *Br. J. Haematol.* **63**, 93–104.

Ell, P. J., Britton, K. E., Farrer-Brown, G., Keeling, D. H., Jelliffe, A. M., and Wood, T. P. (1975) An assessment of the value of spleen scanning in the staging of Hodgkin's disease. *Br. J. Radiol.* **48**, 590–593.

Emile, J. F., Boulland, M. L., Haioun, C., Kanavaros, P., Petrella, T., Delfau-Larue, M. H., et al. (1996) CD5⁻ CD56⁺ T-cell receptor silent peripheral T-cell lymphomas are natural killer cell lymphomas. *Blood* **87**, 1466.

Engelhard, M., Brittinger, G., Huhn, D., Gerhartz, H. H., Meusers, P., Siegert, W., et al. (1997) Subclassification of diffuse large B-cell lymphomas according to the Kiel Classification: distinction of centroblastic and immunoblastic lymphomas is a significant prognostic risk factor. *Blood* **89**, 2291–2297.

Enright, L. P., Trueblood, H. W., and Nelsen, T. S. (1970) The surgical diagnosis of abdominal Hodgkin's disease. *Surg. Gynecol. Obstet.* **130**, 853–858.

Essex, M. E., McLane, M. F., Tachibana, N., Francis, D. P., and Lee, T. H. (1984) Seroepidemiology of human T-cell leukemia virus in relation to immunosuppression and the acquired immunodeficiency syndrome. In: *Human T-cell Leukemia/Lymphoma Virus* (Gallo, R. C. and Cross. D. J., eds.), Cold Spring Harbor Laboratory, Cold Spring Harbor, NY, pp. 355-379.

Estey, E. H., Kurzrock, R., Kantarjian, H. M., O'Brien, S. M., McCredie, K. B., Beran, M., et al. (1992) Treatment of hairy cell leukemia with 2-chlorodeoxyadenosine (2-CdA). *Blood* **79**, 882–887.

Fahey, J. L., Sarna, G., Gale, R. P., and Seeger, R. (1987) Immune interventions in disease. *Ann. Intern. Med.* **106**, 257–274.

Falk, S. and Stutte, H. J. (1990) Primary malignant lymphomas of the spleen: a morphologic and immunohistochemical analysis of 17 cases. *Cancer* **66**, 2612–2619.

Farrer-Brown, G., Bennett, M. H., Harrison, C. V., Millett, Y., and Jelliffe, A. M. (1972) The diagnosis of Hodgkin's disease in surgically excised spleens. *J. Clin. Pathol.* **25**, 294–300.

Fausel, R., Sun, N. C. J., and Klein, S. (1990) Splenic rupture in a human immunodeficiency virus-infected patient with primary splenic lymphoma. *Cancer* **66**, 2414–2416.

Ferry, J. A., Yang, W. I., Zukerberg, L. R., Wotherspoon, A. C., Arnold, A., and Harris, N. L. (1996) CD5+ extranodal marginal zone B-cell (MALT) lymphoma: a low-grade neoplasm with a propensity for bone marrow involvement and relapse. *Am. J. Clin. Pathol.* **105**, 31–37.

Fieschi, A. and Sacchetti, C. (1964) Clinical assessment of granulopoiesis. *Acta Haematol.* **31**, 150–162.

Fisher, R., Gaynor, E., Dahlberg, S., Oken, M., Grogan, T., Urize, E., et al. (1993) Comparison of a standard regimen (CHOP) with three intensive chemotherapy regimens for advanced non-Hodgkin's lymphoma. *N. Engl. J. Med.* **328**, 1002.

Fisher, R. I., Dahlberg, S., Nathwani, B. N., Banks, P. M., Miller, T. P., and Grogan, T. M. (1995) Clinical analysis of two indolent lymphoma entities: mantle cell lymphoma and marginal zone lymphoma (including the mucosa-associated lymphoid tissue and monocytoid B-cell subcategories). A Southwest Oncology Group study. *Blood* **85**, 1075–1082.

Fisher, R. I., Press, O. W., Miller, T. P., and Grogan, T. M. (1996) Clinical course and therapy of mantle cell lymphoma. *PPO Updates* **10**, 1–7.

Flandrin, G., Daniel, M. T., Fourcade, M. and Chelloul, N. (1973) Leucemie à 'tricholeucocyte' (hairy cell leukemia). Etude clinique et cytologique de 55 observations. *Nouv. Rev. Fr. Hematol.* **13**, 609–640.

Flandrin, G., Sigaux, F., Sebahoun, G., and Bouffette, P. (1984) Hairy cell leukemia: clinical presentation and follow-up of 211 patients. *Semin. Oncol.* **11**, 458–471.

Foucar, K. (1992) B cell chronic lymphocytic and prolymphocytic leukemia. In: *Neoplastic Hematopathology* (Knowles, D. M., ed.), Williams & Wilkins, Baltimore, pp. 1181–1208.

Franklin, E. C. (1975) μ-chain disease. *Arch. Intern. Med.* **135**, 71–72.

Franklin, E. C., Lowenstein, J., Bigelow, B., and Meltzer, M. (1964) Heavy chain disease: a new disorder of serum γ-globulins. *Am. J. Med.* **37**, 332–350.

Freedman, A. S., Munro, J. M., Morimoto, C., McIntyre, B. W., Rhynhart, K., Lee, N., and Nadler, L. M. (1992) Follicular non-Hodgkin's lymphoma cell adhesion to normal germinal centers and neoplastic follicles involves very late antigen-4 and vascular cell adhesion molecule-1. *Blood* **79**, 206–212.

Frick, M. P., Feinberg, S. B., and Loken, M. K. (1981) Noninvasive spleen scanning in Hodgkin's disease and non-Hodgkin's lymphoma. *Comput. Tomogr.* **5**, 73–80.

Gall, E. A. and Mallory, T. B. (1942) Malignant lymphoma: a clinicopathologic survey of 618 cases. *Am. J. Pathol.* **18**, 381–415.

Gallo, R. C. (1981) Kyoto workshop on some specific recent advances in human tumor virology (meeting report). *Cancer Res.* **41**, 4738–4739.

Gallo, R. C. (1984) Human T-cell leukemia-lymphoma virus and T cell malignancies in adults. *Cancer Surv.* **3**, 113–159.

Gallo, R. C. and Wong-Staal, F. (1982) Retroviruses as etiologic agents of some animal and human leukemias and lymphomas and as tools for elucidating the molecular mechanisms of leukemogenesis. *Blood* **60**, 545–557.

Gallo, R. C., Kalyanaraman, V. S., Sarngadharan, M. G., Sliski, A., Vonderheid, E. C., Maeda, M., et al. (1983) Association of the human type C retrovirus with a subset of adult T-cell cancers. *Cancer Res.* **43**, 3892–3899.

Galton, D. A., Catovsky, D., and Wiltshaw, E. (1978) Clinical spetrum of lymphoproliferative diseases. *Cancer* **42**, 901–910.

Galton, D. A. G., Goldman, J. M., Wiltshaw, E., Catovsky, D., Henry, K., and Goldenberg, G. J. (1974) Prolymphocytic leukaemia. *Br. J. Haematol.* **27**, 7–23.

Gaynor, E. R. and Fisher, R. I. (1998) CHOP therapy: has shorter-course therapy had an impact on lymphomas? *Cancer Invest.* **16**, 26–32.

Gentile, T. C., Uner, A. H., Hutchison, R. E., et al. (1994) CD3⁺, CD56⁺ aggressive variant of large granular lymphocyte leukemia [see comments]. *Blood* **84**, 2315.

Gibbs, W. N., Lofters, W. S., Campbell, M., Hanchard, B., LaGrenade, L., Cranston, B., et al. (1987) Non-Hodgkin lymphoma in Jamaica and its relation to adult T-cell leukemia-lymphoma. *Ann. Intern. Med.* **106**, 361–368.

Giffin, H. Z. (1921) Present status of splenectomy as a therapeutic measure. *Minn. Med.* **4**, 132–138.

Gill, P. G., Souter, R. G., and Morris, P. J. (1980) Results of surgical staging in Hodgkin's disease. *Br. J. Surg.* **67**, 478–481.

Gill, P. G., Souter, R. G., and Morris, P. J. (1981) Splenectomy for hypersplenism in malignant lymphomas. *Br. J. Surg.* **68**, 29–33.

Gilliland, B. C., Baxter, E., and Evans, R. S. (1971) Red-cell antibodies in Coombs'-negative hemolytic anemia. *N. Engl. J. Med.* **285**, 252–256.

Glatstein, E., Guernsey, J. M., Rosenberg, S. A., and Kaplan, H. S. (1969) The value of laparotomy and splenectomy in the staging of Hodgkin's disease. *Cancer* **24**, 709–718.

Glatstein, E., Trueblood, H. W., Enright, L. P., Rosenberg, S. A., and Kaplan, H. S. (1970) Surgical staging of abdominal involvement in unselected patients with Hodgkin's disease. *Radiology* **97**, 425–432.

Glazer, G. M., Axel, L., Goldberg, H. I., and Moss, A. A. (1981) Dynamic CT of the normal spleen. *Am. J. Roentgenol.* **137**, 343–346.

Glees, J. P., Barr, L. C., and McElwain, T. J. (1982) The changing role of staging laparotomy in Hodgkin's disease: a personal series of 310 patients. *Br. J. Surg.* **69**, 181–187.

Glees, J. P., Taylor, K. J., Gazet, J. C., Peckham, M. J., and McCready, V. R. (1977) Accuracy of grey-scale ultrasonography of liver and spleen in Hodgkin's disease and the other lymphomas compared with isotope scans. *Clin. Radiol.* **28**, 233–238.

Goffinet, D. R., Castellino, R. A., and Kim, H. (1973) Staging laparotomies in unselected previously untreated patients with non-Hodgkin's lymphomas. *Cancer* **32**, 672–681.

Goffinet, D. R., Glatstein, E., Fuks, Z., and Kaplan, H. S. (1976) Abdominal irradiation in non-Hodgkin's lymphomas. *Cancer* **37**, 2797–2806.

Goffinet, D. R., Warnke, R., Dunnick, N. R., Castellino, R., Glatstein, E., Nelson, T. S., et al. (1977) Clinical and surgical (laparotomy) evaluation of patients with non-Hodgkin's lymphomas. *Cancer Treat. Rep.* **61**, 981–992.

Golde, D. W. (1982) Therapy of hairy-cell leukemia. Editorial. (1982) *N. Engl. J. Med.* **307**, 495–496.

Goldthorn, J. F. and Schwartz, A. D. (1978) Poor protective effect of unregenerated splenic tissue to pneumococcal challenge after subtotal splenectomy. *Surg. Forum* **29**, 469–470.

Golomb, H. M. (1987) The treatment of hairy cell leukemia. *Blood* **69**, 979–983.

Golomb, H. M. and Vardiman, J. W. (1983) Response to splenectomy in 65 patients with hairy cell leukemia: an evaluation of spleen weight and bone marrow involvement. *Blood* **61**, 349–352.

Golomb, H. M., Catovsky, D., and Golde, D. W. (1978) Hairy cell leukemia. A clinical review based on 71 cases. *Ann. Intern. Med.* **89**, 677–683.

Golomb, H. M., Ratain, M. J., and Vardiman, J. W. (1986) Sequential treatment of hairy cell leukemia: a new role for interferon. In: *Important Advances in Oncology 1986* (DeVita, V. T., ed.), Lippincott, Philadelphia, pp. 311–321.

Goodman, G. E., Jones, S. E., Villar, H. V., Silverstein, M. E., Dabich, L., and Newcome, S. R. (1982) Surgical restaging of Hodgkin's disease. *Cancer Treat. Rep.* **66**, 751–757.

Goonewardene, A., Bourke, J. B., Ferguson, R., and Toghill, P. J. (1979) Splenectomy for undiagnosed splenomegaly. *Br. J. Surg.* **66**, 62–65.

Gootenberg, J. E., Ruscetti, F. W., Mier, J. W., Gazdar, A., and Gallo, R. C. (1981) Human cutaneous T-cell lymphoma and leukemia cell lines produce and respond to T-cell growth factor. *J. Exp. Med.* **154**, 1403–1418.

Gosselin, G. R., Hanlon, D. G., and Pease, G. L. (1956) Leukaemic reticuloendotheliosis. *Can. Med. Assoc. J.* **74**, 886–891.

Greaves, M. F. (1975) Clinical applications of cell surface markers. In: *Progress in Hematology* (Brown, E. B., ed.), Grune and Stratton, New York, pp. 255–303.

Greenall, M. J., Gough, M. H., and Kettlewell, M. G. (1983) Laparotomy in the investigation of patients with pyrexia of unknown origin. *Br. J. Surg.* **70**, 356–357.

Greenberger, J. S., Come, S. E., and Weichselbaum, R. R. (1979) Issues of controversy in radiation therapy and combined modality approaches to Hodgkin's disease. *Clin. Haematol.* **8**, 611–624.

Grever, M., Kopecky, K., Foucar, M. K., Head, D., Bennett, J. M., Hutchison, R. E., et al. (1995) Randomized comparison of pentostatin versus interferon alfa-2 in previously untreated patients with hairy cell leukemia: an intergroup study. *J. Clin. Oncol.* **13**, 974–981.

Griem, M. L., Moran, E. M., Ferguson, D. J., Mettler, F. A., and Griem, S. F. (1975) Staging procedures in mycosis fungoides. *Br. J. Cancer* **31(Suppl. II)**, 362–367.

Grillot-Courvalin, C., Vinci, G., Tsapis, A., Dokhelar, M. C., Vainchenker, W., and Brouet, J. C. (1986) The syndrome of T8 hyperlymphocytosis: variation in phenotype and cytotoxic activities of granular cells and evaluation of their role in associated neutropenia. *Blood* **69**, 1204–1210.

Gruss, H. J., Pinto, A., Duyster, J., Poppema, S., and Herrmann, F. (1997) Hodgkin's disease: a tumor with disturbed immunological pathways. *Immunol. Today* **18**, 156–163.

Hacker, J. F. III, Richter, J. E., Pyatt, R. S., and Fink, M. P. (1982) Hemorrhagic ascites: an unusual presentation of primary splenic lymphoma. *Gastroenterology* **83**, 470–473.

Halie, M. R., Thiadens, J., Eibergen, R., and van den Broek, A. A. (1978) Hodgkin's disease in the spleen: investigation of Hodgkin foci and areas for the immune response. *Virchows Arch.* **27**, 39–48.

Hamilton, P. J., Richmond, J., Donaldson, G. W., Williams, R., Hutt, M. S., and Lugumba, V. (1967) Splenectomy in 'big spleen disease'. *Br. Med. J.* **iii**, 823–825.

Hanaoka, M., Sasaki, M., Matsumoto, H., Tankawa, H., Yamabe, H., Tomimoto, K., et al. (1979) Adult T-cell leukemia. Histological classification and characteristics. *Acta Pathol. Jpn.* **29**, 723–738.

Hansen, M. M. (1973) Chronic lymphocytic leukaemia. Clinical studies based on 189 cases followed for a long time. *Scand. J. Haematol.* **18 (Suppl.)**, 3–286.

Hanson, C. A., Gribbin, T. E., Schnitzer, B., Schlegelmilch, J. A., Mitchell, B. S., and Stoolman, L. M. (1990) CD11c (LEU-M5) expression characterizes a B-cell chronic lymphoproliferative disorder with features of both chronic lymphocytic leukemia and hairy cell leukemia. *Blood* **76**, 2360–2367.

Harris, I. M., McAlister, J. M., and Prankerd, T. A. J. (1958) Splenomegaly and the circulating red cell. *Br. J. Haematol.* **4**, 97–102.

Harris, J. M. Jr., Tang, D. B., and Weltz, M. D. (1978) Diagnostic tests and Hodgkin's disease. *Cancer* **41**, 2388–2392.

Harris, N. L., Jaffe, E. S., Stein, H., Banks, P. M., Chan, J. K., Cleary, M. L., et al. (1994) A revised European-American classification of lymphoid neoplasms: a proposal from the International Lymphoma Study Group. *Blood* **84**, 1361–1392.

Haskell, C. M. (1981) Significance of splenic vascular invasion in Hodgkin's disease. [Letter]. *Lancet* **i**, 195–196.

Hattori, T., Uchiyama, T., Toibana, T., Takatsuki, K., and Uchino, H. (1981) Surface phenotype of Japanese adult T-cell leukemia cells characterized by monoclonal antibodies. *Blood* **58**, 645–647.

Haynes, B. F., Telen, M. J., Hale, L. P., and Denning, S. M. (1989) CD44-A molecule involved in leukocyte adherence and T cell activation. *Immunol. Today* **10**, 423.

Heifetz, L. J., Fuller, L. M., and Rodgers, R. W. (1980) Laparotomy findings in lymphangiogram-staged I and II non-Hodgkin's lymphomas. *Cancer* **45**, 2778–2786.

Henry-Amar, M., Friedman, S., Hayat, M., Somers, R., Meerwaldt, J.H., Carde, P., et al. EORTC Lymphoma Cooperative Group (1991) Erythrocyte sedimentation rate predicts early relapse and survival in early-stage Hodgkin disease. *Ann. Intern. Med.* **114**, 361–365.

Hermreck, A. S., Kofender, V. S., and Bell, C. (1975) The staging of Hodgkin's disease: preoperative clinical assessment versus operative evaluation. *Am. J. Surg.* **130**, 639–642.

Hiddemann, W., Longo, D. L., Coiffier, B., Fisher, R. I., Cabanillas, F., Cavalli, F., et al. (1996) Lymphoma classification: the gap between biology and clinical management is closing. *Blood* **88**, 4085–4089.

Hodgson, W. J. B. and McElhinney, A. J. (1982) Ultrasonic partial splenectomy. *Surgery* **91**, 346–348.

Hoffman, M. A., Janson, D., Rose, E., and Rai, K. R. (1997) Treatment of hairy-cell leukemia with cladribine: response, toxicity, and long-term follow-up. *J. Clin. Oncol.* **15**, 1138–1142.

Hofmann, V. (1985) Ultrasonic diagnosis of the spleen. *Progr. Pediatr. Surg.* **18**, 150–154.

Hollema, H., Visser, L., and Poppema, S. (1991) Small lymphocytic lymphomas with predominant splenomegaly: a comparison of immunophenotypes with cases of predominant lymphadenopathy. *Modern Pathol.* **4**, 712–717.

Hoppe, R. T., Horning, S. J., and Rosenberg, S. A. (1985) The concept, evolution and preliminary results of the current Stanford clinical trials for Hodgkin's disease. *Cancer Surv.* **4**, 459–475.

Hoppe, R. T., Cox, R. S., Rosenberg, S. A., and Kaplan, H. S. (1982) Prognostic factors in pathologic stage III Hodgkin's disease. *Cancer Treat. Rep.* **66**, 743–749.

Horn, N. L., Ray, G. R., and Kriss, J. P. (1976) Gallium-67 citrate scanning in Hodgkin's disease and non-Hodgkin's lymphoma. *Cancer* **37**, 250–257.

Hubbard, S. M., Chabner, B. A., DeVita, V. T., Simon, R., Berard, C. W., Jones, R. B., et al. (1982) Histologic progression in non-Hodgkin's lymphoma. *Blood* **59**, 258–264.

Imamura, N., Kusunoki, Y., Kawa-Ha, K., Yumura, K., Hara, J., Oda, K., et al. (1990) Aggressive natural killer cell leukaemia/lymphoma: report of four cases and review of the literature. Possible existence of a new clinical entity originating from the third lineage of lymphoid cells [see comments]. *Br. J. Haematol.* **75**, 49.

Ioachim, H. L., Cooper, M. C., and Hellman, G. C. (1985) Lymphomas in men at high risk for acquired immune deficiency syndrome (AIDS). *Cancer* **56**, 2831–2842.

Isaacson, P. and Wright, D. (1983) Malignant lymphoma of mucosa associated lymphoid tissue: a distinctive B cell lymphoma. *Cancer* **52**, 1410.

Jackson, H. Jr. and Parker, F. Jr. (1947) *Hodgkin's Disease and Allied Disorders.* Oxford University Press, New York.

Jaffe, E. S. (1996) Classification of natural killer (NK) cell and NK-like T-cell malignancies. *Blood* **87**, 1207–1210.

Jaffe, N., Paed, D. and Bishop, Y. M. M. (1970) The serum iron level, haematocrit, sedimentation rate and leucocyte alkaline phosphatase level in paediatric patients with Hodgkin's disease. *Cancer* **26**, 332–337.

Jaiyesimi, I. A., Kantarjian, H. M., and Estey, H. (1993) Advances in therapy for hairy cell leukemia. A review. *Cancer* **72**, 5–16.

Janicek, M., Kaplan, W., Neuberg, D., Canellos, G. P., Shulman, L. N., and Shipp, M. A. (1997) Early restaging gallium scans predict outcome in poor-prognosis patients with aggressive non-Hodgkin's lymphoma treated with high-dose CHOP chemotherapy. *J. Clin. Oncol.* **15**, 1631–1637.

Jansen, J. and Hermans, J. (1981) Splenectomy in hairy cell leukaemia: a retrospective multicenter analysis. *Cancer* **47**, 2066–2076.

Johnson, C. S., Rosen, P. J., and Sheehan, W. W. (1979) Acute lymphocytic leukemia manifesting as splenic rupture. *Am. J. Clin. Pathol.* **72**, 118–121.

Johnston, G., Benua, R. S., Teates, C. D., Edwards, C. L., and Kniseley, R. M. (1974) 67Ga-citrate imaging in untreated Hodgkin's disease: preliminary report of cooperative group. *J. Nucl. Med.* **15**, 399–403.

Johnston, J. B., Glazer, R. I., Pugh, L., and Israels, L. G. (1986) The treatment of hairy cell leukemia with 2-deoxycoformycin. *Br. J. Haematol.* **63**, 525–534.

Jones, P. A. E., Miller, F. M., Worwood, M., and Jacobs, A. (1972) Ferritinaemia in leukaemia and Hodgkin's disease. *Br. J. Cancer* **27**, 212–217.

Jones, S. E., Tobias, D. A., and Waldman, R. S. (1978) Computed tomographic scanning in patients with lymphoma. *Cancer* **41**, 480–486.

Jonsson, V., Videbaek, A., Axelsen, N. H., and Harboe, M. (1976) Mu chain disease in a case of chronic lymphocytic leukaemia and malignant histiocytoma. I. Clinical aspects. *Scand. J. Haematol.* **16**, 209–217.

Juliusson, G. and Lilliemark, J. (1992) Rapid recovery from cytopenia in hairy cell leukemia after treatment with 2-chloro-2-deoxyadenosine (2-CdA): relation to opportunistic infections. *Blood* **79**, 888–894.

Juliusson, G., Christiansen, I., Hansen, M. M., et al. (1996) Oral cladribine as primary therapy for patients with B-cell chronic lymphocytic leukemia. *J. Clin. Oncol.* **14**, 2160–2166.

Kadin, M. E., Glatstein, E., and Dorfman, R. F. (1971) Clinicopathologic studies of 117 untreated patients subjected to laparotomy for the staging of Hodgkin's disease. *Cancer* **27**, 1277–1294.

Kager, P. A., Rees, P. H., Manguyu, F. M., Bhatt, K. M., and Bhatt, S. M. (1983) Splenic aspiration: experience in Kenya. *Trop. Geogr. Med.* **35**, 125–131.

Kalter, S. P., Riggs, S. A., Cabanillas, F., Butler, J. J., Hagemeister, F. B., Mansell, P. W., et al. (1985) Aggressive non-Hodgkin's lymphomas in immunocompromised homosexual males. *Blood* **66**, 655–659.

Kalyanaraman, V. S., Sarngadharan, M. G., Robert-Guroff, M., Miyoshi, I., Golde, D., and Gallo, R. C. (1982) A new subtype of human T-cell leukemia virus (HTLV-II) associated with a T-cell variant of hairy cell leukemia. *Science* **218**, 571–573.

Kanzler, H., Kuppers, R., Hansmann, M. L., and Rajewsky, K. (1996) Hodgkin and Reed-Sternberg cells in Hodgkin's disease represent the outgrowth of a dominant tumor clone derived from (crippled) germinal center B cells. *J. Exp. Med.* **184**, 1495–1505.

Kaplan, H. S. (1970) On the natural history, treatment, and prognosis of Hodgkin's disease. *Harvey Lectures, 1968-9.* Academic, New York, pp. 215–259.

Kaplan, H. S. (1972) *Hodgkin's Disease*, Harvard University Press, Cambridge, MA.

Kaplan, H. S. (1980) Hodgkin's disease: unfolding concepts concerning its nature, management and prognosis. *Cancer* **45**, 2439–2474.

Katayama, I. and Finkel, H. E. (1974) Leukemic reticuloendotheliosis. A clinicopathologic study with review of the literature. *Am. J. Med.* **57**, 115–126.

Katz, S. and Schiller, M. (1980) Partial splenectomy in staging laparotomy for Hodgkin's disease. *Isr. J. Med. Sci.* **16**, 669–671.

Kawarada, Y., Goldberg, L., Brady, L., Pavlides, C., and Matsumoto, T. (1976) Staging laparotomy for Hodgkin's disease. *Am. Surg.* **42**, 332–345.

Kay, D. N. and McCready, V. R. (1972) Clinical isotope scanning using Ga citrate in the management of Hodgkin's disease. *Br. J. Radiol.* **45**, 437–444.

Kehoe, J. and Strauss, D. J. (1988) Primary lymphoma of the spleen: clinical features and outcome after splenectomy. *Cancer* **62**, 1433–1438.

Kettle, P., Morris, T. C. M., Markey, G. M., Alexander, H. D., Curry, R. C., Hayes, D., Cameron, C. H. S., and Toner, P. G. (1990) Tartrate resistant acid phosphatase positive splenic lymphoma: a relatively benign condition occurring in a time-space cluster? *J. Clin. Pathol.* **43**, 714–718.

Kim, H. and Dorfman, R. F. (1974) Morphological studies of 84 untreated patients subjected to laparotomy for the staging of the non-Hodgkin's lymphomas. *Cancer* **33**, 657–674.

King, D. J., Dawson, A. A., and Bayliss, A. P. (1985) The value of ultrasonic scanning of the spleen in lymphoma. *Clin. Radiol.* **36**, 473–474.

Kirschner, R. H., Abt, A. B., O'Connell, M. I. J., Sklansky, B. D., Greene, W. H., and Wiernik, P. H. (1974) Vascular invasion and hematogenous dissemination of Hodgkin's disease. *Cancer* **34**, 1159–1162.

Klaue, P., Eckert, P., and Kern, E. (1979) Incidental splenectomy: early and late postoperative complications. *Am. J. Surg.* **138**, 296–300.

Knowles, D. M., Chamulak, G. A., Subar, M., Burke, J. S., Dugan, M., Wernz, J., et al. (1988) Lymphoid neoplasia associated with the Acquired Immunodeficiency Syndrome (AIDS). *Ann. Intern. Med.* **108**, 744–753.

Kobrin, C. B., and Kwak, L. W. (1997) Development of vaccine strategies for the treatment of B-cell malignancies. *Cancer Invest.* **15**, 577–587.

Koga, T. and Morikawa, Y. (1975) Ultrasonographic determination of the splenic size and its clinical usefulness in various liver diseases. *Radiology* **115**, 157–161.

Kosmo, M. A. and Gale, R. P. (1987) Plasma cell leukemia. *Semin. Hematol.* **24**, 202–208.

Kraut, E. H., Bouroncle, B. A., and Grever, M. R. (1986) Low-dose deoxycoformycin in the treatment of hairy cell leukemia. *Blood* **68**, 1119–1122.

Krikorian, J. G., Portlock, C. S., and Mauch, P. M. (1986) Hodgkin's disease presenting below the diaphragm: a review. *J. Clin. Oncol.* **4,** 1551–1562.

Kung, P. C., Berger, C. L., Goldstein, G., LoGerfo, P., and Edelson, R. L. (1981) Cutaneous T-cell lymphomas: characterization by monoclonal antibodies. *Blood* **57,** 261–266.

Kuppers, R., Rajewsky, K., Zhao, M., Simons, G., Laumann, R., Fischer, R., and Hansmann, M. L. (1994) Hodgkin's disease: Hodgkin and Reed-Sternberg cells picked from histological sections show clonal immunoglobulin gene rearrangements and appear to be derived from B cells at various stages of development. *Proc. Natl. Acad. Sci. USA* **91,** 10,962–10,966.

Kurlander, R., Stein, R. S., and Roth, D. (1975) Hyperkalemia complicating splenic irradiation of chronic lymphocytic leukemia. *Cancer* **36,** 926–930.

Kyle, R. A. and Garton, J. P. (1987) The spectrum of IgM monoclonal gammopathy in 430 cases. *Mayo Clin. Proc.* **62,** 719–731.

Lampert, I. A. (1983) Splenectomy as a diagnostic technique. *Clin. Haematol.* **12,** 535–563.

Lampert, I., Catovsky, D., Marsh, G. W., Child, J. A., and Galton, D. A. (1980) The histopathology of prolymphocytic leukemia with particular reference to the spleen: a comparison with chronic lymphocytic leukemia. *Histopathology* **4,** 3–19.

Lampert, I. A., Pizzolo, G., Thomas, A., and Janossy, G. (1980) Immunohistochemical characterization of cells involved in dermatopathic lymphadenopathy. *J. Pathol.* **131,** 145–156.

Lamy, T. and Loughran, T. P. (1998) Large granular lymphocyte leukemia. *Cancer Control,* **5,** 25–33.

Lanzkowsky, P., Shende, A., Karayalcin, G., and Aral, I. (1976) Staging laparotomy and splenectomy: treatment and complications of Hodgkin's disease in children. *Am. J. Hematol.* **1,** 393–404.

Lardelli, P., Bookman, M. A., and Sundeen, J. (1990) Lymphocytic lymphoma of intermediate differentiation: morphologic, immunophenotypic sprectrum and clinical correlations. *Am. J. Surg. Pathol.* **14,** 752.

Larson, R. A. and Ultmann, J. E. (1982) The strategic role of laparotomy in staging Hodgkin's disease. *Cancer Treat. Rep.* **66,** 767–774.

Lauria, F., Benefenati, D., Zinzani, P. L., et al. (1991) 2-chlorodeoxyadenosine in the treatment of hairy cell leukemia patients relapsed after alpha interferon. *Blood* **78(Suppl. 1),** 34a (Abstract).

Le Bourgeois, J. P. and Tubiana, M. (1977) The erythrotyte sedimentation rate as a monitor for relapse in patients with previously treated Hodgkin's disease. *Int. J. Radiat. Oncol. Biol. Phys.* **2,** 241–247.

Le Bourgeois, J. P., Meignan, M. D., Parmentier, C., and Tubiana, M. (1979) Renal consequences of irradiation of the spleen in lymphoma patients. *Br. J. Radiol.* **52,** 56–60.

Leibenhaut, M. H., Hoppe, R. T., Varghese, A., and Rosenberg, S. A. (1987) Subdiaphragmatic Hodgkin's disease: laparotomy and treatment results in 49 patients. *J. Clin. Oncol.* **5,** 1050–1055.

Lennert, K. (1967) Classification of malignant lymphomas (European concept). In: *Progress in Lymphology* (Ruttimann, A., ed.), Thieme, Stuttgart, pp. 103–109.

Lennert, K. (1978) *Malignant Lymphomas Other Than Hodgkin's Disease: Histology, Cytology, Ultrastructure, Immunology.* Springer-Verlag, New York.

Leroux, D., Le Marc'hadour, F., and Gressin, R. (1991) Non-Hodgkin's lymphomas with t(11;14)(q13;q32): a subset of mantle zone/intermediate lymphocytic lymphoma? *Br. J. Haematol.* **77,** 346.

Letoquart, J. P., La Gamma, A., Kunin, N., Grosbois, B., Mambrini, A., and Leblay, R. (1993) Splenectomy for splenomegaly exceeding 1000 grams: analysis of 47 patients. *Br. J. Surg.* **80,** 334–335.

Levi, J. A. and Wiernik, P. H. (1977) The therapeutic implications of splenic involvement in stage IIIA Hodgkin's diease. *Cancer* **39,** 2158–2165.

Levi, J. A., O'Connell, M. J., Murphy, W. L., Sutherland, J. C., and Wiernik, P. H. (1975) Role of ^{67}gallium citrate scanning in the management of non-Hodgkin's lymphoma. *Cancer* **36,** 1690–1701.

Levine, A. M. and Gill, P. S. (1987) AIDS-related malignant lymphoma: clinical presentation and treatment approaches. *Oncology* **1,** 41–46.

Levine, A. M., Meyer, P. R., Begandy, M. K., Parker, J. W., Taylor, C. R., Irwin, L., and Lukes, R. J. (1984) Development of B-cell lymphoma in homosexual men. *Ann. Intern. Med.* **100,** 7–13.

Lewis, S. M., Catovsky, D., Hows, J. M., and Ardalan, B. (1977) Splenic red cell pooling in hairy cell leukaemia. *Br. J. Haematol.* **35,** 351–357.

Ligler, F. S., Smith, R. G., Kettman, J. R., Hernandez, J. A., Himes, J. B., Vitetta, E. S., Uhr, J. W., and Frenkel, E. P. (1980) Detection of tumor cells in the peripheral blood of nonleukemic patients with B cell lymphoma: analysis of 'clonal excess'. *Blood* **55,** 792–801.

Lindfors, K. K., Meyer, J. E., Palmer, E. L., and Harris, N. L. (1984) Scintigraphic findings in large-cell lymphoma of the spleen: concise communication. *J. Nucl. Med.* **25,** 969–971.

Lindgren, P. G., Hagberg, H., Eriksson, B., Glimelius, B., Magnusson, A., and Sundström, C. (1985) Excision biopsy of the spleen by ultrasonic guidance. *Br. J. Radiol.* **58,** 853–857.

LoBuglio, A. F., Cotran, R. S., and Jandl, J. H. (1967) Red cells coated with immunoglobulin C: binding and sphering by mononuclear cells in man. *Science* **158,** 1582–1585.

Long, J. C. and Aisenberg, A. C. (1974) Malignant lymphoma diagnosed at splenectomy and idiopathic splenomegaly. A clinicopathological comparison. *Cancer* **33,** 1054–1061.

Long, J. C. and Mihm, M. C. (1974) Mycosis fungoides with extracutaneous dissemination: a distinct clinicopathologic entity. *Cancer* **34,** 1745–1755.

Longo, D. L. (1995) The REAL classification of lymphoid neoplasms: one clinician's view. *PPO Updates* **9,** 1–12.

Lotz, M. J., Chabner, B., DeVita, V. T., Johnson, R. E., and Berard, C. W. (1976) Pathological staging of 100 consecutive untreated patients with non-Hodgkin's lymphomas. *Cancer* **37,** 266–270.

Loughran, T. (1993) Clonal diseases of large granular lymphocytes. *Blood* **82,** 1.

Loughran, T. P., Kadin, M. E., Starkebaum, G., Abkowitz, L., Clark, E. A., Dietsche, C., Lum, L. G., and Slichter, S. J. (1985) Leukemia of large granular lymphocytes: association with clonal chromosomal abnormalities and autoimmune neutropenia, thrombocytopenia and hemolytic anemia. *Ann. Intern. Med.* **102,** 169–175.

Lukes, R. J. (1971) Criteria for involvement of lymph node, bone marrow, spleen and liver in Hodgkin's disease. *Cancer Res.* **31,** 1755–1767.

Lukes, R. J. and Collins, R. D. (1974) Immunologic characterization of human malignant lymphomas. *Cancer* **34,** 1488–1503.

Lukes, R. J., Butler, J. J., and Hicks, E. B. (1966) Natural history of Hodgkin's disease as related to its pathologic picture. *Cancer* **19,** 317–344.

Lukes, R. J., Tindle, B. H., and Parker, J. W. (1969) Reed-Sternberg-like cells in infectious mononucleosis. [Letter]. *Lancet* **ii,** 1003–1004.

Lutzner, M., Edelson, R., Schein, P., Green, I., Kirkpatrick, C., and Ahmed, A. (1975) Cutaneous T-cell lymphomas: the Sezary syndrome, mycosis fungoides, and related disorders. Edited transcript of 1974 NIH conference. *Ann. Intern. Med.* **83,** 534–552.

MacDonald, H. R. (1995) NK1.1+ T cell receptor α/β + cells: new clues to their origin, specificity, and function. *J. Exp. Med.* **182,** 633.

MacKenzie, M. R. and Fudenberg, H. H. (1972) Macroglobulinemia: an analysis for forty patients. *Blood* **39,** 874–889.

Macon, W. R., Williams, M. E., Greer, J. P., Hammer, R. D., Glick, A. D., Collins, R. D., and Cousar, J. B. (1996) Natural killer-like T-cell lymphomas: aggressive lymphomas of T-large granular lymphocytes. *Blood* **87,** 1474.

MacRae, H. M., Yakimets, W. W., and Reynolds, T. (1992) Perioperative complications of splenectomy for hematologic disease. *Can. J. Surg.* **34,** 432–436.

Majlis, A., Pugh, W. C., Rodriguez, M. A, Benedict, W. F., and Cabanillas, F. (1997) Mantle cell lymphoma: correlation of clinical outcome and biologic features with three histologic variants. *J. Clin. Oncol.* **15,** 1664–1671.

Maloney, D. G., Grillo-Lòpez, A. J., White, C. A., Bodkin, D., Schilder, R. J., Neidhart, J. A., et al. (1997) IDEC-C2B8 (Rituximab) anti-CD20 monoclonal antibody therapy in patients with relapsed low-grade non-Hodgkin's lymphoma. *Blood* **90,** 2188–2195.

Mangan, K. F., Chikkappa, G., and Farley, P. C. (1982) T gamma cells suppress growth of erythroid colony-forming units in vitro in the pure red cell aplasia of B cell chronic lymphocytic leukemia. *J. Clin. Invest.* **70,** 1148–1156.

Mann, J. L., Hafez, G. R., and Longo, W. L. (1986) Role of the spleen in the transdiaphragmatic spread of Hodgkin's disease. *Am. J. Med.* **81,** 959–961.

Manoharan, A., Catovsky, D., Goldman, J. M., Lauria, F., Lampert, I. A., and Galton, D. A. G. (1980) Significance of splenomegaly in childhood acute lymphoblastic leukaemia in remission. *Lancet* **i,** 449–452.

Mason, D., Bastard, C., Rimokh, R., Dastugue, N., Huret, J. L., Kristoffersson, U., et al. (1990) CD30-positive large cell lymphomas ("Ki-1 lymphoma") are associated with a chromosomal translocation involving 5q35. *Br. J. Haematol.* **74,** 161–168.

Matas, A. J., Hertel, B. F., Rosai, J., Simmons, R. L., and Najarian, J. S. (1976) Post-transplant malignant lymphoma: distinctive morphologic features related to pathogenesis. *Am. J. Med.* **61,** 716–720.

Matutes, E., Morilla, R., Owusu-Ankomah, K., Houlihan, A., and Catovsky, D. (1994) The immunophenotype of splenic lymphoma with villous lymphocytes and its relevance to the differential diagnosis with other B-cell disorders. *Blood* **83,** 1558–1562.

Mauch, P., Greenberg, H., Lewin, A., Cassady, J. R., Weichselbaum, R., and Hellman, S. (1983) Prognostic factors in patients with subdiaphragmatic Hodgkin's disease. *Hematol. Oncol.* **1,** 205–214.

Maurer, R. (1985) The role of the spleen in leukemias and lymphomas including Hodgkin's disease. *Experientia* **41,** 215–222.

McCallister, B. D., Bayrd, E. D., Harrison, E. G. Jr., and McGuckin, W. F. (1967) Primary macroglobulinemia: a review with a report on thirty-one cases and notes on the value of continuous chlorambucil therapy. *Am. J. Med.* **43,** 394–434.

McCann, S. R., Whelan, C. A., Breslin, B., and Temperley, I. J. (1982) Lymphocyte subpopulations following splenic irradiation in patients with chronic lymphocytic leukaemia. *Br. J. Haematol.* **50,** 225–229.

McKenna, R. W., Arthur, D. C., Gajl-Peczalska, K. J., Flynn, P., and Brunning, R. D. (1985) Granulated T cell lymphocytosis with neutropenia: malignant or benign chronic lymphoproliferative disorder. *Blood* **66,** 259–266.

McKenna, W., Lampert, I., Oakley, C., and Goldman, J. (1979) Pel-Ebstein fever coinciding with cyclical haemolytic anaemia and splenomegaly in a patient with Hodgkin's disease. *Scand. J. Haematol.* **23,** 378–380.

Meijer, C. J. L. M., Albeda, F., van der Valk, P. Spaander, P. J., and Jansen, J. (1984) Immunohistochemical studies of the spleen in hairy-cell leukaemia. *Am. J. Pathol.* **115,** 266–274.

Melnyk, A., Rodriguez, A., Pugh, W. C., and Cabannillas, F. (1997) Evaluation of the revised European-American lymphoma classification confirms the clinical relevance of immunophenotype in 560 cases of aggresive non-Hodgkin's lymphoma. *Blood* **89,** 4514–4520.

Melo, J., Catovsky, D., and Galton, D. (1986) The relationship between chronic lymphocytic leukaemia and prolymphocytic leukaemia: I. clinical and laboratory features of 300 patients and characterization of an intermediate group. *Br. J. Haematol.* **63,** 377–387.

Melo, J. V., Hedge, U., Parreira, A., Thompson, I., Lampert, I. A., and Catovsky, D. (1987) Splenic B-cell lymphoma with circulating villous lymphocytes: differential diagnosis of B cell leukaemias with large spleens. *J. Clin. Pathol.* **40,** 642–651.

Mercieca, J., Matutes, E. Dearden, C., MacLennan, K., and Catovsky, D. (1994) The role of pentostatin in the treatment of T-cell malignancies: analysis of response rate in 145 patients according to disease subtype. *J. Clin. Oncol.* **12,** 2588–2593.

Merl, S. A., Theodorakis, M. E., Goldberg, J., and Gottlieb, A. J. (1983) Splenectomy for thrombocytopenia in chronic lymphocytic leukemia. *Am. J. Hematol.* **15,** 253–259.

Meugè, C., Hoerni, B., and De Mascarel, A. (1978) Non-Hodgkin malignant lymphomas. Clinicopathologic correlations with the Kiel classification. Retrospective analysis of a series of 274 cases. *Eur. J. Cancer* **14,** 587–592.

Milder, M. S., Larson, S. M., Bagley, C. M., DeVita, V. T., Johnson, R. E., and Johnston, G. S. (1973) Liver-spleen scan in Hodgkin's disease. *Cancer* **31,** 826–834.

Mintz, U. and Golomb, H. M. (1979) Splenectomy as initial therapy in 26 patients with leukemic reticuloendotheliosis (hairy cell leukemia). *Cancer Res.* **39,** 2366–2370.

Mitchell, A. and Morris, P. J. (1983) Surgery of the spleen. *Clin. Haematol.* **12,** 565–590.

Moeschlin, S. (1957) *Spleen Puncture.* Heinemann, London.

Mollejo, M., Menàrguez, J., Lloret, E., Sànchez, A., Campo, E., Algara, P., et al. (1995) Splenic marginal zone lymphoma: a distinctive type of low-grade B-cell lymphoma: a clinicopathological study of 13 cases. *Am. J. Surg. Pathol.* **19,** 1146–1157.

Moore, G. E., Stevens, R. E., Moore, E. E., and Aragon, G. E. (1983) Failure of splenic implants to protect against fatal postsplenectomy infection. *Am. J. Surg.* **146,** 413–414.

Moran, E. M., Ultmann, J. E., Ferguson, D. J., Hoffer, P. B., Ranniger, K., and Rappaport, H. (1975) Staging laparotomy in non-Hodgkin's lymphoma. *Br. J. Cancer* **31(Suppl. 2),** 228–236.

Moriarty, A. T., Schwenk, G. R., and Chua, G. (1993) Splenic fine needle aspiration in the diagnosis of lymphoreticular diseases: a report of four cases. *Acta Cytol.* **37,** 191–196.

Morris, P. J., Cooper, I. A., and Madigan, J. P. (1975) Splenectomy for haematological cytopenias in patients with malignant lymphomas. *Lancet* **ii,** 250–253.

Mulligan, S. P., Matutes, E., Dearden, C., and Catovsky, D. (1991) Splenic lymphoma with villous lymphocytes: natural history and response to therapy in 50 cases. *Br. J. Haematol.* **78,** 206–209.

Myers, T. J., Ikeda, Y., Schwartz, S., Pharmakidis, A. B., and Baldini, M. G. (1981) Primary splenic hairy cell leukemia: remission for 21 years following splenectomy. *Am. J. Hematol.* **11,** 299–303.

Naeim, F. and Smith, G. S. (1974) Leukemic reticuloendotheliosis. *Cancer* **34,** 1813–1821.

Nagasawa, A., Abe, T., and Nakagawa, T. (1981) Pure red cell aplasia and hypogammaglobulinemia associated with T cell chronic lymphocytic leukemia. *Blood* **57,** 1025–1031.

Nanba, K., Soban, E. J., and Bowling, M. C. (1977) Splenic pseudo sinuses and hepatic angiomatous lesions. *Am. J. Clin. Pathol.* **67,** 415–426.

Neal, T. F. Jr., Tefferi, A., Witzig, T. E., Su, J., Phyliky, R. L., and Nagorney, D. M. (1992) Splenectomy in advanced chronic lymphocytic leukemia: a single institution experience with 50 patients. *Am. J. Med.* **93,** 435–440.

Neubauer, A., Thiede, C., Morgner, A., Alpen, B., Ritter, M., Neubauer, B., et al. (1997) Cure of *Helicobacter pylori* infection and duration of remission of low-grade gastric mucosa-associated lymphoid tissue lymphoma. *J. Natl. Cancer Inst.* **89,** 1350–1355.

Newell, J. (1963) Splenic irradiation. *Clin. Radiol.* **14,** 20–27.

Newland, A. C., Catovsky, D., Linch, D., Cawley, J. C., Beverley, P., San Miguel, J. F., et al. (1984) Chronic T cell lymphocytosis: a review of 21 cases. *Br. J. Haematol.* **58,** 433–446.

Ngan, B. Y., Warnke, R. A., Wilson, M., Takagi, K., Cleary, M. L., and Dorfman, R. F. (1991) Monocytoid B-cell lymphoma: a study of 36 cases. *Hum. Pathol.* **22,** 409–421.

Nizze, H., Cogliatti, S., von Schilling, C., Feller, A. C., and Lennert, K. (1991) Monocytoid B-cell lymphoma: morphological variants and relationship to low-grade B-cell lymphoma of the mucosa-associated lymphoid tissue. *Histopathology* **18,** 403–414.

Norton, A. J., Matthews, J., Pappa, V., Shamash, J., Love, S., Rohatiner, A. Z. S., and Lister, T. A. (1995) Mantle cell lymphoma: natural history defined in a serially biopsied population over a 20-year period. *Ann. Oncol.* **6,** 249-256.

O'Connell, M. J., Schimpff, S. C., Kirschner, R. H., Abt, A. B., and Wiernik, P. H. (1975) Epithelioid granulomas in Hodgkin disease. *JAMA* **233,** 886–890.

Ohno, T., Smir, B. N., Weisenburger, D. D., Gascoyne, R. D., Hinrichs, S. D., and Chan, W. C. (1998) Origin of the Hodgkin/Reed-Sternberg cells in chronic lymphocytic leukemia with "Hodgkin's transformation". *Blood* **91,** 1757–1761.

Osadchaya, T. I., Vasilo, N. I., and Baisogolov, G. D. (1980) Diagnosis of splenic involvement in Hodgkin's disease by radionuclide evaluation of splenic contraction in response to adrenaline. *J. Nucl. Med.* **21,** 384–386.

Oscier, D. G., Matutes, E., Gardiner, A., Glide, S., Mould, S., Brito-Babapulle, V., Ellis, J., and Catovsky, D. (1993) Cytogenetic studies in splenic lymphoma with villous lymphocytes. *Br. J. Haematol.* **85,** 487–491.

Palutke, M., Eisenberg, L., Narang, S., Han, L. L., Peeples, T. C., Kukuruga, D. L., and Tabaczka, P. M. (1988) B lymphocytic lymphoma (large cell) of possible splenic marginal zone origin presenting with prominent splenomegaly and unusual cordal red pulp distribution. *Cancer* **62,** 593–600.

Pandolfi, F., Mandelli, F., Semenzato, G., Ranucci, A., and Aiuti, F. (1984) Classification of patients with T-cell chronic lymphocytic leukemia and expansions of granular lymphocytes: heterogeneity of Italian cases by a multiparameter analysis. *J. Clin. Immunol.* **4,** 174.

Pandolfi, F., Loughran, T. P., Starkebaum, G., Chisesi, T., Barbui, T., Chan, W. C., et al. (1990) Clinical course and prognosis of the lymphoproliferative disease of granular lymphocytes: a multicenter study. *Cancer* **65,** 341–348.

Parmentier, C., Chauvel, P., Hayat, M., Bok, B., and Tubiana, M. (1974) La radiothérapie dans la leucémie lymphoide chronique: l'irradiation splenique. *Nouv. Rev. Fr. Hématol.* **14,** 735–754.

Paule, B. and Cosset, J. M. (1985) Radiosensitivity of lymphocytes. Possible therapeutic impact. *Biomed. Pharmacother.* **39,** 467–472.

Paule, B., Cosset, J. M., and Le Bourgeois, J. P. (1985) The possible role of radiotherapy in chronic lymphocytic leukaemia. A critical review. *Radiother. Oncol.* **4,** 45–54.

Pearson, H. A. (1980) Splenectomy: its risks and its roles. *Hosp. Pract.* **15,** 85–94.

Penn, I. (1990) Principles of tumor immunity: immunocompromised patients. *AIDS Updates* **6,** 1–14.

Picker, L. J., Nakache, M., and Butcher, E. C. (1989) Monoclonal antibodies to human lymphocyte homing receptors define a novel class of adhesion molecules on diverse cell types. *J. Cell. Biol.* **109,** 927.

Piekarski, J., Federle, M. P., Moss, A. A., and London, S. S. (1980) Computed tomography of the spleen. *Radiology* **135,** 683–689.

Pilon, V. A., Davey, F. R., and Gordon, G. B. (1981) Splenic alterations in hairy cell leukemia. *Arch. Pathol. Lab. Med.* **105,** 577–581.

Pilon, V. A., Davey, F. R., and Gordon, G. B. (1982) Splenic alterations in hairy cell leukemia: an electron microscopic study. *Cancer* **49,** 1617–1623.

Pinto, R. G. W., Rocha, P. D., and Vernekar, J. A. (1995) Fine needle aspiration of the spleen in hairy cell leukemia: a case report. *Acta Cytol.* **39,** 777–780.

Piro, L. D., Carrera, C. J., Carson, D. A., Beutler, E. (1990) Lasting remissions in hairy cell leukemia induced by a single transfusion of 2-chlorodeoxyadenosine. *N. Engl. J. Med.* **322,** 1117–1121.

Pirofsky, B. (1969) In: *Autoimmunization and the Autoimmune Hemolytic Anemias,* Williams & Wilkins, Baltimore, p. 37.

Pittaluga, S., Wlodarska, I., Stul, M. S., Thomas, J., Verhoef, G., Cassiman, J. J., Van den Berghe, H., and De Wolf-Peeters, C. (1995) Mantle cell lymphoma: a clinicopathological study of 55 cases. *Histopathology* **26,** 17–24.

Pittaluga, S., Verhoef, G., Criel, A., Wlodarska, I., Dierlamm, J., Mecucci, C., Van den Berghe, H., and De Wolf-Peeters, C. (1996) "Small" B-cell non-Hodgkin's lymphomas with splenomegaly at presentation are either mantle cell lymphoma or marginal zone cell lymphoma. *Am. J. Surg. Pathol.* **20,** 211–223.

Plenderleith, I. H. (1970) Hairy cell leukaemia. *Can. Med. Assoc. J.* **102,** 1056–1060.

Plesnicar, S., Sumi-Kriznik, T., and Golouh, R. (1975) Abdominal lymphoma with alpha heavy chain disease. *Isr. J. Med. Sci.* **11,** 832–837.

Poiesz, B. J., Ruscetti, F. W., Gazdar, A. F., Bunn, P. A., Minna, J. D., and Gallo, R. C. (1980) Detection and isolation of type C retrovirus particles from fresh and cultured lymphocytes of a patient with cutaneous T-cell lymphoma. *Proc. Natl. Acad. Sci. USA* **77,** 7415–7419.

Praz, F., Karsenty, G., Binet, J. L., and Lesavre, P. (1984) Complement alternative pathway activation by chronic lymphocytic leukemia cells: its role in their hepatosplenic localization. *Blood* **63,** 463–467.

Prince, H. M., Bashford, J., and van der Weyden, M. B. (1992) CD5[+], CD11C[+], trap-positive chronic lymphocytic leukemia/prolymphocytic leukemia. *Blood* **80,** 1095–1096.

Rai, K. R., Sawitsky, A., Cronkite, E. P., Chanana, A. D., Levy, R. N., and Pasternack, B. S. (1975) Clinical staging of chronic lymphocytic leukemia. *Blood* **46,** 219–234.

Raich, P. C., Carr, R. M., Meisner, L. F., and Korst, D. R. (1975) Acute granulocytic leukemia in Hodgkin's disease. *Am. J. Med. Sci.* **269,** 237–241.

Ray, G. R., Wolf, P. H., and Kaplan, H. S. (1973) Value of laboratory indicators in Hodgkin's disease: preliminary results. *Nat. Cancer Inst. Monogr.* **36,** 315–323.

Redman, H. C., Glatstein, E., Castellino, R. A., and Federal, W. A. (1977) Computed tomography as an adjunct in the staging of Hodgkin's disease and non-Hodgkin's lymphomas. *Radiology* **124,** 381–385.

Risdall, R., Hoppe, R. T., and Warnke, R. (1979) Non-Hodgkin's lymphoma: a study of the evolution of the disease based upon 92 autopsied cases. *Cancer* **44,** 529–542.

Rogers, J. S. II and Shah, S. (1980) Spontaneous splenic rupture in plasma cell leukemia. *Cancer* **46,** 212–214.

Roggero, E., Zucca, E., and Cavalli, F. (1997) Gastric mucosa-associated lymphoid tissue lymphomas: more than a fascinating model (editorial). *J. Natl. Cancer Inst.* **89,** 1328–1330.

Rosen, P. R., Lasher, J. C., Weiland, R. L., and Kopp, D. T. (1982) Predicting splenic abnormality in Hodgkin disease using volume response to epinephrine administration. *Radiology* **143,** 627–629.

Rosenberg, S. A. (1988) Exploratory laparotomy and splenectomy for Hodgkin's disease: a commentary. *J. Clin. Oncol.* **6,** 574–575.

Rosenberg, S. A. and Kaplan, H. S. (1966) Evidence for an orderly progression in the spread of Hodgkin's disease. *Cancer Res.* **26,** 1225–1231.

Rosenberg, S. A. and Kaplan, H. S. (1970) Hodgkin's disease and other malignant lymphomas. *Calif. Med.* **113,** 23–38.

Rosenberg, S. A., Ribas-Mundo, M., and Goffinet, D. R. (1978) Staging in adult non-Hodgkin's lymphomas. *Rec. Res. Cancer Res.* **65,** 51–57.

Rosenberg, S. A., Diamond, H. D., Jaslowitz, B., and Craver, L. F. (1961) Lymphosarcoma: a review of 1269 cases. *Medicine* **40,** 31–84.

Rosenberg, S. A., Berard, C. W., Brown, B. W., Burke, J., Dorfman, R. F., Glatstein, E., Hoppe, R. T., and Simon, R. (1982) NC1-sponsored study of classification of non-Hodgkin's lymphomas: summary and description of a working formulation for clinical usage. *Cancer* **49,** 2112–2135.

Rosier, R. P. and Lefer, L. G. (1977) Spontaneous rupture of the spleen in hairy cell leukemia. Letter to the Editor. *Arch. Pathol. Lab. Med.* **101,** 557.

Rosove, M. H., Naeim, F., Harwig, S., and Zighelboim, J. (1980) Severe platelet dysfunction in hairy cell leukemia with improvement after splenectomy. *Blood* **55,** 903–906.

Rosso, R., Neiman, R. S., Paulli, M., Boveri, E., Kindl, S., Magrini, U., and Barosi, G. (1995) Splenic marginal zone cell lymphoma: report of an indolent variant without massive splenomegaly presumably representing an early phase of the disease. *Hum. Pathol.* **26,** 38–46.

Rubin, A. D., Douglas, S. D., Chessin, L. N., Glade, P. R., and Dameshek, W. (1969) Chronic reticulolymphocytic leukemia. Reclassification of 'leukemic reticuloendotheliosis' through functional characterization of the circulating mononuclear cells. *Am. J. Med.* **47,** 149–162.

Sacks, E. L., Donaldson, S. S., Gordon, J., and Dorfman, R. F. (1978) Epithelioid granulomas associated with Hodgkin's disease. *Cancer* **41,** 562–567.

Sagar, V. V., DelDuca, V. Jr., and Mecklenburg, R. L. (1979) Spleen scan in histiocytic lymphoma: response to therapy. *Clin. Nucl. Med.* **4,** 18–19.

Salgado, C., Feliu, E., Montserrat, E., Villamor, N., Ordi, J., Aguilar, J. L., Vives-Corrons, J. L., and Rozman, C. (1993) B-type large-cell primary splenic lymphoma with massive involvement of the red pulp. *Acta Haematol.* **89,** 46–49.

Salloum, E., Brandt, D. S., Caride, V. J., Cornelius, E., Zelterman, D., Schubert, W., Mannino, T., and Copper, D. L. (1997) Gallium scans in the management of patients with Hodgkin's disease: a study of 101 patients. *J. Clin. Oncol.* **15,** 518–527.

Salzman, J. R. and Kaplan, H. S. (1971) Effect of prior splenectomy on hematologic tolerance during total lymphoid radiotherapy of patients with Hodgkin's disease. *Cancer* **27,** 471–478.

Sander, C. A., Yano, T. Clark, H. M., Harris, C., Longo, D. L., Jaffe, E. S., and Raffeld, M. (1993) P53 mutation is associated with progression in follicular lymphomas. *Blood* **82,** 1994–2004.

Satoh, T., Yamada, T., Nakano, S., Tokunaga, O., Kuramochi, S., Kanai, T., Ishikawa, H., and Ogihara, T. (1997) The relationship between primary splenic malignant lymphoma and chronic liver disease associated with hepatitis C virus infection. *Cancer* **80,** 1981–1988.

Saven, A., Piro, L. D., Carrera, C. J., Carson, D. A., Beutler, E. (1993) Hairy cell leukemia: new understanding of biology and treatment. *Cancer Treat. Res.* **64,** 15–34.

Saven, A., Emanuele, S., Kosty, M., Koziol, J., Ellison, D., and Piro, L. (1995) 2-chlorodeoxyadenosine activity in patients with untreated, indolent non-Hodgkin's lymphoma. *Blood* **86,** 1710–1716.

Sawamura, M., Yamaguchi, S., Murakami, H., Amagai, H., Matsushima, T., Tamura, J., Naruse, T., and Tsuchiya, J. (1994) Multiple autoantibody production in a patient with splenic lymphoma. *Ann. Hematol.* **68,** 251–254.

Schaefer, H. E., Hellriegel, K. P., Zach, J., and Fischer, R. (1975) Zytochemischer Polymorphismus der sauren phosphatase bei Haarzell-Leukamie. *Blut* **31,** 365–370.

Schiffer, C. A., Levi, J. A., and Wiernik, P. H. (1975) The significance of abnormal circulating cells in patients with Hodgkin's disease. *Br. J. Haematol.* **31,** 177–183.

Schmid, C., Kirkham, N., Diss, T., and Isaacson, P. G. (1992) Splenic marginal zone cell lymphoma. *Am. J. Surg. Pathol.* **16,** 455–466.

Schmitt, G. T., Mathiot, C., and Louvel, A. (1981) Rupture spontanée de rate au cours des leucémies a tricholeucocytes. Deux observations. *Nouv. Presse Med.* **10,** 257–259.

Schrek, R. and Donnelly, W. J. (1966) Hairy cells in blood in lymphoreticular neoplastic disease and flagellated cells of normal lymph nodes. *Blood* **27,** 199–211.

Scott, J. L., McMillan, R., Davidson, J. G., and Marino, J. V. (1971) Leukocyte labelling with 51-chromium. II. Leukocyte kinetics in chronic myelocytic leukemia. *Blood* **38,** 162–173.

Seabold, J. E., Votaw, M. L., Keyes, J. W., Foley, W. D., Balachandran, S., and Gill, S. P. (1976) Gallium citrate (Ga 67) scanning. *Arch. Intern. Med.* **136,** 1370–1374.

Seligmann, M., Preud'Homme, J. L., and Brouet, J. C. (1973) B and T cell markers in human proliferative blood diseases and primary immunodeficiencies, with special reference to membrane bound immunoglobulins. *Transplant. Rev.* **16,** 85–113.

Seligmann, M., Danon, F., Hurez, D., Mihaesco, E., and Preud'Homme, J. L. (1968) Alpha chain disease: a new immunoglobulin abnormality. *Science* **162,** 1396–1397.

Semenzato, G., Zambello, R., Starkebaum, G., Oshimi, K., and Loughran, T. P. (1997) Lymphoproliferative disease of granular lymphocytes: updated criteria for diagnosis. *Blood* **89,** 256–260.

Senn, N. (1903) Case of spleno-medullary leukemia successfully treated by use of roentgen ray. *Med. Rec. New York* **63,** 281.

Sextro, M., Lieberz, D., Tesch, H., and Diehl, V. (1997) Liver involvement in Hodgkin's disease (Hodgkin's disease). An analysis of 99 consecutive cases. *Proc. ASCO* **16,** 8a.

Seymour, J. F., Cusack, J. D., Lerner, S. A., Pollock, R. E., and Keating, M. J. (1997) Case/control study of the role of splenectomy in chronic lymphocytic leukemia. *J. Clin. Oncol.* **15,** 52–60.

Sharp, R. A. and MacWalter, R. S. (1983) A role for splenic irradiation in the treatment of hairy-cell leukaemia. *Acta Haematol.* **70,** 59–62.

Shimoyama, M., Abe, T., Miyamoto, K., Minato, K., Tobinai, K., Nagoshi, H., et al. (1987) Chromosome aberrations and clinical features of adult T cell leukemia-lymphoma not associated with human T cell leukemia virus type I. *Blood* **69,** 984–989.

Shimoyama, M., Minato, K., Tobinai, K., Nagai, M., Setoya, T., Watanabe, S., et al. (1983) Anti-ATLA (antibody to adult T-cell leukemia-lymphoma virus-associated antigen)-negative adult T-cell leukemia-lymphoma. *Jpn. J. Clin. Oncol.* **13(Suppl. 2),** 245–376.

Shipley, W. U., Piro, A. J., and Hellman, S. (1974) Radiation therapy of Hodgkin's disease: significance of splenic involvement. *Cancer* **34,** 223–229.

Siler, J., Hunter, T. B., Weiss, J., and Haber, K. (1980) Increased echogenicity of the spleen in benign and malignant disease. *Am. J. Roentgenol.* **134,** 1011–1014.

Silverman, S., DeNardo, G. L., Glatstein, E., and Lipton, J. J. (1972) Evaluation of the liver and spleen in Hodgkin's disease. II. The value of splenic scintigraphy. *Am. J. Med.* **52,** 362–366.

Singer, D. B. (1973) Postsplenectomy sepsis. In: *Perspectives in Pediatric Pathology* (Rosenberg, H. S. and Bolande, R. P., eds.), Year Book, Chicago, pp. 285–305.

Singh, A. K., Bates, T., and Wetherley-Mein, G. (1986) A preliminary study of low-dose splenic irradiation for the treatment of chronic lymphocytic and prolymphocytic leukaemias. *Scand. J. Haematol.* **37,** 50–58.

Skarin, A. T. and Dorfman, D. M. (1997) Non-Hodgkin's lymphomas: current classification and management. *Ca. Cancer J. Clin.* **47,** 351–372.

Skarin, A. T., Davey, F. R., and Moloney, W. C. (1971) Lymphosarcoma of the spleen. Results of diagnostic splenectomy in 11 patients. *Arch. Intern. Med.* **127,** 259–265.

Smith, F. W. (1984) Prospects for tumour monitoring by nuclear magnetic resonance. *Rev. Endocr-Related Cancer* **17,** 25–30.

Smith, S. R., Martin, P. A., Davies, J. M., and Edwards, R. H. T. (1989) Characterization of the spleen by *in vivo* image guided ^{31}P magnetic resonance spectroscopy. *NMR Biomed.* **2,** 172–178.

Smithers, D. W. (1970) Spread of Hodgkin's disease. *Lancet* **i,** 1262–1267.

Smithers, D. W., Lillicrap, S. C., and Barnes, A. (1974) Patterns of lymph node involvement in relation to hypotheses about the modes of spread of Hodgkin's disease. *Cancer* **34,** 1779–1786.

Soederstroem, N. (1970) Cytologie der Milz in Punktaten. In: *Der Milz* (Lennert, K. and Harms, D., eds.), Springer-Verlag, Berlin.

Soederstroem, N. (1979) Cytology of infradiaphragmatic organs. 9. Spleen. *Monogr. Clin. Cytol.* **7,** 224–247.

Solal-Celigny, P., Brice, P., Brousse, H., Caspard, H., Bastion, Y., Haioun, C., et al. (1996) Phase II trial of fludarabine monophosphate as first-line treatment in patients with advanced follicular lymphoma: a multicenter study by the Group d'Etude des Lymphomes de l'Adulte. *J. Clin. Oncol.* **14,** 514–519.

Solbiati, L., Bossi, M. C., Bellotti, E., Ravetto, C., and Montali, G. (1983) Focal lesions in the spleen: sonographic patterns and guided biopsy. *Am. J. Roentgenol.* **140,** 59–65.

Spencer, R. P. and Knowlton, A. H. (1975) Radiocolloid scans in evaluating splenic response to external radiation. *J. Nucl. Med.* **16,** 123–126.

Spiegel, R. J. (1987) The alpha interferons: clinical overview. *Semin. Oncol.* **14(Suppl. 2),** 1–12.

Spiers, A. S. D., Parekh, S. J., and Bishop, M. B. (1984) Hairy cell leukemia: induction of complete remission with pentostatin (2-deoxycoformycin). *J. Clin. Oncol.* **2,** 1336–1342.

Spiers, A. S. D., Parekh, S. J., Ramnes, C. R., Cassileth, P. A., and Oken, M.M. (1985) Hairy cell leukemia (HCL): pentostatin (dcf, 2-deoxycoformycin) is effective both as initial treatment and after failure of splenectomy and alpha interferon. *Blood* **66,** 208.

Spiro, S., Galton, D. A., Wiltshaw, E., and Lohmann, R. C. (1975) Follicular lymphoma: a survey of 75 cases with special reference to the syndrome resembling chronic lymphocytic cell leukaemia. *Br. J. Cancer* **31(Suppl. 11),** 60–72.

Stahel, R. A., Maurer, R., and Cavalli, F. (1982) Idiopathische Splenomegalie: Vorstufe eines malignen Lymphoms? Bericht ueber zwei Falle. *Schweiz. Med. Wochenschr.* **112,** 725–730.

Stamenkovic, I., Amiot, M., Pesando, J. M., and Seed, B. (1989) A lymphocyte molecule implicated in lymph node homing is a member of the cartilage link protein family. *Cell* **56,** 1057.

Stansfeld, A. G., Diebold, J., Noel, H., Kapanci, Y., Rilke, F., Kelenyi, G., et al. (1988) Updated Kiel classification for lymphomas. *Lancet* **i,** 292–293.

Stein, R. S., Hilborn, R. M., Flexner, J. M., Bolin, M., Stroup, S., Reynolds, V., and Krantz, S. (1978) Anatomic substages of stage II Hodgkin's disease: implications for staging, therapy and experimental design. *Cancer* **42,** 429–436.

Stein, R. S., Golomb, H. M., Wiernik, P. H., Mauch, P., Hellman, S., Ultmann, J. E., Rosenthal, D. S., and Flexner, J. M. (1982) Anatomic substages of stage IIIA Hodgkin's disease: followup of a collaborative study. *Cancer Treat. Rep.* **66**, 733–741.

Stephens, P. J. T. and Hudson, P. (1969) Spontaneous rupture of the spleen in plasma cell leukemia. *Can. Med. Assoc. J.* **100**, 31–34.

Sterchi, J. M. and Myers, R. T. (1980) Staging laparotomy in Hodgkin's disease. *Ann. Surg.* **191**, 570–575.

Sterchi, J. M., Buss, D. H., and Beyer, F. C. (1984) The risk of improperly staging Hodgkin's disease with partial splenectomy. *Am. Surg.* **50**, 20–22.

Strauch, G. O. (1979) Accessory spleen in Hodgkin's disease. [Letter]. *JAMA* **241**, 1792–1793.

Straus, D. J., Filippa, D. A., and Lieberman, P. H. (1983) The non-Hodgkin's lymphomas. A retrospective clinical and pathologic analysis of 499 cases diagnosed between 1958 and 1969. *Cancer* **51**, 101–109.

Strijk, S. P., Wagener, D. J. T., Bogman, M. J. J. T., de Pauw, B. E., and Wobbes, T. (1985) The spleen in Hodgkin disease: diagnostic value of CT. *Radiology* **154**, 753–757.

Stroup, R. M., Burke, J. S., Sheibani, K., Ben-Ezra, J., Brownell, M., and Winberg, C. D. (1992) Splenic involvement by aggressive malignant lymphomas of B-cell and T-cell types. *Cancer* **69**, 413-420.

Strum, S. B., Allen, L. W., and Rappaport, H. (1971) Vascular invasion in Hodgkin's disease: its relationship to involvement of the spleen and other extranodal sites. *Cancer* **28**, 1329–1334.

Strum, S. B., Park, J. K., and Rappaport, H. (1970) Observation of cells resembling Sternberg-Reed cells in conditions other than Hodgkin's disease. *Cancer* **26**, 176–190.

Strumia, M. M., Strumia, P. V., and Bassert, D. (1966) Splenectomy in leukemia: hematologic and clinical effects on 34 patients and review of 299 published cases. *Cancer Res.* **26**, 519–528.

Sugarbaker, E. D. and Craver, L. F. (1940) Lymphosarcoma. Study of 196 cases with biopsy. *JAMA* **115**, 17–23.

Sun, T., Brody, J., Susin, M., Marino, J., Teichberg, S., Koduru, P., et al. (1993) Aggressive natural killer cell lymphoma/leukemia. A recently recognized clinicopathologic entity [see comments]. *Am. J. Surg. Pathol.* **17**, 1289.

Sutcliffe, S. B., Katz, D., Stansfeld, A. G., Shand, W. S., Wrigley, P. F. M., and Malpas, J. S. (1978) Post-treatment laparotomy in the management of Hodgkin's disease. *Lancet* **i**, 57–59.

Sutcliffe, S. B., Wrigley, P. F. M., Timothy, A. R., Dorreen, M. A., Shand, W. S., Stansfeld, A.G., et al. (1982) Post-treatment laparotomy as a guide to management in patients with Hodgkin's disease. *Cancer Treat. Rep.* **66**, 759–765.

Swerdlow, S. H., Habeshaw, J. A., Murray, L. J., Dhaliwal, H. S., Lister, T. A., and Stansfeld, A. G. (1983) Centrocytic lymphoma: a distinct clinicopathologic and immunologic entity: a multiparameter study of 18 cases at diagnosis and relapse. *Am. J. Pathol.* **113**, 181.

Swerdlow, S. H., Habeshaw, J. A, Rohatiner, A. Z., Lister, T. A., and Stansfeld, A. G. (1984) Caribbean T-cell lymphoma/leukemia. *Cancer* **54**, 687–696.

Swinnen, L. J., Costanzo-Nordin, M. R., Fisher, S. G., O'Sullivan, E. J., Johnson, M. R., Heroux, A. L., et al. (1990) Increased incidence of lymphoproliferative disorder after immunosuppression with the monoclonal antibody OKT3 in cardiac-transplant recipients. *N. Engl. J. Med.* **323**, 1723–1728.

Takatsuki, K., et al. (1982) Adult T-cell leukemia: proposal as a new disease and cytogenic, phenotypic, and functional studies of leukemic cells. *Gann Monogr.* **28**, 13–22.

Takatsuki, K., Yamaguchi, K., Kawano, F., Hattori, T., Nishimura, H., Tsuda, H., et al. (1985) Clinical diversity in adult T-cell leukemia lymphoma. *Cancer Res.* **45(Suppl.)**, 4644s–4645s.

Tallman, M. and Hakimian, D. (1995) Purine nucleoside analogs: emerging roles in indolent lymphoproliferative disorders. *Blood* **86**, 2463–2474.

Tallman, M. S., Hakimian, D., Variakojis, D., Koslow, D., Sisney, G. A., Rademaker, A. W., Rose, E., and Kaul, K. (1992) A single cycle of 2-chlorodeoxyadenosine results in complete remission in the majority of patients with hairy cell leukemia. *Blood* **80**, 2203–2209.

Terol, M. J., López-Guillermo, A., Bosch, F., Villamor, N., Cid, M. C., Rozman, C., Campo, E., and Montserrat, E. (1998) Expression of the adhesion molecule ICAM-1 in non-Hodgkin's lymphoma: relationship with tumor dissemniation and prognostic importance. *J. Clin. Oncol.* **16**, 35–40.

Non-Hodgkin's Lymphoma Classification Project (1982) National Cancer Institute sponsored study of non-Hodgkin's lymphomas: summary and description of a Working Formulation for clinical usage. *Cancer* **49**, 2112.

Non-Hodgkin's Lymphoma Classification Project (1997) Effect of age on the characteristics and clinical behavior of non-Hodgkin's lymphoma patients. *Ann. of Oncol.* **8**, 973–978.

Thieblemont, C., Bastion, Y., Berger, F., Rieux, C., Salles, G., Dumontet, C., Felman, P., and Coiffier, B. (1997) Mucosa-associated lymphoid tissue gastrointestinal and nongastrointestinal lymphoma behavior: analysis of 108 patients. *J. Clin. Oncol.* **15**, 1624–1630.

Thompson, J. A. and Fefer, A. (1987) Interferon in the treatment of hairy cell leukemia. *Cancer* **59(Suppl. 1)**, 605–609.

Traetow, D., Fabri, P. J., and Carey, L. C. (1980) Changing indications for splenectomy. *Arch. Surg.* **115**, 447–451.

Traub, A., Giebink, G. S., Smith, C., Kuni, C. C., Brekke, M. L., Edlund, D., and Perry, J. F. (1987) Splenic reticuloendothelial function after splenectomy, spleen repair, and spleen autotransplantation. *N. Engl. J. Med.* **317**, 1559–1564.

Tubiana, M., Hayat, M., Henry-Amar, M., Breur, K., van der Werf Messing, B., and Burgers, M. (1981) Five-year results of the E.O.R.T.C. randomized study of splenectomy and spleen irradiation in clinical stages I and II of Hodgkin's disease. *Eur. J. Cancer* **17**, 355–363.

Uchiyama, T., Yodoi, J., Sagawa, K., Takatsuki, K., and Uchino, H. (1977) Adult T-cell leukemia: clinical and hematologic features of 16 cases. *Blood* **50**, 481–492.

Uchiyama, T., Sagawa, K., Takatsuki, K., and Uchino, H. (1978) Effect of adult T-cell leukemia cells on pokeweed mitogen-induced normal B-cell differentiation. *Clin. Immunol. Immunopathol.* **10**, 24–34.

Uckun, F. M. (1990) Regulation of human B-cell ontogeny. *Blood* **76**, 1908–1923.

Uddstroemer, M. (1934) On the occurrence of lymphogranulomatosis (Sternberg) in Sweden, 1915-1931 and some considerations as to its relation to tuberculosis. *Acta Tuberc. Scand.* **(Suppl. 1)**, 1–225.

Urba, W. J. and Longo, D. L. (1985) Clinical spectrum of human retroviral-induced diseases. *Cancer Res.* **45(Suppl.)**, 4637s–4643s.

van Leeuwen, F. E., Somers, R., and Hart, A. A. M. (1987) Splenectomy in Hodgkin's disease and second leukemias. *Lancet* **ii**, 210–211.

Vandenberghe, E. (1994) Mantle cell lymphoma. *Blood Rev.* **8**, 79–87.

Variakojis, D., Rosas-Uribe, A., and Rappaport, H. (1974) Mycosis fungoides: pathologic findings in staging laparotomies. *Cancer* **33**, 1589–1600.

Videbaek, A. A., Christensen, B. E., and Jonsson, V. (1982) *The Spleen in Health and Disease*. FADL's FORLAG AS Yearbook, Copenhagen, Denmark.

Vincent, A. M., Burthem, J., Brew, R., and Cawley, J. C. (1996) Endothelial interactions of hairy cells: the importance of $\alpha 4\beta 1$ in the unusual tissue distribution of the disorder. *Blood* **88**, 3945–3952.

Vincent, P. C. (1977) Granulocyte kinetics in health and disease. *Clin. Haematol.* **6**, 695–717.

Waldman, I. and Suissa, L. (1978) Lymphosarcoma in an ectopic pelvic spleen. *Clin. Nucl. Med.* **3**, 417–419.

Wano, Y., Hattori, T., Matsuoka, M., Takatsuki, K., Chua, A. O., Gubler, U., and Greene, W. C. (1987) Interleukin 1 gene expression in adult T cell leukemia. *J. Clin. Invest.* **80**, 911–916.

Wedelin, C., Björkholm, M., Holm, G., Askergren, J., and Johansson, B. (1981) Routine laboratory tests in relation to spleen size and tumour involvement in untreated Hodgkin's disease. *Acta Med. Scand.* **209**, 309–313.

Weintraub, J. and Warnke, R. A. (1982) Lymphoma in cardiac allotransplant recipients. *Transplantation* **33**, 347–351.

Weisenburger, D. D. (1984) Mantle-zone lymphoma: an immunohistologic study. *Cancer* **53**, 1073.

Weisenburger, D. D. and Armitage, J. O. (1996) Mantle cell lymphoma: an entity comes of age. *Blood* **87,** 4483–4494.

Weisenburger, D. D., Kim, H., and Rappaport, H. (1982) Mantle-zone lymphoma: a follicular variant of intermediate lymphocytic lymphoma. *Cancer* **49,** 1429.

Weisenburger, D. D., Nathwani, B. N., and Diamond, L. W. (1981) Malignant lymphoma, intermediate lymphocytic type: a clinicopathologic study of 42 cases. *Cancer* **48,** 1415.

Weisenburger, D. D., Sanger, W. G., and Armitage, J. O. (1987) Intermediate lymphocytic lymphoma: immunophenotypic and cytogenetic findings. *Blood* **69,** 1617.

Westling, P. (1965) Studies of the prognosis in Hodgkin's disease. *Acta Radiol.* **245(Suppl.),** 5–125.

Wetherley-Mein, G., et al. (1952) Follicular lymphoma. *Q. J. Med.* **21,** 327–351.

Whang-Peng, J., Bunn, P., Knutsen, T., Schechter, G. P., Gazdar, A. F., Matthews, M.J., and Minna, J. D. (1979) Cytogenic abnormalities in patients with cutaneous T-cell lymphomas. *Cancer Treat. Rep.* **63,** 575–580.

Willemze, R., Kerl, H., Sterry, W., Berti, E., Cerroni, L., Chimenti, S., et al. (1997) EORTC classification for primary cutaneous lymphomas: a proposal from the Cutaneous Lymphoma Study Group of the European Organization for Research and Treatment of Cancer. *Blood* **90,** 354–371.

Winter, A. J., Obeid, D., and Jones, E. L. (1995) Long survival after splenic immunoblastic transformation of Waldenström's macroglobulinaemia. *Br. J. Haematol.* **91,** 412–414.

Wong, K. F., Chan, J. K., Ng, C. S., Lee, K. C., Tsang, W. Y., and Cheung, M. M. (1992) CD56 (NKH1)-positive hematolymphoid malignancies: an aggressive neoplasm featuring frequent cutaneous/mucosal involvement, cytoplasmic azurophilic granules, and angiocentricity. *Hum. Pathol.* **23,** 798.

Wong-Staal, F. and Gallo, R. C. (1985) The family of human T-lymphotropic leukemia viruses: HTLV-1 as the cause of adult T cell leukemia and HTLV-III as the cause of acquired immunodeficiency syndrome. *Blood* **65,** 253–263.

Wormsley, S. B., Baird, S. M., Gadol, N., Rai, K. R., and Sobol, R. E. (1990) Characteristics of CD11c[+], CD5[+] B-cell leukemias and the identification of novel peripheral blood B-cell subsets with chronic lymphoid leukemia immunophenotypes. *Blood* **76,** 123–130.

Worthy, T. S. (1981) Evaluation of diagnostic laparotomy and splenectomy in Hodgkin's disease. Report no. 12. *Clin. Radiol.* **32,** 523–526.

Wotherspoon, A. C., Doglioni, C., Diss, T. C., Pan, L., Moschini, A., de Boni, M., and Isaacson, P. G. (1993) Regression of primary low-grade B-cell gastric lymphoma of mucosa-associated lymphoid tissue type after eradication of *Helicobacter pylori. Lancet* **342,** 575–577.

Wright, D. H. (1970) Gross distribution and haematology. In: *Burkitt's Lymphoma* (Burkitt D. P. and Wright, D. H., eds.), Livingstone, Edinburgh, pp. 64–81.

Wu, C. D., Jackson, C. L., and Medeiros, L. J. (1996) Splenic marginal zone cell lymphoma: an immunophenotypic and molecular study of five cases. *Am. J. Clin. Pathol.* **105,** 277–285.

Yam, L. T. and Crosby, W. H. (1974) Early splenectomy in lymphoproliferative disorders. *Arch. Intern. Med.* **133,** 270–274.

Yam, L. T. and Crosby, W. H. (1979) Spontaneous rupture of spleen in leukemic reticuloendotheliosis. *Am. J. Surg.* **137,** 270–273.

Yam, L. T. and Li, C. Y. (1976) Histogenesis of splenic lesions in Hodgkin's disease. *Am. J. Clin. Pathol.* **66,** 976–985.

Yam, L. T., Li, C. Y., and Finkel, H. E. (1972) Leukemic reticuloendotheliosis. *Arch. Intern. Med.* **130,** 248–256.

Yamazaki, K., Shimizu, S., Negami, T., Sawada, K., Nanasawa, H., Ohta, M., Konda, S., and Okuda, K. (1994) Leukemic meningitis in a patient with splenic lymphoma with villous lymphocytes (SLVL). *Cancer* **73,** 61–65.

Yousem, S., Weiss, L., and Warnke, R. (1985) Primary mediastinal non-Hodgkin's lymphomas: a morphologic and immunologic study of 19 cases. *J. Clin. Pathol.* **83,** 676–680.

Zeppa, P., Vetrani, A., Luciano, L., Fulciniti, F., Troncone, G., Rotoli, B., and Palombini, L. (1994) Fine needle aspiration biopsy of the spleen: a useful procedure in the diagnosis of splenomegaly. *Acta Cytol.* **38,** 299–309.

Zhang, B. and Lewis, S. M. (1989) The splenomegaly of myeloproliferative and lymphoproliferative disorders: splenic cellularity and vascularity. *Eur. J. Haematol.* **43,** 63–66.

Zhu, D., Oscier, D. G., and Stevenson, F. K. (1995) Splenic lymphoma with villous lymphocytes involves B cells with extensively mutated Ig heavy chain variable region genes. *Blood* **85,** 1603–1607.

Ziegler, J. L. (1981) Burkitt's lymphoma. *N. Engl. J. Med.* **305,** 735–745.

Ziegler, J. L., Beckstead, J. A., Volberding, P. A., Abrams, D. I., Levine, A. M., Lukes, R. J., et al. (1984) Non-Hodgkin's lymphoma in 90 homosexual men. *N. Engl. J. Med.* **311,** 565–570.

Zinzani, P. L., Bendandi, M., Martelli, M., Falini, B., Sabattini, E., Amadori, S., et al. (1996) Anaplastic large-cell lymphoma: clinical and prognostic evaluation of 90 adult patients. *J. Clin. Oncol.* **14,** 955–962.

Zucker-Franklin, D. (1974) Properties of the Sezary lymphoid cell: an ultrastructural analysis. *Mayo Clin. Proc.* **49,** 567–574.

15 The Spleen in Sickle Cell Disease

GRAHAM R. SERJEANT, CMG, CD(HON), MD, FRCP

15.1. INTRODUCTION

The spleen is central to much of the early pathology in children with homozygous sickle cell disease (SS), and abnormal splenic function secondary to the defective erythrocytes in SS is a major determinant of the morbidity and mortality of the disease in childhood.

Early observations in patients with SS presented a confusing picture of splenomegaly in some patients and splenic atrophy in others. The sequence of splenic pathology in these patients was first recognized in detail by Diggs (1935), who noted that splenomegaly developed in young patients, then gradually disappeared with age as a result of a progressive splenic fibrosis.

The rate of progression of this process varies markedly among individuals with SS, and the basic pattern may be complicated by episodes of acute splenic enlargement (acute splenic sequestration) or sustained enlargement, with or without hypersplenism. Furthermore, splenic immune function is frequently compromised early in life, even in the presence of splenomegaly (functional asplenia), and this loss of splenic function predisposes to overwhelming infections, especially with encapsulated organisms, such as the pneumococcus (*see also* Chapters 10 and 11).

15.2. THE PREVALENCE OF SPLENOMEGALY

Most patients with SS develop palpable splenomegaly early in life. The Jamaican cohort study followed from birth 311 children with SS disease detected among 100,000 consecutive newborns. Analysis of the incidence of splenomegaly revealed that the spleen had become palpable in 82% by the age of 6 months and in 93% by the age of 1 year. Because splenomegaly may be appearing in some patients while disappearing in others, its prevalence at any individual age is lower than the cumulative incidence. Palpable splenomegaly in surviving cohort children without splenectomy occurred in 35% at 6 months, 43% at 1 year, and in 10% at 10 years (Fig. 1). These figures may be biased by the exclusion of 33 children who underwent splenectomy, and in whom splenomegaly may have been more likely to persist. With the assumption that splenomegaly would have persisted in all these patients, the maximum expected prevalence of splenomegaly is 48% at 2 years, 29% at 5 years, and 16% at 10 years. This prevalence may be modified, in different geographic areas, by the frequency of other genetic factors (*see* Subheading 3.), and by environmental factors, such as malaria.

From: *The Complete Spleen: A Handbook of Structure, Function, and Clinical Disorders* Edited by: A. J. Bowdler © Humana Press Inc., Totowa, NJ

The higher levels of fetal hemoglobin (HbF) and the greater frequency of α-thalassemia in some Saudi and Indian populations with SS, result in a greater prevalence of splenomegaly among these groups (Gelpi, 1970; Kar et al., 1986; Padmos et al., 1991). The effect of malaria on the pattern of splenomegaly in SS is unclear, although the reduction in spleen size with malaria chemoprophylaxis (Hendrickse, 1965) suggests that malaria may contribute to more frequent and more marked splenomegaly in SS.

The splenomegaly is usually modest in size, commonly measuring 1–2 cm from the left costal margin, although a spleen measuring 4 cm or more occurred at some time in 118 (38%) cohort-study children (38%). In 51 of these children, the splenomegaly was transient, and represented an episode of acute splenic sequestration, in the remaining 67 children, the splenomegaly persisted for more than 1 month. There are no hematological consequences to be recognized with the moderate splenomegaly characteristic of most patients with SS, although marked hematologic changes may be associated with acute or chronic splenic enlargement.

15.3. DETERMINANTS OF SPLENOMEGALY

15.3.1. DEVELOPMENT OF SPLENOMEGALY
The splenomegaly typical of most children with SS in the first year of life probably results from their relatively rigid red blood cells, which have difficulty in negotiating the interendothelial slits in the basement membrane, as these cells pass from the cordal tissue to the vascular sinus lumen. The elegant studies of Weiss et al. (Weiss and Tavassoli, 1970; Weiss, 1983) have illustrated the extreme deformability needed by erythrocytes (Fig. 2), and those containing intracellular HbS polymer cannot deform to the required extent. Sickled erythrocytes, therefore, obstruct passage through the reticular network and the interendothelial slits (de Boisfleury Chevance and Allard, 1982), resulting in passive splenic engorgement.

Indirect evidence for this process is available from the observation that fetal hemoglobin (HbF), which inhibits HbS polymer formation, is significantly correlated with the age at which splenomegaly develops (Stevens et al., 1981): Patients with rapidly declining HbF levels tend to develop splenomegaly early; those with high levels of HbF, and less intravascular sickling, tend to develop splenomegaly late.

15.3.2. DISAPPEARANCE OF SPLENOMEGALY
The gradual disappearance of splenomegaly, which is associated pathologically with progressive splenic fibrosis, is probably also a sequel of splenic microvascular obstruction. The early development of intravascular sickling would therefore be expected to lead to the early

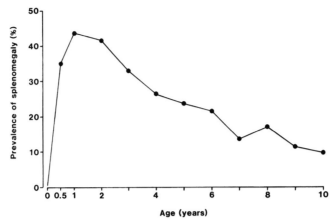

Fig. 15.1. Prevalence of splenomegaly among children with SS in Jamaican cohort study.

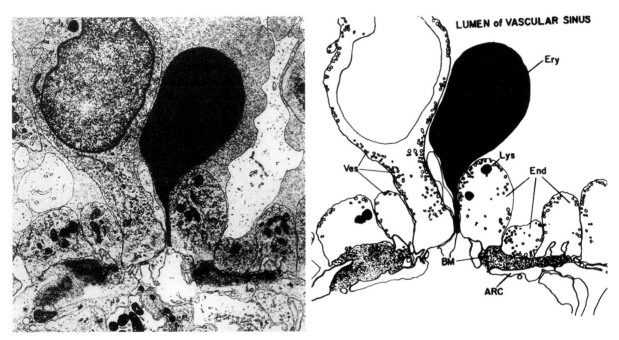

Fig. 15.2. Red blood cell (Ery) traversing an interendothelial slit, from the cordal tissue below to the vascular sinus above, demonstrating the extreme deformability required. BM, basement membrane; ARC, adventitial reticular cell; End, endothelium; Lys, lysosome; Ves, vesicles (Adapted with permission from Weiss, 1983.)

appearance of splenomegaly and to its early disappearance. Factors inhibiting sickling should therefore favor the persistence of splenomegaly, and this is supported by findings in patients with high levels of HbF or with α-thalassemia.

The presence of high levels of HbF at later ages is associated with persistence of splenomegaly (Serjeant, 1970), and there is a simple relationship between HbF level and the proportion of patients with splenomegaly at each age (Fig. 3). In individuals, splenomegaly still tends to disappear with age but the process occurs at a later age, in patients with higher HbF levels.

α-thalassemia also influences persistence of splenomegaly. Heterozygous α+ thalassemia, in which one of a pair of linked α globin genes is deleted, occurs in approx 35% of populations of West African ancestry. The homozygous form, which occurs in 3–4%, affects the hematological expressions of SS, lowering the mean cell hemoglobin concentration (MCHC) and inhibiting HbS poly-

merization. Consequently, there is a lower hemolytic rate, higher hemoglobin levels, amelioration of some clinical complications, and persistence of splenomegaly (Higgs et al., 1982).

The association of genetic factors known to inhibit sickling with the persistence of splenomegaly, suggests that this clinical feature may be used as a tool in the search for other factors inhibiting intravascular sickling.

15.4. SPLENIC FUNCTION IN SS

15.4.1. FUNCTIONAL ASPLENIA
The reduced red blood cell deformability of patients with SS compromises the processing functions of the spleen, and influences not only the development of splenomegaly and later splenic atrophy, but also produces other abnormalities of splenic function. These abnormalities develop early, even while splenomegaly persists, and have given rise to the concept of "functional asplenia" (Pearson et al., 1969). The ability

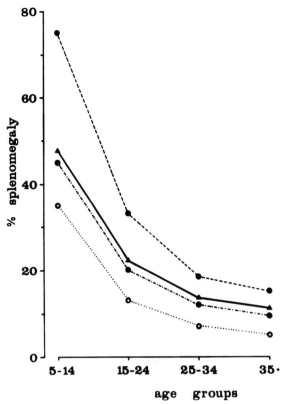

Fig. 15.3. Prevalence of splenomegaly with relation to HbF level. Whole group (▲——▲), HbF < 4% (○......○), HbF 4–7.9% (●-.-.-.●), HbF ≥ 8% (●———●). (Adapted with permission from Serjeant, 1970.)

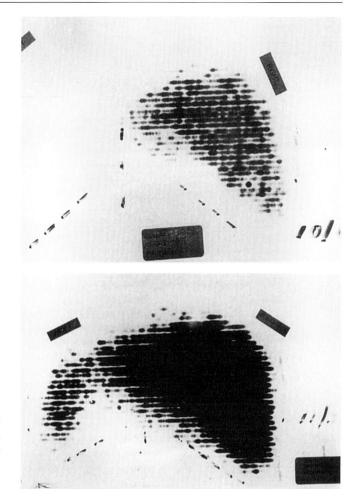

Fig. 15.4. ^{99m}Tc-sulfur colloid scan (posterior view) in a 2-year-old child with SS and splenomegaly, showing (**A**) hepatic uptake, but absence of splenic uptake; and (**B**) restoration of splenic uptake 6 days after transfusion. (Adapted with permission from Pearson et al., 1970.)

of the spleen to take up ^{99m}Tc-sulfur colloid was abnormal in 8/9 children with SS and splenomegaly (Fig. 4), but could be restored by transfusion in some young children (Pearson et al., 1970; Pearson et al., 1979), suggesting that red blood cells diverted through intrasplenic shunts could once again traverse the interendothelial slits and be normally processed. At later ages, this defect becomes irreversible.

15.4.2. PITTING FUNCTION The early impairment in splenic function is also reflected in the loss of the normal "pitting" function of the spleen, and the proportion of pitted red blood cells rises early to levels characteristic of asplenic patients (Fig. 5; *see also* Chapter 10).

15.4.3. OVERWHELMING INFECTIONS The clinical consequence of this loss of processing and phagocytic function of the spleen is a susceptibility to overwhelming infections, especially by encapsulated organisms such as the pneumococcus and *Haemophilus influenzae* b (*see also* Chapter 11). This susceptibility appears to be greatest in the first year of life, and, in the Jamaican cohort study, 80% of pneumococcal septicemias were observed before the age of 2 yr (John et al., 1984). This observation, and the effectiveness of prophylactic penicillin in the prevention of pneumococcal septicemia (Gaston et al., 1986), has led to its widespread use in all children with SS, commencing at 4 months and continuing at least until 4 years of age.

15.4.4. PREDICTION OF INFECTIONS Since the appearance of splenomegaly in SS is believed to signal the onset of splenic dysfunction, a relationship might be expected between early splenomegaly and the subsequent development of overwhelming septicemia. This hypothesis was tested by dividing children in the

cohort study into three groups, according to the age at the time of appearance of palpable splenomegaly: before 6 months, between 6 and 12 months, and after 12 months or not at all (Rogers et al., 1978). The frequency of subsequent overwhelming septicemias or meningitis in the three groups indicated a highly significant association with early splenomegaly (Table 1). These observations are clearly of practical importance, because effective prophylactic programs may be concentrated in the highest risk group, which comprises only one-third of the entire SS population.

15.5. ACUTE SPLENIC SEQUESTRATION

Acute splenic sequestration is a syndrome of sudden splenic enlargement associated with trapping of red blood cells, a decrease in hemoglobin in the peripheral blood, and often reticulocytosis. There is a spectrum of severity, which, at its most severe, results in peripheral circulatory failure, shock, and death (Seeler and Shwiaki, 1972). A useful working definition is the combination of a sudden increase in splenic size (usually ≥3 cm below the costal margin), a fall in hemoglobin (by >2 g/dL, and usually below 4.5 g/dL), and an increase in reticulocyte count (usually 2–3× steady-state values), with decrease in splenomegaly following transfusion or spontaneous resolution of the attack.

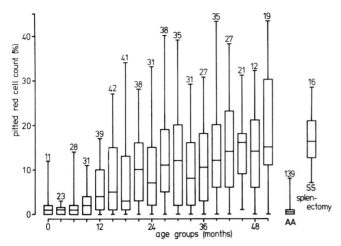

Fig. 15.5. Pitted red blood cells (mean, quartiles, range) and age in children with SS, AA controls, and SS postsplenectomy. Figures above bars indicate numbers in each group. (Adapted with permission from Rogers et al., 1982.)

Table 15.1
First Severe Infections by Spleen Group

Group	Age when spleen first palpable	No. children	Observed infections	Expected infections	Observed/ expected
I	Up to 6 mo	50	12	4.88	2.46
II	7–12 mo	38	2	3.84	0.52
III	Over 12 mo or not at all	47	0	5.27	0

Expected number of first infections calculated from log-rank test (Adapted with permission from Rogers et al., 1978.)

15.5.1. ETIOLOGY

The etiology is unknown. Nonspecific symp-toms and fever are common, but there is no specific symptom complex or associated bacteriology (Topley et al., 1981), and this complication probably represents a nonspecific response to increased intravascular sickling. There is no epidemiological evidence to support an infective etiology, although the behavior of the two sets of twins with SS disease was of interest. In the first set (nonidentical twins), one twin developed acute splenic sequestration at 11 and the other at 19 months, before the spleen became impalpable in both at the age of 21 months. In the other set (identical twins), the first attacks of acute splenic sequestration occurred simultaneously at 366 days, and the third attacks were separated in time by only 3 days (Fig. 6). A fourth attack occurred in twin II while awaiting splenectomy. The virtually simultaneous occurrences argue for an environmental factor that perhaps requires very close personal contact.

15.5.2. RISK FACTORS

Patients prone to acute splenic sequestration have significantly lower HbF levels (Stevens et al., 1981; Emond et al., 1985; Bailey et al., 1992), although no differences are apparent in the total hemoglobin, MCV, MCHC, or reticulocyte counts among patients with and without histories of acute splenic sequestration. Patients with homozygous α-thalassemia appear less likely to develop acute splenic sequestration (Emond et al., 1985), although this possibility was not statistically proved, perhaps because of the small numbers of patients in the study.

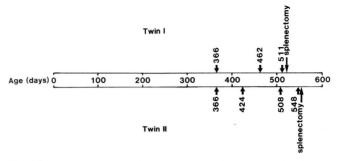

Fig. 15.6. Pattern of attacks of acute splenic sequestration in one pair of twins in Jamaican cohort study.

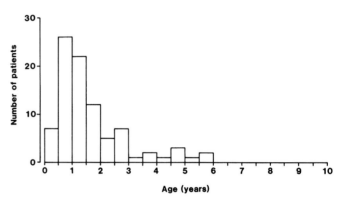

Fig. 15.7. Age at first attack of acute splenic sequestration for 89 affected children in the cohort study. (Adapted with permission from Emond et al., 1985.)

15.5.3. PREVALENCE

Estimates of the prevalence of acute splenic sequestration depend on the definition adopted for inclusion. Topley et al. (1981) argued for the recognition of minor episodes characterized by a fall in the Hb of at least 2 g/dL, because these may have prognostic significance, identifying patients at risk for proceeding to severe or fatal attacks. However, since such mild attacks frequently pass unrecognized, accurate assessment of their prevalence is not possible. When analysis is confined to attacks that are clinically apparent either to the physician or the parent, the cumulative probability is 0.225 by 2 years, 0.265 by 3 years, and 0.297 by 5 years (Emond et al., 1985). Approximately 30% of Jamaican children with SS, therefore, experience episodes of acute splenic sequestration by the age of 5 years.

15.5.4. AGE OF ONSET

Fatal episodes of acute splenic sequestration have been reported to occur as early as 4 months of age (Walterspiel et al., 1984). The distribution of age at first attack, among 89 affected children in the cohort study, indicated the period of highest risk to be the second 6 months of life (Fig. 7), and that 75% of first attacks (67/89) occurred before the age of 2 years. First attacks of acute splenic sequestration are rare after the age of 6 years, although these occasionally occur in adolescents, and may be seen in adults with SS with α-thalassemia (De Ceulaer and Serjeant, 1991), sickle cell–hemoglobin C disease or sickle cell–β° thalassemia.

Attacks tend to be recurrent (Fig. 8), 49% of patients at risk after the first attack proceeding to a second attack, and 21% of those at risk after the second attack proceeding to a third attack. There is also a tendency for attacks to recur at progressively shorter intervals (Emond et al., 1985).

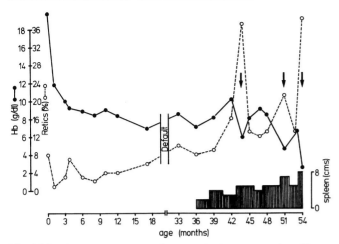

Fig. 15.8. Recurrent pattern of acute splenic sequestration. Hemoglobin, reticulocyte count, and spleen size during three episodes of acute splenic sequestration (marked by arrows), in a child dying in the third attack. (Adapted with permission from Topley et al., 1981.)

Table 15.2
Incidence and Case Fatality Rate for Acute Splenic Sequestration Before and After Parental Education Program

	Preceding	*Succeeding*
Standardized incidence rates/100 patient years	4.6	11.3
Case fatality rate per 100 events	29.4	3.1

15.5.5. CLINICAL FEATURES The clinical features of attacks are dominated by anemia and associated clinical symptoms. In one study (Topley et al., 1981), the mean hemoglobin level was 4.8 g/dL (range 0.8–7.3), with an average fall from steady-state values of 3.2 g/dL. The mean hemoglobin level in fatal cases was 2.6 g/dL (range 0.8–4.8). Mean reticulocyte counts were elevated at 19% (range 4–43%); in particularly acute episodes, the reticulocyte count may not have had time to rise, but normoblasts are usually present in the peripheral blood. The average spleen size was 4 cm from the costal margin. Clinically, the worst-affected patients have signs of peripheral circulatory failure, with tachycardia, tachypnoea, and shock, and the time-course may be precipitate, with patients passing from apparently normal health to gross pallor and shock within as little as 6 hours.

Associated clinical features are common, and in 132 events of acute splenic sequestration in the Jamaican cohort study, these included upper respiratory tract infection in 27 (20%), acute chest syndrome in 27 (20%), gastroenteritis in 7 (5%) and dactylitis in 7 (5%). In 25% of events, there were no other clinical findings.

Bacteriological investigations do not suggest a common etiology. Review of 97 blood cultures in 132 Jamaican episodes indicated growth of *Streptococcus pneumoniae* in two, *H. influenzae* in two, *Klebsiella pneumoniae* in two, and *Escherichia coli* in two. However, prophylactic penicillin did not reduce the prevalence of acute splenic sequestration, implying that penicillin-sensitive organisms are not a common cause of acute splenic sequestration.

15.5.6. TREATMENT The treatment of acute splenic sequestration is both corrective and prophylactic. Treatment of the acute episode requires immediate transfusion and correction of any underlying pathology. Early detection and presentation to hospital

in such episodes is vital, if therapy is to be effective. The education of parents or guardians in the methods of diagnosis and the significance of acute splenic sequestration has had a profound impact on the outcome of this complication, in Jamaica. Comparing the results of the 5 years before and after this education program (Table 2) reveals that, although the apparent incidence of acute splenic sequestration has risen by 2.5×, representing parental detection of mild attacks not normally observed by physicians, the mortality rate has fallen by 90%.

Mortality associated with recurrent attacks may be prevented by prophylactic splenectomy, which, in the Jamaican environment, is usually performed after two attacks, and this has likewise been recommended in the United States (Seeler and Shwiaki, 1972). Occasionally, with adverse social circumstances, splenectomy may be performed after the first attack, or, if social circumstances are good, may be delayed until the third attack. Elective splenectomy has been well-tolerated at this age, in Jamaican patients (Emond et al., 1984), and, over a median follow-up of 8 years in 130 splenectomized patients, there was no evidence of an increased risk of infection or death, compared to age- and sex-matched SS controls (Wright et al., 1999). Effective prophylaxis against *S. pneumoniae* infections may be provided by parenteral (John et al., 1984) or oral penicillin (Gaston et al., 1986) and it is common practice in Jamaica to continue such prophylaxis for approx 3 years after splenectomy. The alternative to splenectomy in the prophylaxis of recurrent attacks of acute splenic sequestration is a chronic transfusion program, which may have the desirable side effect of restoring or improving splenic function at this age (Pearson et al., 1970). However, it is unclear how to monitor, or when to stop, such a transfusion program, and episodes of acute splenic sequestration may recur on cessation of transfusion, even at an age when acute splenic sequestration is no longer expected (Rao and Pang, 1982). Therefore, transfusion therapy may delay, but not abolish, the natural history of acute splenic sequestration.

15.6. HYPERSPLENISM

In some patients, splenomegaly persists, causing a sustained pathological hemolysis accompanied by reactive erythropoietic expansion. A new equilibrium is reached at lower hemoglobin levels and higher reticulocyte counts than had characterized the patient previously. There is a spectrum of severity: the most severe cases present with a spleen measuring 10–15 cm below the costal margin, hemoglobin levels of 2–3 g/dL, and reticulocyte counts of 40–50% (Fig. 9). Estimates of mean red blood cell survival may be as short as 1–2 days and the erythropoietic expansion leads to skeletal changes, with diploic widening, expansion of the zygoma and maxillary bones, and a generalized osteoporosis with cortical thinning.

15.6.1. RISK FACTORS The risk factors for hypersplenism in SS in Jamaica appear to include high levels of HbF (unpublished observations, Sergeant, G. K.) and homozygous α+ thalassemia (Higgs et al., 1982). Approximately one-half the affected children with hypersplenism in the Jamaican cohort study developed this complication, acutely, with a clinical picture similar to an attack of acute splenic sequestration that did not resolve, and was attended by increasing bone marrow compensation.

15.6.2. PREVALENCE The frequency of hypersplenism is unclear, partly because there has not been a clear definition. In the Jamaican cohort study, children in whom splenectomy was considered clinically indicated for hypersplenism had in common a spleen

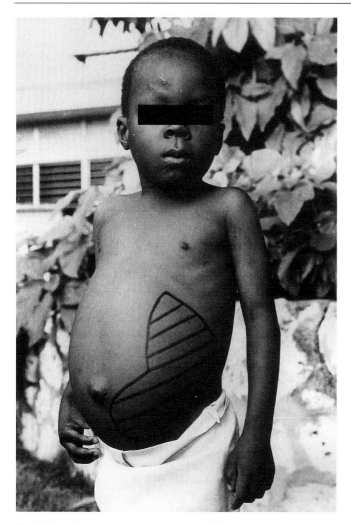

Fig. 15.9.   Hypersplenism in Jamaican child, aged 5 years. The spleen measured 16 cm and weighed 460 g at splenectomy. At the time of photograph, blood values included Hb 2.6 g/dL and reticulocytes 38%. (Adapted with permission from Serjeant, 1985.)

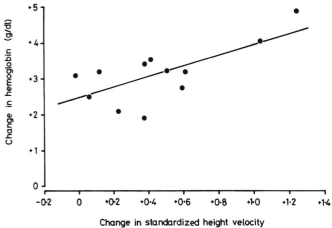

Fig. 15.10.   Relationship between postsplenectomy change in hemoglobin level and change in standard height velocity.

size of at least 4 cm, a hemoglobin of less than 6.5 g/dL, a fall in hemoglobin of at least 2 g/dL from previous steady-state levels, and a platelet count below 260×10^9/L. Using this definition, hypersplenism occurred in 17 (6%) children in the cohort study. Comparable data elsewhere are unavailable, although there is a clinical impression that hypersplenism may be more common among Indian patients with SS in Orissa (Kar et al., 1986).

15.6.3. AGE OF ONSET   Hypersplenism is essentially a pediatric complication, and is rare after the age of 15 years in Jamaican patients. In the cohort study, hypersplenism developed at a median age of 3.1 years with a range from 0.7 to 8.0 years.

15.6.4. CLINICAL FEATURES   The clinical features of hypersplenism result from the low hemoglobin, bone marrow expansion, and growth failure. The low hemoglobin necessitates a hyperdynamic circulation, maintained by tachycardia and increased cardiac work. The increased erythropoietic activity is associated with increased requirements for hematinics, and of amino acids and calories, which compete with the demands for normal growth. Growth failure is common, and a marked growth spurt generally follows splenectomy (Singhal et al., 1995; Badaloo et al., 1996). Splenectomy is associated with reductions of 23–47% in protein

turnover (Badaloo et al., 1991, 1996). The postsplenectomy increase in height velocity was significantly related to the increase in hemoglobin (Fig. 10), and impaired height velocity consistently occurred when the hematological changes persisted for more than 6 months.

15.6.5. OUTCOME   The outcome of untreated hypersplenism is unknown, because severe cases are generally treated by splenectomy or a transfusion program. Hypersplenism is rare among Jamaican adults with SS, and it must be assumed that spontaneous resolution occurs in many mildly affected cases. Untreated severe cases manifest a vicious hemolytic process, with a mean red blood cell survival of 1–2 days and extreme metabolic demands of the grossly expanded erythropoietic marrow. With such short red blood cell survival, serious morbidity might be anticipated from superimposed acute sequestration or coincidental aplastic crisis, and two Jamaican patients have died while awaiting splenectomy, one from superimposed acute splenic sequestration, and another from torrential epistaxis associated with low platelet counts. More information is urgently needed on the natural history of hypersplenism in SS.

15.6.6. TREATMENT   Treatment of hypersplenism is based on removal of splenic tissue (either by splenectomy or splenic embolization), or alleviation of the hematological effects by chronic transfusion, while awaiting the expected spontaneous splenic regression. Chronic transfusion avoids the surgical and anesthetic risks of operation, but may inhibit the tendency to spontaneous regression in SS, by allowing hypersplenism to recur at the end of the transfusion program. The necessary duration of transfusion is unknown, and there are also the customary problems of chronic transfusion programs, which include iron overload, the risk of hepatitis, problems with venous access, transfusion reactions, and the increased destruction of transfused blood by hypersplenism. Splenic embolization (Politis et al., 1987), advocated in the treatment of hypersplenism in β-thalassemia, theoretically allows a controlled splenic ablation, leaving some residual functional splenic tissue. However, it is unclear whether any immune function persists in the hypersplenic spleen in SS, and the procedure has been associated with marked pain and infection (*see also* Chapter 17). Elective splenectomy is well-tolerated, and has the advantage of rectifying the underlying pathology immediately; it has generally been used in Jamaica, where conditions do not favor conservative management.

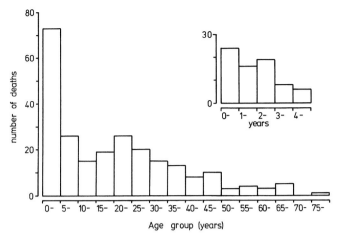

Fig. 15.11. Distribution of age at death in Jamaican patients with SS. (Adapted with permission from Thomas et al., 1982.)

15.7. SIGNIFICANCE OF SPLENIC PATHOLOGY

The role of the spleen is central to much of the early morbidity and mortality in SS. The first year of life carries the highest risk of death of any period in the life of a child with SS (Fig. 11), and much of this early mortality is attributable either to acute splenic sequestration or pneumococcal septicemia (Thomas et al., 1982). Hypersplenism adds significant morbidity, through its effects on the blood picture and growth and development of the child.

Conversely, the persistence of splenomegaly is frequently a manifestation of mild disease, and reflects a splenic microvasculature that has not been destroyed by the vaso-occlusive processes of the disease. The behavior of the spleen in SS is, therefore, not only a cause of severe complications, but also a valuable indicator of the pathological processes active in this disease.

REFERENCES

Badaloo, A. V., Emond, A., Venugopal, S., Serjeant, G., and Jackson, A, A. (1991) The effect of splenectomy on whole body protein turnover in homozygous sickle cell disease. *Acta Paediatr. Scand.* **80,** 103–105.

Badaloo, A. V., Singhal, A., Forrester, T. E., Serjeant, G. R., and Jackson, A. A. (1996) The effect of splenectomy for hypersplenism on whole body protein turnover, resting metabolic rate and growth in sickle cell disease. *Eur. J. Clin. Nutr.* **50,** 672–675.

Bailey, K., Morris, J. S., and Serjeant, G. R. (1992) Fetal haemoglobin and early manifestations of homozygous sickle cell disease. *Arch. Dis. Child.* **67,** 517–520.

de Boisfleury Chevance, A. and Allard, C. (1982) Scanning electron microscopy of the spleen in a case of sickle cell anemia. *Blood Cells* **8,** 467–470.

De Ceulaer, K. and Serjeant, G. R. (1991) Acute splenic sequestration in Jamaican adults with homozygous sickle cell disease: a role of alpha thalassaemia. *Br. J. Haematol.* **77,** 563,564.

Diggs, L. W. (1935) Siderofibrosis of the spleen in sickle cell anemia. *JAMA* **104,** 538–541.

Emond, A. M., Morais, P., Venugopal, S., Carpenter, R. G., and Serjeant, G. R. (1984) Role of splenectomy in homozygous sickle cell disease in childhood. *Lancet* **i,** 88–91.

Emond, A. M., Collis, R., Darvill, D., Higgs, D. R., Maude, G. H., and Serjeant, G. R. (1985) Acute splenic sequestration in homozygous sickle cell disease: natural history and management. *J. Pediatr.* **107,** 201–206.

Gaston, M. H., Verter, J. I., Woods, G., et al. (1986) Prophylaxis with oral penicillin in children with sickle cell anemia. A randomized trial. *N. Engl. J. Med.* **314,** 1593–1599.

Gelpi, A. P. (1970) Sickle cell disease in Saudi Arabs. *Acta Haematol.* **43,** 89–99.

Hendrickse, R. G. (1965) The effect of malaria chemoprophylaxis on spleen size in sickle-cell anemia. In: *Abnormal Haemoglobins in Africa* (Jonxis, J. H. O., ed.), Blackwell, Oxford, pp. 445–449.

Higgs, D. R., Aldridge, B. E., Lamb, J., et al. (1982) The interaction of alpha-thalassemia and homozygous sickle-cell disease. *N. Engl. J. Med.* **306,** 1441–1446.

John, A. B., Ramlal, A., Jackson, H., Maude, G. H., Sharma, A. W., and Serjeant, G. R. (1984) Prevention of pneumococcal infection in children with homozygous sickle cell disease. *Br. Med. J.* **288,** 1567–1570.

Kar, B. C., Satapathy, R. K., Kulozik, A. E., et al. (1986) Sickle cell disease in Orissa State, India. *Lancet* **ii,** 1198–1201.

Padmos, M. A., Roberts, G. T., Sackey, K., et al. (1991) Two different forms of homozygous sickle cell disease occur in Saudi Arabia. *Br. J. Haematol.* **79,** 93–98.

Pearson, H. A., Spencer, R. P., and Cornelius, A. E. (1969) Functional asplenia in sickle-cell anemia. *N. Engl. J. Med.* **281,** 923–926.

Pearson, H. A., Cornelius, E. A., Schwartz, A. D., Zelson, J. H., Wolfson, S. L., and Spencer, R. P. (1970) Transfusion-reversible functional asplenia in young children with sickle-cell anemia. *N. Engl. J. Med.* **283,** 334–347.

Pearson, H. A., McIntosh, S., Ritchey, A. K., Lobel, J. S., Rooks, Y., and Johnston, D. (1979) Developmental aspects of splenic function in sickle cell disease. *Blood* **53,** 358–365.

Politis, C, Spigos, D. G., Georgiopoulou, P., et al. (1987) Partial splenic embolisation for hypersplenism of thalassaemia major; five year follow up. *Br. Med. J.* **294,** 665–667.

Rao, S. and Pang, E. (1982) Transfusion therapy for subacute splenic sequestration in sickle cell disease. *Blood* **60(Suppl.),** 48a.

Rogers, D. W., Vaidya, S., and Serjeant, G. R. (1978) Early splenomegaly in homozygous sickle-cell disease: an indicator of susceptibility to infection. *Lancet* **ii,** 963–965.

Rogers, D. W., Serjeant, B. E., and Serjeant, G. R. (1982) Early rise in 'pitted' red blood cell count as a guide to susceptibility to infection in childhood sickle cell anaemia. *Arch. Dis. Child.* **57,** 338–342.

Seeler, R. A. and Shwiaki, M. Z. (1972) Acute splenic sequestration crises (ASSC) in young children with sickle cell anemia. *Clin. Pediatr.* **11,** 701–704.

Serjeant, G. R. (1970) Irreversibly sickled cells and splenomegaly in sickle-cell anaemia. *Br. J. Haematol.* **19,** 635–641.

Singhal, A., Thomas, P., Kearney, T., Venugopal, S., and Serjeant, G. (1995) Acceleration in linear growth after splenectomy for hypersplenism in homozygous sickle cell disease. *Arch. Dis. Child.* **72,** 227–229.

Stevens, M. C. G., Vaidya, S., and Serjeant, G. R. (1981) Fetal hemoglobin and clinical severity of homozygous sickle cell disease in early childhood. *J. Pediatr.* **98,** 37–41.

Thomas, A. N., Pattison, C., and Serjeant, G. R. (1982) Causes of death in sickle-cell disease in Jamaica. *Br. Med. J.* **285,** 633–635.

Topley, J. M., Rogers, D. W., Stevens, M. C., and Serjeant, G. R. (1981) Acute splenic sequestration and hypersplenism in the first five years in homozygous sickle cell disease. *Arch. Dis. Child.* **56,** 765–769.

Walterspiel, J. N., Rutledge, J. C., and Bartlett, B. L. (1984) Fatal acute splenic sequestration at 4 months of age. *Pediatrics* **73,** 507,508.

Weiss, L. (1983) The red pulp of the spleen: structural basis of blood flow. *Clin. Haematol.* **12,** 375–393.

Weiss, L. and Tavassoli, M. (1970) Anatomical hazards to the passage of erythrocytes through the spleen. *Semin. Hematol.* **7,** 370–380.

Wright, J. G., Hambleton, I. R., Thomas, P. W., Duncan, N. D., Venugopal, S., and Sergeant, G. R. (1998) Post splenectomy course in homozygous sickle cell disease? (submitted for publication).

16 Imaging of Spleen Disorders

Mark R. Paley, md, frcr and Pablo R. Ros, md, facr

16.1. INTRODUCTION

In the past, the spleen had been considered radiologically an "orphan" abdominal organ, because of its relative inaccessibility with available imaging techniques. With recent advances in cross-sectional imaging, including computed tomography (CT), ultrasonography (US), and magnetic resonance imaging (MRI), the spleen can now be imaged with ease, and a wide spectrum of disease entities affecting it can be identified and potentially diagnosed. The purpose of this chapter is to describe the role of imaging in the study of the spleen, and to present the radiographical manifestations of normal and pathological conditions, using the various imaging modalities currently available.

16.1.1. PLAIN FILM

The simplest and most nonspecific means of imaging the spleen is by plain film. The presence of perisplenic fat often makes visualization of the spleen possible on plain film, because of the difference in density between fat and adjacent splenic tissue. Furthermore, the presence and approximate size of the spleen can sometimes be inferred from the position of normal gas-filled structures, such as the stomach and splenic flexure of the colon (Fig. 1). However, the ability to see the spleen on plain radiographs is variable, depending on such factors as body habitus and film technique. Although the spleen is frequently seen more easily in an individual having an average or moderately increased amount of body fat than in an asthenic person, excessively increased body fat, as in morbid obesity, will usually obscure most intra-abdominal organs.

Visualization of the spleen on plain films is typically seen only in ~20% of cases (Shirkhoda, 1993), and detection of splenic pathology by this modality is therefore limited. Because of normal variations in the size, shape, and location of the spleen, only moderate or massive splenomegaly can be appreciated. The spleen normally does not extend below the left costal margin; if it projects below this level, splenomegaly can usually be diagnosed. Plain films are, however, useful in detecting calcifications within the spleen; these are frequently found in granulomatous disease (such as tuberculosis and histoplasmosis), aneurysms of the splenic artery, chronic hematomata, healed abscesses, and cysts. Occasionally, in abscesses, gas may be identified within the spleen, on plain films.

16.1.2. NUCLEAR SCINTIGRAPHY

Nuclear scintigraphy has for many years been considered a conventional means of studying the spleen, radiographically. Although CT and US have come to occupy much of the field of splenic imaging, the radionuclide scan still provides a sensitive, but nonspecific, means for identifying structural and functional pathology, particularly with the use of state-of-the-art γ cameras and optimized technique. In addition, the use of single photon emission computed tomography (SPECT) can increase both spatial and contrast resolution, and improve the sensitivity for focal lesion detection. Splenic scintigraphy demonstrates the entire spleen in one image; the newer modalities offer only a cross-sectional view. The most common application of splenic scintigraphy is in conjunction with hepatic scintigraphy for hepatocellular dysfunction. Other indications include the detection of congenital abnormalities and focal space-occupying lesions, the evaluation of splenomegaly, and suspected asplenia.

The preferred radionuclide for splenic scintigraphy is 99m-technetium sulfur colloid because of its optimal energy emission for imaging, and its short (6-h) half-life, which minimizes patient radiation exposure. 99m-Technetium sulfur colloid is a suspension of sulfur colloid particles labeled with 99m-Technetium. The average particle diameter is 0.3–1.0:m (Mettler, 1986). These particles are filtered out and trapped by the reticuloendothelial cells in the liver, spleen, and bone marrow. Normally, 80–90% of the particles injected are taken up by the liver, and 5–10% by the spleen, with the remainder trapped by the bone marrow. 99m-Technetium sulfur colloid scintigraphy produces simultaneous imaging of both the liver and the spleen. Imaging of the spleen alone is possible, using heat damaged red blood cells labeled with 99m-Technetium, with images being obtained a few hours after dose administration.

The normal spleen scan demonstrates a homogeneous distribution of radionuclide activity in the left upper quadrant, which is equal to or less than the hepatic activity (Fig. 2). A reversal of this distribution, with spleen activity greater than that of the liver, suggests hepatocellular disease with associated portal hypertension, or an intrinsic splenic abnormality. The following factors should be considered when observing a spleen scan: size, position, configuration, and amount and distribution of radionuclide uptake. In patients with congenital and postsurgical asplenia, a search for ectopic or accessory splenic tissue should be made.

Normal variations in size, shape, and position should be taken into consideration before describing an abnormality, because these normal variations may be demonstrable on nuclear scintigraphy. One such normal variant is the so-called "upside-down" spleen, in which the hilum is identified as a concave defect superiorly, rather than in its usual location, toward the inferior aspect of the spleen. Another is the presence of splenic lobulation, seen as small extensions of redundant, normally functioning spleen, usually at

From: *The Complete Spleen: A Handbook of Structure, Function, and Clinical Disorders* Edited by: A. J. Bowdler © Humana Press Inc., Totowa, NJ

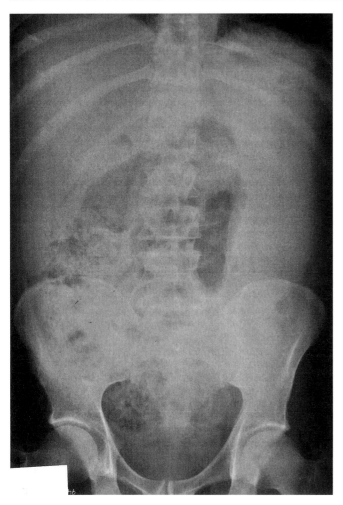

Fig. 16.1. Plain film demonstrating splenomegaly with the spleen tip visible at the level of the left iliac crest and medial displacement of the gas-filled stomach and splenic flexure of the colon.

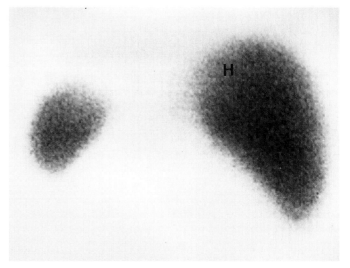

Fig. 16.2. Normal liver-spleen scan ^{99m}Tc sulfur colloid scintigraphy). On this posterior view, the spleen is located on the left. Note the homogeneous distribution of radionuclide activity in the spleen, which is slightly less than the hepatic activity (H). The spleen is best imaged from the posterior direction, since the spleen lies in the posterior abdomen. The spleen is not well-visualized on anterior projections because of overlying stomach and bowel. (Image courtesy of W. Drane, M.D.)

the anterior or inferior margin. This redundant tissue can cause a relative hot spot, when imaged in an overlapping fashion. A wandering spleen can also be easily identified by scintigraphy.

Other pitfalls in the interpretation of splenic radionuclide studies exist. A false focal defect in the spleen may be caused by barium retained in the colon from a previous barium enema study (Rao et al., 1979). Significant enlargement of the left lobe of the liver may also create a false defect in the splenic contour. In addition, following surgical splenectomy, radionuclide uptake in the left lobe of the liver may mimic a normal or accessory spleen.

16.1.3. ANGIOGRAPHY AND SPLENOPORTOGRAPHY

The role of angiography in the diagnosis of splenic disorders has been reduced significantly by the development of cross-sectional imaging techniques, and is usually now only performed prior to vascular intervention, such as embolization. On arteriography, the splenic parenchymal phase, or "blush," is seen as a region of homogeneous or slightly speckled contrast density. Large infarcts, hematomas, avascular or cystic masses, and other nonperfused space-occupying lesions may sometimes be detected as defects in the parenchymal blush. The splenic vein can be visualized approx 7 seconds after arterial injection, during the venous phase. Immediate filling of the vein after arterial injection suggests arteriovenous shunting. Delayed filling raises the possibility of portal venous hyperten-

sion, whereas absent filling indicates splenic vein thrombosis or occlusion, or severe portal venous hypertension. In the presence of portal venous hypertension, gastric varices can frequently be identified. Evaluating all phases of the arteriogram is important, when performing splenic angiography.

16.1.4. ULTRASONOGRAPHY

US is the most widely available and least expensive method of effectively evaluating the spleen. Ade-quate visualization of the spleen on US is occasionally difficult, because of the location of the spleen high in the left upper abdominal quadrant, since it is obscured by the adjacent ribs. In addition, air is a poor conductor of the beam, and the air-filled stomach and colon may further reduce sonographic access. The spleen may be visualized for most purposes by scanning intercostally, but these obstacles may create blind areas within the spleen, especially in those portions adjacent to the dome of the left hemidiaphragm. Improved visualization, especially of the peridiaphragmatic portion of the spleen, can sometimes be obtained, in the cooperative patient, by using varying degrees of inspiration to move the nonvisualized portions into view. For scanning in the supine position, it may be useful to have the stomach filled with fluid, which provides an excellent transmitter of ultrasound energy. Using a variety of these techniques, the best images of the spleen are usually obtained with the patient in the left anterior oblique position, or left-side-up decubitus. Both transverse and longitudinal (sagittal or coronal) views should be obtained.

On ultrasound, the parenchyma of the spleen produces a homogeneous pattern of echoes having a fine texture, with scattered echogenic foci representing blood vessels (Fig. 3). The general pattern is similar to that of the liver, but the overall echogenicity is slightly greater. The size and shape of the spleen are easily evaluated, and its relationship to other organs and the position of the hilum can be defined during the examination. Color Doppler is useful in identifying the course of the splenic artery and vein, and to differentiate vascular from nonvascular structures. Ultrasound is also the

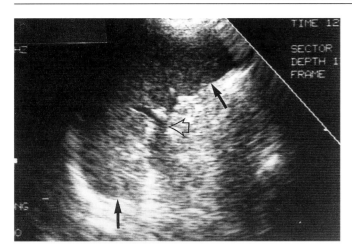

Fig. 16.3. Normal spleen on ultrasound. Axial or transverse view demonstrates normal size and shape of the spleen (black arrows). Note the fine, homogeneous echo pattern of the parenchyma. Tubular, hypoechoic structures in the hilum of the spleen (open arrow) represent blood vessels.

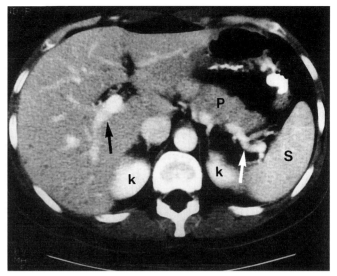

Fig. 16.4. Normal spleen on contrast-enhanced CT. Axial or transverse section through the midportion of the spleen (S) demonstrates homogeneous contrast enhancement. The splenic hilar vessels are well-visualized, because of the presence of perisplenic fat (which appears black on this image). The branching vessel demonstrating marked contrast enhancement in the splenic hilum (white arrow) is the splenic artery. The splenic vein would be seen on a lower slice, and would be much straighter in its course. Note the intense enhancement of the superior poles of the kidneys (K) and the branching portal vein (black arrow). The pancreas (P) is also well seen.

best method of imaging guidance for the occasional percutaneous biopsy of focal splenic lesions, when cytologic diagnosis is needed.

16.1.5. COMPUTED TOMOGRAPHY CT has revolutionized the examination of the spleen, as it has in evaluating other areas of the abdomen. The spleen is usually well-visualized on CT, unless technical artifacts or respiratory motion obscure the area (Federle, 1983). Beam-hardening is perhaps the most common technical artifact, and is seen with barium in the stomach or colon, or in the presence of multiple metallic surgical clips.

CT of the spleen is usually performed as part of a more generalized examination of the upper abdomen. At our institution, contiguous 7-mm slices are obtained from the dome of the diaphragm, down to the top of the pelvis, in a single breath-hold. Oral contrast agent is administered prior to the scan, to opacify loops of bowel that might otherwise lead to interpretive difficulties.

CT provides an excellent evaluation of the size, shape, and position of the spleen, as well as identifying focal or diffuse intrasplenic pathology. In addition, the relationship to adjacent organs is well-demonstrated, particularly with respect to the pancreatic tail, diaphragm, left kidney, and stomach.

On CT obtained without intravenous (iv) contrast, the spleen appears homogeneous, and of slightly lower density than the liver. The capsule and hilar vessels are often sharply delineated by surrounding perisplenic fat. The splenic artery may appear curvilinear, and, when tortuous, may be seen coursing in and out of the plane of section. The splenic vein usually pursues a straighter course, and is of slightly greater diameter than the artery (Fig. 4).

Use of iv contrast is necessary to evaluate optimally for splenic pathology, as many splenic lesions are isodense with spleen on unenhanced scans. With the increasing use of helical CT, the routine method of iv contrast enhancement is now with a rapid dynamic or bolus injection, typically 100–150 mL iodinated contrast material injected via a pump injector, at a rate of 2–4 mL/s. This, together with the rapid breath-hold scanning capability of helical CT, enables the entire spleen to be imaged in different phases of enhancement, the early or arterial and the late or venous phases, providing useful diagnostic information on the differential enhancement patterns of

the spleen, associated lesions, and adjacent structures. This dynamic technique may result in heterogeneous splenic enhancement in the early phase, which is thought to be related to variable flow rates of contrast through the red pulp, and it is important to avoid misinterpreting this appearance for focal splenic disease (Fig. 5). If in doubt, homogeneous enhancement should normally be seen within 2 minutes of the bolus injection (Glazer et al., 1981), and persistent areas of heterogeneity beyond this point should be considered pathological.

The relative CT density of the liver and spleen is often useful in determining the presence of abnormalities, e.g., when hepatic density is less than that of spleen, it may indicate fatty change in the liver. Lobulation of the spleen is a normal variant frequently appreciated on CT, and it is usually more prominent inferiorly. An unusually prominent lobulation secondary to a deep fissure may give the appearance of a band or waist in the spleen (Wilson and Lieberman, 1983).

16.1.6. MAGNETIC RESONANCE A number of factors have, until recently, limited the role of MRI in imaging the spleen. Motion-induced artifact from respiration, cardiac and vascular pulsation, and bowel peristalsis have significantly limited MRI of the abdomen, in general. In addition, unlike the liver, the normal spleen has T1 and T2 relaxation times that are similar to those of solid malignant lesions, which results in poor contrast and lesion conspicuity (Torres et al., 1995). The recent development of fast scanning techniques, which enables a complete scan of the upper abdomen to be obtained in a single breath-hold of 15–20 seconds has minimized motion-induced artifact, and this can be combined with the dynamic injection of iv contrast material, such as gadolinium-DTPA, with significant improvement in lesion conspicuity.

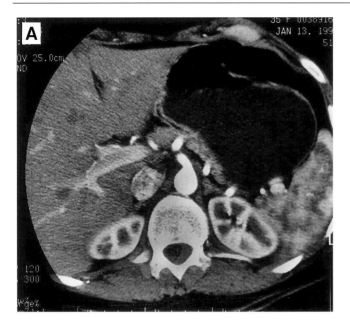

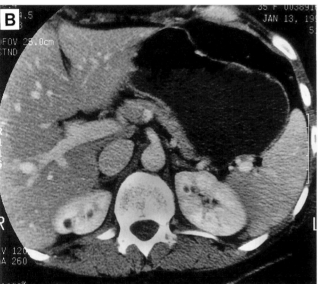

Fig. 16.5. Enhanced CT showing, (**A**) heterogeneous enhancement of the spleen, mimicking multiple focal lesions, in the early arterial phase; (**B**) but a normal homogeneous appearance is seen in the later portal phase.

A further area of much research has been in the use of tissue-specific contrast agents, particularly ferumoxides (superparamagnetic iron oxides) and ultrasmall superparamagnetic iron oxides, which are actively taken up by reticuloendothelial cells in normal spleen, but not by tumor cells (Weissleder et al., 1988). These agents significantly reduce the signal from normal spleen on T2-weighted images, while tumor remains of high signal intensity, thus improving lesion contrast and detection. As yet, there is no consensus on the optimum MRI technique for studying the abdomen, the choice of appropriate pulse sequence depending on the particular clinical question to be answered and the type of pathology to be identified, but the basic protocol will consist of both T1- and T2-weighted images in the axial plane. The ability of MRI to image in the coronal and sagital planes is of value, when assessing lesions adjacent to the diaphragm, but these are not usually acquired

routinely. Optional additional sequences available include fat suppression, to improve lesion detection and MR angiography, which is being found to be an increasingly useful noninvasive method of evaluating the splenic and perisplenic vasculature. The normal spleen is hypointense or isointense on T1-weighted images, compared with the liver, and is hyperintense on T2-weighted images. On MRI, fat is seen as areas of high-intensity, and fat in the splenic hilum and surrounding the spleen can thus be distinguished. Vessels, because of the blood flow within, are seen as low-intensity tubular structures surrounded by high-intensity fat. Although the appearance of fat and vessels on MRI is constant, the appearance of the splenic parenchyma may vary, depending on the pulse sequences chosen for imaging.

16.1.7. PERCUTANEOUS DRAINAGE, BIOPSY, AND SPLENIC EMBOLIZATION
There has traditionally been a reluctance to biopsy the spleen, and to provide percutaneous drainage for splenic lesions; this has been related principally to the vascular nature of the spleen and the consequent risk of hemorrhage, as well as the concern about potentially traversing lung, pleura, or bowel with a needle or catheter. However, there has been an increased interest in performing such procedures with the use of CT, and particularly ultrasound guidance, encouraged by the established success and safety of these techniques in other regions of the body.

Percutaneous drainage of solitary splenic abscesses has been performed using small-bore drainage catheters, without complications. This may be the procedure of choice when the abscess is very large, or when the patient is a poor surgical candidate and surgical splenectomy is not feasible. In addition, puncture of a splenic fluid collection makes the definitive diagnosis, identifies the infective organism, and aids in planning therapy. Percutaneous needle aspiration of other splenic lesions for cytologic diagnosis has also been performed without complications, using a 22-gage needle, and this procedure can be useful in diagnosing lymphoma, metastases, and other malignancies involving the spleen. Such percutaneous drainage and biopsy procedures can aid materially in the clinical management of patients, and should be considered in appropriate circumstances.

Splenic artery embolization has been usefully employed in a variety of clinical situations: This consists of placing one or more of a variety of materials into an artery via a selectively placed catheter, in order to induce thrombosis. Materials used for embolization include Gelfoam (small particles of a synthetic substance), detachable balloons, steel coils, and bucrylate (Goldman et al., 1981). Embolization can be performed at the level of the small branch arteries, or in the main splenic artery. In carefully selected groups, it can be used to stop bleeding in cases of trauma, without inducing hyposplenism with the risk of postsplenectomy infection, and avoiding the need for laparotomy. It can also be performed to produce a "medical splenectomy," e.g., to alleviate thrombocytopenia and anemia in hypersplenism, or to reduce the risk of bleeding from gastric varices secondary to splenic vein thrombosis or portal hypertension. Embolization in such cases reduces or eliminates the risk of surgery, and reduces transfusion requirements. However, the complications of splenic embolization are not infrequent, particularly if complete splenic infarction occurs, and include pain, splenic and subphrenic abscess formation, splenic rupture, and partial infarction of stomach or pancreas. Preoperative splenic embolization has also been advocated as a means of reducing the risk of bleeding during splenectomy of patients at risk with splenomegaly, adhesions, hypersplenism-induced thrombocytopenia, or varices. Another potential role for embolization is in the treatment of splenic artery pseudoaneurysms arising in patients with chronic pancreatitis, as a viable alternative to surgery.

16.2. ANOMALIES AND CONGENITAL DISORDERS

16.2.1. WANDERING SPLEEN "Wandering spleen" is the term usually applied to a spleen that is not located in the left upper quadrant of the abdomen. It may also be known as ectopic spleen, aberrant spleen, floating spleen, or splenic ptosis. It is thought to occur as a result of abnormal fusion of the dorsal mesogastrium, leading to ligamentous laxity and hypermobility. The incidence is less than 0.2% of the population, but its clinical importance lies in its potential for torsion and infarction. Supine and upright plain radiographs of the abdomen may demonstrate a mass in the left lower quadrant or midabdomen, which can mimic a renal or intestinal mass. There may be a marked difference in position of the mass on supine film, compared to the upright view, with bowel loops filling the left upper quadrant. Extrinsic compression of various intra-abdominal structures, especially the colon, may be detected by plain films or barium studies, and the splenic flexure of the colon may be interposed between the diaphragm and the spleen (Gordon et al., 1977; Salomonowitz et al., 1984). In addition, the vascular pedicle of a wandering spleen may cause a linear impression across the bowel in barium studies (Gordon et al., 1977).

Nuclear scintigraphy using 99m-Technetium sulfur colloid is a frequently performed study for diagnosing wandering spleen (McArdle, 1980), which may be seen to migrate with different patient positioning. Torsion can be diagnosed in the patient with acute abdominal pain, if there is absent or diminished radionuclide uptake at the site of a previously demonstrated wandering spleen (Rosenthall et al., 1974). Angiography also demonstrates the spleen definitively, and, in anticipation of surgery, can indicate the site of a vascular torsion, and define abdominal vasculature. In the presence of chronic torsion or splenic vein compression, solitary gastric varices may be seen (Smulewicz and Clement, 1975).

By ultrasound, an echogenic mass is identified lying away from the left upper quadrant, with a peripheral indentation representing the splenic hilum. The left kidney may be elevated in position, and lack the normal splenic hump. Color Doppler can demonstrate the absence of blood flow in torsion, although, often, collaterals develop from the short gastric and pancreatic arteries. Decreased echogenicity of the spleen may be seen with infarction and necrosis secondary to torsion, and a complex mass may be seen with superimposed infection (Kelly et al., 1982).

On CT or MRI, the spleen will be seen in an abnormal position, and a portion of the spleen or the entire organ may appear of low density on CT or low signal intensity on T1-weighted MRI, in the presence of torsion with infarction (Toback et al., 1984). In chronic torsion, a thick, enhancing pseudocapsule may develop, resulting from the formation of adhesions.

Overall, nuclear scintigraphy or ultrasound are probably the studies of choice for the diagnosis of a suspected wandering spleen. If there is no uptake of radionuclide on nuclear scan, as in torsion, ultrasound will identify the spleen. CT may be necessary, if the spleen is obscured by bowel gas on ultrasound (Sheflin et al., 1984).

16.2.2. ACCESSORY SPLEEN Accessory spleen refers to a small body of splenic tissue of congenital origin, which is separate from the main body of the spleen, and which may be ectopic in location. It results from failure of embryologic splenic buds to unite in the dorsal mesogastrium. It may be seen in 20% of the population,

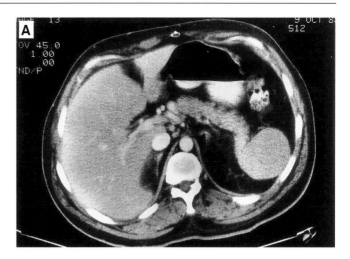

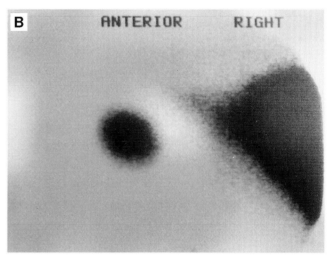

Fig. 16.6. Accessory spleen. (**A**) CT scan in a patient, with a previous splenectomy and left nephrectomy, shows a spherical mass related to the tail of the pancreas; (**B**) uptake of tracer on the ^{99m}Tc sulfur colloid scan, similar to that of the liver.

usually occurring near the splenic hilum, but can be found anywhere in the abdomen or retroperitoneum. It is frequently discovered incidentally on radiological examination, particularly on CT. Accessory splenic tissue may be discovered by nuclear scintigraphy and ultrasound, especially when hypertrophied following splenectomy (Fig. 6), when it may be the source of recurrent disease, such as lymphoma. In subjects with intact spleens, accessory spleens are usually less than 2.5 cm in diameter, as measured by CT and ultrasound (Beahrs and Stephens, 1980; Subramanyam et al., 1984). When hypertrophied following splenectomy, they may measure 3–5 cm in size.

Differential diagnosis of an accessory spleen on CT and ultrasound depends on its location. Diagnosis can usually be made with confidence when the patient is asymptomatic, and the tissue is located in the splenic hilus. However, location of the nodule of splenic tissue elsewhere in the left upper quadrant or abdomen may simulate a mass, and further diagnostic studies may be indicated to exclude the presence of a neoplasm. In such cases, nuclear scintigraphy using 99m-Technetium sulfur colloid is diagnostic, demonstrating the presence of functioning splenic tissue in the area of concern.

On MRI, the signal characteristics of the accessory spleen are the same as for the normal spleen, and there is normally a smooth, round or oval shape (Torres et al., 1995). MRI with ferumoxides is an excellent way to confirm an accessory spleen, because of the marked signal loss on T2-weighted images, indicating normal splenic uptake of the agent. The vascular supply was formerly demonstrated using arteriography (Clark et al., 1972; Kaude, 1973), but ultrasound can demonstrate the relationship of the accessory spleen to a splenic artery and vein, in a large number of cases (Subramanyam et al., 1984).

16.2.3. SPLENIC CLEFT   A splenic cleft is a fissure, easily identified on CT, usually occurring in the diaphragmatic surface of the spleen, in contrast to normal splenic lobulation, which is typically on the inferior surface. It may traverse the spleen, giving rise to a waist, and should not be mistaken for a laceration, in a patient presenting with a history of trauma.

16.2.4. SPLENIC GONADAL FUSION   This is a rare congenital anomaly, usually found in males, which consists of ectopic splenic tissue in close association with the left gonad, sometimes with an abnormal connection between the left gonad and the spleen. The diagnosis is usually made postoperatively, following surgery for suspected gonadal neoplasm (Bearss, 1980; Ceccacci and Tosi, 1981). Ultrasound is frequently performed as an early study of a scrotal mass, and, in the appropriate clinical setting, it is possible to suspect the diagnosis on the basis of this study. The mass has the sonographic characteristics of splenic tissue, such as accessory spleen, and [99m]-Technetium sulfur colloid scintigraphy may be diagnostic, demonstrating a focal area of uptake in close association with the left testicle (Mandell et al., 1983; Guarin et al., 1975).

16.2.5. ASPLENIA AND POLYSPLENIA SYNDROMES   In asplenia, or congenital absence of the spleen, there is usually a wide range of other congenital abnormalities, principally taking the form of situs ambiguous with bilateral right-sidedness. It occurs predominantly in males. Solitary absence of the spleen, caused by vascular occlusion or thrombosis, is an acquired abnormality, which is usually found without other associated anomalies (Monie, 1982).

Radiographically, manifestations of asplenia are as wide-ranging as the associated congenital abnormalities. Plain films of the chest and abdomen may demonstrate evidence of bilateral right-sidedness, with ultrasound, CT, and MRI providing more definitive findings. Features on a chest film include bilateral eparterial right-sided bronchial pattern and minor fissures, and widening of the superior mediastinum caused by bilateral superior vena cava. Nuclear scintigraphy may be useful in demonstrating absence of the spleen, using [99m]-Technetium sulfur colloid and tagged red blood cells (Rao et al., 1982; Piepsz et al., 1977). If the [99m]-Technetium sulfur colloid scan is equivocal for absence of the spleen, because of the presence of bilaterally symmetrical hepatic tissue or a prominent left lobe, a hepatobiliary tract scan can be added to find the full extent of the liver. Angiography is useful for defining the cardiac anomalies and detecting absence of the splenic artery. The entire celiac axis may be absent, with the hepatic artery rising from the superior mesenteric artery (27). Ultrasound, CT, and MRI can demonstrate abnormal situs with absence of the spleen, and may also show the abdominal aorta and inferior vena cava lying on the same side of the abdomen, usually the right.

In contrast to asplenia, polysplenia takes the form of multiple small masses of splenic tissue, with absence of an identifiable normal spleen, and features of bilateral left-sidedness. It is seen predominantly in females. Like asplenia, polysplenia is associated with anomalies of other systems (Van Mierop et al., 1972). Radiographic findings are variable, depending on the congenital anomalies present. On plain chest films, there is a bilateral hyparterial bronchial pattern, cardiac abnormalities, and a prominent azygous vein resulting from azygous continuation of the inferior vena cava may be seen. Again, radionuclide imaging can be used to demonstrate the multiple splenunculi, ranging in number from a few to as many as 16 (Peoples et al., 1983). However, CT, MRI, and ultrasound may be the best imaging methods for demonstrating the multiple features of this syndrome.

16.3. SPLENIC TRAUMA

The spleen is the most commonly injured organ in cases of blunt trauma to the abdomen. The main concern following trauma to the spleen is the possibility of splenic rupture, which is associated with a mortality in >75% of cases, if surgery is not performed promptly (Delaney and Jason, 1981). Radiology, particularly CT, has come to play a key role in the early diagnosis of splenic injury. Because of the important role of the spleen in preventing infection, it has become important to determine not only the presence of injury, but also the exact extent of the injury, to allow conservative surgical management whenever possible. Although blunt abdominal trauma is the most common cause of splenic injury, iatrogenic injury is not uncommon, including injury during surgery, thoracocentesis, and left renal biopsy (Pachter et al., 1981; Rauch et al., 1983).

16.3.1. PLAIN FILM   With intraparenchymal or subcapsular bleeding, plain radiographs may demonstrate evidence of splenic enlargement, with medial displacement of the gastric air bubble and inferior displacement of the splenic flexure of the colon. Elevation of the left hemidiaphragm may also be seen. Significant splenic injury, such as laceration and rupture, is frequently associated with rib fracture and left pleural effusion. Hemoperitoneum caused by splenic rupture may lead to an appearance of the abdomen simulating ascites, with diffusely increased density throughout. However, because of frequently poor visualization of the spleen, even in normal patients, plain films may usually only be suggestive of splenic trauma, and additional radiographic examination must be performed for definitive diagnosis. Evidence of previous splenic trauma may be detected on plain films, in the form of calcification of old hematomas.

16.3.2. ULTRASOUND   Ultrasound and CT have come to assume much of the role of imaging in splenic trauma previously played by angiography and nuclear scintigraphy. Ultrasound, when performed by a skilled operator, can be accurate in the diagnosis of splenic trauma, and may be very useful in situations in which a CT scanner is not immediately available, particularly as a screening tool for the presence of hemoperitoneum to decide who needs to go to surgery and who requires further imaging. Ultrasound can also be used to follow patients who are clinically stable and being managed conservatively. The limitations of ultrasound in the acute trauma setting may be technical, as when rib fractures, chest tubes, and dressings are present, limiting the available acoustic window. It also is limited in its ability to evaluate concurrent trauma in the retroperitoneum, bowel, and mesentery.

The appearance of a collection of blood on ultrasound, whether intracapsular or extracapsular, depends on the time of the examination, relative to the time of injury. Immediately following trauma, a collection of blood is still liquid, and may be easily differentiated from splenic tissue. However, after the blood clots, it may be very similar in echogenicity to the normal spleen, for up to 48 hours or

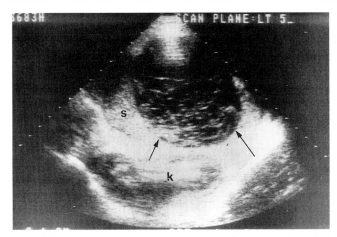

Fig. 12.7. Splenic hematoma on ultrasound. Scan through the left upper quadrant in a coronal plane demonstrates a large area of mixed echogenicity, measuring approx 7 cm in diameter (arrows), at the inferior margin of the spleen (S). This region of mixed echogenicity represents a hematoma in the subacute stage of evolution. Irregular anechoic, hypoechoic, and hyperechoic areas are seen within the hematoma, which has a well-defined margin. These anechoic areas will coalesce to form a relatively anechoic, cystic structure on follow-up scans. The left kidney (K) is also seen.

more. After several days, the blood collection begins to reliquefy, and may again become more apparent (Cooperberg, 1987).

In the presence of an intraparenchymal or subcapsular hematoma of the spleen, without rupture of the capsule, the appearance on subacute examination is that of a focal heterogeneous area within or at the periphery of the spleen (Fig. 7). Subsequent scans may show clearing of this heterogeneity, leading to the presence of a relatively anechoic, cystic structure representing the resolving hematoma (Lupien and Sauerbrei, 1984). These anechoic fluid collections may then decrease in size, and disappear, or leave a small scar manifested as an echogenic line.

Rupture of the splenic capsule leads to intraperitoneal bleeding, which may be found as massive hemoperitoneum in the seriously injured patient, or as a more focal perisplenic hematoma. With a free hemoperitoneum, a fluid collection may be found distant from the spleen, in the left upper quadrant, or elsewhere. Free intraperitoneal spread of blood is common, but the blood occasionally becomes walled-off in the left upper quadrant, and is seen as a large fluid collection or mass having irregular echogenicity. A smaller perisplenic hematoma may be seen as a focal area of inhomogeneous echogenicity adjacent to the spleen. Again, these fluid collections will undergo evolution, and may appear on subsequent scans as cystic structures adjacent to the spleen. A focal perisplenic hematoma can mimic a perisplenic abscess.

16.3.3. COMPUTED TOMOGRAPHY CT has become established as the imaging modality of choice in evaluating splenic trauma in the stable patient, determining not only the presence of splenic injury, but also its extent and the presence of injury in other organs. With the information obtained from CT, the surgeon can better decide between splenectomy and splenorrhaphy or splenic reimplantation. A 96% accuracy for CT in diagnosing splenic trauma was observed by Jeffrey et al. (1981) in a prospective study: A normal CT virtually excludes significant splenic injury.

The severity of the injury determines whether radiological studies, such as CT, can be performed prior to surgery. With severe injury, in which surgery seems necessary immediately, peritoneal lavage may be used to confirm hemoperitoneum, prior to surgery. However, if there is time to perform CT, peritoneal lavage should be omitted or delayed; CT can identify a hemoperitoneum, as well as define other organ injury, and CT performed after peritoneal lavage may lead to uncertainty as to whether the intraperitoneal fluid is caused by the trauma or the lavage.

As with ultrasound, the appearance of hematoma on CT changes with time (Korobkin et al., 1978; Moss et al., 1979). Immediately following injury, the hematoma is usually isodense with the spleen, on noncontrast scan, and may only be detectable by causing abnormality of the splenic contour. Such hematomas become apparent on a contrast-enhanced scan, as focal areas lacking contrast enhancement. With evolution of the hematoma, the blood components are broken down, leading to a decrease in hemoglobin content, and the hematoma becomes hypodense. Occasionally, a hematoma may have an onion skin appearance, as the result of alternating layers of clotted and unclotted blood.

Clearly, evaluation of acute splenic trauma requires iv administration of contrast material. Subcapsular hematomas, on contrast-enhanced CT, are seen as peripheral crescentic areas of lower density, and may cause flattening of the splenic contour. If there is active bleeding, this will appear as an area of higher density, representing contrast-enhanced blood, within the lower-density hematoma. Perisplenic hematomas are identified as low-density fluid collections surrounding the spleen. The final sequelae of many splenic hematomas are thought to be the formation of false or nonepithelialized cysts, which are of water density, and may remain unchanged in size for several years.

Splenic lacerations are usually more variable and subtle in appearance than hematomas. They appear as low-density bands, linear or stellate in configuration, with associated parenchymal defects, usually involving the lateral aspect of the spleen, and having associated free intraperitoneal blood or a sentinel clot of higher attenuation than splenic parenchyma (Jeffrey et al., 1981; and Fig. 8). Splenic fractures are lacerations that extend across the parenchyma, and may result in devascularized segments, typically in the upper and lower poles; a shattered spleen represents severe disruption. Pedicle injuries are associated with extensive hemoperitoneum, but these patients are often unstable, and seldom have a CT scan, rather going straight to surgery.

A number of CT grading systems for splenic trauma have been suggested, in an effort to improve CT evaluation of splenic injury and help clinical decision-making. These are based on the morphology of splenic injury and the size of any associated hematoma. The success of these systems is rather limited, and factors such as the hemodynamic stability of the patient and the presence and type of other injuries are better management indicators (Mirvis et al., 1989).

With the increasing trend toward conservative management of splenic injuries, follow-up CT plays an important role in the detection of complications, particularly delayed splenic rupture (Mirvis et al., 1989). In the normal uncomplicated resolution following injury, hematomas will reduce in density toward that of water, but they may initially increase slightly in size, lacerations may develop smoother borders, and capsular thickening may occur, because of fibrosis.

Anatomical variants of splenic anatomy may cause pitfalls in the evaluation of splenic trauma, as with the splenic cleft mentioned previously. An otherwise normal appearance of the spleen,

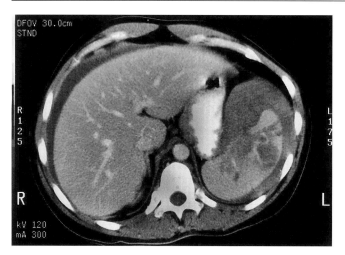

Fig. 16.8. Splenic trauma. CT scan shows a stellate laceration of the spleen, with a large perisplenic hematoma of mixed attenuation within an intact splenic capsule. Fluid is also seen around the liver.

with a thin, linear configuration to the cleft and absence of intraperitoneal fluid, will usually lead to the correct diagnosis (Jeffrey et al., 1981). Extension of the left lobe of the liver, and unopacified segments of bowel, can sometimes mimic a lacerated or fragmented spleen. Heterogeneous splenic enhancement, in the early phase following dynamic iv contrast administration, can also mimic a laceration, but again there will be no associated features, such as hematoma or hemoperitoneum. Several technical artifacts may occur in CT scanning, which can cause interpretation problems, including motion artifact, especially arising from the interface of oral contrast and water in the stomach, streak artifact caused by the presence of tubes, lines, and leads, and beam hardening, arising from the ribs. Careful patient preparation prior to scanning, and an awareness of these artifacts, help to minimize the problem.

16.3.4. ANGIOGRAPHY With the advent of CT and ultrasound, angiography has become less important to the diagnosis of splenic trauma, and is no longer appropriate as a screening modality. Angiography, however, continues to play an important role in identifying the exact sites of vascular injury and bleeding in the spleen. Splenectomy can be avoided, in many instances, by employing the various methods of angiographic occlusion of bleeding sites, including vasopressin infusion and therapeutic embolization using steel coils or Gelfoam particles. In this way, surgical morbidity can be avoided, and functioning splenic tissue retained.

Linear or wedge-shaped defects in the parenchymal phase may be seen with splenic laceration and distal arterial occlusion, respectively. Displacement of the spleen from the chest wall, by a lens-shaped peripheral avascular zone, suggests the presence of subcapsular hematoma (Osborn et al., 1973). Following penetrating injury, vascular occlusion and parenchymal defects predominate, rather than extravasation (Haertel and Ryder, 1979). In addition, angiography may reveal pseudoaneurysm formation or rupture, or formation of arteriovenous fistulae, as late complications of splenic trauma.

16.3.5. NUCLEAR MEDICINE Like angiography, nuclear scintigraphy has also yielded to CT and ultrasound in the diagnosis of splenic trauma. Formerly, nuclear scintigraphy, using [99m]-Technetium sulfur colloid was the procedure of choice in splenic trauma (Lutzker et al., 1973). Subcapsular hematoma may be seen as a concave defect along the splenic contour (Nesbesar et al., 1974).

The fractured spleen may show a linear defect, or a portion of splenic tissue may be displaced from the main body of the spleen. The limitations of scintigraphy are its nonspecificity, i.e., it cannot differentiate trauma from congenital variants and other splenic diseases, and its inability to detect hemoperitoneum.

16.3.6. MAGNETIC RESONANCE IMAGING With the accepted high sensitivity of CT, MRI is seldom employed in the acute setting of splenic trauma, although it is recognized to be a highly sensitive tool for the detection of blood and blood breakdown products. The signal intensity of hematomas depends on the age of the extravascular bleed. During the first 48 hours following extravasation, blood undergoes transformation into deoxyhemoglobin and other paramagnetic products. With high-field-strength magnets, deoxyhemoglobin within red blood cells may be identified on T2-weighted images, within a few hours after trauma. Subacute hematomas are of high signal on T1-weighted images, because of the paramagnetic effect of the extracellular methemoglobin, which shortens T1 relaxation times (Gomori et al., 1985).

16.3.7. SPLENOSIS Splenosis is the result of autotransplantation of splenic tissue to ectopic sites, following splenic rupture or penetrating injuries, such as a gunshot wound. The nodules of splenic tissue may implant almost anywhere in the peritoneum, and may be found in the thorax following diaphragmatic penetration or tear (Dalton et al., 1971; Dillion et al., 1977; Nielson, 1981). Patients having this condition are virtually all asymptomatic, with the splenosis frequently detected incidentally during radiological evaluation for an unrelated problem. For example, splenosis in the abdomen may be detected as multiple small masses on CT, or as extrinsic masses on examination of the GI tract. In the thorax, CT or plain chest film may demonstrate the presence of a small, pleural-based, soft tissue nodule. The nodules are usually multiple and small, ranging from several millimeters to several centimeters in size, and rarely larger than 3 cm (Nielsen, 1981). Differential diagnosis includes metastases in both the chest and abdomen, as well as endometriosis, hemangiomas, and accessory spleens in the abdomen.

On CT scan, detection of multiple masses in the chest or abdomen, demonstrating contrast enhancement similar to splenic tissue, may suggest the diagnosis. In patients with a known history of splenic trauma or surgery, in whom the diagnosis is suspected, confirmation can be obtained by radionuclide scan, using either [99m]-Technetium sulfur colloid or tagged, damaged red blood cells. On MRI, the signal characteristics are the same as for normal spleen, and, in a reported case in which ferumoxide was given, the signal intensity of the ectopic splenic tissue decreased following contrast administration, indicating the presence of functioning reticuloendothelial cells (Torres et al., 1995).

16.4. FOCAL DISEASE

16.4.1. CYSTS Cystic lesions of the spleen have a varied etiology, and include the true cyst containing an epithelial lining, and believed to be congenital in origin; the false cyst, which is probably posttraumatic; and other less common lesions, such as cystic neoplasms and parasitic cysts. True cysts account for 20% of splenic cystic lesions, and are usually incidental findings, unless size leads to the development of symptoms, or complications such as infection, hemorrhage, or rupture occur. Radiographically, it is often difficult to differentiate true from false cysts. On radiographic examination, a large, usually solitary, splenic mass is identified in the left upper quadrant of the abdomen. Although these are most commonly found in patients in the second or third decade (Sirinek and Evans, 1973), they may also be discovered in children (Griscom et al., 1977). Plain film may demonstrate evidence of a large left upper quadrant mass, with displacement of the gastric air bubble or elevation of the left hemidiaphragm, basilar atelectasis, and flaring of the ipsilateral lower ribs. Curvilinear calcification may suggest the presence of a cystic structure, and has been found to occur in up to 25% of posttraumatic cysts. It is less common in true cysts (Propper et al., 1979).

On ^{99m}-Technetium sulfur colloid scintigraphy, a splenic cyst will be seen as a large photopenic zone, representing the mass, often partially surrounded by a crescent of normal but compressed spleen. Barium study of the gastrointestinal tract may demonstrate displacement of the stomach, and occasionally inferior displacement of the splenic flexure of the colon. Such displacement of adjacent organs is common, because splenic cysts have been found in recent studies to average 10 cm in diameter (Garvin and King, 1981).

On CT, a splenic cyst appears as a large, well-defined, near-water-density lesion having a smooth, thin, nonenhancing wall; however, there are few reports of the CT characteristics of these lesions (Davidson et al., 1980; Cooperberg, 1987; Piekarski et al., 1980; Shin and Ho, 1983). It is usually found in a subcapsular location, but approximately one-third are located deep within the spleen. Although approx 80% are solitary and unilocular, 20% are multiple or multilocular (Delaney and Jason, 1981), and the septa may be visible on CT. The cyst walls are often trabeculated pathologically, and this trabeculation may also be seen (Dachman et al., 1986) more often in true cysts. The cyst may have the classic appearance on CT of a low-density structure, but the presence of blood or debris within the cyst may give it a more complex appearance, and this is more typical of false cysts (Dawes and Malangoni, 1986). The differential diagnosis, on the basis of CT, should include a large abscess or hematoma, cystic neoplasm (e.g., lymphangioma or hemangioma), or even echinococcal cyst, if multiseptated. Splenic echinococcal cyst, caused by *Echinococcus granulosus*, occurs in less than 2% of patients with hydatid disease, and there are usually concurrent liver cysts to aid the diagnosis. Pancreatic pseudocyst, directly adjacent to, or within, the splenic parenchyma, is also a possibility. Intrasplenic fluid collections, in association with pancreatitis, is reported in 1–5% of patients with pancreatitis (Lankisch, 1990), presumably resulting from direct extension of digestive enzymes along the splenorenal ligament, or because of infarction and liquefaction secondary to splenic thrombosis. CT is particularly useful in demonstrating both the fluid collection and associated changes of pancreatitis, as well as any precipitating conditions, such as biliary calculi or calcification of chronic pancreatitis (Fig. 9).

Ultrasound is also useful for identifying the splenic origin of the cyst, as well as in distinguishing cystic from solid or complex lesions (Wright and Williams, 1974). On ultrasound, a simple cyst is seen as a focal, usually well-defined, area containing no echoes (Fig. 10). Occasionally, the presence of debris or hemorrhage may account for the presence of some fine internal echoes. In addition, it demonstrates excellent transmission of the ultrasound waves to structures deep to the cyst, and increased echogenicity of the cyst wall furthest from the ultrasound transducer, or so-called "back wall enhancement." As on CT, trabeculation of the wall or septation may be seen, as well as wall calcification (Dachman et al., 1986).

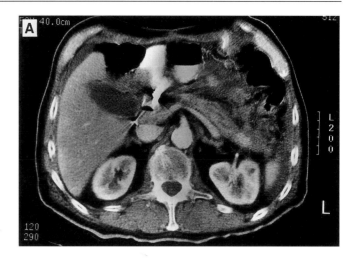

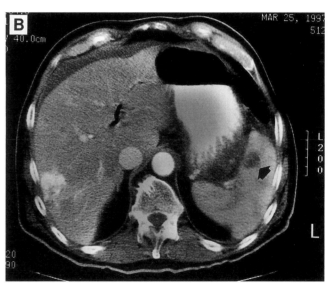

Fig. 16.9. Intrasplenic pseudocyst secondary to acute pancreatitis. (**A**) CT shows extensive inflammation around the pancreas; and (**B**) within the spleen is a well-circumscribed fluid density (arrow) consistent with a pseudocyst.

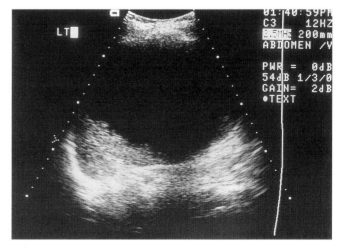

Fig. 16.10. A false (posttraumatic) cyst. Ultrasound demonstrates a large, anechoic area within the spleen, which shows through-transmission of the sound with posterior enhancement.

MRI of splenic cysts typically shows a well-defined mass, with low signal on T1-weighted images and high signal on T2-weighted images, equal to that of water. The presence of protein and hemorrhage can cause considerable variation in signal, particularly on T1-weighted images, which may become quite high (Rabushka et al., 1994).

Angiography shows a large avascular zone, with draping or stretching of vessels around the cyst. The splenic vessels are intrinsically normal in appearance, with no evidence of neovascularity in benign cysts (Bron and Hoffman, 1971). The parenchymal phase may demonstrate compression of the normal splenic tissue. However, CT and ultrasound usually make angiography unnecessary (Davidson et al., 1980).

Although CT and ultrasound will usually provide the most revealing imaging studies, thin-needle aspiration of cystic lesions in the spleen can be performed for diagnosis in equivocal cases, using a 22-gage needle. However, caution should be used in selecting this procedure, when there is the possibility of an echinococcal cyst. Frequently, a clinical history of trauma will help differentiate a true cyst from a false cyst, but past trauma may not be reliably recalled by the patient.

16.4.2. SPLENIC ABSCESS　Splenic abscess is relatively uncommon overall, but it is more frequent in the chronically debilitated or immunosuppressed, such as patients with malignancies, hematological disorders, diabetes, and AIDS, as well as those on aggressive chemotherapy regimes. Immunosuppressed patients account for some 25% of patients with splenic abscess (Caslowitz et al., 1989), usually occurring as part of a more generalized infection. Commonly, hematogenous seeding from a distant site of infection creates multiple small abscesses throughout the spleen and other organs. Perhaps less common is a solitary splenic abscess seen with hematogenous seeding of a splenic hematoma or infarct, or rarely with inadvertent iatrogenic embolization of the spleen during angiography. Penetrating trauma may also cause a solitary septic lesion.

Plain film findings in splenic abscess are often nonspecific, but findings are present in the majority of patients with this condition. Standard frontal and lateral chest radiographs may demonstrate elevation of the left hemidiaphragm, left pleural effusion, and left lower lobe infiltrates or atelectasis (Freund et al., 1982; Pawar et al., 1982). A focal adynamic ileus is frequently present in the left upper quadrant. The presence of gas or gas-fluid levels in the spleen is uncommon, but is more specific for the diagnosis, if present (Fig. 11). When splenic abscess is complicated by rupture, fistula formation, or bowel obstruction, plain films may be altered accordingly.

Like plain films, contrast studies of the gastrointestinal tract usually demonstrate only indirect evidence of splenic abscess. When splenic abscess is suspected, CT provides a much higher diagnostic yield, and is more specific. Furthermore, prior gastrointestinal studies may compromise further evaluation by CT, particularly if barium is used.

On [99m]-Technetium sulfur colloid scintigraphy, splenomegaly is a common but nonspecific finding. If multiple abscesses are present, patchy, inhomogeneous splenic uptake of radionuclide may be seen. A solitary abscess produces a focal defect within the spleen. In either ease, there are multiple differential diagnostic possibilities, and clinical correlation with fever or sepsis aids in the diagnosis.

67-Gallium citrate has been used as an additional radionuclide for the detection of splenic abscess, often as a secondary study to

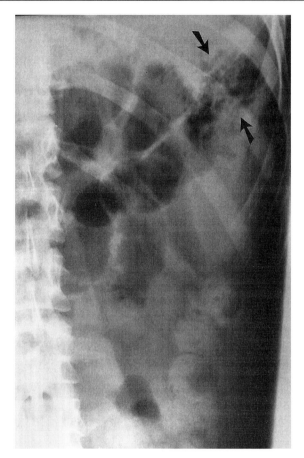

Fig. 16.11.　Splenic abscess on plain film. Localized view of the left upper quadrant, in this supine film of the abdomen, demonstrates extraluminal gas in the region of the spleen (arrows). Although extraluminal air in the left upper quadrant is not specific for splenic abscess, when present, this diagnosis should be considered, and CT of the upper abdomen should be performed to confirm the presence of a splenic abscess.

increase the specificity of the diagnosis (Henkin, 1975). Gallium will localize at the site of infection, permitting the detection of lesions that may be equivocal or not apparent in other studies. Since gallium also localizes in a variety of tumors, particularly lymphoma, distinction between tumor and abscess may at times be difficult.

Ultrasound, together with CT, has become one of the principal imaging modalities in suspected splenic abscess. Early in its evolution, a splenic abscess may produce only subtle alterations in the echogenicity of splenic tissue. In the presence of multiple small abscesses, ill-defined patchy areas of increased and decreased echogenicity may be seen diffusely throughout the spleen; these may coalesce and become more well-defined with time. With a solitary abscess, similar changes will be seen in a single area. Later in its development, a focal abscess will be seen as an irregular area of decreased echogenicity. Septations and scattered internal echoes, representing necrotic tissue, blood, and other debris, are often seen. Through-transmission is therefore less than that found with simple cyst (Pawar et al., 1982; Ralls et al., 1982). Distinguishing an abscess from a resolving hematoma may present difficulties.

The presence of multiple intrasplenic gas collections may compromise ultrasound examination of a splenic abscess, because gas

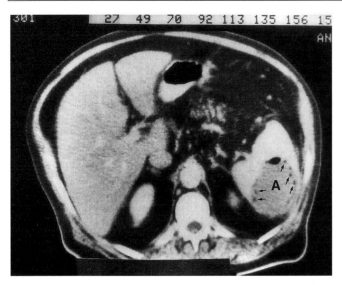

Fig. 16.12. Splenic abscess: CT demonstrates the presence of a solitary lesion in the spleen. Note the presence of small bubbles of gas (arrows) in the periphery of a low-density mass, A, which corresponded with a focal defect on [99m]Technetium sulfur colloid scintigraphy.

appears intensely echogenic, and blocks through-transmission of the ultrasound beam. As mentioned previously, bowel gas in the left upper quadrant may also interfere with the examination, making CT scanning necessary (Moss et al., 1980). In addition, very small lesions, or lesions in the superior portion of the spleen, may be missed.

CT is an excellent means of demonstrating splenic abscess, especially when ultrasound is equivocal or difficult, because of the presence of surrounding bowel gas. It is highly sensitive, can reveal areas of concurrent infection, and may help in identifying the underlying source. On CT, a splenic abscess is seen as an irregular, rounded area of low density, which may be localized, but which frequently replaces most of the normal splenic parenchyma. Gas is present in only a small number of splenic abscesses, but it is easily detected on CT, and may even be seen in the splenic or portal vein (Fig. 12). Evidence of inflammatory changes is frequently seen in tissues surrounding the abscess. The abscess wall is usually thick, and enhances following iv contrast. Although splenic abscesses are often poorly defined, use of iv contrast, and appropriate CT-imaging technique, will frequently accentuate the subtle findings. Opacification of stomach and bowel with contrast is also crucial for accurate diagnosis, because nonopacified bowel loops in a perisplenic location may lead to false-positive diagnoses or confusion in diagnosis.

CT has become the imaging modality of choice at many institutions for the diagnosis of abscess in any part of the body, and it provides a reliable method for follow-up. However, considerable overlap can occur between the CT appearances of an abscess and those of hematoma, infarct, lymphoma, and metastases, so fine-needle aspiration to confirm the diagnosis, followed, if necessary, by percutaneous drainage using CT or ultrasound guidance, has been increasingly accepted and performed in recent years.

MRI is seldom performed to diagnose splenic abscess, and its application for interventional procedures, such as percutaneous drainage, is yet to be established. When present, an abscess ap-

pears, of low signal intensity, on T1-weighted images, with a high signal on T2-weighted images, and may have some low signal representing necrotic debris (Shirkhoda, 1993).

16.4.3. LYMPHOMA Lymphomatous involvement of the spleen, as a manifestation of systemic lymphoma, is common; primary splenic lymphoma, without evidence of nodal disease, is uncommon, although on the increase, as the result of the increasing prevalence of AIDS. Lymphoma in the spleen characteristically involves the white pulp, frequently appearing as nodules. In advanced disease, the entire spleen may be replaced by tumor (Kim and Dorfman, 1974). Ahmann et al. (1966) described four categories of splenic lymphoma on gross pathology: homogeneous enlargement without masses, miliary masses, 2–10 cm masses, and a large, solitary mass. However, the spleen may be entirely normal in both cut-section and size, with tumor cells seen only microscopically.

Determining splenic involvement in lymphoma is a challenge, because this may affect the management and choice of therapy. The radiographic diagnosis of splenic lymphoma is often difficult, because of the wide range of presentation, and the possibility of a normal appearance of the spleen, despite the presence of tumor. No single imaging modality, including ultrasound, CT (Glazer et al., 1981), or MRI, has proved to be very accurate in diagnosis: More than 50% of lesions are manifest as either diffuse infiltration or subcentimeter lesions.

As a rule, splenomegaly is not a reliable sign of lymphomatous involvement. Although splenomegaly in most patients with non-Hodgkin's lymphoma indicates splenic involvement, up to one-third of patients with splenomegaly have no evidence of splenic lymphoma on histologic examination (Shirkhoda, 1993). In addition, up to one-third of patients with lymphoma of any kind will have histologic involvement of the spleen in the absence of splenomegaly. Thus, radiographic demonstration of splenomegaly can only suggest or support a diagnosis of splenic involvement. Greater accuracy in the diagnosis of splenic lymphoma can be obtained with both CT and ultrasound by demonstrating adenopathy in the splenic hilum or focal splenic defects, in addition to splenomegaly (Carroll and Ta, 1980). Furthermore, demonstration of liver involvement indicates a high probability of splenic involvement, even if no splenic abnormalities can be identified radiographically.

On ultrasound, lymphomatous involvement of the spleen is usually seen as single or multiple heterogeneous, hypoechoic, nodular lesions of variable size (Carroll and Ta, 1980). These lesions are often poorly defined. As described above, a single, large lesion involving most of the spleen or multiple smaller lesions may be seen. Lymphoma appearing as focal anechoic or hypoechoic defects can simulate an abscess (Bloom et al., 1981; Castellino et al., 1972; Cunningham, 1978), and may cause diagnostic difficulty in the individual with clinical features of abscess. Hyperechoic lesions have also been described (Carroll and Ta, 1980).

CT is the current modality of choice for diagnosis, staging, and monitoring response to treatment. As described earlier, CT is susceptible to the same difficulties as ultrasound and other modalities, in identifying microscopic or diffuse splenic disease. The overall accuracy of CT in detecting splenic lymphoma is about 65% (Glazer et al., 1981). In diagnosing lymphoma at any site in the body, CT is least effective in identifying early disease, because microscopic infiltration may be seen in nodes of normal size or borderline enlargement. In more-advanced disease, the nodes may be unequivocally enlarged (Fig. 13). In lymphomatous involvement of the spleen, the CT appearances mirror various pathological appearances.

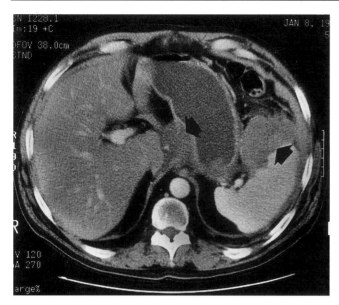

Fig. 16.13. Lymphoma. CT scan shows extensive nodal disease in the gastrohepatic and gastosplenic ligaments (arrows), the latter involving the spleen.

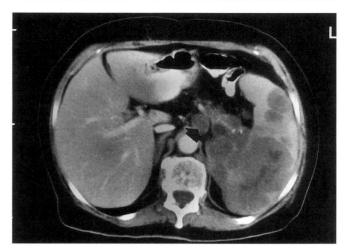

Fig. 16.15. Lymphoma. CT scan shows multiple, smaller, low-density masses within the spleen, but also some evidence of nodal disease (arrow).

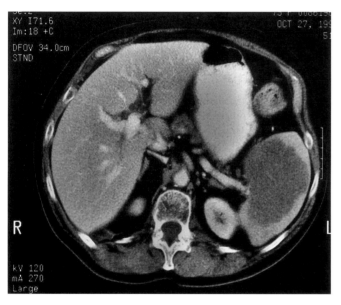

Fig. 16.14. Lymphoma. CT scan shows a large, solitary, homogeneous, low-density mass in the spleen, which may mimic an abscess.

Contrast-enhanced CT usually demonstrates heterogeneous lesions of decreased density and variable size, either solitary (Fig. 14) or multiple (Fig. 15). As with ultrasound, the appearance may mimic an abscess, and the distinction may have to depend on clinical findings. Calcification is rare, and probably represents dystrophic change secondary to necrosis, hemorrhage, or fibrosis, and so is more commonly seen following treatment.

If the spleen is diffusely involved, some focal areas of low density may represent infarcts or hematomas. Some authors feel that abnormality of the spleen on CT is more likely to occur in non-Hodgkin's lymphoma (Koehler, 1983), with high-grade more likely to have focal lesions, and low-grade more likely to show diffuse involvement. Primary splenic lymphoma, when it does occur, may be bulky, transgress the capsule, and invade adjacent

organs, such as pancreas, stomach, diaphragm, and abdominal wall (Meyer et al., 1983).

The detection of splenic lymphoma, particularly diffuse disease, is not reliable on unenhanced MRI, because of the similarity in T1 and T2 relaxation times of tumor and normal spleen, which results in poor lesion-to-spleen contrast (Shirkhoda, 1993). The presence of necrosis, hemorrhage, and cystic change will result in increased conspicuity. Nodules are easier to identify on T2-weighted images, because as they have a longer T2 relaxation. Gadolinium can increase the conspicuity of nodules on T1-weighted images; the role of ferumoxides remains to be determined, but initial studies concentrating on lesions in the liver appear promising (Weissleder et al., 1989).

16.4.4. HEMANGIOMA   Although rare, the hemangioma is the most common benign tumor of the spleen; it is usually asymptomatic, and infrequently presents as splenomegaly or as a mass in the left upper abdominal quadrant, although it may be associated with the potential life-threatening complication of rupture, in up to 25% of cases (Ros et al., 1987). However, it is more often discovered incidentally at autopsy, or radiologically during studies performed for other purposes. Although usually solitary, it may be multiple, as in splenic hemangiomatosis, and occasionally is seen as part of a more generalized angiomatosis.

There are in fact few reports in the literature of splenic hemangioma. When present, the radiographical appearance is similar to that of hemangiomas found elsewhere in the body. Calcification is occasionally present, and usually appears either peripherally, in curvilinear form, or centrally and punctate, on plain film (Ros et al., 1987).

On sonography, two patterns have been identified. One is a predominantly echogenic mass, corresponding to a solid hemangioma; the other is that of a complex, echodense mass containing anechoic areas representing blood pools within proliferating vascular channels.

CT also demonstrates two patterns: One is that of a homogeneous, well-marginated solid mass, which is either hypodense or isodense on nonenhanced studies, in relation to the normal splenic parenchyma (Fig. 16); the other pattern is that of a multicystic mass. The cystic areas demonstrate a density similar to water, and

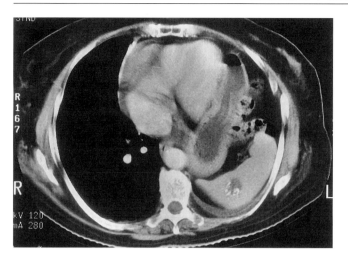

Fig. 16.16. Hemangioma. A solitary, hypodense, intrasplenic lesion is seen on this CT, with peripheral calcification.

lie within a mass that is isodense with normal spleen (Ros et al., 1987). Peripheral enhancement with iv contrast, with delayed central enhancement, similar to that of hepatic hemangioma, has been observed (Paivansalo and Siniluoto, 1983; Fig. 17A). In the multicystic type of lesion, the solid portions will enhance following iv contrast.

The pattern of splenic hemangioma on angiography is variable and nonspecific. Solid hemangiomas or cystic spaces may be seen as hypovascular areas; hypervascularity, tumor vessels, and pooling of contrast medium may also be seen. On MRI, a round mass of homogeneous signal intensity is seen. The lesions demonstrate low signal intensity on T1-weighted (Fig. 17B), and very high signal intensity on T2-weighted, images, with respect to the spleen, similar in appearance to hepatic hemangioma (Ros et al., 1987). Occasionally, T1-weighted images will show high signal, corresponding with hemorrhage or high protein content, and T2-weighted images may appear heterogeneous, with mixed cystic and solid components. Gadolinium can help distinguish solid from cystic areas, by its enhancement (Fig. 17C).

The radiographical appearance of splenic hemangioma ranges from a solid to a predominantly cystic tumor, and includes a variety of solid and cystic splenic masses in its differential diagnosis. The radiographical findings most suggestive of the diagnosis of splenic hemangioma are a large, asymptomatic mass in the left upper abdominal quadrant; peripheral curvilinear or central punctate calcification in a left upper quadrant mass; and a solid or combined solid and cystic intrasplenic mass seen on ultrasound or CT. The ability to diagnose this tumor radiographically is important: Needle biopsy is not indicated, because of the location and vascular nature of the tumor, and unnecessary splenectomy may be avoided (Ros et al., 1987).

16.4.5. ANGIOSARCOMA Primary angiosarcoma of the spleen is a rare pathological entity, with less than 100 cases reported in the literature (Garvin and King, 1981; Arbona et al., 1982; Chen et al., 1979, Kishikawa et al., 1977; Sordillo et al., 1981). Splenic angiosarcoma may be a primary lesion, but it is frequently associated with hepatic lesions (Chen et al., 1979; Locker et al., 1979), in which case the primary site cannot be definitely identified. Although many hepatic angiosarcomas are associated with toxic exposure (such as vinyl chloride or arsenic) or ionizing radiation (thorium), primary splenic angiosarcoma may not show such an association

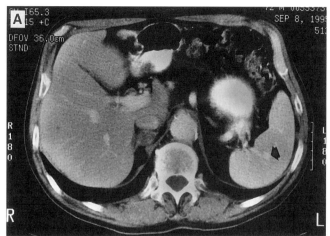

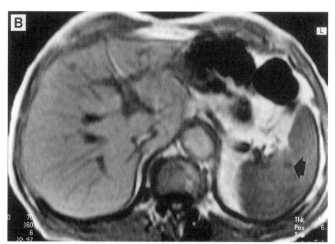

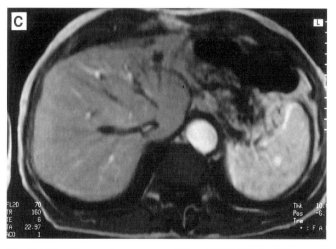

Fig. 16.17. Hemangioma seen on CT and MRI. (**A**) On CT, a small lesion, which enhances uniformly, to the same degree as adjacent vessels, is identified in the midpole of the spleen (arrow). (**B**) Unenhanced TI-weighted scan shows a small, hypointense lesion (arrow), which enhances homogeneously following iv gadolinium, (**C**).

(Mahoney et al., 1982). Radiographical evaluation usually demonstrates no specific abnormality. Presentation frequently consists of abdominal pain, a left upper quadrant mass, and anemia. ^{99m}-Technetium sulfur colloid scintigraphy, performed on a patient with left upper quadrant symptoms, may show an enlarged spleen containing single or multiple photopenic defects. Ultrasound and CT demonstrate an enlarged spleen with nodules of varying size, frequently involving the liver, as well (Arbona et al., 1982), but differentiation from other tumors cannot be made on the basis of these studies. The nodules have a mixed echogenicity on US, and may be of high attenuation on CT, because of hemorrhage or hemosiderin deposition. Peripheral enhancement is variable, and there may be high attenuation to the background spleen, if thorotrast is present. MRI may show multiple nodular masses with low signal rims, caused by hemosiderin deposition (Rabushka et al., 1994). The signal on T1-weighted images varies, depending on the degree of necrosis and hemorrhage.

16.4.6. HAMARTOMA
Splenic hamartomas are usually solitary, but may be multiple, and are usually an incidental finding. White pulp or red pulp tissue, or a mixture thereof, may predominate (Iozzo et al., 1980). As in many other splenic abnormalities, plain films are either normal or may show some degree of splenomegaly. Calcifications found in splenic hamartomas have ranged from punctate to stellate in configuration, and have been found to lie in the fibrotic portions of the lesions, rather than within the vascular channels. There has been limited CT experience with this lesion, but the solid lesion may appear hypo- or isodense on unenhanced CT, and nearly isodense with the spleen on contrast-enhanced CT (Dachman et al., 1986). Large hamartomas may have a central area of necrosis or scar formation, with punctate calcification. Ultrasound typically shows a well-defined homogeneous echogenic mass, which may contain cystic areas. Cystic hamartomas demonstrate both solid and cystic components on CT and ultrasound (Brinkley and Lee, 1981). MRI shows a well-defined mass, isointense on T1-weighted, and low signal on T2-weighted, images, with respect to the spleen. Linear low signal strands may be seen representing fibrotic cords. Prolonged enhancement following gadolinium has been observed, because of stagnant blood flow within sinusoids (Ohtomo et al., 1992). However, it is again true that accurate differentiation of splenic hamartoma from other splenic masses cannot be made on the basis of these studies.

16.4.7. SPLENIC LYMPHANGIOMATOSIS
Splenic lymphangiomatosis is a rare entity, with approx 90 cases reported in the literature (Pistoia and Markowitz, 1988). The lesion is characteristically diffuse, and involves almost the entire spleen, but solitary cystic lesions can be found (Asch et al., 1974; Tuttle and Minielly, 1978). The lesion is composed of single or multiple cysts of varying sizes, which are lined by endothelium and filled with proteinaceous fluid (Asch et al., 1974; Pearl and Nassar, 1979). Simultaneous involvement of other organ systems, including skin, lungs, bones, or other viscera, is occasionally present. Curvilinear calcification in cyst walls has been described (Rao et al., 1981).

Plain films may demonstrate splenomegaly, with mass effect on adjacent structures. On [99m]-Technetium sulfur colloid scintigraphy, single or multiple photopenic defects in the spleen are present (Dachman et al., 1986; Novetsky and Epstein, 1982). On ultrasound, a single, well-defined cyst may be seen, which may be difficult to differentiate from other solitary cystic lesions. More commonly, in diffuse lymphangiomatosis, multiple well-defined hypoechoic masses (cysts) of various sizes will be seen throughout an enlarged spleen (Enzinger and Weiss, 1983). Septations or proteinaceous debris can sometimes be seen within these cystic masses, as internal echoes (Rao et al., 1981).

CT scanning may demonstrate an enlarged spleen containing single or multiple areas of low density. These lesions have thin walls, are sharply marginated, and do not enhance after administration of iv contrast material. Small, marginal, linear calcifications may be more easily detected than on plain film (Pistoia and Markowitz, 1988; Pyatt et al., 1981). On MRI, lymphangiomas appear bright on both T1- and T2-weighted images, because of the proteinaceous nature of the fluid within the lesions.

16.4.8. METASTASES
Metastasis to the spleen is usually seen only late in the course of metastatic disease, common primaries being the breast, lung, and melanoma, and such patients generally have multiorgan involvement. However, solitary splenic metastases have been described, without evidence of involvement of other organs (Federle and Moss, 1983), and this can alter the patient's staging and subsequent therapy. Most splenic metastases are of hematogenous origin, but direct invasion from adjacent organs (including the stomach, left colon, left kidney, and pancreas) and peritoneal seeding are also seen.

Plain films are usually normal. However, diffuse metastases may result in splenomegaly, which preserves the normal contour of the spleen. [99m]-Technetium sulfur colloid scintigraphy may show single or multiple photopenic defects within the spleen, if macroscopic disease is present. Extensive splenic metastases may cause partial or complete nonvisualization of the spleen, possibly by encasing or invading the splenic vessels, and, in effect, causing autosplenectomy.

On ultrasound, metastatic lesions in the spleen, as elsewhere, have a varied appearance. They can be homogeneously hypoechoic or hyperechoic. No correlation has been found between lesion echogenicity and the primary tumor type. In addition, lesions having mixed hypoechoic and hyperechoic areas are seen, because of solid masses having cystic or necrotic components. Larger lesions tend to be more complex than smaller ones, and diffuse involvement of the spleen may be seen in 10% of cases.

By CT, metastatic lesions usually have a lower density, or are isodense, compared to surrounding normal spleen, prior to iv contrast administration. Following injection of iv contrast, the low-density lesions become accentuated against the enhancing normal splenic tissue (Fig. 18). Cystic lesions may show peripheral enhancement. Frequently, isodense lesions, not apparent on noncontrast CT, are detectable only after contrast injection, since the normal splenic tissue enhances to a greater degree than the metastatic disease (Piekarski et al., 1980). As on ultrasound, mixed-density lesions, having cystic or necrotic components, are also seen. Frequently, metastatic lesions in the liver and other organs are also present. Evidence of necrosis is usually seen in the larger metastases. Calcification is rare, unless the primary is a mucinous adenocarcinoma. CT-guided percutaneous needle biopsy can be performed on splenic lesions, for definitive diagnosis.

On MRI, metastases may be hard to see without administering iv contrast, but are typically of low signal on T1-weighted, and higher signal on T2-weighted, images. If old hemorrhage has occurred, then the signal on T2-weighted images will be low, because of the presence of hemosiderin. Melanoma metastases have a characteristic high signal on T1-weighted images, because of the paramagnetic effect of melanin, which shortens T1 relaxation. The use of ferumoxides has been shown to be better than CT for determining the size and number of splenic metastases (Weissleder et al., 1989).

16.5. DIFFUSE DISEASE

16.5.1. SPLENOMEGALY
Splenomegaly is probably the most common finding in the presence of diffuse splenic disease. Although the differential diagnosis of splenomegaly is extensive, the degree

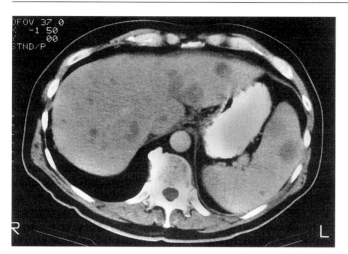

Fig. 16.18. Melanoma metastases involving liver and spleen. CT scan shows multiple nonenhancing focal lesions of varying size.

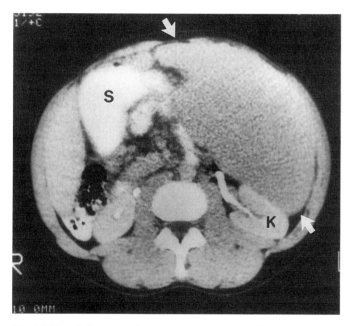

Fig. 16.19. Splenomegaly secondary to leukemia on CT. Enhanced CT of the upper abdomen at the level of the left kidney demonstrates a markedly enlarged spleen (white arrows). This marked splenomegaly was caused by chronic lymphocytic leukemia. Note that the spleen is homogeneous in density. There is compression of the left kidney, posteriorly (K), and of the stomach (S) to the right of the midline.

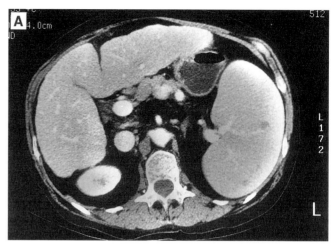

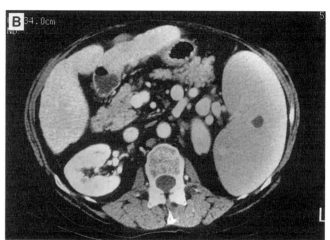

Fig. 16.20. Splenomegaly caused by portal hypertension. (**A**) CT scans show a cirrhotic liver architecture with multiple varices; (**B**) diffuse splenomegaly and several focal, low-density lesions consistent with infarcts.

of splenomegaly and associated findings may help in differentiating the various causes (*see also* Chapter 9). However, many diseases, causing splenomegaly without specific characteristics, can be diagnosed only on the basis of clinical or laboratory data. Some of the causes of diffuse splenic disease are discussed briefly here. The myeloproliferative group of disorders, including certain leukemias and myelofibrosis, are often associated with massive splenomegaly (Fig. 19), and are discussed in Chapter 13. Such splenomegaly can be detected by almost any imaging modality. Diagnosis is made on the basis of hematological findings. Lymphoma was discussed previously, under focal diseases (*see* Subheading 4.3.), but may also present as diffuse splenic involvement (*see also* Chapter 14).

Marked splenomegaly may be seen in cases of chronic passive congestion, which is commonly secondary to portal hypertension or congestive heart failure. The spleen is enlarged, but uniform in texture. Dilatation of the splenic vein or associated varices may be identified by imaging studies (Fig. 20). On MRI, the T1 and T2 relaxation times of the spleen are increased, probably because of its increased blood content, resulting in lower-than-normal intensity on T1-weighted images, and higher-than-normal on T2-weighted images (Stark et al., 1984). In patients with portal hypertension, multiple low-signal-intensity spots may be identified within the spleen, relating to siderotic nodules (Gandy-Gamna bodies). These are best seen at high field strength, and using gradient echo sequences, which are more sensitive to the dephasing effect of hemosiderin (Minami et al., 1989).

In sarcoidosis, the radiological features in the abdomen are non-specific, usually suggesting lymphoma or metastases. Splenomegaly may be found, even when few lesions are present elsewhere: Up to one-fourth of cases show mild hepatosplenomegaly. With ultrasound a diffusely increased echogenicity of the splenic parenchyma is found, and focal hypoechoic or mixed echogenicity lesions may be present. CT shows irregularly distributed low-density focal areas within the spleen, and abdominal or pelvic lymph nodes are often present. A pattern of multifocal defects on [99m]-Technetium sulfur colloid scan, apparently secondary to sarcoid granulomas, has been reported (Iko et al., 1982). On MRI, the spleen shows a diffuse, mottled heterogeneous reduction in signal, as the result of the presence of fibrosis (Torres et al., 1995).

Many storage diseases cause splenomegaly. Gaucher's disease is one of the more common lipid storage diseases, caused by accumulation of glucocerebroside in macrophages of the spleen, liver, and bone marrow. Massive hepatosplenomegaly results, and is associated with characteristic skeletal lesions. Ultrasound, CT, and MRI all show marked splenomegaly. On CT, the spleen may have abnormally low attenuation, and ultrasound may reveal discrete hypoechoic lesions, representing focal clusters of Gaucher cells. On MRI, there is increased signal on T1-weighted images, because the shortening of the T1 relaxation time, as a result of accumulation of glucocerebroside (Lanir et al., 1986). Unlike most infiltrations, the spleen in Gaucher's disease often retains its shape, because the Gaucher cells and fibrosis prevent tissue collapse.

16.5.2. QUANTITATIVE MEASUREMENT OF SPLEEN SIZE AND VOLUME

As discussed previously and in Chapter 9, splenomegaly is a nonspecific finding caused by many different disorders of the spleen. Measurement of spleen volume is, in some instances, useful both in the initial assessment and the later follow-up of patients with splenomegaly. One of the earliest approaches to predicting spleen weight radiologically was devised by Whitley et al. (1966), in which a computer-based system was used to predict spleen weight from routine films of the abdomen. However, for routine use without the aid of a computer, plain films can only give an approximate estimate of spleen size, with only marked changes being detectable. More recently, with the use of CT and ultrasound, determination of spleen size has become increasingly accurate.

Sonography has been used by many for volume determination, calculated by the summation of multiple, parallel, cross-sectional areas (Koga et al., 1972). Pietri and Boscaini (1984) proposed sonographic calculation of a splenic volumetric index, using measurements of the maximum breadth, thickness, and height of the spleen. However, measurement of the spleen, using sonography, is hampered by the inaccessibility of those portions of the spleen that are hidden by overlying bowel gas or ribs, and by the difficulty of scanning under the left hemidiaphragm. In addition, the manual nature of sonography and its extreme operator dependency make reproducibility of measurements problematic.

The easiest and most accurate method of measuring spleen size is by CT. Several authors have described computer analysis of CT sections (Heymsfield et al., 1979; Henderson et al., 1981), using complex mathematical formulae. Breiman et al. (1982) simplified and refined this method, obtaining contiguous sections through the spleen at 2-cm intervals, and calculating volume using a summation-of-areas technique. The area of the spleen on each CT section is calculated by tracing the spleen outline with a cursor, then using a computer program. The mean percentage error of volume measurements, using this technique, is ~3.6%. The advantages of the summation-of-areas technique, using CT, are: The CT scans are completely automated, reproducible, and easily obtainable; the boundaries of the spleen are easily recognized by CT; and the method does not require the use of complex mathematical formulae. Three-dimensional reconstruction techniques, using CT, allow the most accurate volumetric evaluation of the spleen.

Although an accurate determination of spleen size and volume can be obtained by CT, in routine daily practice, an experienced observer can judge spleen size and volume by simple study of the CT scans. Typically, the craniocaudal length of the normal spleen is less than 15 cm, and the inferior tip does not usually extend to the level of the tip of the right lobe of the liver. In addition, the anterior edge of the spleen usually does not extend anteriorly beyond the midaxillary line (Federle, 1983). Splenomegaly may be strongly suspected, if either of these boundaries is transgressed.

16.5.3. INFECTIONS

Infection involving the spleen may result simply in diffuse splenomegaly, as is found frequently in malaria, mononucleosis, leishmaniasis, trypanosomiasis (Chaga's disease), histoplasmosis, schistosomiasis, echinococcosis, and AIDS. Splenic infection may also take the form of multiple microabscesses or granulomas. Radiological manifestations of focal splenic abscess were discussed in Subheading 4.2. Infectious mononucleosis causes mild splenomegaly in the second week of illness in 75% of patients, but marked splenomegaly may occasionally occur. Splenic rupture and hemoperitoneum are rare complications, and CT or ultrasound can be used to evaluate the spleen for suspected rupture.

In schistosomiasis, splenomegaly is produced secondary to the characteristic cirrhosis, which produces perisplenic vein fibrosis and splenic vein thrombosis. Thrombosis of the portal or splenic can be detected by ultrasound (Mousa et al., 1967). Other findings on ultrasound in patients with schistosomiasis include periportal fibrosis, thickening of the gallbladder wall, echogenic hepatic nodules, and hypertrophy of the left lobe of the liver, with associated atrophy of the right lobe (Cerri et al., 1984).

Splenic infection by echinococcus is usually associated with liver and/or lung involvement; this is the only parasite to produce splenic cysts. The cysts, solitary or multiple, may cause a focal mass effect or splenic enlargement, which may be detected on plain films. These cysts may demonstrate peripheral, ring-like calcification, as is seen with other types of cysts. However, the presence of multiple cysts, the appearance of daughter cysts within a larger cyst, and similar calcified cystic structures in the liver or lung, help to differentiate echinococcal cysts from other forms. On ultrasound, solitary or multiple anechoic cysts are identified, sometimes with a cyst-within-a-cyst pattern (Wurtele et al., 1982). Extensive echoes may be seen within the cyst, representing internal debris, infolded membranes, scolices, or hydatid sand (Schulman et al., 1983). Similar findings are seen on CT, in which the cysts are near water density, but may increase in density, because of debris or sand. Concurrent liver echinococcal cysts are usually present.

Granulomatous disease of the spleen is most commonly secondary to tuberculosis or histoplasmosis, and is usually found with generalized disease. Mild-to-moderate splenomegaly may be present acutely, along with focal areas of low attenuation on CT. Calcified granulomas are frequently seen at a later stage. These calcifications are small and round in appearance, are frequently identified on plain film, and may be associated with similar calcifications in the lungs or liver. On ultrasound, the calcified granulomas are seen as small, bright echogenic foci with shadowing.

Pneumocystis carinii infection is becoming more common, with the increasing prevalence of an immunosuppressed population, and there is an increasing incidence of extrapulmonary disease. On CT, there is mild splenomegaly, and the spleen contains multiple low attenuation areas that may enlarge and progressively calcify in a rim or punctate fashion (Rabushka et al., 1994). Ultrasound characteristically shows tiny, highly reflective, nonshadowing foci and hypoechoic lesions. In later stages, calcification develops and acoustic shadowing is seen.

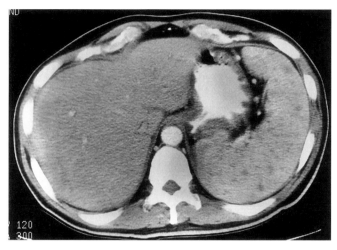

Fig. 16.21. Candidiasis. CT shows splenomegaly with multiple, small, low-density lesions throughout the spleen.

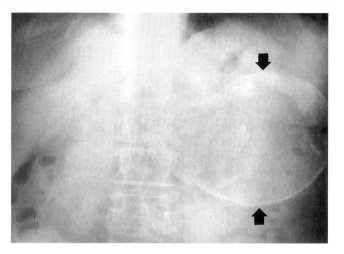

Fig. 16.22. Splenic artery aneurysm on plain films. Localized view of the upper abdomen, from a supine abdominal radiograph, demonstrates a large ring-like calcification (arrows) characteristic of an aneurysm.

As discussed earlier, splenic abscess is usually a solitary focal lesion, but diffuse microabscesses may also be seen, typically with a fungal etiology. The most common cause of microabscesses is *Candida albicans*, usually in immunocompromised patients, particularly in patients on therapy for leukemia. Ultrasound may demonstrate a diffusely hypoechoic spleen, or multiple small hypoechoic or anechoic foci. The small hypoechoic lesions may contain an echogenic center (target lesions), which may represent fungus and inflammatory cells within the microabscess (Sumner et al., 1983). With healing, the lesions become uniformly hypoechoic. CT demonstrates similar findings, with multiple, small, low-density lesions in the spleen and/or liver, some having a target appearance that does not enhance with contrast media (Fig. 21). Although seldom performed, MRI shows small intermediate signal lesions in both liver and spleen, with slightly higher signal on T2-weighted images. Lesions may be more conspicuous, if the patient has hemosiderosis caused by repeated blood transfusions, when the background spleen will have a diffusely low signal intensity (Shirkhoda, 1993). The use of fat saturation with T2-weighted images may improve detection of these small lesions, as may the use of gadolinium.

16.6. VASCULAR DISEASE

16.6.1. ARTERIOSCLEROSIS AND SPLENIC ARTERY ANEU-
RYSMA   As with many arteries affected by arteriosclerosis, involve-ment of the splenic artery leads to calcification of the wall and tortuosity. These changes principally affect the main splenic artery and its major divisions, and tend to become more apparent with age, although severe stenosis is unusual. Although aneurysms of visceral arteries are uncommon, the splenic artery is the most commonly affected (Cobos et al., 1982). Splenic artery aneurysm is usually diagnosed by the presence of ring calcification in the left upper quadrant on plain film (Fig. 22), CT, or ultrasound. The aneurysms are cystic in appearance on ultrasound but the use of Doppler will confirm their vascular nature. They demonstrate contrast enhancement on CT, which may be partially caused by the presence of blood clot. Because of the presence of flowing blood, a low-signal round mass is seen on MRI. Angiography is useful for demonstrating splenic artery aneurysms, as well as associated findings, such as rupture or fistula formation. Transcatheter embolization may be utilized for treatment of a bleeding aneurysm (Probst

et al., 1978). Pseudoaneurysms of the splenic artery may also be seen, especially following trauma, or in association with chronic pancreatitis; the findings are similar to those of true aneurysms.

Most arteriovenous fistulas involving the splenic vessels are secondary to rupture of a splenic aneurysm, but they also occur as a result of penetrating (stab or gunshot) wounds. In the presence of splenic arteriovenous fistula, splenomegaly is often present, with portal hypertension, esophageal varices and ascites. These findings may be detected by a variety of imaging studies: angiography with selective splenic artery injection, yields the definitive diagnosis. Early filling of the splenic vein is seen, often in association with the presence of a splenic artery aneurysm. In addition, the splenic vein may appear dilated secondary to increased pressure, and gastroesophageal varices may be present. Surgery is usually regarded as the treatment of choice, both transcatheter embolization of the involved splenic artery may be considered.

16.6.2. SPLENIC VEIN THROMBOSIS   The pathophysiology of splenic vein thrombosis includes compression, encasement, and inflammation about the splenic vein. In most cases, thrombosis is related to pancreatic carcinoma or chronic pancreatitis; however, the list of causes is long, and includes trauma and large masses causing compression.

Radiographical findings may demonstrate evidence of the underlying cause of the splenic vein thrombosis, e.g., pancreatic calcification on plain film, in a patient with chronic pancreatitis, or a large pancreatic mass seen on CT. A primary finding is the presence of solitary gastric varices, which can be seen on contrast-enhanced CT scan, angiography, or barium study. Such varices are usually located in the region of the gastric fundus or cardia, but they may also occur in the body and antrum, especially along the greater cuvature (Itzchak and Glickman, 1977). Splenomegaly may or may not be present.

Angiography demonstrates splenic vein thrombosis definitively, following injection of the celiac or splenic artery. Percutaneous transhepatic portography can also be used. Diagnostic findings on angiography include partial or complete nonopacification of the splenic vein, with visualization of venous collaterals.

Ultrasound has also been used to diagnose splenic vein thrombosis, and is being increasingly utilized for this purpose (Weinberger et al., 1982). On ultrasound, echogenic material may be seen within the splenic vein, with absent flow on Doppler ultrasound. CT scans may demonstrate lack of patency of the splenic vein on dynamic contrast enhanced scans, in association with gastric varices. CT and ultrasound are also useful in discovering the underlying cause of splenic vein thrombosis.

16.6.3. SPLENIC INFARCTION Splenic parenchymal arterial branches are endarteries that do not intercommunicate; therefore, occlusion of the splenic artery or its branches leads to infarction. Causes of splenic artery occlusion include sickle cell disease (SCD), embolic disease, atherosclerosis, arteritis, splenic artery aneurysm, splenic torsion, and a mass lesion, such as pancreatic carcinoma (Cohen et al., 1984; Anderson and Kissane, 1977).

Findings on plain film may include splenomegaly, an elevated left hemidiaphragm, and left pleural effusion, but these are infrequently seen (Balcar et al., 1984). Despite the advent of newer imaging modalities, nuclear scintigraphy is probably still the best method for diagnosing splenic infarction. On ^{99m}-Technetium sulfur colloid scintigraphy, the area of infarction creates a defect that is classically wedge-shaped and peripheral, with the apex directed toward the splenic hilum (Fig. 23; Lin and Donati, 1981). However, the infarct may be irregular in shape, or even multiple, but these findings are less specific for infarction. SPECT imaging is useful in equivocal cases, and may detect an infarct not seen on planar images.

Sonographically, splenic infarct has been described as a sharply demarcated, hypoechoic area in an enlarged spleen (Yeh et al., 1981), correlating pathologically with edema and necrosis. A similar appearance has been described following transcatheter therapeutic embolization of the spleen (Nunez et al., 1978). However, echogenicity varies with the age of the infarct, being hypoechoic in the acute stages, and becoming more echogenic with time.

As with ultrasound, the CT appearance of a splenic infarct depends on the period that has elapsed since the acute event. Four phases of splenic infarction have been demonstrated (Balcar et al., 1984): hyperacute (d 1), acute (d 2–4), subacute (d 4–8), and chronic (2–4 wk). In the hyperacute phase, an area of decreased density (compared to normal spleen) is usually seen on unenhanced scans, which shows a diffusely mottled pattern, on contrast enhancement. However, a large, focal hyperdense lesion may be seen on unenhanced scans in the hyperacute stage. In the acute and subacute stages, focal well-defined areas of low density are seen, which become better demarcated, and which demonstrate no contrast enhancement. Again, infarcts may be wedge-shaped, irregular, or multiple. Density of the infarcted area may return to normal in the chronic stage, on both pre- and postcontrast scans. The infarct gradually decreases in size, and may completely disappear. Frequently, however, a residual contour defect, representing scarring, is seen at the site of infarction.

16.6.4. SPLENORENAL SHUNT Splenorenal shunts are seen in patients with chronic portal hypertension, and are most often secondary to cirrhosis: The definitive diagnosis may be made angiographically, with reverse flow in the splenic vein, dilated collaterals communicating with the left renal vein, and opacification of the inferior vena cava (Nunez et al., 1978). Enlarged perisplenic veins and left renal vein, and splenomegaly, are seen on CT and ultrasound. Postoperative patency of splenorenal shunts, created surgically for treatment of portal hypertension may also be evaluated angiographically.

16.6.5. SPLENIC VASCULAR CHANGES IN PANCREATIC DISEASE The pancreas is intimately associated with the splenic

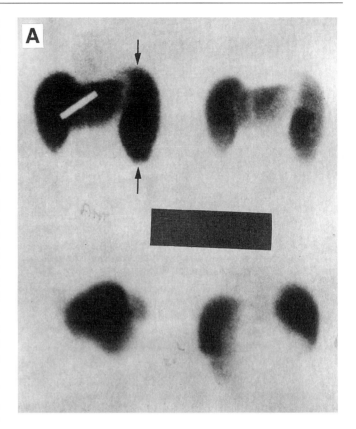

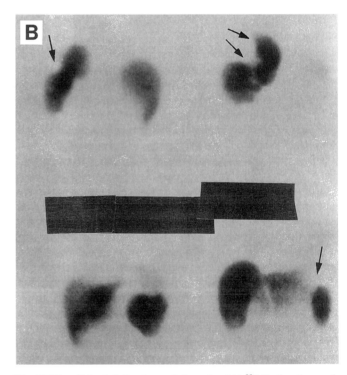

Fig. 16.23. Splenic infarct on scintigraphy. (**A**) ^{99m} Technetium-sulfur colloid scintigraphy, in this patient with polycythemia vera, demonstrates a large spleen with increased uptake (arrows). (**B**) 1 month later, in the same patient, a large, wedge-shaped defect can be identified in the spleen (arrows), in different projections. This defect represents an infarct, commonly seen in polycythemia vera. Splenic infarcts appear, on scintigraphy, as a defect, wedge-shaped and peripherally based, with the apex directed toward the splenic hilus.

vessels, along their entire course. A mass in the tail of the pancreas may cause displacement of these vessels, without intrinsic damage to them. However, pancreatic carcinoma may cause encasement of the splenic artery, resulting in stenosis or complete occlusion. Occasionally, this stenosis mimics atherosclerotic disease, in which case evaluation of the splenic vein may help differentiate benign from malignant disease. The splenic vein is normal in the presence of atherosclerosis; involvement or obstruction of the splenic vein suggests pancreatic adenocarcinoma. Pancreatitis can also cause narrowing of the splenic vessels as the result of fibrosis, mimicking, angiographically, the findings seen in adenocarcinoma.

16.7. MISCELLANEOUS DISORDERS

16.7.1. SICKLE CELL DISEASE   SCD has widespread manifestations, with frequent involvement of the spleen secondary to slow blood flow through the organ (*see also* Chapter 15). Sickled cells lodge in endarteries, causing occlusion and infarction. Repetitive splenic infarction gradually causes autosplenectomy in homozygous subjects, resulting in complete loss of splenic function, usually by the age of 5. In heterozygous patients with sickle cell trait, there are fewer, and less severe, episodes of vaso-occlusion, and the spleen may be damaged without being functionally destroyed (*see* Chapter 10; Fig. 3). Unlike the homozygous patient who has undergone vaso-occlusive autosplenectomy, continued function of the spleen in heterozygous patients provides the continuing potential for complications, such as abscess formation and rupture. Because of their frequent episodes of crisis, with abdominal pain and other symptoms, sicklers often require medical care and concomitant imaging.

Splenomegaly may be seen at any age, on plain film, in the heterozygous population, but is usually seen only to about the age of 5 years in homozygous patients. An acute and marked increase in spleen size may indicate splenic sequestration of red blood cells. In addition, splenic enlargement may be secondary to abscess or infarction. Likewise, nonspecific perisplenic inflammatory changes may be detected, including left pleural effusion, an elevated left hemidiaphragm, and left lower-lobe atelectasis.

In older homozygous patients, the fibrotic, end-stage spleen may contain diffuse or patchy punctate or stippled calcification. By the time these are seen on plain film, splenic function is usually greatly impaired or lost.

[99m]-Technetium sulfur colloid scintigraphy may show multiple infarcts prior to autosplenectomy, in the homozygous patient. In addition, there is progressively decreasing uptake on serial scans, secondary to declining splenic function. Following autosplenectomy, the spleen is not visualized on sulfur colloid scans. Radionuclide uptake may be impaired in doubly heterozygous patients, but at least partial splenic uptake persists into adult life, and frequently the uptake is normal. Such changes in the heterozygous population are usually proportional to the amount of abnormal hemoglobin.

With ultrasound, sickle cell-related splenomegaly is easily imaged, and permits the detection of infarction, abscess, and other complications of the disease. In the homozygous patient with a small, fibrotic, end-stage spleen, adequate visualization is often impossible, because of the location of the spleen high up under the rib cage and the presence of bowel gas in the left upper quadrant. However, this is seldom important, since active splenic disease is unlikely, following autosplenectomy.

CT is probably the most reliable means of imaging the spleen in the patient with SCD (Magid et al., 1984). Because these patients frequently present with abdominal pain, the entire abdomen can be imaged easily. The study is first performed without iv contrast, to allow demonstration of splenic calcification. The spleen in SCD, even if normal or enlarged, is frequently of higher density than normal. This is thought to be secondary to the presence of diffuse and sometimes microscopic calcification, and also because of increased iron deposition caused by hemolysis and red blood cell transfusions.

With MRI in SCD, the spleen has a diffusely reduced signal, initially because of hemosiderin deposition, and subsequently because of calcification and fibrosis, as the patient progresses to autosplenectomy. In sequestration, areas of abnormally high signal, with a dark rim, may be seen on T1-weighted images, as the result of the presence of subacute hemorrhage. Areas of infarction are seen as peripheral wedge-shaped areas of increased signal, on T2-weighted images, against the background low-intensity spleen (Adler et al., 1986).

16.7.2. DENSE OR OPACIFIED SPLEEN   There are several causes of a radiographically dense spleen. Abnormal iron deposition, in secondary hemochromatosis, causes increased density in the spleen, as well as in the liver. This is evident, on CT, as a diffuse increase in attenuation, but is rarely seen on plain film (Mitnick et al., 1981). Intracellular iron has a characteristic appearance on MRI, because of shortening of T2 relaxation time, resulting in a diffuse low signal intensity, most apparent on T2-weighted images. Focal lesions within the spleen become more conspicuous, analogous to the effect of administration of ferumoxide contrast agents.

Increased density of the spleen, caused by the prior use of Thorotrast, is also occasionally seen. Thorotrast, a solution containing thorium dioxide, was introduced in 1930 as a radiographic contrast medium, and was most commonly used for cerebral angiography until the mid-1950s. It was subsequently withdrawn, because of the high radiation dose emitted during the decay of thorium to lead, and because of its biological half-life of 400 yr. Thorotrast particles are phagocytosed by reticuloendothelial cells, and, therefore, the radiation dose is highest in the spleen, liver, and bone marrow. Thorotrast causes the spleen to shrink in size, and to undergo fibrous replacement, sometimes resulting in functional asplenia (Burroughs et al., 1982). Thorotrast-induced splenic angiosarcoma has been described, but splenic neoplasms are rare following use of this contrast material (Levy et al., 1986), compared to the incidence of hepatic neoplasms, such as angiosarcoma, hepatocellular carcinoma, and cholangiocarcinoma.

On plain films and CT, the post-Thorotrast spleen is small and dense, and contains diffusely scattered punctate opacities (Fig. 24). Opacification of the liver, lymphatics, and peripancreatic nodes may also be seen. If a splenic mass is present, a filling defect may be identified within the dense spleen (Levy et al., 1986). Dense calcification of the spleen, mimicking Thorotrast, may be seen in diffuse splenic infarction, most commonly in SCD. However, in this case, the pattern of splenic opacification is less dense, and is limited to the spleen, and high density in the liver or perisplenic lymph nodes is lacking.

16.7.3. HYPOSPLENISM (FUNCTIONAL ASPLENIA)   Hyposplenism is the functional condition that follows autosplenectomy and other causes of splenic atrophy. Splenic atrophy, with a small or dense spleen, results from inflammatory bowel diseases, dermatitis herpetiformis, celiac disease, thyrotoxicosis, and the post-

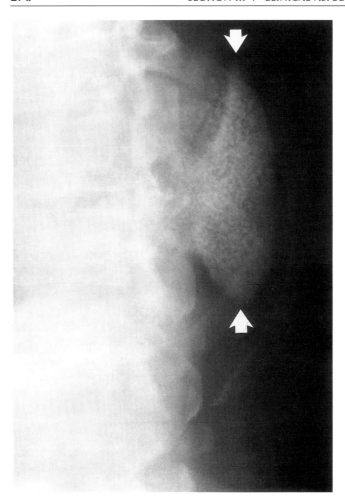

Fig. 16.24. Thorotrast spleen on plain films. Oblique plain film of the left upper quadrant demonstrates a spleen with diffusely scattered punctate opacities (arrows). This fine, dense, well-delineated network pattern is typical of Thorotrast deposition (white arrows) in the reticuloendothelial system of the spleen.

Thorotrast spleen (Corozza and Gasbarrini, 1983; Eichner, 1979; *see also* Chapter 10). Hyposplenism associated with a normal or enlarged spleen may be seen in sarcoidosis, amyloidosis, SCD, and possibly with administration of high-dose corticosteroids (Eichner, 1979).

Nuclear scintigraphy, using heat damaged red blood cells, is a useful technique for confirming the presence of hyposplenism. The half-life for the blood clearance of heat damaged red blood cells is 10–16 min, for normal subjects, and is increased to the range of 35 min to several hours, in functionally asplenic patients.

16.8. SUMMARY

This chapter has attempted to demonstrate the imaging appearance of the normal spleen, as well as congenital anomalies, trauma, focal and diffuse diseases, vascular disorders, and the miscellaneous processes involving the spleen. A systematic approach reviewing the radiological findings by modality has been used, covering plain film, ultrasound, CT, scintigraphy, angiography, and MRI. Although a specific diagnosis may be difficult to achieve, the information provided by imaging, coupled with clinical and labora-

tory data, is capable, in many instances, of providing information affecting clinical management. Surgery, percutaneous intervention, medical therapy, or simple observation may then be pursued, with greater assurance, because of the radiological findings.

REFERENCES

Adler, D. D., Glazer, G. M., and Aisen, A. M. (1986) MRI of the spleen: normal appearance and findings in sickle-cell anemia. *Am. J. Roentgenol.* **147,** 843–845.

Anderson, W. A. D. and Kissane, J. M., eds. (1977) *Pathology*, 7th ed., vol. 2, Mosby, St. Louis, MO, pp. 1489–1513.

Ahmann, D. L., Kiely, J. M., Harrison, E. G. Jr., and Payne, W. S. (1966) Malignant lymphoma of the spleen. A review of 49 cases in which the diagnosis was made at splenectomy. *Cancer* **19,** 826–834.

Arbona, G. L., Lloyd, T. V., Lucas, J., and Sharma, H. M. (1982) Computed tomographic demonstration of angiosarcoma of the spleen. *South Med. J.* **75,** 348–350.

Asch, M. J., Cohen, A. H., and Moore, T. C. (1974) Hepatic and splenic lymphangiomatosis with skeletal involvement: report of a case and review of the literature. *Surgery* **76,** 334–339.

Avigad, S., Jaffe, R., Frand, M., Izhak, Y., and Rotem, Y. (1976) Lymphangiomatosis with splenic involvement. *JAMA* **236,** 2315–2317.

Balcar, I., Seltzer, S. E., Davis, S., and Geller, S. (1984) CT patterns of splenic infarction: a clinical and experimental study. *Radiology* **151,** 723–729.

Beahrs, J. R. and Stephens, D. H. (1980) Enlarged accessory spleens: CT appearance in postsplenectomy patients. *Am. J. Roentgenol.* **135,** 483–486.

Bearss, R. W. (1980) Splenic-gonadal fusion. *Urology* **16,** 277–279.

Bloom, R. A., Freund, U., Perkes, E. H., and Weiss, Y. (1981) Acute Hodgkin disease masquerading as splenic abscess. *J. Surg. Oncol.* **17,** 279–282.

Breiman, R. S., Beck, J. W., Korobkin, M., Glenny, R., Akwari, O. E., Heaston, D. K., Moore, A. V., and Ram, P. C. (1982) Volume determinations using computed tomography. *Am. J. Roentgenol.* **138,** 329–333.

Brinkley, A. A. and Lee, J. K. T. (1981) Cystic hamartoma of the spleen: CT and sonographic findings. *J. Clin. Ultrasound* **9,** 136–138.

Bron, K. M. and Hoffman, W. J. (1971) Preoperative diagnosis of splenic cysts. *Arch. Surg.* **102,** 459–461.

Burroughs, A. K., Bass, N. M., Wood, J., and Sherlock, S. (1982) Absence of splenic uptake of radiocolloid due to Thorotrast in a patient with Thorotrast-induced cholangiocarcinoma. *Br. J. Radiol.* **55,** 598–600.

Carroll, B. A. and Ta, H. N. (1980) The ultrasonic appearance of extranodal abdominal lymphoma. *Radiology* **135,** 419–425.

Caslowitz, P. L., Labs, J. D., Fishman, E. K., and Siegelman, S. S. (1989) The changing spectrum of splenic abscess. *Clin. Imaging* **13,** 201–207.

Castellino, R. A., Silverman, J. F., Glatstein, E., Blank, N., and Wexler. L. (1972) Splenic arteriography in Hodgkin's disease: a roentgenographic-pathologic study of 33 consecutive untreated patients. *Am. J. Roentgenol.* **114,** 574–582.

Ceccacci, L. and Tosi, S. (1981) Splenic-gonadal fusion: case report and review of the literature. *J. Urol.* **126,** 558,559.

Cerri, G. G., Alves, V. A. F., and Magalhaes, A. (1984) Hepatosplenic schistosomiasis mansoni: Ultrasound manifestation. *Radiology* **153,** 777–780.

Chen, K. T. K., Bolles, J. C., and Gilbert, E. F. (1979) Angiosarcoma of the spleen. *Arch. Pathol. Lab. Med.* **103,** 122–124.

Clark, R. E., Korobkin, M., and Palubinskas, A. J. (1972) Angiography of accessory spleens. *Radiology* **102,** 41–44.

Cobos, J. M., Hisano, K., Matsumori, M., Okada, M., and Nakamura, K. (1982) Multiple calcified aneurysms of splenic artery, hypersplenism and concomitant cholelithiasis. *Jpn. J. Surg.* **12,** 448–452.

Cooperberg, P. L. (1987) Ultrasonography of the spleen. In: *Diagnostic Ultrasound, Text and Cases* (Sarti, D. A., ed.), Year Book, Chicago, p. 312.

Corozza, G. R. and Gasbarrini, G. (1983) Defective splenic function and its relation to bowel disease. *Clin. Gastroenterol.* **12,** 651–669.

Cunningham, J. J. (1978) Ultrasonic findings in isolated lymphoma of the spleen simulating splenic abscess. *J. Clin. Ultrasound* **6**, 412–414.

Dachman, A. H., Ros, P. R., Murari, P. J., Olmsted, W. W., and Lichtenstein, J. E. (1986) Nonparasitic splenic cysts: a report of 52 cases with radiologic-pathologic correlation. *Am. J. Roentgenol.* **147**, 537–542.

Dalton, M. L. Jr., Strange, W. H., and Downs, E. A. (1971) Intrathoracic splenosis: case report and review of the literature. *Am. Rev. Resp. Dis.* **103**, 827–830.

Davidson, E. D., Campbell, W. G., and Hersh, T. (1980) Epidermoid splenic cyst occurring in an intrapancreatic accessory spleen. *Dig. Dis. Sci.* **25**, 964–967.

Dawes, L. G. and Malangoni, M. A. (1986) Cystic masses of the spleen. *Ann. Surg.* **52**, 333–336.

Delaney, H. M. and Jason, R. S. (1981) *Abdominal Trauma: Surgical and Radiological Diagnosis*, Springer-Verlag, New York.

Dillion, M. L., Koster, J. K., and Coy, J. (1977) Intrathoracic splenosis. *South Med. J.* **70**, 112.

Eichner, E. R. (1979) Splenic function: normal, too much and too little. *Am. J. Med.* **66**, 331–320.

Enzinger, F. M. and Weiss, S. W. (1983) *Soft Tissue Tumors*, Mosby, St. Louis, p. 485.

Federle, M. P. (1983) Computed tomography of the spleen. In: *Computed Tomography of the Body* (Moss, A. A., Gamsu, G., and Genant, H. K., eds.), Saunders, Philadelphia, p. 879.

Federle, M. P. and Moss, A. A. (1983) Computed tomography of the spleen. *CRC Crit. Rev. Diagn. Imaging* **19**, 1–16.

Freund, R., Pichl, J., Heyder, N., Rodl, W., and Riemann, J. F. (1982) Splenic abscess- clinical symptoms and diagnostic possibilities. *Am. J. Gastroenterol.* **77**, 35–38.

Garvin, D. E. and King, F. M. (1981) Cysts and nonlymphomatous tumors of the spleen. *Pathol. Ann.* **16**, 61–80.

Glazer, G. M., Axel, L., Goldberg, H. I., and Moss, A. A. (1981) Dynamic CT of the normal spleen. *Am. J. Roentgenol.* **137**, 343–346.

Goldman, M. L., Philip, P. K., Sarrafizadeh, M. S., Sarfeh, I. J., Salam, A. A., Galambos, J. T., Powers, S. R., Balint, J. A. (1981) Intra-arterial tissue adhesive for medical splenectomy in humans. *Radiology* **140**, 341–349.

Gomori, J. M., Grossman, R. I., Goldberg, H. I., Zimmerman, R. A., and Bilaniuk, L. T. (1985) Intracranial hematomas: imaging by high field MR. *Radiology* **157**, 87–93.

Gordon, D. H., Burrell, M. I., Levin, D. C., Mueller, C. F., and Becker, J. A. (1977) Wandering spleen — the radiological and clinical spectrum. *Radiology* **125**, 39–46.

Griscom, N. T., Hargreaves, H. K., Schwartz, M. Z., Reddish, J. M., and Colodny, A. H. (1977) Huge splenic cyst in a newborn: comparison with 10 cases in later childhood and adolescence. *Am. J. Roentgenol.* **129**, 889–891.

Guarin, U., Dimitrieva, Z., and Ashley, S. (1975) Spleno-gonadal fusion: a rare congenital anomaly demonstrated by 99mTc-sulfur colloid imaging. *J. Nucl. Med.* **16**, 992.

Haertel, M. and Ryder, D. (1979) Radiologic investigation of splenic trauma. *Cardiovasc. Radiol.* **2**, 27–33.

Henderson, J. M., Heymsfield, S. B., Horowitz, J., and Kutner, M. H. (1981) Measurements of liver and spleen volume by computed tomography. Assessment of reproducibility and changes found following a selective distal splenorenal shunt. *Radiology* **141**, 525–527.

Henkin, R. E. (1975) Selected topics in intraabdominal imaging via nuclear medicine techniques. *Radiol. Clin. North Am.* **17**, 39–54.

Iozzo, R. V., Haas, J. E. R., and Chard, R. L. (1980) Symptomatic splenic hamartoma: a report of two cases and review of the literature. *Paediatrics* **66**, 261–265.

Heymsfield, S. B., Fulenwider, T., Nordlinger, B., Barlow, R., Sones, P., and Kutner, M. (1979) Accurate measurement of liver, kidney and spleen volume and mass by computerized axial tomography. *Ann. Intern. Med.* **90**, 185–187.

Itzchak, Y. and Glickman, M. G. (1977) Splenic vein thrombosis in patients with a normal size spleen. *Invest. Radiol.* **12**, 158–163.

Jeffrey, R. B., Laing, F. C., Federle, M. P., and Goodman, P. C. (1981) Computed tomography of splenic trauma. *Radiology* **141**, 729–732.

Kaude, J. (1973) Accessory spleens as demonstrated by celiac angiography. *Radiology* **13**, 53–56.

Kelly, K. J., Chusid, M. J., and Camitta, B. M. (1982) Splenic torsion in an infant associated with secondary disseminated Haemophilus influenza infection. *Clin. Paediatr.* **21**, 365,366.

Kim, H. and Dorfman, F. R. (1974) Morphological studies of 84 untreated patients subjected to laparotomy for staging of non-Hodgkins lymphomas. *Cancer* **33**, 557–647.

Kishikawa, T., Numaguchi, Y., Tokunaga, M., and Matsuura, K. (1977) Hemangiosarcoma of the spleen and liver metastases: angiographic manifestations. *Radiology* **123**, 31–35.

Koehler, R. E. (1983) Spleen. In: *Computed Body Tomography* (Lee, J. K. and Sagel, S. R. J., eds.), Raven, New York, pp. 243–256.

Koga, T. M., et al. (1972) Ultrasonic tomography of the spleen. VII. Ultrasonic determination of the spleen volume from parallel sectional areas. *Med. Ultrason.* **10**, 2–14.

Korobkin, M., Moss, A. A., Callen, P. W., DeMartini, W. J., and Kaiser, J. A. (1978) Computed tomography of subcapsular splenic hematoma. Clinical and experimental studies. *Radiology* **129**, 441–445.

Lanir, A., Hader, H., Cohen, I., Tal, E., Benmair, J., Schreiber, R., and Clouse, M. E. (1986) Gaucher disease: assessment with MR imaging. *Radiology* **161**, 239–244.

Lankisch, P. G. (1990) Spleen in inflammatory pancreatic disease. *Gastroenterology* **98**, 509–516.

Levy, D. W., Rindsberg, S., Friedman, A. C., Fishman, E. K., Ros, P. R., Radecki, P. D., Siegelman, S. S., Goodman, Z. D., Pyatt, R. S., and Grumbach, K. (1986) Thorotrast-induced hepatosplenic neoplasia: CT identification. *Am. J. Roentgenol.* **146**, 997–1004.

Lin, M. S. and Donati, R. M. (1981) Wedged appearance of splenic infarcts on scans. *Clin. Nucl. Med.* **11**, 556.

Locker, G. Y., Doroshow, J. H., Zwelling, L. A., and Chabner, B. A. (1979) The clinical features of hepatic angiosarcoma: a report of four cases and a review of the English literature. *Medicine* **58**, 48–64.

Lupien, C. and Sauerbrei, E. E. (1984) Healing in the traumatized spleen: sonographic investigation. *Radiology* **151**, 181–185.

Lutzker, L., Koenigsberg, M., Meng, C. H., Freeman, L. M. (1974) The role of radionuclide imaging in spleen trauma. *Radiology* **110**, 419–425.

Magid, D., Fishman, E. K., and Siegelmann, S. S. (1984) Computed tomography of the spleen and liver in sickle cell disease. *Am. J. Roentgenol.* **143**, 245–249.

Mahoney, B., Jeffrey, R. B., and Federle, M. P. (1982) Spontaneous rupture of hepatic and splenic angiosarcoma demonstrated by CT. *Am. J. Roentgenol.* **138**, 965,966.

Mandell, J. A., et al. (1983) A case of microgastria with splenic-gonadal fusion. *Paediatr. Radiol.* **13**, 95–98.

McArdle, C. (1980) Case of the winter season. Diagnosis: torsion of a wandering spleen. *Semin. Roentgenol.* **15**, 7–8.

Mettler, F. A. (1986) *Essentials of Nuclear Medicine Imaging*, Grune and Stratton, Orlando, FL.

Meyer, J. E., Harris, N. L., Elman, A., and Stomper, P. C. (1983) Large cell lymphoma of the spleen: CT appearances. *Radiology* **148**, 199–202.

Minami, M., Itai, Y., Ohtomo, K., Ohnishi, S., Niki, T., Kokubo, T., Yoshikawa, K., and Iio, M. (1989) Siderotic nodules in the spleen: MR imaging of portal hypertension. *Radiology* **172**, 681–684.

Mirvis, S. E., Whitley, N. O., Glens, D. R. (1989) Blunt splenic trauma in adults: CT-based classification and correlation with prognosis and treatment. *Radiology* **171**, 33–39.

Mitnick, J. S., Bosniak, M. A., Megibow, A. J., Karpatkin, M., Feiner, H. D., Kutin, N., Van Natta, F., and Piomelli, S. (1981) CT in B-thalassemia: iron deposition in the liver, spleen and lymph nodes. *Am. J. Roentgenol.* **136**, 1191–1194.

Monie, I. W. (1982) The asplenia syndrome: an explanation for absence of the spleen. *Teratology* **25**, 215–219.

Moss, M. L., Kirschner, L. P., Peereboom, G., and Ferris, R. A. (1980) CT demonstration of a splenic abscess not evident at surgery. *Am. J. Roentgenol.* **135**, 159,160.

Moss, A. A., Korobkin, M., Price, D., and Brito, A. C. (1979) Computed tomography of splenic subcapsular hematomas: an experimental study in dogs. *Invest. Radiol.* **1**, 60–64.

Mousa, A. H., et al. (1967) Hepatosplenic schistosomiasis. In: *Bilharziasis* (Mostofi, F. K., ed.), Springer-Verlag, New York, p. 15.

Nesbesar, R. A., Rabinov, K. R., and Potsaid, M. S. (1974) Radionuclide imaging of the spleen and suspected splenic injury. *Radiology* **110**, 609–614.

Nielsen, J. L. (1981) Splenosis on the right kidney and diaphragmatic surface following traumatic rupture of the spleen. *Acta Chir. Scand.* **147**, 721–724.

Novetsky, G. S. and Epstein, A. J. (1982) Cystic lymphangiomatosis: an unusual cause of splenic scintigraphic defects. *Clin. Nucl. Med.* **7**, 416–417.

Nunez, D., Russell, E., Yrizarry, J., Pereiras, R., and Viamonte, M. Jr. (1978) Portosystemic communications studied by transhepatic portography. *Radiology* **127**, 75–79.

Ohtomo, K., Fukuda, H., Mori, K., Minami, M., Itai, Y., and Inoue, Y. (1992) CT and MR appearances of splenic hamartoma. *J. Comput. Assist. Tomogr.* **16**, 425–428.

Osborn, D. J., Glickman, M. G., Grnja, V., and Ramsby, G. (1973) The role of angiography in abdominal nonrenal trauma. *Radiol. Clin. North Am.* **11**, 579–592.

Pachter, H. L., Hofstetter, S. R., and Spencer, F. C. (1981) Evolving concepts in splenic surgery. Splenography versus splenectomy and post-splenectomy drainage: experience in 105 patients. *Ann. Surg.* **194**, 262–267.

Paivansalo, M. and Siniluoto, T. (1983) Cavernous hemangioma of the spleen. *Fortschr. Roentgenstr.* **142**, 228–230.

Pawar, S., Kay, C. J., Gonzalez, R., Taylor, K. J., and Rosenfield, A. T. (1982) Sonography of splenic abscess. *Am. J. Roentgenol.* **138**, 259–262.

Pearl, G. S. and Nassar, V. H. (1979) Cystic lymphangioma of the spleen. *South. Med. J.* **72**, 667–669.

Peoples, W. M., Moller, J. H., and Edwards, J. E. (1983) Reviews: polysplenia, a review of 146 cases. *Paediatr. Cardiol.* **4**, 129–137.

Piekarski, J., Federle, M. P., and Moss, A. A. (1980) Computed tomography of the spleen. *Radiology* **135**, 683–689.

Pietri, H. and Boscaini, M. (1984) Determination of a splenic volumetric index by ultrasound scanning. *J. Ultrasound Med.* **3**, 319–323.

Piepsz, A., Viart, P., Szymusik, B., and Jeghers, O. (1977) A real clinical indication for selective spleen scintigraphy with 99mTc-labeled red blood cells. *Radiology* **123**, 407,408.

Pistoia, F. and Markowitz, S. K. (1988) Splenic lymphangiomatosis: CT diagnosis. *Am. J. Roentgenol.* **150**, 121,122.

Probst, P., Castenada-Zuniga, W. R., Gomes, A. S., Yonehiro, E. G., Delaney, J. P., and Amplatz, K. L. (1978) Nonsurgical treatment of splenic-artery aneurysms. *Radiology* **128**, 619–623.

Propper, R. A., Weinstein, B. J., Skolnick, M. L., and Kisloff, B. (1979) Ultrasonography of hemorrhagic splenic cysts. *J. Clin. Ultrasound* **7**, 18–20.

Pyatt, R. S., Williams, E. D., Clark, M., and Gaskins, R. (1981) Case report. CT diagnosis of splenic cystic lymphangiomatosis. *J. Comput. Assist. Tomogr.* **5**, 446–448.

Rabushka, L. S., Kawashima, A., and Fishman, E. K. (1994) Imaging of the spleen: CT with supplemental MR examination. *RadioGraphics* **14**, 307–332.

Ralls, P. W., Quinn, M. F., Colletti, P., Lapin, S. A., and Halls, J. (1982) Sonography of pyogenic splenic abscess. *Am. J. Roentgenol.* **138**, 523–525.

Rao, B. K., AuBuchon, J., Lieberman, L. M., and Polcyn, R. E. (1981) Cystic lymphangiomatosis of the spleen: a radiologic-pathologic correlation. *Radiology* **141**, 781,782.

Rao, B. K., Shore, R. M., Lieberman, L. M., and Polcyn, R. E. (1982) Dual radiopharmaceutical imaging in congenital asplenia syndrome. *Radiology* **145**, 805–810.

Rao, B. K., Winebright, J. W., and Dresser, T. P. (1979) Splenic artifact caused by barium in the colon. *Clin. Nucl. Med.* **4**, 249.

Rauch, R. F., Korobkin, M., Silverman, P. M., and Moore, A. V. (1983) CT detection of iatrogenic percutaneous splenic injury. *J. Comput. Assist. Tomogr.* **7**, 1018–1021.

Ros, P. R., Moser, R. P. Jr., Dachman, A. H., Murari, P. J., and Olmsted, W. W. (1987) Hemangioma of the spleen: radiologic-pathologic correlation in ten cases. *Radiology* **162**, 73–77.

Rosenthall, L., Lisbona, R., and Banerjee, K. (1974) A nucleographic and radioangiographic study of a patient with torsion of the spleen. *Radiology* **110**, 427,428.

Salomonowitz, E., Frick, M. P., and Lund, G. (1984) Radiologic diagnosis of wandering spleen complicated by splenic nodules and infarction. *Gastroint. Radiol.* **9**, 57–59.

Schulman, A., van Jaarsveld, J., Loxton, A. J., and Grove, W. H. (1983) Pseudolipid appearance of simple and echinococcal cysts on ultrasonography. A report of 2 cases. *S. Afr. Med. J.* **63**, 905,906.

Shanser, J. D., Moss, A. A., Clark, R. E., and Palubinskas, A. J. (1973) Angiographic evaluation of cystic lesions of the spleen. *Am. J. Roentgenol.* **119**, 166–174.

Sheflin, J. D., Chung, M. L., and Kretchmar, K. A. (1984) Torsion of the wandering spleen and distal pancreas. *Am. J. Roentgenol.* **142**, 100–101.

Shin, M. S. and Ho, K. (1983) Mesodermal cyst of the spleen: computed tomographic characteristics and pathogenetic considerations. *J. Comput. Tomogr.* **7**, 295–299.

Shirkhoda, A. (1993) Spleen. In: *Abdominal Magnetic Resonance Imaging* (Ros, P. R. and Bidgood, W. D. Jr., eds.), Mosby-Year Book, St. Louis, MO.

Sirinek, K. R. and Evans, W. E. (1973) Nonparasitic splenic cysts: case report of epidermoid cyst with review of the literature. *Am. J. Surg.* **126**, 8–13.

Smulewicz, J. J. and Clement, A. R. (1975) Torsion of the wandering spleen. *Dig. Dis. Sci.* **20**, 274–279.

Sordillo, E. M., Sordillo, P. P., and Hajdu, S. I. (1981) Primary hemangiosarcoma of the spleen: report of four cases. *Med. Pediatr. Oncol.* **9**, 314–324.

Stark, D. D., Goldberg, H. I., Moss, A. A., and Bass, N. M. (1984) Chronic liver disease: evaluation by magnetic resonance. *Radiology* **150**, 149–151.

Subramanyam, B. R., Balthazar, E. J., and Horii, S. C. (1984) Sonography of the accessory spleen. *Am. J. Roentgenol.* **143**, 47–49.

Sumner, T. E., Volberg, F. M., Chauvenet, A. R., Abramson, J. S., Turner, C. S., and Young, L. W. (1983) Radiological case of the month. Hepatic and splenic candidiasis in acute leukemia. *Am. J. Dis. Child.* **137**, 1193–1194.

Toback, A. C., Steece, D. M., and Kaye, M. D. (1984) Case report. Splenic torsion: an unusual cause of splenomegaly. *Dig. Dis. Sci.* **29**, 868–871.

Torres, G. M., Terry, N. L., Mergo, P. J., and Ros, P. R. (1995) MR imaging of the spleen. *MRI Clin. North Am.* **3**, 39–50.

Tuttle, R. J. and Minielly, J. A. (1978) Splenic cystic lymphangiomatosis. *Radiology* **126**, 47,48.

Van Mierop, L. H. S., Gessner, J. H., and Sciebler, G. L. (1972) Asplenia and polysplenia syndromes. *Birth Defects* **8**, 36–44.

Weinberger, G., Mitra, S. K., and Yoeli, G. (1982) Case report: ultrasound diagnosis of splenic vein thrombosis. *J. Clin. Ultrasound* **10**, 345,346.

Weingarten, M. J., Fakhry, J., McCarthy, J., Freeman, S. J., and Bisker, J. S. (1984) Sonography after splenic embolization: the wedge shaped acute infarct. *Am. J. Roentgenol.* **142**, 957–959.

Weissleder, R., Elizondo, G., Stark, D. D., Hahn, P. F., Marfil, J., Gonzalez, J. F., et al. (1989) The diagnosis of splenic lymphoma by MR imaging: value of superparamagnetic iron oxide. *Am. J. Roentgenol.* **152**, 175–180.

Weissleder, R., Hahn, P. F., Stark, D. D., Elizondo, G., Saini, S., Todd, L. E., Wittenberg, J., and Ferrucci, J. T. (1988) Superparamagnetic iron oxide; enhanced detection of focal splenic tumors with MR imaging. *Radiology* **169**, 399–403.

Wilson, D. G. and Lieberman, L. M. (1983) Unusual splenic band appearence on liver-spleen scan. *Clin. Nucl. Med.* **8**, 270.

Whitley, J. E., Maynard, C. D., and Rhyne, A. L. (1966) A computer approach to the prediction of spleen weight from routine films. *Radiology* **86**, 73–76.

Wright, F. W. and Williams, F. W. (1974) Large post-traumatic splenic cyst diagnosed by radiology, isotope scintigraphy and ultrasound. *Br. J. Radiol.* **47**, 454.

Wurtele, L. H., Tondreau, R. L., and Pollack, H. (1982) Ultrasonographic appearance of splenic echinococcal cyst. *Penn. Med.* **85**, 55,56.

Yeh, H.-C., Zacks, J., and Jurado, R. A. (1981) Ultrasonography of splenic infarct. *Mt. Sinai Med. NY* **48**, 446–448.

17 Surgery of the Spleen

*CAROL E. H. SCOTT-CONNER, MD, PhD, ANNE T. MANCINO, MD,
AND JOHN LAWRENCE, MD*

17.1. INTRODUCTION

Laparoscopic splenectomy, nonoperative management of splenic trauma, and the increasing use of partial splenectomy, in cases in which total splenectomy is not obligatory, are among the significant trends in splenic surgery that have emerged since publication of the first edition of this text. As recently as 30 yr ago, splenectomy was routinely performed for even minor splenic injuries. Now the emphasis is on preserving, whenever possible, splenic mass and function by a variety of surgical options.

In this chapter, the most common indications for splenic surgery are reviewed. Surgical options, including laparoscopic splenectomy, partial splenectomy, and splenic biopsy are considered. Techniques of partial and total splenectomy (both laparoscopic and "open") are detailed, and measures to avoid or manage surgical complications are discussed. Surgical anatomy (formerly included in this chapter) is reviewed in Chapter 1.

17.2. HEMATOLOGICAL INDICATIONS FOR SURGERY

Most elective splenic surgery is performed for diagnosis, palliation, or definitive management of hematological disorders. A review of 1240 splenectomies, performed at the University of Mississippi Medical Center (UMMC) from 1955 to 1992, was recently completed by two of the authors. In the UMMC series, 37% of elective splenectomies were performed for this purpose (Table 1). Within the category of hematologic disorders, treatment of cytopenias is the most common indication (Coon, 1991; Flowers et al., 1996; Jameson et al., 1996; Schwartz, 1996). Total splenectomy, with a careful search for and removal of accessory splenic tissue, is the usual surgical strategy, because residual splenic tissue is apt to cause recurrence of cytopenia. Laparoscopic splenectomy is a safe and effective alternative, in carefully selected patients (Silvestri et al., 1995; Flowers et al., 1996; Smith, 1996). The management of specific disorders is discussed in this subheading. Technical issues related to both open and laparoscopic splenectomy are discussed in more detail later in this chapter.

17..1. HEMOLYTIC ANEMIAS   When accelerated destruction of erythrocytes results from increased reticuloendothelial clearance or extravascular hemolysis, splenectomy may improve red blood cell survival. Increased reticuloendothelial clearance occurs when surface properties, such as membrane-bound immunoglobu-

lin G (IgG), or physical abnormalities of the erythrocyte (such as shape of the erythrocyte or impaired deformability of the red blood cell membrane) render it unable to survive passage through the spleen. Hemolysis may be caused by trauma to the erythrocytes, exogenous toxins, or the fixation of complement to the erythrocytes with subsequent lysis. When the spleen is the major cause of abnormal erythrocyte destruction, either by splenic destruction of red blood cells or by production of antibody or opsonizing factors, splenectomy may be indicated. Partial splenectomy has been used for some of these disorders, in the hope of preserving splenic immune function (Tchernia et al., 1993), but late results are variable. Accurate diagnosis of the nature and site of the hemolysis is important.

The hemolytic anemias may be usefully considered as the congenital hemolytic anemias (including hereditary spherocytosis and the thalassemias) and the acquired hemolytic anemias (including autoimmune hemolytic anemia). In the congenital anemias, structural abnormalities of the erythrocyte membrane or hemoglobin render the erythrocyte more vulnerable to destruction in the spleen. Splenectomy may significantly lengthen erythrocyte survival in these cases, even though the underlying red blood cell defect remains unchanged. In contrast, the acquired anemias are generally immunologically mediated, the site of red blood cell destruction is frequently intravascular, and the response to splenectomy is variable.

The increased bilirubin load associated with chronic hemolysis leads to pigment gallstone formation in a significant percentage of patients. The stones contain a black, insoluble pigment composed of polymerized hemoglobin breakdown products (Bissel, 1986). The incidence varies with the duration and severity of hemolysis, and is highest in adult patients with congenital hemolytic anemias. In adults with hereditary spherocytosis, the reported incidence of biliary tract disease is 30–55%. Thus, gallbladder ultrasound evaluation should be performed as part of the preoperative evaluation of patients with hemolytic anemia, supplemented by careful intraoperative assessment of the gallbladder (which may disclose small stones not noted on ultrasound). Cholecystectomy and operative cholangiography, with common duct exploration, if needed, may then be performed at the time of elective splenectomy (whether performed by an open or laparoscopic approach). In a representative series, concomitant cholecystectomy was performed in 9/113 patients undergoing splenectomy for congenital or acquired hemolytic anemia, with no adverse effects (Coon, 1985c). In some patients, hemolysis is reduced, but not eliminated, by splenectomy, and pigment gallstones may occasionally form after splenectomy. The

From: *The Complete Spleen: A Handbook of Structure, Function, and Clinical Disorders* Edited by: A. J. Bowdler © Humana Press Inc., Totowa, NJ

281

Table 17.1
Indications for Elective Splenectomy,
University of Mississippi Medical Center
1955–1992

Hematologic disorders	
Idiopathic Thrombocytopenic Purpura	107
Hodgkin's Lymphoma	152
Other hematologic disorder	196
Cancer[a]	71
Other[b]	124

[a]Cancer includes splenectomies performed as a planned part of radical cancer surgery, e.g., total gastrectomy with splenectomy. Incidental (unplanned) splenectomies, which occurred as a result of surgical trauma, were not included.

[b]Includes all other elective conditions, e.g., splenic cyst or abscess.

incidence of subsequent gallstone formation does not appear to justify prophylactic removal of an essentially normal gallbladder.

17.2.1.1. Hereditary Spherocytosis and Related Disorders
The hemolytic anemia resulting from hereditary spherocytosis is the type most commonly and predictably responsive to splenectomy. The incidence of hereditary spherocytosis is 1/4500 of the general population. Although, in most cases, an autosomal dominant pattern of inheritance can be demonstrated, approx 20% of cases arise sporadically. The characteristic triad of anemia, splenomegaly, and acholuric jaundice is initially mild, and the illness may escape detection until adult life. The level of jaundice fluctuates, being less pronounced in early childhood. Similarly, the degree of anemia varies from slight to moderate, depending on the balance between hemolysis and red blood cell production. A precarious state of compensation may be disrupted by systemic infection, resulting in jaundice and profound anemia.

An abnormality in red blood cell membrane structure, related to a deficiency of spectrin synthesis, causes the characteristic spheroidal shape of the erythrocytes. This abnormality of red blood cell structure renders it susceptible to loss of membrane by fragmentation, especially when incubated in adverse metabolic conditions, such as are postulated to occur in the red blood cell pool of the red pulp of the spleen (Weed and Bowdler, 1966; Smedley and Bellingham, 1991). Splenectomy corrects the anemia, by allowing the abnormal erythrocytes to survive longer within the circulation. Correction of the anemia of hereditary spherocytosis by splenectomy is highly predictable, although the abnormality of the red blood cells remains unchanged by the surgery. Study of the mechanism of hemo-lysis in this disorder has been instrumental in uncovering the mechanisms of culling of abnormal red blood cells by the spleen.

The differential diagnosis of hereditary spherocytosis includes spherocytic hemolytic anemias associated with anti-erythrocyte antibodies, in which the direct antiglobulin (Coombs') test is positive. A negative Coombs' test supports the diagnosis of hereditary spherocytosis, but does not exclude all other causes of sphering. Spherocytes are also seen in patients with hepatic cirrhosis, chronic infections, and, occasionally, in other hematologic disorders.

Most, but not all, patients with hereditary spherocytosis require splenectomy. In young children, the surgery should be delayed at least until after the age of 4, when the risk of postsplenectomy sepsis is decreased. Generally, surgery can be postponed until early

adulthood; however, it is unwise to defer surgery indefinitely, because continued hemolysis leads to gallstone formation. In the most severe form of hereditary spherocytosis, splenectomy may be required in infancy (Croom et al., 1986). In severely affected individuals under age 5, partial splenectomy has been used to decrease the risks of postsplenectomy sepsis. Tchernia et al. (1993) reported on 11 children treated by partial splenectomy; an acceptable increase in hemoglobin (with a mean increase of 3 g/dL) was accompanied by preservation of splenic function. Older children and adults are more appropriately managed by total splenectomy, which is increasingly being performed laparoscopically (Yee and Akpata, 1995).

The spleen is generally slightly-to-moderately enlarged. Accessory spleens should be sought diligently, since their subsequent enlargement can produce significant recurrence of hemolysis. The biliary tract should be assessed prior to surgery, so that any associated biliary tract disease can be dealt with at the time of elective splenectomy (either open or laparoscopic). The postoperative course in these otherwise healthy patients is usually uncomplicated, and the hematologic response to splenectomy is gratifying.

Hereditary elliptocytosis is a related but milder disorder, which is also transmitted as an autosomal dominant trait. The incidence is between 1/4000 and 1/5000. In approx 10–15% of cases, significant hemolysis warrants splenectomy. Other less common congenital defects of erythrocyte membrane structure include hereditary pyropoikilocytosis and hereditary stomatocytosis. In hereditary pyropoikilocytosis, a spectrin structural abnormality causes red blood cells to assume bizarre shapes. In vitro thermal disruption occurs at 44–45°C, rather than at the normal 49°C. Severe hemolysis is characteristic of the disorder; in contrast to hereditary spherocytosis, splenectomy only partially corrects the hemolytic tendency. In hereditary stomatocytosis, anemia is generally mild. The indications for splenectomy are similar to those for hereditary spherocytosis. Splenectomy decreases the rate of hemolysis, but does not halt it completely. The molecular basis for the clinical and morphologic heterogeneity of these disorders is an area of active research (Lecomte et al., 1993).

17.2.1.2. Thalassemia   The thalassemias constitute a group of congenital disorders characterized by greatly decreased production of one or another of the subunits of hemoglobin, with the intra-erythrocytic accumulation of unmatched α or β globin chains, and significant hemolysis (Yuan et al., 1995).

The most common disorder is β-thalassemia. The gene frequency of this condition approaches 0.1 in southern Italy and some of the islands of the Mediterranean. It is also commonly encountered in regions of central Africa, southern China, southeast Asia, the South Pacific, and parts of India. Individuals who are homozygous are said to have β-thalassemia major (Cooley's anemia).

In β-thalassemia major, severe anemia is accompanied by hemolysis, iron overload, and hyperactive erythropoiesis, including extramedullary sites. The expanded vasculature of the marrow spaces produces a dilutional component to the anemia (*see* below). Hemolysis is improved to a variable extent by splenectomy. Affected individuals develop skeletal abnormalities, from the increased mass of the highly erythropoietic marrow; cardiomegaly, often with congestive heart failure; and hepatosplenomegaly. A regular program of transfusion therapy can be highly effective in reversing the anemia and suppressing extramedullary hematopoiesis, but hemolysis continues and iron overload frequently becomes a problem. The decision to recommend splenectomy is based on transfusion requirements; in one series, splenectomy was successful in decreasing transfusion requirement to between 150 and 180 mL/kg/yr (Piomelli, 1995).

Blendis et al. (1974) studied the effects of splenectomy in seven patients with thalassemia syndromes: these were almost all untransfused patients. Autologous red blood cell life-span increased in all patients, but without a proportionate rise in red blood cell mass. Plasma volume was greatly increased before splenectomy, and, in two patients, was twice the expected volume. However, the volume excess was unrelated to spleen size, and, unlike the effect of splenectomy on plasma volume in most patients with splenomegaly, plasma volumes were little affected by the procedure. It was considered that the plasma volume excess was related to the increase in total blood volume induced by the gross expansion of the vasculature of the expanded bone marrow. Furthermore, it was noted that long-term, high-volume blood transfusion therapy prevents or reverses the skeletal changes and the expansion of plasma volume.

Patients with thalassemia major (particularly children) are considered to be at high risk of septic complications after splenectomy. Some of the earliest observations of overwhelming postsplenectomy infection (OPSI) were made in children who underwent splenectomy for Cooley's anemia. In an attempt to balance the potential benefits of splenectomy against the risks in this condition, both partial splenic embolization and partial splenectomy have been used. Politis et al. (1987) reported a 5-yr follow-up of six patients with thalassemia major, who were treated with partial splenic embolization, and compared their clinical course to that of seven patients who underwent total splenectomy. Partial splenic embolization successfully reduced transfusion requirements, and no infectious complications were noted during the 5-yr follow-up. In contrast, two patients in the splenectomized group subsequently suffered recurrent infections. As patients have been followed longer after partial splenectomy or partial splenic embolization, however, increasing numbers of treatment failures, resulting from recurrent hypersplenism, have been recorded (Piomelli, 1995). Current therapeutic recommendations therefore center around carefully optimized transfusion regimens. Total splenectomy is performed, when indicated, to decrease transfusion requirements. Partial splenic embolization is reserved for the rare patient who is considered to be a high anesthetic risk (Piomelli, 1995).

17.2.1.3. Sickle Cell Disease   An abnormal hemoglobin (sickle hemoglobin [HbS]), which polymerizes when deoxygenated, causes the diverse clinical manifestations characteristic of the condition (*see also* Chapter 15). Approximately 8% of black Amer-icans have the heterozygous variant of the disorder (sickle cell trait). The incidence of the trait is substantially higher in certain regions of Africa, and exceeds 30% in Nigeria. In America, 0.15% of black children are homozygous for the disorder.

The erythrocytes of homozygous individuals tend to assume a rigid, sickled configuration when the HbS is desaturated. Sickled erythrocytes are destroyed in the spleen, and lodge in the microvasculature of various organs. In the microcirculation, a vicious cycle of microthrombosis, interruption of blood flow, local decrease in oxygen tension, and further sickling of more erythrocytes causes progressive infarction of the spleen and kidneys, and produces the characteristic periodic vaso-occlusive crises. Between crises, anemia and hemolysis continue. The spleen is enlarged in the early stages in childhood, but later shrinks as sequential infarction occurs (*see* Subheading 3.6.).

Acute splenic sequestration crises (ASSC), characterized by sudden enlargement of the spleen and worsening anemia, may

occur. Thrombocytopenia and signs of hypovolemia may be present. Transient splenic vein obstruction with sickled erythrocytes results in distention of the spleen and sequestration of a significant, and sometimes massive, amount of blood (Solanki et al., 1986). ASSC is most common in patients under the age of 6 yr, because, with time, progressive splenic infarction renders the spleen fibrotic and incapable of acute distention. Splenectomy may be needed (al-Salem et al., 1996). Partial splenectomy was employed by Svarch et al. (1996) in 25 children with recurrent splenic sequestration crises. No recurrent splenic sequestration crises occurred subsequently, and the transfusion requirement was significantly decreased in all.

ASSC has been reported in adolescents and adults with mixed sickle-cell syndromes, including sickle-cell hemoglobin C disease and sickle cell thalassemia, in which splenic infarction is less likely to occur (Solanki et al., 1986). Homozygotes (HbSS), with high levels of fetal hemoglobin, may similarly be at risk (Moll and Orringer, 1996). Transfusion and hydration generally lead to resolution of ASSC in these individuals, but occasionally splenectomy is performed for recurrent crises, or in patients in whom transfusion is difficult, because of erythrocyte alloantibodies.

Even before splenic atrophy develops, splenic function is diminished in homozygous individuals with HbS, and a hyposplenic state, in which bacterial clearance is decreased, can be detected. Occasionally, splenic abscesses (*see* Subheading 3.3.) form within the parenchyma of an infarcted spleen, requiring drainage or splenectomy (al-Salem et al. 1996).

17.2.1.4. Other Hemolytic Anemias   Many forms of hereditary hemolytic anemia associated with erythrocyte enzyme deficiency have been identified. The two major forms of surgical importance are pyruvate kinase (PK) deficiency and glucose-6-phosphate dehydrogenase (G-6-PD) deficiency. Most patients with enzyme deficiencies maintain an adequate hemoglobin level, and do not require splenectomy. The spleen is generally enlarged in PK deficiency, and splenectomy may be required in severe forms. In contrast, splenectomy is rarely indicated in G-6-PD deficiency (Ravindranath and Beutler, 1987).

Autoimmune hemolytic anemia is an acquired disorder, which, in later life especially, tends to be secondary to other disorders. A positive direct antiglobulin (Coombs') test is characteristic, although in some cases the surface antibody is below the threshold of detection by this method. The condition may be secondary to an underlying lymphoproliferative, autoimmune, or myeloproliferative disorder that must be excluded. Hemolytic anemia may complicate the course of lymphoproliferative disorders, including chronic lymphatic leukemia (CLL) and (rarely) Hodgkin's disease.

In some instances, other cytopenias may be superimposed, and splenectomy may be required. Approximately 75% of patients with autoimmune hemolytic anemia will respond, at least temporarily, to corticosteroid therapy. Patients who do not respond after 6–8 wk of steroid therapy, or those in whom a contraindication to steroid use exists, may be referred for splenectomy. Careful evaluation to exclude other causes of hemolysis, particularly acute self-limited forms, is essential. Chromium-51-tagged erythrocyte sequestration studies may be helpful, if carefully standardized.

Paroxysmal nocturnal hemoglobinuria is an acquired erythrocyte membrane disorder, in which red blood cells become inordinately sensitive to complement. The sensitivity to complement also involves neutrophils and platelets, and is thought to arise from a change in the pluripotent stem cell, which gives rise to all three cell lines. Splenectomy is usually not recommended, because of its limited therapeutic value and inordinately high operative risk.

Severe aplastic anemia has been treated with splenectomy, with results comparable to antilymphocyte globulin (ALG) administration. Speck et al. (1996) reviewed 80 patients with severe aplastic anemia, who were treated with ALG and splenectomy, and compared them with an additional 52 patients who were treated with ALG, but not splenectomized. Splenectomy resulted in an increase in neutrophils, reticulocytes, and platelets within 2 wk, but there was no difference in long-term outcome (including late survival) between the two groups. Those authors concluded that splenectomy should be considered only in selected patients who are not candidates for bone marrow transplantation, and who have continued major transfusion requirements, despite optimal therapy.

17.2.2. DISORDERS ASSOCIATED WITH THROMBOCY-TOPENIA One large series showed that 81% of elective splenectomies were performed for cytopenias, especially thrombocytopenia (Dotevall et al., 1987). The most common disorder for which splenectomy is recommended is idiopathic thrombocytopenic purpura, and this accounted for 16% of elective splenectomies in the UMMC series.

The profound thrombocytopenia, which is present in most of these patients, renders bleeding complications more likely at the time of surgery. In addition, many patients have been on corticosteroid treatment preoperatively, necessitating perioperative steroid therapy, and resulting in diminished wound healing.

Accurate diagnosis is important. Response to previous therapy, as discussed in subsequent subheading, is the most important predictor of response to splenectomy in ITP. Neither platelet sequestration studies with chromium-5-tagged platelets nor antiplatelet antibody levels are routinely recommended, at present, to better define the selection of patients for splenectomy. Because human immunodeficiency virus (HIV) infection has emerged as a major cause of thrombocytopenia, often preceding other clinical manifestations of acquired immunodeficiency syndrome (AIDS), serologic testing for HIV is recommended (George et al., 1996).

An incision that does not require muscle transection is recommended, to minimize wound bleeding and hematoma formation. Initial control of the splenic artery in the lesser sac, as described in Subheading 4.1.2., allows dissection to proceed under controlled conditions. Laparoscopic splenectomy has been safely performed in this patient population. Platelet transfusions are rarely necessary, because the autologous circulating platelets, although decreased in number, are young and hemostatically highly effective, and because the platelet count rises rapidly after surgery. If platelet transfusions are used, they should be given after control of the splenic artery has been achieved, to avoid platelet destruction in the spleen. Reperitonealization of raw surfaces after splenectomy, and the use of topical hemostatic agents, helps to control oozing from the splenic bed, in profoundly thrombocytopenic patients.

17.2.2.1. Idiopathic Thrombocytopenic Purpura Idiopathic thrombocytopenic purpura is a hemorrhagic disorder characterized by a decreased platelet count, despite the presence of normal or increased megakaryocytes in the bone marrow. Definitive diagnosis depends on ruling out other causes of thrombocytopenia, such as systemic illness or drug ingestion. Systemic lupus erythematosus, hepatitis, cytomegalovirus, Epstein-Barr virus, toxoplasmosis, and HIV infection are all in the differential diagnosis. ITP is categorized into two forms: acute and chronic.

Acute ITP is seen most commonly in children, following a viral illness or upper respiratory tract infection. Over 80% of affected individuals recover spontaneously within 3–6 mo, and only a minority proceeds to the chronic form. Conversely, in adults, only 10% of cases of ITP are of the self-limited acute form. The majority evolves into the chronic form, so that, after a period of temporizing therapies and observation of the course of the disease, the more permanently effective therapy of splenectomy should be considered. The present tendency is to minimize the duration of medical therapy, in favor of early surgery.

The typical adult patient with chronic ITP is a woman between the ages of 20 and 40 years, who presents with the typical petechial rash and/or bleeding from the gingivae, vagina, gastrointestinal tract, or urinary tract. The platelet count is generally less than 50,000/mm^3. Bone marrow examination, to confirm the presence of normal or increased numbers of megakaryocytes, and to identify possible hematologic malignancy, is required. Treatment may not be necessary unless the platelet count is below 20,000/mm^3, or there is extensive bleeding.

The basic cause is the production of autoantibodies, which react against platelets. This leads to destruction of the less heavily antibody-coated platelets in the spleen; those more heavily sensitized tend to be destroyed in the liver. Platelet survival (autologous or infused) is markedly diminished, and platelet turnover increased. Splenectomy not only removes the major site of platelet destruction, but may also abolish a major site of antiplatelet antibody production.

Initial therapy of ITP consists of corticosteroid treatment for 6 wk–2 mo. Patients who respond to corticosteroids are subsequently tapered in dosage; a significant percentage will subsequently remain in remission. Patients who respond to steroids, but relapse after steroid withdrawal, are candidates for splenectomy, as are those patients who do not respond satisfactorily to steroid treatment. Emergency splenectomy may be necessary, if serious bleeding complications, particularly intracranial hemorrhage, occur, and the condition is unresponsive to medical therapy, including IgG administration (George et al., 1996; Stiemer et al., 1996).

Of 216 patients who underwent splenectomy for ITP, Coon (1987) reported a satisfactory response, with platelet counts over 150,000/mm^3, in 72%. This result is similar to those of other reported series. Patients who responded favorably to steroids were more likely to respond to splenectomy, but no other predictive factors were identified. In more recent series, the response to IgG, as well as corticosteroids, have been predictive (*see* below). Naouri et al. (1993) reported that 90% of 72 patients, who underwent splenectomy for ITP, maintained platelet counts over 120,000 at long-term follow-up. Chirletti et al. (1992) reported a series of 70 patients splenectomized for ITP, 63 of whom achieved platelet counts over 150,000; 2/7 nonresponders were subsequently found to have accessory spleens. Patients who do not respond to splenectomy may require long-term treatment with immunosuppressive agents. Several therapeutic options exist for nonresponders, and the natural history of the disease is quite variable. Although published treatment guidelines state that data to support the search for, and removal of, accessory spleens in relapsed ITP are lacking (George et al., 1996), most surgical series contain several such patients. Search for accessory spleens should be considered part of the original procedure; in the series from Chirletti et al. (1992), accessory spleens were found in 11 (5.7%) patients at initial exploration, and were the cause of 2/7 treatment failures (*see* above).

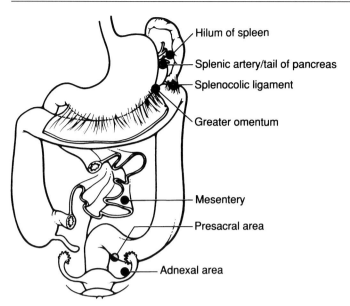

Fig. 17.1. Typical locations for accessory spleens (in approximate order of frequency) include: splenic hilum, tail of pancreas, greater omentum, vicinity of splenic artery, splenocolic ligament, mesentery, and gonads. The majority of accessory spleens are found in the splenic hilum or adjacent to the tail of the pancreas (Skandalakis et al., 1993). (Reproduced with permission from Scott-Conner and Dawson, 1993.)

Figure 1 shows the various locations in which accessory spleens are found.

Spleen size is usually close to normal in ITP. Initial control of the splenic artery, as previously discussed, facilitates splenectomy by allowing platelet transfusion to be performed when necessary. Most patients do not require intraoperative platelet infusion. Administration of preoperative corticosteroids and IgG may result in significant transient increase in platelet count, and are advocated by many surgeons (Chirletti et al., 1992; Law et al., 1997).

Because spleen size is usually normal, and the patients are generally young and otherwise healthy, ITP was one of the first disorders for which laparoscopic splenectomy was performed. Many series have documented safety and effectiveness, although most surgeons occasionally find it prudent to convert patients to open splenectomy, usually for intraoperative bleeding (Lefor et al., 1993; Gigot et al., 1994; Zamir et al., 1996; Friedman et al., 1996; Watson et al., 1997).

The need to search assiduously for accessory spleens is no different with the laparoscopic approach; Gigot et al. (1994) commented that it was difficult to be certain that none was overlooked, and stressed the need for long-term follow-up. To circumvent this issue, some have attempted computed tomography (CT) scan localization of accessory spleens, prior to splenectomy (Gigot et al., 1994) with variable results. In a retrospective review, Watson et al. (1997) found that one accessory spleen had been missed in 13 laparoscopic splenectomies, and one accessory spleen had been missed in 47 open splenectomies. Friedman et al. (1996) succeeded in finding and removing accessory spleens in 6/31 laparoscopic splenectomies. Newer adjunctive methods, such as the use of laparoscopic ultrasound, may facilitate the intraoperative search for accessory spleens. An alternative method for intraoperative localization of accessory spleens, utilizing [99]m-technetium labeled,

autologous, heat-damaged red blood cells and an intraoperative probe, has been described (Pohlson et al., 1994), and may prove to be helpful, if adapted for laparoscopic use. Until more data are available, careful follow-up of patients undergoing laparoscopic splenectomy remains necessary.

Factors predictive of response to splenectomy in recent studies include not only preoperative response to corticosteroids, but also young age and response to preoperative IgG (Naouri et al., 1993; Najean et al., 1991; Chirletti et al., 1992; Shiino et al., 1996; Law et al., 1997). Kinetic study, with radionuclide-labeled platelets, by Najean et al. (1991) documented that splenic sequestration correlated highly with response to splenectomy. In their series, 71/76 patients with splenic sequestration had postoperative platelet counts greater than 100,000, compared to 7/13 with mixed splenic and hepatic sequestration, and 1/14 with predominantly hepatic sequestration. In their series, splenic sequestration was an independent predictor, and did not correlate with age, history, or severity of disease (Najean et al. 1991).

Accessory spleens causing recurrence of thrombocytopenia after splenectomy may be sought with technetium sulfur colloid or technetium-labeled heat-damaged red blood cells (Massey and Stevens, 1991; Facon et al., 1992). In the latter series, five patients with recurrent ITP underwent accessory splenectomy, with only a partial response in the platelet count. In the review by George et al. (1996) of 12 large case series from 12 countries, although essentially all adult patients received glucocorticoid therapy and half underwent splenectomy, 36% of patients had persistent thrombocytopenia at the time of last follow-up.

17.2.2.2. Systemic Lupus Erythematosus Autoimmune thrombocytopenic purpura is the most common indication for splenectomy in systemic lupus erythematosus (SLE). Occasionally, autoimmune hemolytic anemia or hypersplenism, caused by portal hypertension occurs and necessitates removal of the spleen. Thrombocytopenia occurs in approx 20% of patients with SLE, and is related to the presence of antiplatelet antibodies. Medical therapy is similar to that for ITP; corticosteroids are used as first-line therapy; danazol is effective in a significant number of patients refractory to corticosteroid therapy (Cervera et al., 1995). Splenectomy is reserved for failure of medical management (Formiga et al., 1997). In a representative series, Gruenberg et al. (1986) reported that 1.9% of patients diagnosed with SLE required splenectomy during the study period. Of 16 patients, 12 underwent splenectomy for thrombocytopenia. Eight had satisfactory results, with platelet counts being maintained at normal levels without the need for steroids, although these might be required for treatment of other manifestations of SLE. Splenectomy did not accelerate the development of other manifestations of SLE in this series. The spleen is usually normal in size, but may be enlarged. Although the characteristic histologic changes associated with SLE provide important diagnostic confirmation, this was noted in only 2/16 spleens in the Gruenberg et al. series (1986).

17.2.2.3. Thrombotic Thrombocytopenic Purpura Thrombotic thrombocytopenic purpura (TTP) is a multisystem disease of uncertain etiology, which is being recognized with increasing frequency. An abnormal interaction between vascular endothelium and platelets causes diverse clinical manifestations, classically included in a pentad of thrombocytopenic purpura, microangiopathic hemolytic anemia, fluctuating neurological abnormalities, renal disease, and fever. Systemic manifestations are related to the formation of microthrombi within the capillaries and terminal arterioles of many organs, and platelet survival is decreased, because of consumption in the thrombi. Untreated, the mortality rate is between 80 and 90%. With current therapy, survival is the rule, rather than the exception; most patients can achieve remission, although approx 50% will subsequently relapse (Rose et al., 1993). The relapse is generally less severe than the initial episode. Application of a carefully designed protocol led to 91% survival in a series of 108 patients (Bell et al., 1991).

The present treatment of choice is plasma exchange, with the transfusion of fresh-frozen plasma, which is believed to remove a platelet-aggregating agent. Antiplatelet drugs, dextran, and corticosteroids may be used, in addition. Splenectomy is reserved for patients who fail to respond to plasma exchange, and results are variable. Splenectomy was not effective in patients with acute TTP who did not respond to medical therapy in the series of Bell et al. (1991). In contrast, a series of six patients, who failed medical management and underwent splenectomy, was reported by Winslow and Nelson (1995); all survived, and all were without active disease at follow-up. In an earlier series (Schneider et al., 1985), 11 patients with TTP were treated initially with plasma exchange and infusion of fresh-frozen plasma. Six patients who did not respond to plasma exchange underwent splenectomy and treatment with antiplatelet drugs, corticosteroids, and dextran. All patients survived splenectomy, and remained in remission during subsequent observation. The use of additional antiplatelet agents, such as aspirin and dipyridamole, as well as corticosteroids and vincristine, in conjunction with plasma exchange, have significantly decreased the number of treatment failures. There still remains a small subset of patients in whom splenectomy may be necessary to induce remission, when medical therapy fails (Rowe et al., 1985; Liu et al., 1986).

Splenectomy may be indicated in patients who relapse, and is performed (whenever possible) during a disease-free period, after the tendency to relapse has been demonstrated. Although long-term remissions can then be achieved (Veltman et al., 1995; Onundarson et al., 1992; Thompson et al., 1992; Wells et al., 1991; Hoffkes et al., 1995), a note of caution is in order. Splenectomy does not change the von Willebrand's factor multimeric patterns in any consistent fashion (Pereira et al., 1993), and some patients continue to relapse, despite splenectomy (Bowdler, 1987; Crowther et al., 1996).

17.2.2.4. Other Disorders Associated with Thrombocytopenia

17.2.2.4.1. Hematological Malignancies Thrombocytopenia may complicate the course of patients with malignant lymphoma, CLL, and myeloproliferative disorders, but this is rarely an indication for splenectomy in these circumstances (Lehman et al., 1987). These situations are discussed further in Subheading 2.3., and also in Chapters 13 and 14.

17.2.2.4.2. Chronic Liver Disease Thrombocytopenia also occurs in the context of chronic liver disease, and usually results from hypersplenism secondary to portal hypertension. Splenomegaly caused by chronic splenic congestion leads to the splenic sequestration of platelets, leukocytes, and erythrocytes, and may result in neutropenia and anemia, as well as thrombocytopenia. Skootsky et al. (1986) reported two patients who underwent splenectomy for thrombocytopenia associated with chronic liver disease, who had only minimally enlarged spleens (230 and 375 g). They postulated that increased levels of platelet-associated IgG may be important in the pathogenesis of thrombocytopenia in chronic liver disease. Spleen size, measured by ultrasound or radionuclide imaging, correlated inversely with leukocyte count,

but not with hematocrit or platelet count in a recent series, leading Shah et al. (1996) to postulate that other factors must contribute to the thrombocytopenia. The majority of patients are asymptomatic, and do not require treatment, unless bleeding occurs.

Although splenectomy has been used in the past as a means of treating symptomatic hypersplenism in this setting, it is rarely indicated today (Crosby, 1987; El-Khishen et al., 1985). Correction of the portal hypertension by portosystemic shunting (Soper and Rikkers, 1982), transjugular intrahepatic portocaval shunting (TIPS) (Pursnani et al., 1997), distal splenorenal shunting (El-Khishen et al., 1985), or small-diameter, H-graft portocaval shunting (McAllister et al., 1995) improves thrombocytopenia within 1–2 wk.

17.2.2.4.3. AIDS Thrombocytopenic purpura occurs in association with the AIDS and AIDS-related complex, and has been termed "immunodeficiency-associated thrombocytopenic purpura" (Walsh et al., 1985; Schneider et al., 1987). It may be the presenting symptom in a patient not known to be infected with the HIV. Splenomegaly was present clinically in 20% of patients in one series (Schneider et al., 1987).

The condition shares many features with ITP, and treatment with corticosteroids and splenectomy has been patterned empirically after that used for ITP. Of 15 homosexual men treated by splenectomy for immunodeficiency-associated thrombocytopenic purpura, 14 initially responded favorably, with an increase in platelet count to greater than $150,000/mm^3$ (Schneider et al., 1987). In nine of these patients, the clinical response was sustained; with additional therapy (corticosteroids and danazol), the response was sustained in two additional patients. Subsequent series have confirmed that splenectomy is effective, and results in a sustained improvement in the platelet count in most patients (Ravikumar et al., 1989; Tyler et al., 1990; Alonso et al., 1993; Brown et al., 1994; Ajana et al., 1996). Early concerns about infectious complications in these patients have not proven justified, although a high rate of pneumococcal infections was noted in one series (Ajana et al., 1996). The concern that splenectomy might accelerate progress of the disease has also been laid to rest: in two series, there is in fact a suggestion that the disease may progress more slowly after splenectomy (Morlat et al., 1996; Tsoukas et al. 1993).

17.2.3. MYELOPROLIFERATIVE AND LYMPHOPROLIFERATIVE DISORDERS
The indications for splenectomy and staging laparotomy in malignant hematological disorders will be considered in this section (*see also* Chapters 13 and 14). Experience in this field over 10 years was recently reviewed from Roswell Park Cancer Institute (Horowitz et al., 1996), which reiterated the general impression in the surgical literature that these patients fare less well after splenectomy than those with ITP or hemolytic anemia. In this series, the subset of patients with non-Hodgkin's lymphoma, CLL, or chronic myelocytic leukemia fared worst. Because indications for, and outcomes resulting from, splenectomy vary, the major disorders are considered individually here.

17.2.3.1. Myeloid Metaplasia
In myeloid metaplasia (MM), there is extramedullary proliferation of hematopoietic stem cells. Enlargement of the spleen and liver result, and there is progressive replacement of the bone marrow by fibrous tissue (myelofibrosis).

Splenectomy is selectively performed for hypersplenism or symptomatic splenomegaly. At one time, splenectomy was believed to be contraindicated, because of an inordinately high postoperative mortality, and morbidity and mortality rates after splenectomy for MM remain higher than those following any other hematological disorder, with the possible exception of chronic myelogenous leukemia. One literature review and decision analysis quoted an operative mortality of 13.4%, with an early complication rate of 45%, and suggested that this palliative procedure should only be considered in informed, symptomatic patients (Benbassat et al., 1990). Despite these discouraging statistics, splenectomy may be indicated for palliation of massive splenomegaly or excessive transfusion requirements. Compensatory hepatomegaly has been reported to occur after splenectomy, presumably in response to continued extramedullary hematopoiesis (Towell and Levine, 1987).

Subtotal splenectomy has been used to avoid postsplenectomy sepsis, and also to preserve some of the hematopoietic function of the spleen. Petroianu (1996b) reported on three patients undergoing subtotal splenectomy for MM, with preservation of the upper splenic pole supplied by the short gastric vessels; improvement had been maintained at an almost 3-year follow-up.

The spleen is commonly massively enlarged in MM, with spleen weights ranging from 400 to >6000 g. The massively enlarged spleen may be adherent to the abdominal parietes in the left upper quadrant, as the result of previous radiation therapy or infarcts; in these cases, initial control of the splenic artery and splenic vein prior to mobilization of the spleen, may be prudent, to limit blood loss.

17.2.3.2. Chronic Myelogenous Leukemia
In a representative series (Coon, 1985a), 11 patients underwent splenectomy for chronic myelogenous leukemia (CML). Two of these splenectomies were performed as a prelude to bone marrow transplantation; other indications included severe thrombocytopenia, massive splenomegaly, splenic infarction, and impending splenic rupture. 3/11 patients died during the immediate postoperative period. Similar results have been reported by other centers (Wilson et al., 1985). A recent series of 53 patients who underwent splenectomy during the accelerated phase, or "blastic crisis," of acute myelogenous leukemia (AML), at MD Anderson Medical Center, showed minimal morbidity and mortality, with one death within 30 days, excellent palliation, and a decrease in transfusion requirements (Bouvet et al., 1997). Early splenectomy, prior to bone marrow grafting, has been reported to result in more rapid hematological reconstitution (Goldman et al., 1980).

The spleen is usually enlarged (up to 6000 g), especially when splenectomy is performed late in the disease. Histological examination of the spleen almost invariably reveals a diffuse or nodular leukemic infiltration. Extramedullary hematopoiesis, infarction, and fibrosis of the spleen may also be seen (see also Chapter 13).

17.2.3.3. Chronic Lymphocytic Leukemia
Chronic lymphocytic leukemia (CLL) is the most common chronic form of leukemia in the United States and Europe. The clinical course is frequently indolent, and the diagnosis is made on the basis of an incidental finding in an asymptomatic adult, in 25% of cases. The development of symptomatic splenomegaly, anemia, or thrombocytopenia may necessitate treatment.

Splenectomy is sometimes useful in treating cytopenias associated with late-stage, refractory CLL. In the past, splenectomy was performed very late in the course of the disease, and early series produced discouraging results. Recent series demonstrate more acceptable rates of morbidity and mortality (Delpero et al., 1987; Pegourie et al., 1987; Coad et al., 1993; Seymour et al., 1997), leading to a reassessment of the role of splenectomy for splenomegaly with cytopenias associated with CLL. In Delpero et al.'s series (1987), 32 patients underwent splenectomy for CLL. 22/23 patients with thrombocytopenia and 15/19 patients with anemia were improved. No consistent effect on peripheral blood leukocyte

counts was noted. A favorable response to splenectomy was observed in the majority of patients studied by Stein et al. (1987) and Pegourie et al. (1987). In Pegourie et al.'s series, the blood lymphocyte clone disappeared in 4/15 patients after splenectomy and discontinuous high-dose chlorambucil therapy. Seymour et al. (1997) reported on 55 patients who underwent splenectomy from 1971 to 1993: the overall mortality rate was 9%. Thrombocytopenic patients were most likely to benefit, but the majority of patients did achieve some hematologic improvement. The increases in hematocrit and leukocyte count correlated with spleen weight (Seymour et al., 1997).

The spleen is typically enlarged: splenic weight ranged from 1000 to 3572 g in a representative series (Stein et al., 1987). Generally, the histology reflects extensive involvement by leukemic cells (see also Chapter 14).

17.2.3.4. Hairy Cell Leukemia
Hairy cell leukemia is a rare lymphoproliferative disorder of adults, presenting with cytopenias and splenomegaly. A characteristic "hairy cell" is an activated lymphocyte that is seen in the bone marrow and peripheral blood (Platanias and Golomb, 1993). Only 500–600 new cases are reported in the United States each year (Cheson and Martin, 1987). Before effective chemotherapy, splenectomy was virtually the only effective treatment, and resulted in improvement in blood counts in almost all patients (Golomb, 1987; Brochard et al., 1987). Splenectomy does not cure the underlying disease, and, in those early series, almost half the patients subsequently required further treatment, after a median interval of 8.3 mo from splenectomy.

The first medical therapy to offer an alternative to splenectomy was treatment with α-interferon (Cheson and Martin, 1987). In a randomized study of previously untreated patients, 20 individuals with hairy cell leukemia were treated either by splenectomy or with α-interferon; a better response was demonstrated after α-interferon, albeit with more side effects (Smalley et al., 1992). In an Italian cooperative study designed to investigate the role of splenectomy vs α-interferon, 8/12 patients who were splenectomized relapsed, and the study was closed because of low patient accrual (Damasio and Frassoldati, 1994).

Therapeutic options now include chemotherapy (with the nucleosides, 2-deoxycoformycin or 2-chlorodeoxyadenosine), as well as α-interferon and/or splenectomy. The nucleosides are now used as first-line treatment (Platanias and Golomb, 1993; Bouroncle, 1994). In contrast to splenectomy, which is essentially a palliative treatment, these agents hold some promise for cure and long-term survival. Trials continue to define the role of these agents alone and in combination, and to redefine the role of splenectomy. Splenectomy is still indicated in young patients with significant splenomegaly and only minimal bone marrow involvement (Platanias and Golomb, 1993), or in the rapid reversal of severely depressed counts in association with systemic infection (Golomb and Ellis, 1991). The use of hematopoietic growth factors in the latter situation is under investigation.

Splenomegaly is generally moderate, and the pattern of involvement differs from other lymphoproliferative disorders, in that it is the red pulp that is predominantly involved. The mean splenic weight in one series (Van Norman et al., 1986) was 1460 g, with a range of 245-5012 g. The hairy cells show a highly characteristic pattern in the spleen, on histological examination.

17.2.3.5. Hodgkin's Disease and Non-Hodgkin's Lymphomas
The lymphomas are tumors of the lymphoid system, primarily divided into Hodgkin's disease and the non-Hodgkin's lymphomas, and are further subdivided by histological type (see Chapter 14).

The diagnosis of Hodgkin's disease usually requires the presence of characteristic Sternberg-Reed cells, but these are not pathognomonic in themselves. Approximately 90% of cases of Hodgkin's disease arise in lymph nodes, and there is frequently a pattern of contiguous spread to adjacent nodal groups or organs. The involved spleen is frequently normal in size, and the involvement may be nodular or diffuse.

The non-Hodgkin's lymphomas are a heterogeneous group of disorders. Accurate histological classification and staging are important for therapy and prognosis. Only 60% of non-Hodgkin's lymphomas arise in nodal tissue, and the remainder arise in extranodal sites, including the gastrointestinal tract, lung, and skin. Spread is generally noncontiguous in the non-Hodgkin's lymphomas, and many appear to be disseminated at the time of diagnosis (Williams and Golomb, 1986). The incidence of NHL is increasing in the United States.

Splenectomy for lymphoma is most commonly performed as part of a staging laparotomy (discussed in the next subheading). Occasionally, the diagnosis of lymphoma is initially made, when splenectomy is performed for undiagnosed splenomegaly (Spier et al., 1985). Hypersplenism with secondary cytopenias may be an indication for splenectomy in selected patients. These issues are discussed individually.

17.2.3.5.1. Staging Laparotomy
Staging laparotomy was introduced at a time when radiotherapy to clinically involved areas was the principal treatment for Hodgkin's disease with curative intent, and the optimal anatomical extent of radiotherapy needed careful definition. Likewise, the natural history of the disease was still obscure, and noninvasive imaging methods were in an early stage of development. Stage laparotomy is a diagnostic maneuver designed to determine precisely the extent of disease within the abdomen. At the present time, it is performed only when clinical staging is uncertain, or when a difference in stage will affect treatment, and it remains the gold standard against which other methods are judged (Irving, 1985; Mann et al., 1986). In a classic staging laparotomy, total splenectomy is performed for diagnostic purposes, and also to avoid the subsequent need to irradiate the spleen. In a review of the Stanford University Hospital experience (Taylor et al., 1985), the clinical stage was changed in 43.2% of 825 patients who underwent staging laparotomy. In 296 patients (36.1% of all cases), the stage was increased by findings at laparotomy. In 60 patients (7.3%), the stage was decreased. In this series, as in the earlier series, splenic involvement correctly predicted visceral involvement.

There was only one postoperative death, and 37 patients (4.5%) sustained major complications. In recent series, the operation has proven safe in this patient population. In a collective review of more than 1000 patients in reported series, the overall operative mortality rate was less than 0.5%, with a major morbidity rate of 8% (Huang and Urist, 1993).

Long-term sequelae include OPSI (Frezzato et al., 1993), small bowel obstruction, and myocardial infarction. Jockovich et al. (1994) reported 10 episodes of OPSI in 9/133 patients followed for a median of 15 years. The risk was highest for those patients with advanced or recurrent disease. Their series included 13 episodes of small bowel obstruction. Dietrich et al. (1994) reported that splenectomy correlated with an increased risk of secondary acute leukemia. Myocardial infarction was reported in three young patients who had been treated for Hodgkin's disease: two had undergone mediastinal radiotherapy, and the third had had a splenectomy

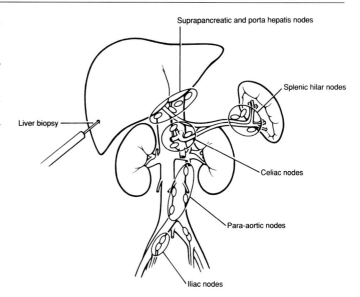

Fig. 17.2. Staging laparotomy for Hodgkin's disease includes splenectomy, liver biopsy (generally both wedge and needle), and biopsy of multiple node groups shown here. The yield is highest for the nodes around the celiac axic (Reproduced with permission from Scott-Conner and Dawson, 1993.)

(with subsequent marked increase in platelet count) (Scholz et al. 1993). In another series of three reported cases, radiation therapy, in addition to splenectomy, was implicated in the possible causation of myocardial infarction in young patients (Putterman and Polliack, 1992).

The technique of staging laparotomy has been carefully designed to maximize diagnostic accuracy. Preoperative evaluation usually includes CT scan of the abdomen (which has mostly replaced earlier diagnostic tests, such as bipedal lymphangiography). A midline or left paramedian incision is used to gain wide exposure and access to all quadrants of the abdomen. A general abdominal exploration is performed. Wedge and needle biopsies of both main lobes of the liver are obtained. Splenectomy, with excision of splenic hilar nodes, is performed next. The spleen is submitted for immediate gross and histological examination. If Hodgkin's disease is confirmed within the spleen, then biopsy of intra-abdominal node groups may be curtailed. Abdominal node sampling should include the left para-aortic nodes, nodes from the small bowel mesentery, from the celiac axis, and the region of the inferior vena cava or iliac region (Fig. 2). Clips may be used to mark the splenic hilum, sites of node sampling, and any gross intra-abdominal disease. Some pediatric surgeons perform incidental appendectomy, generally by an inversion technique, which does not involve opening the lumen of the appendix at the time of staging laparotomy.

Because of the risk of postsplenectomy sepsis, particularly in children (Hays et al., 1986), there has been an interest in the possibility of staging with less than total splenectomy (Lally et al., 1986). Partial splenectomy has been used in children (Hoekstra et al., 1994). Although the pattern of splenic involvement in Hodgkin's disease may be focal rather than diffuse, which raises the possibility of failing to recognize lesions, a recent series reported only a 1% risk of missing abdominal disease, when hemisplenectomy was used during staging laparotomy (Tubbs et al., 1987). Better preoperative imaging may improve results; in a recent series of 12 children, treated from 1982 to 1988, adequate staging with partial splenectomy was achieved in all (Hoekstra et al., 1994). Late recurrence of Hodgkin's disease in a splenic remnant has been reported 13 years after treatment, in one case (Slaiby et al., 1996). The second purpose of splenectomy during staging laparotomy is to avoid the need to radiate the spleen. Splenic irradiation is not a benign therapeutic alternative to surgical splenectomy. Splenic atrophy, hyposplenism, and postsplenectomy sepsis have all been reported to occur (Dailey et al., 1980). Full staging, including splenectomy, has also been performed laparoscopically (Childers et al., 1993; Lefor et al., 1993).

17.2.3.5.2. Splenectomy for Splenomegaly or Hypersplenism Cytopenias in patients with malignant lymphoma may arise from several causes: they are most commonly seen in patients with stage III and stage IV disease. Depression of the bone marrow by chemotherapy, infiltration by tumor cells, effects of radiation therapy, increased splenic pooling of red blood cells, and hypersplenism may all be factors. Selection of patients who benefit from splenectomy is difficult. Tagged erythrocyte or platelet sequestration studies have been of limited value in predicting the response to splenectomy. Bone marrow involvement by lymphoma is not considered a contraindication to surgery, because many of these patients show a good response to splenectomy (Mitchell and Morris, 1985). Splenectomy may allow resumption of chemotherapy, and thus contribute to remission. Removal of a bulky spleen relieves symptoms caused by pressure, and eliminates the risk of rupture with minor trauma. Brodsky et al. (1996) reported on 12 patients with non-Hodgkin's lymphoma, who underwent splenectomy for palliation of splenomegaly or for diagnostic purposes. There were no operative deaths, and 80% had a favorable hematologic result.

17.2.3.5.3. Primary Splenic Lymphoma Primary splenic lymphoma, basically a diagnosis of exclusion, in that no other foci of disease (other than spleen or splenic hilar nodes) can be demonstrated, is effectively treated by splenectomy (Mulligan et al., 1991; Gobbi et al., 1994; Cavanna et al., 1995). When diagnosis, rather than treatment, is the issue, ultrasound-guided percutaneous core biopsy is useful and safe. In a series of 46 patients, only one biopsy was inadequate for diagnosis of lymphoma (Cavanna et al., 1992).

17.2.4. HYPERSPLENISM Hypersplenism is a syndrome in which there is enlargement of the spleen, deficits in one or more cell lines in the peripheral blood, evidence for adequate production of the deficient cells, and (in retrospect) correction of the condition by splenectomy (Coon, 1985b). It is categorized into primary and secondary hypersplenism, and is found in a wide range of disorders, many of which have already been discussed (*see also* Chapter 9). Its presence usually implies abnormal sequestration or destruction of circulating blood cells in the spleen, but the mechanisms involved are diverse, and the term does not, in fact, refer to any specific process by which the cell deficit is generated. Mechanisms that may be involved include production of antierythrocyte, antigranulocyte, or antiplatelet antibodies, abnormal splenic hemodynamics, or maldistribution cytopenias and the effects of expanded blood volume. Individual disorders are discussed in some of the preceding subheading, as well as in Subheading 2.6.

17.2.5. UNDIAGNOSED SPLENOMEGALY The spleen may be palpable in as many as 3% of young adults, on physical examination, and many enlarged spleens are not palpable or are difficult to palpate (*see* Chapter 9). Splenomegaly may be detected by pal-

pation or by percussion of the area of splenic dullness, but radiographic techniques are important to confirm the diagnosis of splenic enlargement (*see* Chapter 16), and to provide a permanent record by which to assess progress with therapy. Radioisotope scan, CT scan, and ultrasound are all useful in delineating splenic size, and to demonstrate lesions, such as cysts and abscesses. Image-guided percutaneous core biopsy and laparoscopy have greatly decreased the need for splenectomy in this situation. Splenectomy is occasionally performed for diagnosis, when a full diagnostic evaluation has otherwise failed to reveal the cause of splenomegaly, particularly when signs of chronic illness are present. Although earlier series emphasized a high incidence of lymphoma in patients with splenomegaly of unknown origin, a more recent review of 28 patients failed to reveal any patient in whom the diagnosis of lymphoma was made at splenectomy, and only one patient developed lymphoma in the postoperative period (Knudson et al., 1982). The cause of splenomegaly was determined at laparotomy in only seven of these 28 patients. Three patients were found to have cirrhosis, three were found to have undiagnosed splenic cysts (CT scanning was not available preoperatively), and one patient was found to have sarcoid of the spleen (*see also* Chapter 9).

In some parts of the world, tropical splenomegaly (usually secondary to infection with malaria, schistosomiasis, or leishmaniasis, but sometimes idiopathic) may affect as many as 60% of the population (Jimmy et al., 1996; el-Shazly et al., 1995). Accurate diagnosis and differentiation from hematologic malignancy can generally be made without surgery. Symptomatic tropical splenomegaly, with associated cytopenias, may require splenic surgery (Cooper and Williamson, 1984; Sigueria-Batista and Quintas, 1994).

Preoperative evaluation of patients with splenomegaly of unknown origin demands close cooperation between surgeon and hematologist. The evaluation will generally require a blood count, bone marrow aspiration and biopsy, serum protein electrophoresis, erythrocyte sedimentation rate, and serological studies for collagen-vascular disorders. Liver function studies and additional tests, such as percutaneous liver biopsy, angiography, or upper gastrointestinal series, may be required to identify hepatic cirrhosis and portal hypertension. Cultures of blood, urine, sputum, and bone marrow aspirates should be performed, and sometimes studies relevant to viral and fungal infections. In the most recent series of patients with undiagnosed splenomegaly, one patient was subsequently shown to have AIDS; hence, testing for HIV antibodies may need to be included in the preoperative evaluation. CT of the abdomen should be included to detect splenic cyst or abscess (Knudson et al., 1982; Coon, 1985b).

If a full evaluation has failed to reveal the cause of splenomegaly, laparotomy with splenectomy may be considered. Although a diagnosis may be made in a significant number of patients, delay in proceeding to laparotomy may still be justified, especially in young asymptomatic patients with a history of recent infection (Knudson et al., 1982; Coon, 1985b).

17.2.6. MISCELLANEOUS CONDITIONS ASSOCIATED WITH SPLENOMEGALY AND/OR HYPERSPLENISM Splenic surgery is occasionally required for the diagnosis or treatment of several other conditions, mostly associated with splenomegaly, hypersplenism, or both; the most common of these are discussed here.

17.2.6.1. Felty Syndrome The characteristic triad of rheumatoid arthritis, splenomegaly, and neutropenia was described by Felty in 1924. Anemia and chronic leg ulcers may also be present. Felty syndrome develops in approx 1/300 patients with rheumatoid arthritis.

Splenectomy has been used for the relief of intractable neutropenia or chronic, nonhealing leg ulcers; however, the response to splenectomy is variable and unpredictable, with an estimated 60–80% of patients having a favorable response (Coon, 1985d).

The pathogenesis of the neutropenia is incompletely understood, at present. Increased levels of serum IgG, which binds to neutrophils, have been measured in patients with Felty syndrome. The spleen is the site of destruction of IgG-coated granulocytes, and may be the site of production of serum granulocyte, binding IgG, as well. Blumfelder et al. (1981) measured serum granulocyte-binding IgG levels in 14 patients, before and after splenectomy for Felty syndrome, in an attempt to identify a subset of patients who might be expected to respond favorably to splenectomy. In this series, a partial or complete response to splenectomy was obtained in nine patients. Markedly elevated amounts of serum granulocyte-binding IgG, preoperatively, and the postoperative fall in serum granulocyte-binding antibody, both correlated with a favorable response to splenectomy.

Treatment with hematopoietic growth factors or methotrexate may produce sustained response in many patients, and is emerging as the preferred initial treatment. Splenectomy is currently reserved for patients in whom therapy with growth factors fails, or those in whom rapid amelioration of neutropenia is needed (Rashba et al., 1996). A better understanding of the pathogenesis of the disorder is needed to define more precisely the characteristics of patients likely to respond favorably to splenectomy.

17.2.6.2. Gaucher's Disease Gaucher's disease is the commonest of the lysosomal storage diseases. It is an autosomal-recessive disorder, in which lysosomal p-glucocerebrosidase is deficient, and consequently the cerebroside P-glucosylceramide accumulates in macrophages in the liver, spleen, and bone marrow. Hypersplenism, with pancytopenia, and progressive, eventually massive, enlargement of the spleen result. Heterogenous changes in the spleen, including intrasplenic lesions, may mimic malignancy, on ultrasound (Neudorfer et al., 1997). Several forms of the disorder have been identified, corresponding to several structural enzyme abnormalities. Effective cure of these disorders requires enzyme replacement (see Chapter 9).

Splenectomy has been used to alleviate the mechanical symptoms caused by the massively enlarged spleen and pancytopenia. However, postsplenectomy sepsis may result, and acceleration of bone destruction has been reported (Fleshner et al., 1991). Whenever possible, splenectomy should be postponed until the second decade of life, in an attempt to minimize infectious and osteolytic complications (Ashkenazi et al., 1986).

Partial splenectomy has been employed at several centers (Rodgers et al., 1987; Guzzetta et al., 1987; Fleshner et al., 1991; Zer and Freud, 1992; Petroianu, 1996a). In one series (Rubin et al., 1986), partial splenectomy was attempted in 11 children with Gaucher's disease, and was successfully performed in seven. Long-term follow-up of these seven children showed improvement in hematological indices, with no episodes of postsplenectomy sepsis or clinical problems related to increased hepatic or bone accumulation of P-glucocerebroside. Partial splenic embolization has also been used in this disorder (Thanopoulos and Frimas, 1982), as has 95% splenectomy, employing the short gastric vessels as the splenic remnant blood supply (Fonkalsrud et al., 1990). Fleshner et al. (1991) reported a 27-year experience, encompassing 35 patients who underwent total, and 13 who underwent partial, splenectomy. They concluded that both were effective forms of therapy,

but that total splenectomy was associated with accelerated progression of bone disease and some increased incidence of malignancy.

Regrowth of the splenic remnant, with recurrence of hypersplenism, has been reported in a significant percentage of patients treated with partial splenectomy (Cohen et al. 1992; Morgenstern et al., 1993; Holcomb and Green, 1993; Bar-Maor, 1993; Zimran et al., 1995). Bar-Maor (1993) noted that partial splenectomy failed to halt progression of bone disease, if that destruction existed prior to surgery. At the present time, enzyme replacement therapy, with Ceredase, appears to be obviating the need for surgical intervention in many cases of Gaucher's disease (Zimran et al., 1995). When splenectomy is required, partial splenectomy with enzyme therapy has theoretic appeal (Bar-Maor, 1993).

17.2.6.3. Wiskott-Aldrich Syndrome This is an X-linked hereditary immunodeficiency disorder characterized by the triad of combined B- and T-cell mediated immunodeficiency, thrombocytopenia with a reduction in mean platelet size, and eczema. Bone marrow transplant is currently the treatment of choice, if a suitable donor is available (Mullen et al., 1993; Litzman et al., 1996). Splenectomy results in a significant increase in platelet size and number, with a significant increase in quality of life for affected individuals for whom bone marrow transplantation is not available (Corash et al., 1985; Mullen et al., 1993; Gaspoz et al., 1995; Litzman et al., 1996). Initial concerns that splenectomy would potentiate the immunodeficiency have not been borne out; in a recent review of 62 patients, treated at the National Institutes of Health between 1966 and 1992, splenectomy and prophylactic antibiotics were determined to be the treatment of choice, when a suitable bone marrow donor was not available (Mullen et al., 1993). In this series, the median survival after splenectomy was 25 years, compared with 5 years without splenectomy.

17.2.6.4. Schistosomiasis Approximately 150 million persons worldwide are infected with Schistosoma mansoni or japonicum. Splenomegaly and hypersplenism result from chronic infestation, and are frequently indications for splenectomy, in endemic areas of the world. Partial splenectomy has been described for this disorder. Fifty-one patients who underwent segmental splenectomy, and 44 patients treated by total splenectomy for schistosomiasis, were followed: the percentage of T-lymphocytes increased after segmental splenectomy, and there was also an increased T-helper: T-suppressor cell ratio after segmental splenectomy (Kamel et al., 1986). Only two patients required conversion from a partial to a total splenectomy, for technical reasons, and no increase in size of the splenic remnant was noted during the subsequent 2–4 years. This is the largest series of elective partial splenectomies reported to date, and provides encouraging data in favor of the concept of partial splenectomy for hypersplenism. Gastrointestinal bleeding caused by varices is best treated with esophagogastric devascularization and splenectomy (Shekhar, 1994; el-Gendi et al., 1994), which is more effective than splenectomy alone.

17.3. OTHER CONDITIONS REQUIRING SPLENIC SURGERY

Surgery is occasionally required for a wide spectrum of other lesions of the spleen. The radiological aspects of these disorders are considered in Chapter 16.

17.3.1. SPLENIC CYST AND PSEUDOCYST Splenic cysts present with symptoms of pressure, secondary infection, or rupture. They may be asymptomatic until much enlarged. Occasionally, a calcified splenic cyst is noted radiographically, in an otherwise asymptomatic individual.

Parasitic cysts are the most common on a worldwide basis: the majority of these are hydatid cysts resulting from infection with *Echinococcus granulosa*. This parasite is epidemic in regions of south-central Europe, South America, Australia, and Alaska. Even in regions of high prevalence of echinococcal disease, splenic involvement is rare, occurring in 1.7–4% of all patients with hydatid disease (Al-Mohaya et al., 1986; Uriarte et al., 1991). Infection of the spleen with *E. granulosa* results in the formation of a unilocular cyst, with a wall composed of several layers, including an outer fibrous membrane. The fluid within the cyst is under pressure, and contains infective scolices and daughter cysts. Splenectomy remains the treatment of choice.

In children with hydatid cysts, concerns regarding the long-term risk of sepsis have led to advocacy for cyst enucleation, instead of splenectomy (Narasimharao et al., 1987; Bhatnagar et al., 1994). Care must be taken at laparotomy to avoid spillage of the cyst contents, not only to prevent infective material from seeding the peritoneal cavity, but also to avoid anaphylactic reactions. Because the cyst fluid is under pressure, dissection may be accomplished more safely if the cyst is first carefully aspirated, then 1% formalin solution or 3% sodium chloride solution instilled to kill the scolices. Mebendazole may be useful as an adjunctive treatment in inoperable cases, in patients with multiple cysts, and in those in whom spillage occurs at laparotomy. Although enucleation is generally not recommended in adults, for fear of spillage of cyst contents, the success of this modality in children, and the development of improved surgical technique, will probably lead to more frequent use of this procedure.

The nonparasitic true cysts are less common. In young patients, epidermoid and dermoid cysts are encountered. Partial splenectomy is a good option for these generally benign lesions, in both adults (Golinsky et al., 1995) and children (Khan et al., 1986; Brown et al., 1989). Accurate preoperative imaging, to localize the cyst within the splenic parenchyma, facilitates operative planning (Williams and Glazer, 1993). Partial splenectomy can be performed by a number of techniques, such as mobilizing the spleen, or identifying a plane external to the cyst and carefully enucleating it, followed by hemostasis in the splenic remnant. By this method, the intact cyst can be removed, and a substantial amount of splenic parenchyma preserved. Alternatively, more formal anatomic resections, based on the segmental blood supply, can be employed. Recurrence of an epidermoid cyst, after an incomplete excision, led Musy et al. (1992) to suggest that frozen-section examination of the cyst wall be obtained, whenever less than total cystectomy (i.e., marsupialization) is contemplated. Other approaches to splenic cysts in children have included partial splenic decapsulation (Toulenkian and Seashore, 1987) and cyst aspiration with sclerosis (Moir et al., 1989); the latter approach has not been proven to provide adequate long-term control of cystic lesions.

Cystic lymphangiomas and true mesothelial cysts also occur. Multiple mesothelial cysts, throughout the spleen, have been reported in familial syndromes. When these lead to symptomatic splenomegaly, total splenectomy is likely to be required (Iwanaka et al., 1995).

Pseudocysts of the spleen are generally related to previous trauma. They are more common in women, and tend to occur in young adults. One review emphasized the minor nature of the antecedent trauma (Pachter et al., 1993). The incidence of these cysts will probably increase as more patients with splenic trauma are treated with splenic conservation techniques, or nonoperatively. Partial splenectomy is recommended, when surgery is required (Pachter et al., 1993; Golinsky et al., 1995). Laparoscopic fenestration or cyst wall excision has been reported, and may become the treatment of choice, as techniques evolve (Posta, 1994; Targarona et al., 1995; Cala et al., 1996). Benign inflammatory pseudotumors may similarly be treated by partial splenectomy (Yeung et al., 1996).

Occasionally, a pseudocyst of the tail of the pancreas will involve the spleen, and needs to be distinguished from a splenic cyst. A history of chronic pancreatitis, or the presence of characteristic pancreatic calcifications, radiographically, indicate this diagnostic possibility. The serum and cyst fluid amylase are generally elevated. Treatment of the underlying pancreatic ductal abnormality is critical: Simple removal of the cyst and the spleen, or marsupialization of the cyst, is likely to result in recurrence or formation of a pancreatic fistula.

17.3.2. SPLENIC NEOPLASMS Both benign and malignant splenic neoplasms are distinctly uncommon. The most common benign neoplasm is the cavernous hemangioma. Small hemangiomas are asymptomatic, and do not require surgery. Larger tumors may cause symptoms by pressure, cytopenias, consumption coagulopathy (Hoeger et al., 1995), or spontaneous rupture. The treatment is splenectomy. The possibility of malignant degeneration to hemangiosarcoma has been suggested, but this remains debatable. Lymphangiomas are less common, and are frequently part of a generalized lymphangiomatosis (*see* the prior discussion). Hamartomas, lipomas, leiomyomas, and fibromas are less common benign tumors (Oguzkurt et al., 1996). Morgenstern et al. (1984) reported a series of hamartomas, many of which were multiple, and expressed the opinion that splenic hamartomas are more common than previously suspected. In a review of 105 cases of "splenomas" reported in the literature, 26% of this heterogeneous group of lesions were hamartomas (Steinberg et al., 1991). Because hamartomas are frequently multiple, and may result in cytopenias, total splenectomy is generally required (Wirbel et al., 1996; Kumar, 1995). Fine-needle aspiration cytology may be misleading, and resulted in an erroneous diagnosis of metastatic tumors in three patients in one series (Kumar 1995).

Primary malignant tumors of the spleen are distinctly uncommon. When patients with splenic involvement from lymphoma, leukemia, and myeloproliferative disorders are excluded, the majority of the remaining malignant tumors are hemangiosarcomas (also called "angiosarcomas" and "hemangioendothelial sarcomas"). These lesions present with splenomegaly, microangiopathic hemolytic anemia, ascites, pleural effusion, and, occasionally, spontaneous rupture. The prognosis is poor (McGinley et al. 1995). In contrast to similar tumors of the liver, etiological factors, such as thorium dioxide, vinyl chloride, and arsenic, are rarely identified, when angiosarcoma occurs as a primary splenic tumor (Morgenstern et al., 1985).

Although it is often stated that the spleen rarely harbors metastatic tumors, tumor cells are frequently found within the splenic sinuses, at autopsy in cancer patients, and gross metastases were found within the spleens of 7% of patients with carcinoma at autopsy (Berge, 1974). The most common primary sites were breast, lung, skin, and colon. Because metastatic disease to the spleen frequently coexists with widespread systemic metastases, splenectomy is rarely recommended. However, when spontaneous rupture occurs, or if splenomegaly is pronounced, resection of the spleen may be required.

Klein et al. (1987) described four patients in whom isolated splenic metastases were identified. All four patients were treated by splenectomy and multimodality treatment of their underlying malignancy. One patient survived for over 12 years, two survived for >2 years, and the remaining patient lived for >1 year after splenic resection for isolated metastatic disease. Thus, it appears that isolated splenic metastases, although rare, should be treated by resection and aggressive therapy directed at the underlying malignancy (Zamora and Halpern, 1987; Klein et al., 1987; Hamy et al., 1995).

Splenectomy has been employed as part of a radical debulking procedure for ovarian carcinoma (Nicklin et al., 1995). Fine-needle aspiration cytology is an effective diagnostic modality, when it is important to confirm the diagnosis of metastatic disease, and splenectomy is not contemplated (Silverman et al., 1993). As previously noted, there are reports of splenic hamartomas being misdiagnosed as metastatic disease on fine-needle aspiration.

17.3.3. SPLENIC ABSCESS

The spleen is rarely the site of intraabdominal abscess formation. In a review of approx 400 cases reported between 1900 and 1986, Ooi and Leung (1997) identified five categories of etiologic factors: bloodborne infection associated with endocarditis or intravenous drug abuse, contiguous spread of infection from an adjacent hollow viscus, secondary infection of a splenic infarct, trauma, and immunodeficiency. Over 30% of reported cases fell into the immunodeficiency category, which includes cases of HIV infection, systemic lupus erythematosus, and Felty syndrome. The association with intravenous drug abuse, noted for some time, and attributed to bacteremia (Nallathambi et al., 1987), is thus strengthened by the additional factor of HIV infection in some of these patients. Splenic abscess secondary to trauma usually involves infection of a splenic hematoma; the incidence of this particular complication may rise as more splenic injuries are treated nonoperatively (Sands et al., 1986). In areas where typhoid fever is endemic, splenic abscesses are occasionally seen as a complication (Kizilcan et al., 1993).

In ambulatory patients, the diagnosis is difficult, because the symptoms of weight loss and fever are nonspecific. Presenting symptoms include any or all of the following: left upper quadrant pain and tenderness, diminished breath sounds, and left pleural effusion. CT and, in some cases, ultrasound of the left upper quadrant usually provide support for the diagnosis (Ooi et al., 1992; Paris et al., 1994). Occasionally, intraperitoneal or transdiaphragmatic rupture may occur, causing generalized peritonitis or empyema, respectively.

Although the majority of abscesses are bacterial in origin, an increasing number of fungal abscesses are being reported, particularly in pediatric patients with malignancies (Keidl and Chusid, 1989). Predominant bacterial organisms include the aerobic microbes, with *Staphylococcus, Streptococcus, Salmonella* and *E. coli* being the most common. *Enterococcus* is being recognized with increasing frequency in the intensive care unit population (Ooi and Leong, 1997), and *Pseudomonas* is also rising in incidence (Ooi et al., 1992). In a recent series of nine critically ill patients, who developed splenic abscesses while in intensive care, enteric organisms were cultured from six, and only three patients had *Staphylococcus* (Ho and Wisner, 1993). Unusual organisms, such as *Clostridium difficile*, have been reported in the elderly (Studemeister et al., 1987).

Helton et al. (1986) reported a series of eight patients with fungal splenic abscesses, and identified several etiological factors, including cytotoxic chemotherapy, long-term corticosteroid administration, neutropenia, treatment with antibiotics for more than 3 weeks, and gastrointestinal colonization with *Candida albicans*. Five patients were treated with splenectomy and antifungal drugs, and three patients received antifungal drugs alone. 7/8 were cured of their splenic abscesses, and five were long-term survivors. Three similar series in pediatric patients with leukemia have shown that treatment of multiple splenic abscesses can be successfully undertaken by splenectomy with antifungal drugs (Marmon et al., 1990; Wald et al., 1981; Hatley et al., 1989). This disorder may come to be recognized with increasing frequency, and should be considered in any patient at risk, who develops fever, tenderness over the left upper quadrant, and a nontoxic appearance. CT and ultrasound can be used as a guide to the diagnosis.

Therapeutic options include splenectomy, splenotomy, and percutaneous drainage, in addition to antibiotic therapy. The treatment of choice is splenectomy and intravenous antibiotic therapy directed at the causative organism. In the past, splenotomy (incision and drainage of the splenic parenchyma) was used as an alternative to splenectomy. This more limited procedure may still be useful in patients in whom intense inflammatory reaction in the left upper quadrant renders splenectomy difficult. Because over 70% of splenic abscesses are solitary (the majority unilocular), percutaneous drainage is a logical therapeutic alternative to splenotomy and drainage in such cases, and may be considered first-line therapy in conjunction with antibiotics, in selected patients (Lerner and Spataro, 1984; Hadas-Halpren et al., 1992; Schwerk et al., 1994; Ooi and Leung, 1997). Splenectomy may be performed, if percutaneous drainage fails, or if multiple abscesses are present. The overall mortality rate has decreased from over 60 to 10%, and most deaths are related to the underlying cause of the sepsis.

17.3.4. SPLENIC ARTERY ANEURYSM

With the solitary exception of the aorta, the splenic artery is the most common site of intra-abdominal aneurysmal disease. During the childbearing years, approximately twice as many women as men present with splenic artery aneurysms. In middle age and beyond, the incidence in men equals that in women. Etiological factors include atherosclerosis and congenital defects in the arterial internal elastic lamina. Trauma, pancreatitis, and arteritis can cause splenic artery aneurysms, and mycotic aneurysms of the splenic artery occur.

Although most splenic artery aneurysms are small (1.5–3.5 cm in diameter), occasionally, aneurysms measuring up to 15 cm in diameter have been recorded. Many aneurysms are asymptomatic, and are identified when the characteristic calcification is noted in an abdominal film. However, a significant number present with intraperitoneal rupture or rupture into the gastrointestinal tract. In a series of 23 pediatric-age patients with aneurysms, two patients with splenic artery aneurysms were identified (Sarkar et al., 1991).

Asymptomatic, nonpregnant patients may be observed, if the aneurysm is small (<1 cm, if noncalcified; or <3 cm, if calcified), or if the risk of operation is high because of severe systemic disease. Symptomatic aneurysms of any size, any aneurysm identified in a pregnant woman, or those pseudoaneurysms caused by pancreatitis or pancreatic pseudocysts should be treated. The preferred management is surgical, with exposure of the aneurysm in the lesser sac, and total excision. Depending on the location of the aneurysm, ligation of the splenic artery, vascular reconstruction, or splenectomy may be required (Trastek et al., 1982; Chakfe et al., 1993). Laparoscopic ligation has been performed: this procedure is easiest with a markedly tortuous splenic artery, in which the aneurysm protrudes into the lesser sac from the normal position behind the pancreas (Hashizume et al., 1993). Recurrence has been reported after ligation and partial aneurysmectomy (Sasada et al., 1995). Endovascular techniques have been employed with good success, but it is essential that a postprocedure study be performed to confirm total obliteration of the aneurysm (Tarazov et al., 1991; McDermott et al., 1994).

17.3.5. SPLENIC VEIN THROMBOSIS Because splenic vein thrombosis causes elevated pressure in the veins of the left upper quadrant, and results in gastric and esophageal varices, most patients with this condition present with gastrointestinal bleeding (Røder, 1984). This potentially curable cause of variceal bleeding is easily excluded by an abdominal ultrasound with Doppler examination of the splenic vein. The thrombosis is generally secondary to pancreatitis, trauma, infection, or a pancreatic pseudocyst (Nishiyama et al., 1986; Hofer et al., 1987). Splenectomy is the treatment of choice. Splenic artery ligation without splenectomy is not recommended, because continued gastrointestinal hemorrhage may occur (Glynn, 1986).

17.3.6. SPLENIC INFARCTION Splenic infarction occurs in several situations: typical autoinfarction of the spleen is associated with sickle cell disease, systemic embolization, and as a surgical complication of partial splenic embolization and splenic artery ligation, performed in an attempt to preserve splenic function. Autoinfarction of the spleen occurs with the progression of sickle cell anemia, and does not require treatment, unless secondary bacterial infection causes abscess formation (*see* Chapter 11). Acute splenic infarction has been reported in association with systemic thromboembolism. The presentation is nonspecific, with fever, left upper quadrant pain, and tachycardia. In a review of 96 cases of thromboembolic splenic infarction, O'Keefe et al. (1986) reported that, although 44% of splenic infarcts had caused significant additional morbidity, only 10% had been suspected clinically. Atheromatous debris from the aorta, mural thrombus from the left ventricle, and vegetations on infected valves in bacterial endocarditis were the three most common sources. The diagnosis may be confirmed by CT scan. Finally, splenic infarction may occur as a complication of partial splenic embolization or splenic artery ligation, which are discussed in subsequent subheadings.

Management of pain, and treatment of the underlying cause, if systemic embolization is suspected, comprise the initial therapeutic approach. If secondary bacterial infection occurs, or signs of sepsis develop, splenectomy may be required.

17.3.7. WANDERING SPLEEN Wandering spleen, or splenoptosis, is an unusual entity that is seen most commonly in childhood and in women of reproductive age (Buehner and Baker, 1992). It most often stems from congenital abnormalities in the dorsal mesogastrium, allowing for excessive splenic mobility. Many are undoubtedly asymptomatic, but some come to surgical attention because of acute or chronic torsion. The sequelae of torsion range from pain and an abdominal mass, to splenic infarction, to left-sided portal hypertension (related to splenic vein thrombosis) (Schmidt et al., 1992; Greig et al., 1994; Melikoglu et al., 1995). Diagnosis can be difficult, but ultrasound, computed tomography, or nuclear scanning may demonstrate the abnormal position of the spleen.

Surgical therapy depends on the status of the spleen at the time of operation. The customary approach of splenectomy is now reserved only for those patients in whom splenic infarction makes salvage impractical. Particularly in children, the need to preserve

functioning splenic tissue has led to advocacy for splenopexy as treatment for wandering spleen (Stringel et al., 1982; Allen and Andrews, 1989). Numerous technical approaches have been employed, including direct suture of the splenic capsule to the subdiaphragmatic region, placement of the spleen in an extraperitoneal pouch (Seashore and McIntosh, 1990), or wrapping the spleen in an absorbable mesh and suturing the mesh to the diaphragm and lateral abdominal wall (Schmidt et al., 1992).

17.3.8. PATHOLOGIC RUPTURE OF THE SPLEEN Rupture of the spleen after minor trauma, is usually called "spontaneous or pathological rupture." Most cases of pathological rupture have occurred in malaria, typhoid fever, infectious mononucleosis, pregnancy, or in patients with splenomegaly caused by hematologic malignancies or coagulation abnormalities (Gordon et al., 1995; Berne et al., 1997). Rapid enlargement of the spleen, and infiltration of the splenic capsule with abnormal cells (as in acute myelogenous leukemia), may predispose to rupture. The inciting trauma may have been so slight as to have been forgotten. There is frequently a delayed presentation, characterized by diffuse or localized abdominal pain, left shoulder pain, and fatigue. Tachycardia, hypotension, and tachypnea may be present, but a significant proportion of patients present with normal vital signs. The diagnosis may be confirmed by ultrasound, CT scan, or diagnostic paracentesis. Prompt recognition of the problem, splenectomy when necessary, and nonoperative management, in selected cases, are crucial for success (Gordon et al., 1995).

17.3.9. ABDOMINAL TRAUMA Although the spleen lies in a protected position, high in the left upper quadrant and sheltered by the costal structures, it is frequently injured by both blunt and penetrating abdominal trauma.

Blunt trauma may cause a variety of injuries, including transverse fracture along an intersegmental plane (especially in children), stellate laceration, avulsion injuries from traction on the upper or lower pole, and subcapsular hematomas. Sometimes, bleeding is initially slight, and there is a variable latent period, before the signs and symptoms of splenic rupture are clinically evident. This has given rise to the term "delayed rupture." This is a misnomer, because the rupture occurs at the time of the initial injury, and is simply delayed in its presentation. It has been speculated that more occurences of this will occur with current trends toward splenic conservation (Deva and Thompson, 1996).

In contrast to the earlier belief that all splenic injuries require splenectomy, many patients with isolated splenic injury are now treated nonoperatively (Rutledge, 1996). When surgery is performed, the current preferred management of many injuries is to use one or more of several techniques of splenorrhaphy, or splenic repair (Seufert and Mitrou, 1985; Kidd et al., 1987), including suture of capsular lacerations, application of topical hemostatic agents, partial splenectomy, or wrapping the spleen with absorbable mesh. The commonly used techniques are described in Subheading 4.3.2. Most require extensive mobilization of the spleen and meticulous, time-consuming control of bleeding. For patients who are hemodynamically unstable, or for those with extensive injuries elsewhere, splenectomy is still the procedure of choice, since it can be accomplished more rapidly, and frequently with less blood loss, than splenic salvage (Mucha et al., 1986). Similarly, nonoperative management and splenorrhaphy are rarely good choices for patients with massive splenomegaly, hematologic malignancies, or portal hypertension (Gordon et al., 1995; Berne et al., 1997).

Nonoperative management of blunt abdominal trauma, despite suspected splenic injury, was introduced after the chance postmortem observation of a child who had died in a motor vehicle accident, and in whom splenic injury had been suspected in the past (Douglas and Simpson, 1971). A well-healed, completely transected spleen was found, providing the first evidence that significant splenic injuries can heal spontaneously.

One advantage of the nonoperative approach includes the avoidance of laparotomy, in which there is the possibility of further injury to the spleen during splenic mobilization, and which could preclude splenic salvage. Against this must be set the potential disadvantages of possibly increased transfusion requirements, conversion of a simple laceration (which might easily be repaired at laparotomy) to a complex subcapsular hematoma, which would necessitate splenectomy, and the possibility of overlooking injury to other organs, such as bowel and kidney. The nonoperative approach to blunt abdominal trauma has gradually been formalized, and is now the standard management of suspected splenic injuries in children. It is estimated from combined series that only 10% of children who are observed under a careful protocol will require laparotomy, and that splenic salvage will still be possible in 25% of those requiring surgical exploration (Luna and Dellinger, 1987; Pranikoff et al., 1994).

There was initial hesitation about extending these results to the adult, in whom stellate lacerations, complex fractures, and fragmentation of the splenic parenchyma are more common, and which stand in contrast to the pattern of transverse fractures along intrasegmental planes seen in children. The importance of strict adherence to a protocol was emphasized by Mucha et al. (1986), who listed three selection criteria: hemodynamic stability, absence of peritoneal signs, and a maximum transfusion requirement of two units of blood for the splenic injury. They also emphasized the importance of using modern imaging techniques (double-contrast CT scan) to exclude other intra-abdominal injuries. From this and several other combined series, it appears that nonoperative management may be successful in as many as 60% of carefully selected patients with isolated splenic injuries (Mucha et al., 1986; Kidd et al., 1987; Splenic Injury Study Group, 1987).

Sequential series from single institutions clearly document a trend away from splenectomy, initially to splenorrhaphy, and increasingly to nonoperative management (Morrell et al., 1995; Smith et al., 1996). In a 10-year retrospective review, Jalovec et al. (1993) stated that, in the last year of the study, 65% of bluntly injured spleens were salvaged (35% by splenorrhaphy and 30% by nonoperative management). Wasvary et al. (1997), managed 55% of their patients with blunt splenic injury nonoperatively, with a >90% success rate. No adverse outcomes have been identified as a result of these trends (Morrell et al., 1995; Coburn et al., 1995).

Which patients with blunt splenic injury are suitable candidates for nonoperative management? Neither ISS scores nor CT grading systems have proven to be accurate predictors (Godley et al., 1996; Umlas and Cronan, 1991; Savoiz et al., 1997). In one detailed study of the value of CT, 56 patients, with documented blunt splenic injury on CT, were analyzed as to outcome (Umlas and Cronan, 1991). 40 patients were managed nonoperatively, with three failures. Two of these three had CT grades that predicted success of nonoperative management; of the 16 patients who went to surgery, 50% had significant discrepancies between CT grade and/or interpretation and operative findings. Success is less likely in older patients undergoing observation, even when CT scan and ISS

scores are similar (Godley et al., 1996). Velanovich (1995) performed decision analysis based on 56 published studies, and concluded that only patients with minor splenic injuries, not requiring transfusion, should be managed nonoperatively. Patients with bleeding sufficient to require transfusion should undergo early exploration, with attempted splenic salvage by splenorrhaphy.

In contrast to the trend toward nonoperative management, Witte et al. (1992) advocate an early operative strategy, utilizing intraoperative autotransfusion to minimize the use of blood transfusions, stating that the spleen, or a large remnant, can usually be salvaged, and blood requirements minimized. Transfusion requirements are consistently highest for splenectomy, intermediate for splenorrhaphy, and least for nonoperative splenic injury (Jalovec et al., 1993; Rutledge 1996), but these numbers must be interpreted in light of the fact that only those with the most severe injuries (or cases in which there are other significant injuries) currently undergo splenectomy. Transfusion significantly increased the risk of infection, respiratory complications, and admission to surgical intensive care, after splenic injury, in a retrospective review by Duke et al. (1993).

Penetrating abdominal trauma requires celiotomy, and the decision whether or not to attempt splenorrhaphy is made on the basis of hemodynamic stability, integrity of hilar vessels, and the severity of associated injuries. In a series of 69 patients with splenic injuries caused by penetrating trauma, Ivatury et al. (1993) achieved an overall 54.5% salvage rate. They stressed the utility of absorbable mesh in the more-severe injuries, and felt that splenorrhaphy should be possible in the great majority of patients with penetrating trauma. Injuries to adjacent organs, such as stomach, pancreas, duodenum, colon, diaphragm, and lung, are common, and must be carefully sought and treated.

Polyvalent pneumococcal vaccine and the selective use of antibiotic prophylaxis are recommended in patients who undergo splenectomy for trauma. Patients in whom nonoperative management or splenorrhaphy has been utilized should avoid strenuous physical activity and contact sports for at least 3 months. They should have follow-up splenic imaging by CT or radioisotope scan 1–2 months after injury (Mucha et al., 1986). Ultrasound may also be efficacious for follow-up studies, particularly in children.

Posttraumatic cysts and splenic abscesses have been reported, following the nonoperative management of splenic injuries, and may require surgical excision, drainage, or splenectomy (Sands et al., 1986).

17.4. SPECIFIC SURGICAL CONSIDERATIONS

In this subheading, techniques of open splenectomy and splenorrhaphy are discussed. Laparoscopic splenectomy is then described. Splenic surgery for trauma is discussed in Subheading 4.3., including a discussion of splenic conservation techniques (including laparoscopic implementation). These techniques are applicable in both trauma and in elective situations, when preservation of some splenic function is desired.

17.4.1. SPLENECTOMY The technique of elective splenectomy performed during formal laparotomy ("open") is described first.

17.4.1.1. Choice of Incision A variety of incisions have been employed for splenic surgery. When the spleen is of normal size, a left subcostal incision provides the best access (Fig. 3A). Extension of the incision vertically, in the midline, may be used to provide additional exposure. As the spleen enlarges, it descends and the hilum is displaced medially. For massively enlarged spleens,

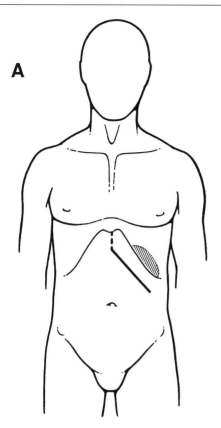
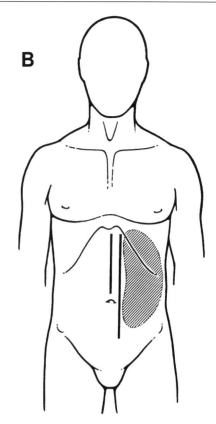

Fig. 17.3. (**A**) When the spleen is normal in size, a left subcostal incision provides good exposure for splenic surgery. The incision may be extended upward in the midline, as indicated by the dotted line. This incision transects the abdominal muscles; persistent oozing, or the development of a wound hematoma, may occur in profoundly thrombocytopenic patients. For this reason, many surgeons prefer a midline or paramedian incision for those cases. (**B**) As the spleen enlarges, it descends, and the hilar structures are displaced medially. A vertical midline or left paramedian incision gives good exposure and access to the hilum. These incisions may be preferred in profoundly thrombocytopenic patients, even when the spleen is small, because no muscle is transected.

a midline or left paramedian incision (Fig. 3B) then provides better exposure. In children, a left subcostal incision, made lateral to the rectus muscle, which is retracted rather than divided, may be used.

In the profoundly thrombocytopenic patient, it may be preferable not to divide the rectus muscle, and, in this situation, a midline or paramedian incision may also be preferred. Splenic surgery for trauma is best performed through a vertical midline incision, which gives excellent access to all quadrants of the abdomen.

17.4.1.2. Preliminary Control of Splenic Artery When difficulty in dissection is anticipated, ligation of the splenic artery in the lesser sac should be performed before the spleen is mobilized (Fig. 4). This allows control of the major blood supply to the spleen, and the effective transfusion of platelets systemically, if necessary, in profoundly thrombocytopenic patients.

Preoperative transcatheter embolization of the splenic artery is sometimes used as a means of decreasing hemorrhage during elective splenectomy, and may be useful in patients who present high operative risks. Successful preoperative splenic infarction may decrease splenic volume, increase the platelet count, and decrease intraoperative bleeding. In most patients, however, this is not necessary, and there is at least one study showing no decrease in blood loss (Hoefer et al., 1991). Total infarction of the spleen by transcatheter embolization has mostly been abandoned as an alternative

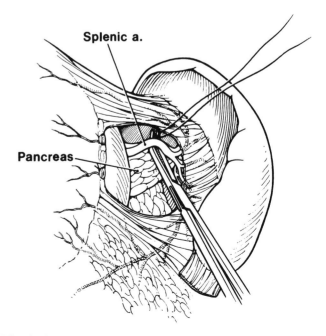

Fig. 17.4. An opening is made in the lesser sac, and the splenic artery encircled with a tape or ligature.

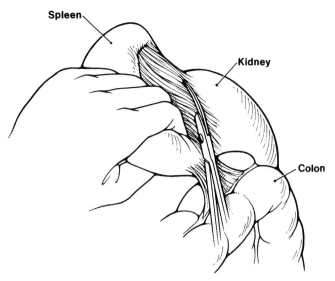

Fig. 17.5. In the initial stage of splenectomy, the spleen is mobilized by incising the lateral peritoneal attachments to abdominal wall, diaphragm, and left kidney.

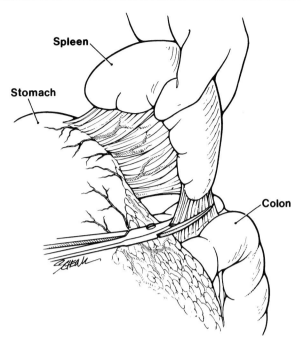

Fig. 17.6. The splenocolic ligament is divided.

to splenectomy, because of its high complication rate (Back et al., 1987; Farid and O'Connell, 1996); however, partial splenic embolization shows promise as a technique of partial splenic ablation, and is discussed in detail later.

17.4.1.3. Technique of Open Splenectomy The patient is positioned supine on the operating table. Additional exposure may be obtained by placing a small roll under the left costal margin. The use of a framework, which can anchor an "upper-hand"-type of retractor, may also facilitate exposure.

During the initial incision and subsequent steps, care is taken to effect meticulous hemostasis, because patients who undergo elective splenic surgery frequently have coagulation or immunological defects that may predispose to hematoma formation, or in whom poor wound healing can be anticipated. Placement of a nasogastric tube, unless contraindicated by extreme thrombocytopenia, facilitates operative exposure, by decompressing the stomach.

The surgeon's hand is passed carefully up over the spleen, to assess the size, consistency, and mobility of the organ. A thorough intra-abdominal exploration is performed. In patients with hemolytic anemia, the gallbladder is carefully palpated. Accessory spleens are best sought at the beginning of the dissection, before blood stains the operative field, and again after mobilization of the spleen and the tail of pancreas.

Preliminary ligation of the splenic artery may be performed by exposing the splenic artery in the lesser sac (Fig. 4).

The spleen is mobilized by incising the lateral peritoneal attachments (Fig. 5). The surgeon's left hand pulls the spleen medially and upwards. The dissection is performed in a plane deep to the tail of the pancreas and splenic vessels, which are mobilized gently out of the retroperitoneum. Further mobilization is limited by the gastrosplenic and splenocolic ligaments. The splenocolic ligament is generally avascular, occasionally a few small vessels may require ligature (Fig. 6). The lower pole of the spleen is further freed by division of several branches of the gastroepiploic vessels (Fig. 7).

The upper pole of the spleen is mobilized by dividing several short gastric vessels, which are carefully ligated (Fig. 8). Care must be taken not to include a small portion of the wall of the

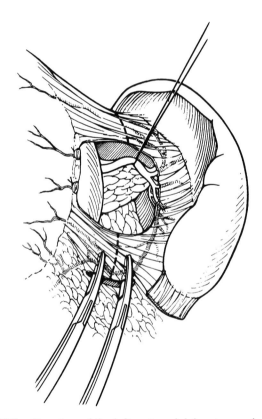

Fig. 17.7. Branches of the left gastroepiploic artery and vein are serially clamped and tied.

stomach in the ligature, which may otherwise induce necrosis and gastric fistula formation.

The spleen is now attached only by the hilum and tail of the pancreas. The dissection of the splenic artery and vein should be performed with care, to avoid damage to the tail of the pancreas,

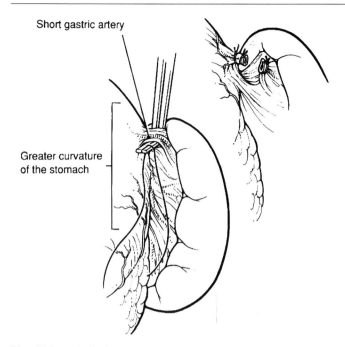

Short gastric artery

Greater curvature
of the stomach

Fig. 17.8. Similarly, the short gastric vessels, which connect the stomach to the spleen, are ligated and divided. Care must be taken not to incorporate the gastric wall in the tie. This can result in necrosis of a small portion of the greater curvature, with delayed perforation, gastric fistula, or subphrenic abscess formation. (Reproduced with permission from Scott-Conner and Dawson, 1993.)

which extends for a variable distance into the hilum of the spleen. In many cases, serial ligation of several branches of the splenic artery and vein is preferable to ligation of the main arterial and venous trunk, because of the proximity to the pancreas. This dissection is most conveniently performed from the underside of the spleen, accessible now because of careful mobilization of spleen and pancreas (Fig. 9). The artery should be ligated before the vein, to avoid sequestration of a significant volume of blood within the spleen.

Ligation of the splenic vein at the juncture with the inferior mesenteric vein (Fig. 10) has been recommended as a means of decreasing the probability of portal vein thrombosis after splenectomy, and may be advisable when massive splenomegaly, with a correspondingly large splenic vein, is encountered.

17.4.1.4. Avoidance and Management of Hemorrhage Blood loss correlates with spleen size. Some surgeons use preliminary control of the splenic artery in the lesser sac (Fig. 4). Preoperative embolization of the splenic artery is an alternative, but is rarely necessary. If the spleen is torn during mobilization or dissection, it is best to control bleeding by direct pressure and continue mobilization. An atraumatic vascular clamp can be placed across the hilar vessels, if necessary, for temporary control while dissection progresses. The major vascular trunks should be suture ligated; a double-clamp technique may be advisable. Occasionally, the splenic vein is so large that oversewing the stump with a running vascular suture is safer than simple ligature or suture ligature.

The short gastric vessels can be the source of troublesome bleeding, which is more easily controlled after the spleen has been removed. If there is any question that a ligature or suture ligature may have encroached on part of the wall of the stomach, the area in question should be imbricated with interrupted Lembert sutures, to avoid the development of a gastric fistula.

The splenic bed is carefully checked for hemostasis. Bleeding from raw peritoneal and diaphragmatic surfaces may be controlled by packing, topical hemostatic agents, or by reperitonealizing the raw area with a running suture. If there is any question of the adequacy of hemostasis, or injury to the tail of the pancreas, a drain should be placed. Closed-suction drains are preferred.

17.4.1.5. The Search for Accessory Spleens When accessory spleens are carefully sought at autopsy, they are found in about 10% of the general population. The most common location is within the splenic hilum, along the course of the splenic artery, or within the tail of the pancreas. Other common locations include the omentum, the gastrosplenic and splenocolic ligaments, and the mesentery of the small bowel (Fig. 1). Occasionally, an accessory spleen is found in a presacral, pelvic, or paratesticular location. The accessory spleen is generally involved in the same pathological process as the primary spleen (Skandelakis et al., 1993).

When total splenectomy is performed for disorders such as hereditary spherocytosis, hereditary elliptocytosis, or idiopathic thrombocytopenic purpura, a careful search should be made, and any accessory spleens present should also be removed. After splenectomy, an accessory spleen may enlarge and cause a recurrence of the condition for which the original surgery was performed (Seufert and Mitrou, 1985). Howell-Jolly bodies normally appear within the erythrocytes after splenectomy; when these are absent, an accessory spleen should be suspected. The combination of CT scan and radionuclide scan provides satisfactory diagnostic accuracy in identifying the location of most accessory spleens. The treatment of choice is surgical removal, which has been performed laparoscopically.

17.4.1.6. Laparoscopic Splenectomy Laparoscopic splenectomy is considered an "advanced laparoscopic procedure" that should only be performed by suitably experienced surgeons (Hunter, 1997). Although operative time is frequently greater than for the comparable open procedure, a shorter postoperative stay, decreased pain, and more rapid return to usual activities make this an attractive modality. In a case-control study, Diaz et al. (1997) showed that laparoscopic splenectomy was associated with an increased operative time and cost, but decreased length of stay and decreased complication rate, compared with open splenectomy. Others have shown comparable blood loss (Brunt et al., 1996; Glasgow et al., 1997) and similar complication rates. One potential limitation with laparoscopic splenectomy, particularly germane to treatment of cytopenia by planned total splenectomy, is the variable success in locating accessory splenic tissue. In a prospective multicenter trial (Gigot et al., 1995), there was a 20% recurrence rate at 8.2 months when laparoscopic splenectomy was performed for immune thrombocytopenia.

Laparoscopic splenectomy was initially performed with the patient supine, in a manner analogous to laparoscopic cholecystectomy (Cuschieri et al., 1992). Many surgeons continue to use this approach. When cholecystectomy is planned at the time of laparoscopic splenectomy, the supine position gives excellent access to both sides of the abdomen (Trias et al., 1994; Katkhouda et al., 1996). The lateral approach described here is an alternate method that is emerging as easier under most circumstances (Trias et al., 1994; Kollias et al., 1995; Delaitre, 1995; Rege et al., 1996; Dexter et al., 1996; Park et al., 1997). The technique is felt to be both safe and effective (Liew and Storey, 1995).

The patient is positioned in the right lateral decubitus position. Trocar placement varies with surgeon preference, spleen size, and

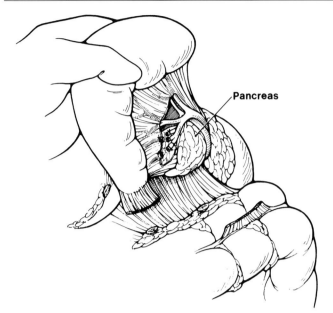

Fig. 17.9. Careful dissection and ligation of the splenic vessels in the hilum, with identification and preservation of the tail of the pancreas, is often easier from the underside. Adequte mobilization of the spleen and tail of pancreas facilitates this maneuver.

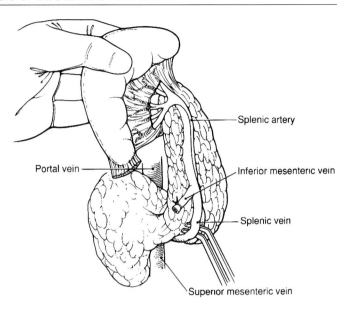

Fig. 17.10. Ligation of the splenic vein close to the confluence of the splenic vein with the superior mesenteric vein and portal vein, can decrease the possibility of thrombus forming within the splenic remnant, propagation of clot, and mesenteric venous thrombosis. (Reproduced with permission from Scott-Conner and Dawson, 1993.)

patient habitus. Generally, four trocars are used (Fig. 11). A 30-degree angled laparoscope gives the best view of the splenic hilum.

In both methods (i.e., the supine position and lateral approach), the dissection progresses from below upward. The attachments of splenic flexure of colon to spleen are first taken down (Fig. 12). After mobilization of the splenic flexure, an additional 5-mm trocar may be placed in a flank position.

The lateral peritoneal attachments are divided, creating a peritoneal cuff, which can be grasped for retraction. Many surgeons leave the spleen attached to the diaphragm, producing a "hanged spleen" configuration that facilitates subsequent exposure. The hilar vessels are divided from below, either with ligatures (Fig. 13) or an endoscopic linear stapling device with a vascular cartridge (Saldinger et al., 1996; Rhodes et al., 1995). The short gastric vessels are divided next, with clips or ligatures. The spleen is placed into a bag (Fig. 14), and may be morcellated and extracted in pieces through a small incision (often placed in the pubic hairline) (Park et al., 1997).

Laparoscopic splenectomy was initially performed for patients with small spleens. The technique has been extended and used in patients with massive splenomegaly. Balloon occlusion of the splenic artery (Yamashita et al., 1996) and preoperative embolization (Poulin and Thibault, 1995) have been used to decrease blood loss in these cases. One surgeon reported that preoperative embolization created perisplenic inflammation, rendering the dissection more difficult (Park et al., 1997).

Laparoscopic partial splenectomy, using the linear stapling device (Uranus et al., 1995), splenorrhaphy, and resection of accessory spleens (Mercan et al., 1996; Diaz et al., 1996), have all been reported.

17.4.1.7. Decision to Drain or Not to Drain the Splenic Bed

Routine drainage of the splenic bed has mostly been abandoned, because of several studies demonstrating an increase in postoperative complications, particularly subphrenic abscess formation,

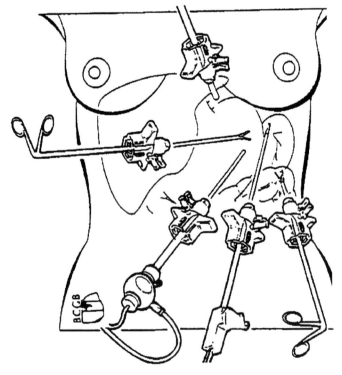

Fig. 17.11. Trocar placement for laparoscopic splenectomy with patient in lithotomy position. (Reproduced with permission from Scott-Conner, 1998.)

when older, passive drainage devices (such as Penrose drains) were left in for prolonged periods of time. A recent study of the results of routine closed-suction drainage, in 282 patients undergoing splenectomy, reported a subphrenic abscess rate of only 0.71% (Ugochukwu and Irving, 1985). In that study, drains were removed

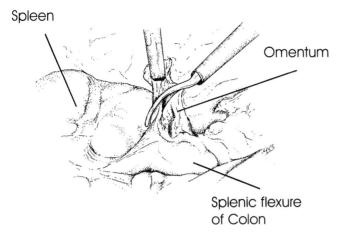

Spleen

Omentum

Splenic flexure
of Colon

Fig. 17.12. Initial division of splenocolic ligament. Dissection progresses from below upward.

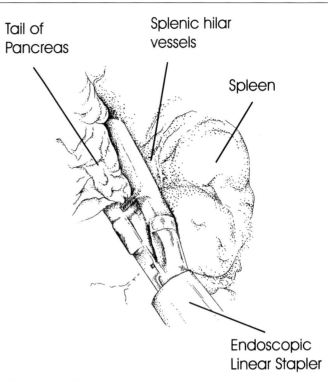

Tail of
Pancreas

Splenic hilar
vessels

Spleen

Endoscopic
Linear Stapler

Fig. 17.13. Control of splenic hilar vessels is done by ligature or endoscopic stapling device.

between the third and fifth postoperative day. Many surgeons utilize selective drainage, employing closed-suction drains, when there are associated injuries in the setting of abdominal trauma, or if there is a possibility of incomplete hemostasis, or of injury to the tail of the pancreas. The role of drains in prevention of subphrenic abscess remains controversial (Irving, 1997).

17.4.2. SPECIAL CONDITIONS AND THEIR EFFECT ON SURGERY

17.4.2.1. Massive Splenomegaly   As the spleen enlarges, the hilum is displaced medially, and the spleen moves inferiorly. In some ways, this facilitates dissection, but adhesions between the spleen and the diaphragm may be more vascular and troublesome. In one series of 49 patients who underwent removal of massively enlarged spleens, perisplenitis with dense adhesions was encountered in more than half (Wobbes et al., 1984). Although the mortality rate was not increased in those patients with massive splenomegaly, the complication rate (principally hemorrhage) was twice that of patients with smaller spleens.

17.4.2.2. Surgery in the Elderly   Deckings and Printen (1977) reviewed a 10-year experience of elective splenectomy in patients over the age of 55 years. During the study period, 55 such patients, comprising 27% of all elective splenectomies, underwent elective splenectomy, with five deaths. The complication rate was similar to that reported in larger series spanning all age groups. The response to splenectomy was comparable to that reported for younger patients with similar preoperative diagnoses. Conservative management of blunt splenic trauma has been less successful in patients over age 55, as previously discussed.

17.4.3. OPERATIVE STRATEGY IN SPLENIC TRAUMA   The nonoperative approach is being used with increasing frequency, as previously described (Subheading 3.9.). This subheading details the specific techniques and strategies used when operative management is to be followed.

17.4.3.1. Laparotomy for Splenic Trauma   Laparotomy for trauma is performed through a long midline incision, which provides excellent access to all quadrants of the abdomen. A rapid and thorough abdominal assessment is performed. The presence of blood and clots within the left upper quadrant confirms the probability of splenic injury. All blood and clots should be evacuated and the abdomen packed in quadrants. Any continuing hemorrhage is dealt with first. If the patient's condition is stable and splenic salvage is to be attempted, the spleen is first carefully mobilized as

described previously. This mobilization must be performed with extreme care to avoid further injury which might preclude successful splenorrhaphy. Occasionally, an isolated capsular avulsion injury of the lower pole of the spleen can be treated without full mobilization of the spleen. The decision to perform splenectomy, rather than splenorrhaphy is based upon the hemodynamic stability of the patient, the severity of associated injuries, the age of the patient, and the severity of the splenic injury. If no blood or hematoma are found in the left upper quadrant, the spleen should not be mobilized, to avoid iatrogenic injury. Splenectomy for trauma is performed in a fashion similar to that described for elective splenectomy. Preliminary ligation of the splenic artery is generally not performed.

17.4.3.2. Splenic Conservation Techniques   Careful, atraumatic mobilization of the spleen is performed. Division of the short gastric vessels and the splenocolic ligament may be required for adequate exposure. Temporary control of the splenic hilum by application of an atraumatic vascular clamp may be used to diminish blood loss while repair is being performed. In dogs, a warm ischemia time of 2 hours was well-tolerated, leading Teperman et al. (1994) to suggest that 1 h should be tolerated in humans, allowing "bloodless" splenic surgery. In practice, this is rarely required.

Minor capsular avulsion injuries may be managed by the application of topical hemostatic agents and pressure.

A simple capsular tear or laceration may be debrided and sutured with interrupted sutures (Fig. 15A,B). Pledgets may be required, to avoid the problem of sutures tearing through the delicate splenic capsule (Fig. 15C). Viable omentum, with an intact vascular pedicle, may be used to buttress the repair (Fig. 15D). Many surgeons prefer the use of a fine monofilament suture on a vascular needle, for these repairs, to avoid injury from a large needle. Others prefer the use of chromic catgut on a gastrointestinal needle, which is less likely to cut through the delicate capsule. Aidonopoulos et al. (1995) prefer 0-chromic on a liver needle, and

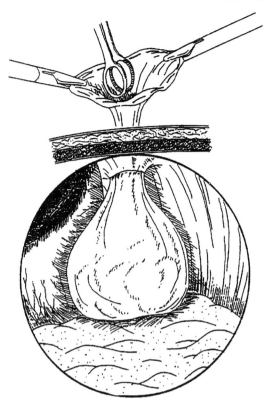

Fig. 17.14.   The spleen is placed in a bag, morcellated, and removed through a trocar site or small incision in the pubic hair line. (Reproduced with permission from Scott-Conner, 1998.)

use large figure-of-eight sutures over pledgets of oxidized cellulose. This approach was successful in 23 patients with lacerations and two patients who underwent partial splenectomy. Whichever suture and needle are chosen, care should be taken to avoid lacerating the capsule as the sutures are placed and tied. The argon beam coagulator can also be used to facilitate capsular hemostasis (Dunham et al., 1991).

When a stellate laceration of one pole of the spleen, or damage to one of the hilar vessels, has occurred, partial splenectomy may be necessary (Fig. 16A). This operation is based on the segmental anatomy of the spleen, which varies from individual to individual, but generally results in avascular planes between segments (Sow et al., 1991; Skandalakis et al., 1993; Farag et al., 1994; Liu et al., 1996). The segmental artery and vein supplying the involved pole are ligated, and the spleen is allowed to demarcate (Fig. 16B). The segment will become dusky, and a line of demarcation will develop. The capsule is divided and the splenic parenchyma opened, by a finger fracture technique. Occasional small vessels will be encountered, and should be ligated or clipped with fine hemostatic clips. Hemostasis is again checked, and the capsule is sutured, to provide some additional compression and hemostasis (Fig. 16C). Omentum may be used to wrap the splenic remnant. Partial splenectomy with a linear stapling device has been described (Uranus et al., 1994). The argon-beam coagulator has been used to attain hemostasis in difficult splenorrhaphies (Dunham et al., 1991; Dowling et al., 1991). Laparoscopic splenorrhaphy, using fibrin glue (Tricarico et al., 1994), and laparoscopic partial splenectomy (after preoperative segmental embolization) have been described, but are not yet routine (Poulin and Mamazza, 1995).

A badly damaged spleen with intact hilar vessels may be salvaged by wrapping it with absorbable synthetic mesh (Fig. 17). The mesh may be applied with several concentric pursestring sutures placed at the splenic hilum. Alternatively, a hole may be cut for the hilum, and the spleen wrapped and the mesh sutured around the front and toward the diaphragmatic surface of the spleen. It is critical that the mesh be sutured in such a manner as to apply firm but gentle compression of the splenic parenchyma, without encroaching on the vascular supply (Rogers et al., 1991; Fingerhut et al., 1992). Mesh splenorrhaphy has been performed laparoscopically (Koehler et al., 1994).

Splenic artery ligation is occasionally performed, to control hemorrhage and allow splenic salvage. Schwalke et al. (1991) studied 20 patients who had undergone splenic artery ligation for blunt trauma, and found that clearance of opsonized red blood cells was no different from the value found in normal volunteers. Partial splenectomy, leaving a substantial remnant nourished by the short gastric vessels alone, has also been described (Farag et al., 1994). Recent experimental work, demonstrating the importance of an intact splenic artery in bacterial clearance by the spleen, raises the possibility that the spleen, even if viable, may no longer be an efficient bacterial filter after splenic artery ligation (Scher et al., 1985; Saxe et al., 1994).

17.5. ALTERNATIVES TO TOTAL SPLENECTOMY

Total splenectomy remains the treatment of choice for patients with hemolytic anemias (with the possible exception of β-thalassemia major, in which partial splenectomy may be preferred), immune thrombocytopenias, and severely injured patients who are hemodynamically unstable and have sustained significant splenic injury. In patients undergoing elective splenectomy for hematological disorders, accessory spleens should be carefully sought and removed, to avoid recurrent symptoms. In contrast, when splenectomy is required because of trauma, accessory spleens are preserved, with the intent that they may provide some protection against the sequelae of hyposplenism (*see also* Chapter 10).

The principal alternatives to total splenectomy are splenic biopsy (which may be performed under laparoscopic guidance), partial splenectomy, and partial splenic embolization. Techniques of splenic preservation during trauma surgery are discussed in Subheadings 3.9. and 4.1.

17.5.1. SPLENIC BIOPSY   Laparoscopic biopsy has been used mainly to determine splenic involvement in Hodgkin's disease; it has been shown to be a safe technique. However, because of the nonuniform involvement of the spleen, it is generally not regarded as a satisfactory alternative to full staging laparotomy with splenectomy.

17.5.2. PARTIAL SPLENECTOMY   Partial splenectomy is being used in an increasing number of situations, to preserve some splenic function. The technique of elective partial splenectomy is essentially the same as that described for trauma (Fig. 16). When partial splenectomy is performed for Gaucher's disease, myeloid metaplasia, schistosomiasis, or for some similar indication, the resection is generally planned so that the remaining splenic remnant is about the size of a normal spleen. This generally means ligating several segmental vessels, and carefully preserving the final segment. In contrast, partial splenectomy for a cyst or benign tumor is planned according to the location of the lesion. In all other respects, the partial resection is performed in the same manner as that performed for trauma.

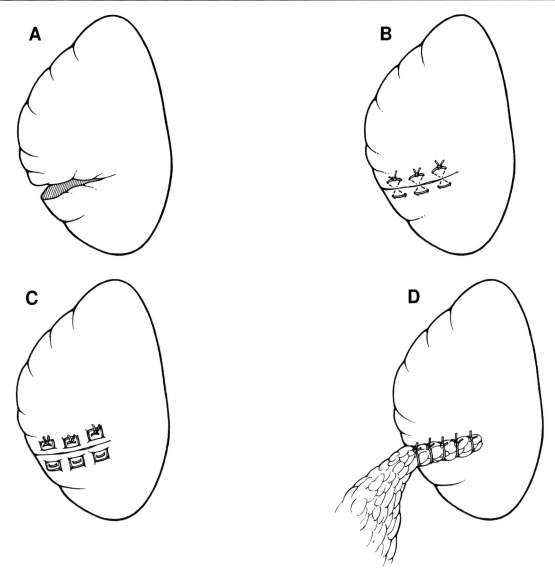

Fig. 17.15. (**A**) A laceration of the spleen, which may be managed by simple repair. (**B**) The laceration may be closed with interrupted sutures placed through the capsule. (**C**) Pledgets may be necessary, to avoid the tendency of sutures to cut through the delicate capsule. (**D**) Buttress of viable omentum, with intact arterial and venous blood supply, may be used to reinforce the repair.

Late postoperative follow-up of patients who have undergone partial splenectomy suggests that the splenic remnant enlarges and provides protection against sepsis. Enlargement may be sufficient to cause recurrence of symptoms; this problem is discussed in detail in prior subheadings. Petroianu et al. (1997) felt that enlargement was less likely to be problematic, if the splenic remnant was planned so that the blood supply was derived from the short gastric vessels, and the splenic hilum was not preserved.

17.5.3. SPLENOSIS The occasional observation of generalized studding of omental and peritoneal surfaces, in patients who undergo laparotomy years after unrecognized splenic injury, led to the speculation that such "born-again spleens" might protect against subsequent sepsis (Pabst and Kamran, 1986). Attempts have been made to reproduce the growth of such splenic tissue as a compensatory maneuver, when the spleen is removed. The spleen is minced, and slices no thicker than 1 cm are placed on the greater omentum, which is then folded over to contain the splenic remnants. The location of these remnants may be marked by fine

hemostatic clips. Such splenic autotransplants have been demonstrated to remain viable, and to achieve a blood supply from the omentum. Subsequent radionuclide scanning will frequently demonstrate uptake of radionuclide within the splenic fragments (Livingstone et al., 1983). However, several studies have failed to demonstrate normal bacterial clearance in experimental animals in the absence of a significant fragment (perhaps one-third) of the spleen, which is supplied by the splenic artery (Scher et al., 1985). OPSI has been documented in a patient found to have approx 25 g of viable splenic tissue in splenosis of the omentum and mesentery (Holmes et al., 1981). Thus, although splenic autotransplantation is feasible, and may be performed with minimal difficulty, it is not clear that such autotransplants provide protection against OPSI. Many surgeons continue to place such autotransplants, when splenectomy for trauma is unavoidable; however, these patients should probably also receive polyvalent pneumococcal vaccine, and be considered for antibiotic prophylaxis, as if they were asplenic.

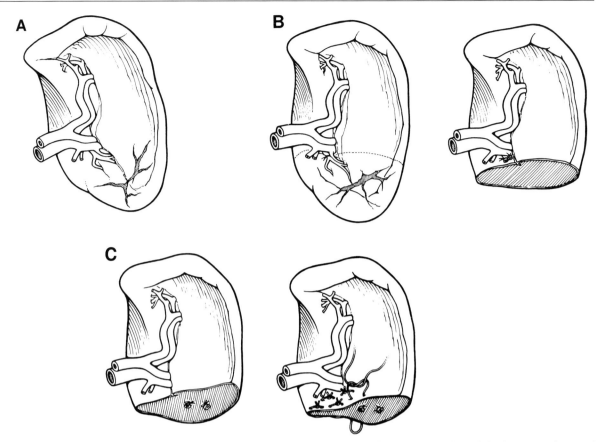

Fig. 17.16. (**A**) A complex stellate fracture of the lower pole of the spleen is typical of the sort of injury for which partial splenectomy is a good form of management. Partial splenectomy may also be utilized when a benign cyst or tumor occupies part of the spleen, or for preservation of some splenic function in selected disorders (such as schistosomiasis or thalassemia major). (**B**) Hilar artery and vein supplying the involved segment are ligated and the pole is allowed to demarcate. Resection is accomplished along the line of demarcation. Occasional intrasplenic branches of vessels may require ligation or control by fine hemostatic clips. (**C**) Sutures are placed to compress the raw surface. These may be placed over pledgets, if desired.

17.5.4. PARTIAL SPLENIC EMBOLIZATION Partial trans-catheter embolization has been used in patients in whom partial ablation of splenic function is desired, and in whom both surgery and the asplenic state carry considerable risk (Yoshioka et al., 1985; Israel et al., 1994). Mozes et al. (1984) conducted a prospective randomized study comparing partial splenic embolization with total splenectomy, in patients requiring splenic ablation prior to renal transplantation. Partial splenic embolization resulted in a mean reduction in splenic mass of 65%. A significant number of patients experienced regeneration of the spleen after partial splenic embolization, and repeated procedures were performed in 11 patients. The immediate complication rate was similar in patients of the two groups, which underwent either partial splenic embolization or splenectomy. Both groups subsequently underwent renal transplantation, with similar results.

Witte et al. (1982) confirmed the importance of occluding the intrasplenic, rather than the extrasplenic, vasculature. The use of large coils to occlude the main splenic artery has generally been associated with a high failure rate. In a series of 136 patients undergoing partial splenic embolization, fever, pain, atelectasis, leukocytosis, hyperamylasemia, and pleural effusion were commonly seen (Jonasson et al., 1985). More serious complications were infrequent; however, two patients developed pancreatitis, two developed pancreatic pseudocysts, and two developed splenic abscesses. Partial splenic embolization shows promise as a relatively safe and

effective technique for partial splenic ablation, in selected patients. However, the risks and relatively high failure rate associated with partial and total splenic embolization, in children, were recently emphasized (Back et al., 1987), and the precise role of these techniques in the management of splenic disorders remains to be defined.

17.6. COMPLICATIONS OF SPLENECTOMY

Careful preoperative preparation and meticulous operative technique have significantly decreased the complication rate associated with elective splenectomy. Improvements in postoperative care have also benefited these patients.

17.6.1. IMMEDIATE COMPLICATIONS Complications and death rates vary with the indication for elective splenectomy and the size of the spleen (Table 2). In general, older patients, those with hematologic malignancies and large spleens, fare worst (MacRae et al., 1992; Horowitz et al., 1996; Irving, 1997). Survival after splenic surgery for trauma is determined by the severity of the original insult and any associated injuries. The discussion in this and subsequent subheadings is limited to the complications of splenectomy and splenic surgery *per se*.

Atelectasis is the most common complication of splenic surgery, because of the upper abdominal incision, and extensive dissection in the left upper quadrant. Careful preoperative pulmonary preparation, with instruction in deep breathing and coughing, as well as meticulous postoperative pulmonary care, can minimize

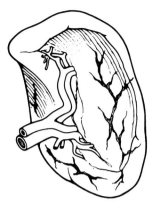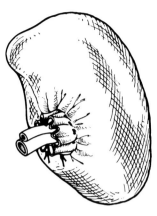

Fig. 17.17. When the spleen has been severely damaged, but the hilar vessels are intact, a synthetic, absorbable mesh wrap may be used to provide hemostasis, by gentle compression. Several pursestring sutures are placed to assure that the mesh provides adequate compression.

Table 17.2
Complications of Splenic Surgery

Immediate complications (within the first week)
    Atelectasis
    Pleural effusion
    Pneumonia
    Bleeding
Early postoperative period (within the first 2 weeks)
    Subphrenic abscess
    Gastric fistula
    Pancreatic fistula
    Pancreatitis
    Thrombocytosis
    Mesenteric vein thrombosis
Late postoperative period (after first 1–2 weeks)
    Mesenteric vein thrombosis
    Overwhelming sepsis

this complication. Pleural effusion is less frequent, occurring in 10% of most series (Ellison and Fabri, 1983).

Pleural effusion was more common when prolonged drainage of the splenic bed with passive drains was employed: This has been one reason for abandoning such drainage. It also occurs when mesh is used to wrap the spleen for splenic repair apparently as a reaction to the mesh in this setting. Pneumonia is generally reported to occur in approx 10% of patients. Atelectasis, pleural effusion, and pneumonia are more common in patients experiencing blunt trauma, in which associated chest wall trauma and rib fractures cause diminished respiratory excursions. The presence of such pulmonary complications after the third postoperative day should alert the surgeon to the possibility of a left subphrenic abscess (Ellison and Fabri, 1983). Subphrenic abscesses can be diagnosed by CT, and drained percutaneously under CT guidance (McNicholas et al., 1995). Surgical drainage may be required if adequate drainage cannot be accomplished under CT guidance.

17.6.1.1. Hemorrhage Postoperative bleeding is most common when splenectomy is performed for hypersplenism, particularly when thrombocytopenia is present. Left shoulder pain from diaphragmatic irritation, hemodynamic instability, and the appearance of blood in drains (if these have been placed) suggest that bleeding is occurring. Prompt reoperation, with evacuation of clot, irrigation of the left upper quadrant, and re-establishment of hemostasis, is advisable. Most postoperative bleeding comes from raw peritoneal and diaphragmatic surfaces. Frequently, no specific bleeding source is found at reoperation, but bleeding from the hilar vessels, short gastric vessels, or the pancreatic surface may also occur (Ellison and Fabri, 1983).

17.6.1.2. Injury to Tail of Pancreas: Pancreatic Fistula Pancreatic injuries are reported to occur in 13% of splenectomies in large series, and are believed to be related to injury during ligation of the splenic artery and vein. Ugochukwu and Irving (1985) measured serum and drain fluid amylase in 10 patients who underwent elective splenectomy. Pancreatic injury was suspected in only one patient; however, all 10 had an elevated level of amylase in the drain fluid, in the early postoperative period. Pancreatic fistula results when the amount of drainage remains elevated, and when a drainage tract becomes established. If there is no path to the skin, a collection of amylase-rich fluid in the left upper quadrant may

predispose to subphrenic abscess formation, or may present as a pseudocyst of the tail of the pancreas. Occasionally, hemorrhagic pancreatitis occurs after splenectomy.

Careful dissection in the splenic hilum, and placement of closed suction drains when pancreatic injury is suspected, should minimize the occurrence of these complications.

17.6.1.3. Injury to Greater Curvature of Stomach: Gastric Fistula Gastrocutaneous fistula is a rare complication of splenectomy. Harrison et al. (1977) reviewed 14 previously reported cases, and four additional ones. They identified several factors as contributing to the development of this complication. Trauma to the greater curvature of the stomach, by instruments or by ligatures placed when the short gastric vessels are controlled, is probably the most important preventable cause of gastric fistula. This is most likely to occur at the extreme upper pole of the spleen, where the distance between the splenic capsule and the stomach may be relatively short and exposure difficult (Fig. 8). The rich anastomotic blood supply of the stomach usually prevents ischemia when these vessels are ligated.

Occasionally, previous gastric surgery or atherosclerosis may contribute to ischemia in the region of the greater curvature. Although this is not thought to be severe enough to result in fistula formation, it may prevent healing of otherwise minor serosal injuries. Gastric injury may result in a subphrenic abscess, which can be confirmed by performing an upper gastrointestinal series with water-soluble contrast medium (Ellison and Fabri, 1983). Adequate drainage, antibiotic treatment of related infection, and prolonged nutritional support are necessary.

The complication can be prevented by careful surgical technique, and by imbricating the greater curvature with interrupted Lembert sutures, when injury is suspected.

17.6.1.4. Subphrenic Abscess The incidence of subphrenic abscess is variable: It is more common when adjacent organs have been injured, either by trauma or iatrogenic injury, and is consistently more common when the splenic bed is drained. More recent studies, using closed-suction drainage, demonstrate much lower rates of subphrenic abscess formation (Ugochukwu and Irving, 1985). However, there may be an element of selection bias in the association of abscess and drainage: Many surgeons employ drainage only when there is concern about the adequacy of hemostasis or injury to the tail of the pancreas. Mesh, and some of the topical hemostatic agents employed during splenorrhaphy, may potentiate the tendency to infection in a contaminated field (Wolf et al., 1996).

Pleural effusion, shoulder pain, singultus, and fever may be signs of a subphrenic abscess. The diagnosis can be confirmed by CT scan, and percutaneous CT-directed drainage may be performed. Adequate drainage and treatment with appropriate antibiotics are necessary.

17.6.2. DELAYED COMPLICATIONS Late complications of splenectomy include OPSI and an increased tendency to develop thromboembolic and ischemic complications (*see* Chapter 10). Failure of the original operation, because of undetected accessory spleens, may also develop late in the postoperative period.

17.6.2.1. Thrombocytosis and Thrombotic Complications
The platelet count will commonly rise by 30–100% after splenectomy, reaching a maximum 7–20 d after surgery. Thrombocytosis developed in 239/318 patients who underwent splenectomy; none of these patients had a myeloproliferative disorder (Boxer et al., 1978). In 72 patients, platelet counts over 1,000,000/mm^3 were encountered. 10 patients developed a thromboembolic complication; however, no correlation with postoperative platelet count, preoperative diagnosis, or medication could be established in this series.

An impression of increased risk persists for splenectomy for myeloid metaplasia or congestive splenomegaly, especially when postoperative platelet counts are high (Malmaeus et al., 1986). Broe et al. (1981) studied 28 patients who underwent splenectomy for myeloid metaplasia, and identified thromboembolic complications in nine. The postoperative platelet count did not predict the occurrence of thrombosis. The incidence of thromboembolic disease reported in this series is considerably higher than the incidence reported when splenectomy is performed for other hematological indications. Antecedent antithrombin III deficiency (e.g., from hepatic dysfunction) may cause thrombosis in the postsplenectomy state, even when platelet counts are normal (Peters et al., 1977).

Mesenteric infarction, secondary to portal vein occlusion, is a particularly lethal complication, which has been reported most commonly in patients who underwent splenectomy for myeloid metaplasia and other myeloproliferative disorders. With massive splenomegaly, splenic vein enlargement occurs; it has been postulated that thrombus forms in the cul-de-sac, which remains when the splenic vein is ligated near the hilum of the spleen. Clot then propagates into the portal vein. Ligation of the splenic vein close to the junction with the inferior mesenteric vein, may diminish the incidence of this complication, by eliminating this cul-de-sac (Broe et al., 1981). Petit et al. (1994) studied 119 patients after splenectomy, using ultrasound or CT, and documented splenic vein thrombosis in 13 (12 patients with hematologic indications for splenectomy, and one patient with trauma). Seven of these were asymptomatic. Early anticoagulation led to resolution in 10, but two went on to cavernous transformation of the portal vein. They suggested that routine Doppler ultrasound examination should be done to detect splenic vein thrombosis early, so that anticoagulation can be undertaken.

Postoperative thrombosis and thromboembolic complications are also found in patients treated for hemolytic anemia who remain anemic after splenectomy (Balz and Minton, 1975). This has been particularly problematic in patients with unstable hemoglobins characterized by high oxygen affinity: deaths have occurred in this population (Phyliky and Fairbanks, 1997). The mechanism of this relationship, if in fact it is valid, continues to be conjectural.

Finally, whole blood viscosity increases significantly after splenectomy, partly because of the increase in platelets, but also because of a decrease in erythrocyte deformability and an increase in circulating protein aggregates normally removed by the spleen (Robertson et al., 1981).

Treatment of postsplenectomy thrombocytosis continues to be debated. Many recommend the use of acetylsalicylic acid and dipyridamole or low-dose heparin, and initiate such therapy when the platelet count exceeds 800,000–1,000,000/mm^3. Chemotherapy, with agents such as phenylalanine mustard, has been used to treat symptomatic postsplenectomy thrombocytosis in patients with myeloproliferative disorders.

Thromboembolic complications remain one of the hazards of splenectomy. Mesenteric venous thrombosis should be considered, when a patient develops abdominal pain or ileus after splenectomy. Surgery is required once thrombosis has occurred.

17.6.2.2. Infectious Complications: OPSI OPSI was originally described as a fulminant, acute illness, frequently progressing to death within 36 hours of first symptoms (*see also* Chapter 11). The organisms most commonly implicated have been *Streptococcus pneumoniae, meningococcus,* and *Haemophilis influenzae* (Hays et al., 1986). Review of large numbers of splenectomized children, by the Surgical Section of the American Academy of Pediatrics, confirmed the existence of the syndrome, and showed a tendency for OPSI to occur more frequently when splenectomy was performed early in life. It also appeared to be more frequent in children with certain disorders, such as thalassemia and sickle cell disease. Initially, it was thought that children splenectomized for trauma rarely developed OPSI (Hays et al., 1986). The risk to adults was thought to be correspondingly lower still. Subsequently, OPSI was recognized in adults (Chaikof and McCabe, 1985). An extensive review, using the Swedish inpatient registry to ensure completeness of the data accrued, identified a small but definite increase in septic deaths in 1297 adults followed more than 1 year after splenectomy for trauma (Linet et al., 1996). The risk is currently thought to relate to the age of the patient, the interval since splenectomy, and the underlying disorder leading to the splenectomy (Lynch and Kapila, 1996). Schilling (1995) developed a model to estimate the risk of sepsis following splenectomy for hereditary spherocytosis, a disorder in which the continuing demands of ongoing hemolysis, and the risk of erythropoietic shutdown with infections, must be balanced against risk of splenectomy, when decisions on the timing of surgery are made.

The incidence of a large number of infections, including OPSI, is now recognized to be increased in previously splenectomized individuals of all ages, especially in those with underlying diseases that affect immune competence (Mower et al., 1986; Green et al., 1986; Willis et al., 1986; Lynch and Kapila, 1996).

Three effective preventive measures have been identified: immunization, antibiotic prophylaxis, and patient education (Williams and Kaur, 1996). Current recommendations for children over age two include the administration of polyvalent pneumococcal vaccine, which should be given at least 2 wk preoperatively, when elective splenectomy is anticipated. Revaccination should be given after 3–5 years in those under 10 years of age. Quadrivalent meningococcal vaccine should also be administered to all asplenic children over the age of 2 yr, and *H. influenzae* type b vaccine should be given to all children at risk for OPSI. Adults are generally given all three vaccines, ideally, at least 2 wk prior to splenectomy. Although the efficacy of antimicrobial prophylaxis, in addition to immunizations, has only been proven in children with sickle cell disease, other asplenic children at particularly high risk for sepsis (those with malignancies, thalassemia, those under age 5 yr) should be strongly considered for prophylaxis. Oral penicillin V is usually recommended (American Academy of Pediatrics, 1997). For older children and adults, considerable debate still exists about the need for, and the useful duration of, antibiotic prophylaxis (Lortan, 1993).

All patients who have undergone splenectomy should be warned of their increased susceptibility to infection; should be instructed to seek medical attention, when signs of infection or systemic illness develop, and should carry a warning card or device that indicates their asplenic state. Such patients should be followed indefinitely, because it is unclear whether risk diminishes with time. In Schilling's review (1995), the risk of fatal infection was estimated at 0.73/1000 patient years; and 3/4 deaths in that series occurred many years after splenectomy. Patients with Wiskott-Aldrich syndrome are unable to produce antibodies to polysaccharide antigens, and should be kept on long-term prophylactic antibiotic therapy (Lum et al., 1980).

17.6.2.3. Miscellaneous Long-Term Complications   Cholesterol and serum low-density lipoprotein levels rise after splenectomy, and this rise is most significant when splenectomy is performed for myeloproliferative disorders (Aviram et al., 1986). Thromboembolic complications were identified as occurring in the Swedish registry study previously cited (Linet et al., 1996). This is discussed in the subheading on Hodgkin's disease, where the association has been most pronounced. In that patient population, splenectomy, and mediastinal irradiation were identified as causative factors.

There have been several suggestions that splenectomy may predispose to the development of cancer, through some unknown, but possibly immunologic mechanism. In a Danish cancer registry study of 1103 patients followed for a mean of 6.8 years after splenectomy, the relative risk of developing an unrelated malignancy was 1.0 (Mellemkjoer et al., 1995).

Splenectomy is no longer routinely advocated during *en bloc* radical cancer operations, particularly total or subtotal gastrectomy, because several series have demonstrated not only an increase in immediate complications (such as subphrenic abscess), but worse long-term survival (Griffith et al., 1995; Kwon, 1997; Wanebo et al., 1997).

17.7. SUMMARY

Increasing recognition of the unique and significant functions of the spleen has stimulated interest in the development of therapeutic alternatives to total splenectomy. Techniques for partial splenic resection and splenic salvage, initially developed for the management of splenic trauma, are being applied to an increasing number of conditions in which reduction, rather than total ablation, of splenic tissue is effective treatment. The precise role of these techniques in the treatment of hematological conditions requiring splenic surgery is still being defined. In patients requiring total splenectomy, careful preoperative evaluation, meticulous surgical technique, and postoperative care can minimize complications and operative mortality. Furthermore, awareness of the longer-term hazards of the hyposplenic state will stimulate a continued search for improved methods of management, and greater attention to the possible complications of those for whom total splenectomy cannot be avoided.

REFERENCES

Aidonopoulos, A. P., Papavramidis, S. T., Goutzamanis, G. D., Filos, G. G., Deligiannidis, N. P., and Vogiatzis, I. M. (1995) Splenorrhaphy for splenic damage in patients with multiple injuries. *Eur. J. Surg.* **161**, 247–251.

Ajana, F., Senneville, E., Valette, M., Bourez, J. M., Chidiac, C., and Mouton, Y. (1996) Pneumococcal infections after splenectomy in HIV+ patients. *Int. Conf. AIDS* **11**, 17 (Abstract).

Aksnes, J., Abdelnoor, M., and Mathisen, O. (1995) Risk factors associated with mortality and morbidity after elective splenectomy. *Eur. J. Surg.* **161**, 253–258.

Allen, K. B. and Andrews, G. (1989) Pediatric wandering spleen—the case for splenopexy: review of 35 reported cases in the literature. *J. Pediatr. Surg.* **24**, 432–435.

Al-Mohaya, S., Al-Awami, M., Vaidya, M. P., and Knox-Macaulay, H. (1986) Hydatid cyst of the spleen. *Am. J. Trop. Med. Hyg.* **35**, 995–999.

Alonso, M., Gossot, D., Bourstyn, E., et al. (1993) Splenectomy in human immunodeficiency virus-related thrombocytopenia. *Br. J. Surg.* **80**, 330–333.

al-Salem, A. H., Qaisaruddin, S., Nasserallah, Z., al Dabbous, I., and al Jam'a, A. (1996) Splenectomy in patients with sickle-cell disease. *Am. J. Surg.* **172**, 254–258.

American Academy of Pediatrics, Active and Passive Immunization. In: *1997 Red Book: Report of the Committee on Infectious Diseases,* 24th ed. (Peter G., ed.), American Academy of Pediatrics, Elk Grove Village, IL, pp. 56–58.

Ashkenazi, A., Zaizov, R., and Matoth, Y. (1986) Effect of splenectomy on destructive bone changes in children with chronic (Type 1) Gaucher disease. *Eur. J. Pediatr.* **145**, 138–141.

Aviram, M., Brook, J. G., Tatarsky, I., Levy, Y., and Carter, A. (1986) Increased low-density lipoprotein levels after splenectomy: a role for the spleen in cholesterol metabolism in myeloproliferative disorders. *Am. J. Med. Sci.* **291**, 25–28.

Back, L. M., Bagwell, C. E., Greenbaum, B. H., and Marchildon, M. B. (1987) Hazards of splenic embolization. *Clin. Pediatr.* **26**, 292–295.

Bar-Maor, J. A. (1993) Partial splenectomy in Gaucher's disease: follow-up report. *J. Pediatr. Surg.* **28**, 686–688.

Balz, J. and Minton, P. (1975) Mesenteric thrombosis following splenectomy. *Ann. Surg.* **181**, 126–128.

Beanes, S., Emil, S., Kosi, M., Applebaum, H., and Atkinson, J. (1995) Comparison of laparoscopic versus open splenectomy in children. *Am. Surg.* **61**, 908–910.

Bell, W. R., Braine, H. G., Ness, P. M., and Kickler, T. S. (1991) Improved survival in thrombotic thrombocytopenic purpura-hemolytic uremic syndrome. Clinical experience in 108 patients. *N. Engl. J. Med.* **325**, 398–403.

Benbassat, J., Gilon, D., and Penchas, S. (1990) The choice between splenectomy and medical treatment in patients with advanced agnogenic myeloid metaplasia. *Am. J. Hematol.* **33**, 128–135.

Berge, T. (1974) Splenic metastases: frequencies and patterns. *Acta Pathol. Microbiol. Scand.* **82**, 499–506.

Berne, J. D., Asensio, J. A., Falabella, A., and Gomez, H. (1997) Traumatic rupture of the spleen in a patient with hereditary spherocytosis. *J. Trauma* **42**, 323–326.

Bhatnagar, V., Agarwala, S., and Mitra, D. K. (1994) Conservative surgery for splenic hydatid cyst. *J. Pediatr. Surg.* **29**, 1570–1571.

Bissel, D. M. (1986) Heme catabolism and bilirubin formation in bile pigments and jaundice. In: *Molecular, Metabolic and Medical Aspects* (Ostrow, J. D., ed.), Marcel Dekker, New York, pp. 133–156.

Blendis, L. M., Modell, C. B., Bowdler, A. J., and Williams, R. (1974) Some effects of splenectomy in thalassaemia major. *Br. J. Haematol.* **28**, 77–87.

Blumfelder, T. M., Logue, G. L., and Shimm, D. S. (1981) Felty's syndrome: effect of splenectomy upon granulocyte count and granulocyte associated IgG. *Ann. Intern. Med.* **94**, 623–628.

Bouroncle, B. A. (1994) Thirty-five years in the progress of hairy cell leukemia. *Leuk. Lymphoma* **14(Suppl. 1)**, 1–12.

Bouvet, M., Babiera, G. V., Termuhlen, P. M., Hester, J. P., Kantarjian, H. M., and Pollock, R. E. (1997) Splenectomy in the accelerated or blastic phase of chronic myelogenous leukemia: a single-institution, 25-year experience. *Surgery* **122**, 20–25.

Bowdler, A. J. and Glick I. W. (1966) Autoimmune hemolytic anemia as the herald state of Hodgkin's disease. *Ann. Intern. Med.* **65**, 761–767.

Bowdler, A. J. (1987) Chronic relapsing thrombotic thrombocytopenic purpura. *South. Med. J.* **80**, 507–510.

Boxer, M. A., Braun, J., and Ellman, L. (1978) Thromboembolic risk of postsplenectomy thrombocytosis. *Arch. Surg.* **113**, 808–809.

Brochard, M., Sigaux, F., Flandrin, G., Bourstyn, E., and Clot, P. (1987) Splenectomy performed upon thirty-seven patients with hairy cell leukemia. *Surg. Gynecol. Obstet.* **165**, 305–308.

Brodsky, J., Abcar, A., and Styler, M. (1996) Splenectomy for non-Hodgkin's lymphoma. *Am. J. Clin. Oncol.* **19**, 558–561.

Broe, P. J., Conley, C. L., and Cameron, J. L. (1981) Thrombosis of the portal vein following splenectomy for myeloid metaplasia. *Surg. Gynecol. Obstet.* **152**, 488–492.

Bronsther, O., Merhav, H., Van Thiel, D., and Starzl, T. E. (1991) Splenic artery aneurysms occurring in liver transplant recipients. *Transplantation* **52**, 723–724.

Brown, M. F., Ross, A. J. III, Bishop, H. C., Schnaufer, L., Ziegler, M. M., and Holcomb, G. W. III (1989) Partial splenectomy: the preferred alternative for the treatment of splenic cysts. *J. Pediatr. Surg.* **24**, 694–696.

Brown, S. A., Majumdar, G., Harrington, C., Bedford, M., Winter, M., O'Doherty, M. J., and Savidge, G. F. (1994) Effect of splenectomy on HIV-related thrombocytopenia and progression of HIV infection in patients with severe haemophilia. *Blood Coagul. Fibrinolysis* **5**, 393–397.

Brunt, L. M., Langer, J. C., Quasebarth, M. A., and Whitman, E. D. (1996) Comparative analysis of laparoscopic versus open splenectomy. *Am. J. Surg.* **172**, 596–601.

Buehner, M. and Baker, M. S. (1992) The wandering spleen. *Surg. Gynecol. Obstet.* **175**, 373–387.

Burchard, G. D., Reimold-Jehle, U., Burkle, V., Kretschmer, H., Vierbuchen, M., Racz, P., and Lo, Y. (1996) Splenectomy for suspected malignant lymphoma in two patients with loiasis. *Clin. Infect. Dis.* **23**, 979–982.

Cala, Z., Cvitanovic, B., Perko, Z., Velnic, D., and Rasic, Z. (1996) Laparoscopic treatment of nonparasitic cysts of spleen and liver. *J. Laparoendosc. Surg.* **6**, 387–391.

Campbell, D. A., Corman, L. C., and Williams, R. C. Jr. (1992) Splenectomy as treatment for nonhealing soft tissue defect after total knee arthroplasty in a patient with Felty's syndrome. *J. Rheumatol.* **19**, 1126–1129.

Cavanna, L., Artioli, F., Vallisa, D., Di Donato, C., Berte, R., Carapezzi, C., et al. (1995) Primary lymphoma of the spleen. Report of a case with diagnosis by fine-needle guided biopsy. *Haematologica* **80**, 241–243.

Cavanna, L., Civardi, G., Fornari, F., Di Stasi, M., Sbolli, G., Buscarini, E., et al. (1992) Ultrasonically guided percutaneous splenic tissue core biopsy in patients with malignant lymphomas. *Cancer* **69**, 2932–2936.

Cervera, H., Jara, L. J., Pizarro, S., Enkerlin, H. L., Fernandez, M., Medina, F., and Miranda, J. M. (1995) Danazol for systemic lupus erythematosus with refractory autoimmune thrombocytopenia or Evans' syndrome. *J. Rheumatol.* **22**, 1867–1871.

Chaikof, E. L. and McCabe, C. J. (1985) Fatal overwhelming postsplenectomy infection. *Am. J. Surg.* **149**, S34–S39.

Chakfe, N., Mantz, F. Kretz, J. G., Gasser, B., Loson, R., and Eisenmann, B. (1993) Treatment of a distal splenic artery aneurysm with splenic conservation. A case report. *J. Cardiovasc. Surg.* **34**, 503–506.

Cheson, B. D. and Martin, A. (1987) Clinical trials in hairy cell leukemia. Current status and future directions. *Ann. Intern. Med.* **106**, 871–878.

Childers, J. M., Balserak, J. C., Kent, T., and Surwit, E. A. (1993) Laparoscopic staging of Hodgkin's lymphoma. *J. Laparoendosc. Surg.* **3**, 495–499.

Chirletti, P., Cardi, M., Barillari, P., Vitale, A., Sammartino, P., Bolognese, A., et al. (1992) Surgical treatment of immune thrombocytopenic purpura. *World J. Surg.* **16**, 1001–1005.

Coad, J. E., Matutes, E., and Catovsky, D. (1993) Splenectomy in lymphoproliferative disorders: a report on 70 cases and review of the literature. *Leuk. Lymphoma* **10**, 245–264.

Coburn, M. C., Pfeifer, J., and DeLuca, F. G. (1995) Nonoperative management of splenic and hepatic trauma in the multiply injured pediatric and adolescent patient. *Arch. Surg.* **130**, 332–338.

Cohen, I. J., Katz, K., Freud, E., Zer, M., and Zaizov, R. (1992) Long-term follow-up of partial splenectomy in Gaucher's disease. *Am. J. Surg.* **164**, 345–347.

Coon, W. W. (1985a) The limited role of splenectomy in patients with leukemia. *Surg. Gynecol. Obstet.* **160**, 291–294.

Coon, W. W. (1985b) Splenectomy for splenomegaly and secondary hypersplenism. *World J. Surg.* **9**, 437–443.

Coon, W. W. (1985c) Splenectomy in the treatment of hemolytic anemia. *Arch. Surg.* **120**, 625–628.

Coon, W. W. (1985d) Felty's syndrome: when is splenectomy indicated? *Am. J. Surg.* **149**, 272–275.

Coon, W. W. (1987) Splenectomy for idiopathic thrombocytopenic purpura. *Surg. Gynecol. Obstet.* **164**, 225–229.

Coon, W. W. (1991) The spleen and splenectomy. *Surg. Gynecol. Obstet.* **173**, 407–414.

Cooper, M. J. and Williamson, R. C. N. (1984) Splenectomy: indications, hazards and alternatives. *Br. J. Surg.* **71**, 173–180.

Corash, L., Shafer, B., and Blaese, R. M. (1985) Platelet-associated immunoglobulin, platelet size, and the effect of splenectomy in the Wiskott Aldrich syndrome. *Blood* **65**, 1439–1443.

Croom, R. D. III, McMillan, C. W., Orringer, E. P., and Sheldon, G. F. (1986) Hereditary spherocytosis. Recent experience and current concepts of pathophysiology. *Ann. Surg.* **203**, 34–39.

Crosby, W. H. (1987) Splenectomy for thrombocytopenia in chronic liver disease. *Arch. Intern. Med.* **147**, 195–197.

Crowther, M. A., Heddle, N., Hayward, C. P., Warkentin, T., and Kelton, J. G. (1996) Splenectomy done during hematologic remission to prevent relapse in patients with thrombotic thrombocytopenic purpura. *Ann. Int. Med.* **125**, 294–296.

Cuschieri, A., Shimi, S., Banting, S., and Vander Velpen, G. (1992) Technical aspects of laparoscopic splenectomy: hilar segmental devascularization and instrumentation. *J. R. Coll. Surg. Edinb.* **37**, 414–416.

Dailey, M. O., Coleman, C. N., and Kaplan, H. S. (1980) Radiation-induced splenic atrophy in patients with Hodgkin's disease and non-Hodgkin's lymphomas. *N. Engl. J. Med.* **302**, 215–217.

Dalton, M. L. and West, R. L. (1965) Fate of the dearterialized spleen. *Arch. Surg.* **91**, 541–544.

Damasio, E. E. and Frassoldati, A. (1994) Splenectomy following complete response to alpha interferon (IFN) therapy in patients with hairy cell leukemia (HCL): results of the HCL88 protocol. Italian Cooperative Group for the Study of Hairy Cell Leukemia (ICGHCL). *Leuk. Lymphoma* **14(Suppl. 1)**, 95–98.

Dawson, D. L., Molina, M. E., and Scott-Conner, C. E. H. (1986) Venous segmentation of the human spleen: a corrosion cast study. *Am. Surg.* **52**, 253–256.

Deckings, B. G. and Printen, K. J. (1977) Elective splenectomy in the elderly patient. *Am. Surg.* **43**, 195–199.

Delaitre, B. (1995) Laparoscopic splenectomy. The "hanged spleen" technique. *Surg. Endosc.* **9**, 528–529.

Delpero, J. R., Gastaut, J. A., Letreut, Y. P., Caamano, A., Mathieu-Tubiana, N., Maraninchi, D., et al. (1987) The value of splenectomy in chronic lymphocytic leukemia. *Cancer* **59**, 340–345.

Deva, A. K. and Thompson, J. F. (1996) Delayed rupture of the spleen 5½ years after conservative management of traumatic splenic injury. *Aust. NZ J. Surg.* **66**, 494–495.

Dexter, S. P., Martin, I. G., Alao, D., Norfolk, D. R., and McMahon, M. J. (1996) Laparoscopic splenectomy. The suspended pedicle technique. *Surg. Endosc.* **10**, 393–396.

Diaz, J., Eisenstat, M., and Chung, R. S. (1996) Laparoscopic resection of accessory spleen for recurrent immune thrombocytopenic purpura 19 years after splenectomy. *J. Laparoendosc. Surg.* **6**, 337–339.

Diaz, J., Eisenstat, M., and Chung, R. (1997) A case-controlled study of laparoscopic splenectomy. *Am. J. Surg.* **173**, 348–350.

Dietrich, P. Y., Henry-Amar, M., Cosset, J. M., Bodis, S., Bosq, J., and Hayat, M. (1994) Second primary cancers in patients continuously disease-free from Hodgkin's disease: a protective role for the spleen? *Blood* **84**, 1209–1215.

Dotevall, A., Kutti, J., Wadenvik, H., Westin, J., Angeras, U., and Darle, N. (1987) A retrospective analysis of a consecutive series of patients splenectomized for various haematologic disorders. *Acta Haematol.* (Basel), **77**, 38–44.

Douglas, G. L. and Simpson, J. S. (1971) The conservative management of splenic trauma. *J. Pediatr. Surg.* **6**, 565–570.

Dowling, R. D., Ochoa, J., Yousem, S. A., Peitzman, A., and Udekwu, A. O. (1991) Argon beam coagulation is superior to conventional techniques in repair of experimental splenic injury. *J. Trauma* **31**, 717–721.

Duke, B. J., Modein, G. W., Schecter, W. P., and Horn, J. K. (1993) Transfusion significantly increases the risk for infection after splenic injury. *Arch. Surg.* **128**, 1125–1132.

Dunham, C. M., Cornwell, E. E. III, and Militello, P. (1991) The role of the argon beam coagulator in splenic salvage. *Surg. Gynecol. Obstet.* **173**, 179–182.

el-Gendi, M. A., Azzam, Z. A., Karara, K., el-Rakshy, T., el-Hammadi, H. A., Abu-Nasr, A., and Mosimann, R. (1994) Effect of gastro-esophageal decongestion on variceal pressure in patients with schistosomal hepatic fibrosis. *Int. Surg.* **79**, 68–71.

El-Khishen, M. A., Henderson, J. M., Millikan, W. J. Jr., Kutner, M. H., and Warren, W. D. (1985) Splenectomy is contraindicated for thrombocytopenia secondary to portal hypertension. *Surg. Gynecol. Obstet.* **160**, 234–238.

Ellison, E. C. and Fabri, P. J. (1983) Complications of splenectomy: etiology, prevention and management. *Surg. Clin. North Am.* **63**, 1313–1330.

el-Shazly, M., Okello, D. O., and Kawooya, M.G. (1995) Non-invasive diagnosis of tropical splenomegaly syndrome. *Trop. Doct.* **25**, 128–130.

Facon, T., Caulier, M. T., Fenaux, P., Plantier, I., Marchandise, X., Ribet, M., Jouet, J. P., and Bauters, F. (1992) Accessory spleen in recurrent chronic immune thrombocytopenic purpura. *Am. J. Hematol.* **41**, 184–189.

Farag, A., Shoukry, A., and Nasr, S. E. (1994) A new option for splenic preservation in normal sized spleen based on preserved histology and phagocytic function of the upper pole using upper short gastric vessels. *Am. J. Surg.* **168**, 257–261.

Farid, H. and O'Connell, T. X. (1996) Surgical management of massive splenomegaly. *Am. Surg.* **62**, 803–805.

Fingerhut, A, Oberlin, P., Cotte, J. L., et al. (1992) Splenic salvage using an absorbable mesh: feasibility, reliability and safety. *Br. J. Surg.* **79**, 325–327.

Fitzgerald, P. G., Langer, J. C., Cameron, B. H., et al. (1996) Pediatric laparoscopic splenectomy using the lateral approach. *Surg. Endosc.* **10**, 859–861.

Fleshner, P. R., Aufses, A. H. Jr., Grabowski, G. A., and Elias, R. (1991) 27-year experience with splenectomy for Gaucher's disease. *Am. J. Surg.* **161**, 69–75.

Flowers, J. L., Lefor, A. T., Steers, J., Heyman, M., Graham, S. M., and Imbembo, A. L. (1996) Laparoscopic splenectomy in patients with hematologic diseases. *Ann. Surg.* **224**, 19–28.

Fonkalsrud, E. W., Philippart, M., and Feig, S. (1990) Ninety-five percent splenectomy for massive splenomegaly: a new surgical approach. *J. Pediatr. Surg.* **25**, 267–269.

Formiga, F., Mitjavila, F., Pac, M., and Moga, I. (1997) Effective splenectomy in agranulocytosis associated with systemic lupus erythematosus. *J. Rheumatol.* **24**, 234–235.

Frezzato, M., Castaman, G., and Rodeghiero, F. (1993) Fulminant sepsis in adults splenectomized for Hodgkin's disease. *Haematologica* **78 (Suppl. 2)**, 73–77.

Friedman, R. L., Fallas, M. J., Carroll, B. J., Hiatt, J. R., and Phillips, E. H. (1996) Laparoscopic splenectomy for ITP. The gold standard. *Surg. Endosc.* **10**, 991–995.

Gaspoz, J. M., Waldvogel, F., Cornu, P., Gugler, E., and Dayer, J. M. (1995) Significant and persistent improvement of thrombocytopenia after splenectomy in an adult with the Wiskott-Aldrich Syndrome and intra-cerebral bleeding. *Am. J. Hematol.* **48**, 182–185.

George, J. N., Woolf, S. H., Raskob, G. E., Wasser, J. S., Aledort, L. M., Ballem, P. J., et al. (1996) Idiopathic thrombocytopenic purpura: a practice guideline developed by explicit methods for the American Society of Hematology. *Blood* **88**, 3–40.

Gigot, J. F., Healy, M. L., Ferrant, A., Michaux, J. L., Njinou, B., and Kestens, P. J. (1994) Laparoscopic splenectomy for idiopathic thrombocytopenic purpura. *Br. J. Surg.* **81**, 1171–1172.

Gigot, J. F., Legrand, M., Cadiere, G. B., Delvaux, G., de Ville de Goyet, J., de Neve de Roden, A., et al. (1995) Is laparoscopic splenectomy a justified approach in hematologic disorders? Preliminary results of a prospective multicenter study. *Int. Surg.* **80**, 299–303.

Glasgow, R. E., Yee, L. F., and Mulvihill, S. J. (1997) Laparoscopic splenectomy. The emerging standard. *Surg. Endosc.* **11**, 108–112.

Glynn, M. J. (1986) Isolated splenic vein thrombosis. *Arch. Surg.* **121**, 723–725.

Gobbi, P. G., Grignani, G. E., Pozzetti, U., Bertoloni, D., Pieresca, C., Montagna, G., and Ascari, E. (1994) Primary splenic lymphoma: does it exist? *Haematologica* **79**, 286–293.

Godley, C. D., Warren, R. L., Sheridan, R. L., and McCabe, C. J. (1996) Nonoperative management of blunt splenic injury in adults: age over 55 years as a powerful indicator for failure. *J. Am. Coll. Surg.* **183**, 133–139.

Goldman, J. M., Johnson, S. A., Islam, A., Catovsky, D., and Galton, D. A. (1980) Haematological reconstitution after autografting for chronic granulocytic leukemia in transformation: the influence of previous splenectomy. *Br. J. Haematol.* **45**, 223–231.

Golinsky, D., Freud, E., Steinberg, R., and Zer, M. (1995) Vertical partial splenectomy for epidermoid cyst. *J. Pediatr. Surg.* **30**, 1704–1705.

Golomb, H. M. (1987) The treatment of hairy cell leukemia. *Blood* **69**, 979–983.

Golomb, H. M. and Ellis, E. (1991) Treatment options for hairy-cell leukemia. *Semin. Oncol.* **18(Suppl. 7)**, 7–11.

Gordon, M. K., Rietveld, J. A., and Frizelle, F. A. (1995) The management of splenic rupture in infectious mononucleosis. *Aust. NZ J. Surg.* **65**, 247–250.

Govrin-Yehudain, J. and Bar-Maor, J. A. (1980) Partial splenectomy in Gaucher's disease. *Isr. J. Med. Sci.* **16**, 665–668.

Green, J. B., Shackford, S. R., Sise M. J., and Fridlund, P. (1986) Late septic complications in adults after splenectomy for trauma: a prospective analysis in 144 patients. *J. Trauma* **26**, 999–1004.

Greig, J. D., Sweet, E. M., and Drainer, K. K. (1994) Splenic torsion in a wandering spleen, presenting as an acute abdominal mass. *J. Pediatr. Surg.* **29**, 571–572.

Griffith, J. P., Sue-Ling, H. M., Martin, I., Dixon, M. F., McMahon, M. J., Axon, A. T., and Johnston, D. (1995) Preservation of the spleen improves survival after radical surgery for gastric cancer. *Gut* **36**, 684–690.

Grossbard, M. L. (1996) Is laparoscopic splenectomy appropriate for the management of hematologic and oncologic diseases? *Surg. Endosc.* **10**, 387–388.

Gruenberg, J. C., Van Slyck, E. J., and Abraham, J. P. (1986) Splenectomy in systemic lupus erythematosus. *Am. Surg.* **52**, 366–370.

Guzzetta, P. C., Connors, R. H., Fink, J., and Barranger, J. A. (1987) Operative technique and results of subtotal splenectomy for Gaucher disease. *Surg. Gynecol. Obstet.* **164**, 359–362.

Hadas-Halpren, I., Hiller, N., and Dolbert, M. (1992) Percutaneous drainage of splenic abscesses: an effective and safe procedure. *Br. J. Radiol.* **65**, 968–970.

Hamy, A., Letessier, E., Guillard, Y., Paineau, J., and Visset, J. (1995) Splenectomy for isolated splenic metastasis from endometrial carcinoma. *Acta Obstet. Gynecol. Scand.* **74**, 745–746.

Hansen, M. S., Christensen, B. E., and Jonsson, V. (1979) The effect of acetylsalicylic acid and dipyridamole on thromboembolic complications in splenectomised patients with myelofibrosis. *Scand. J. Haematol.* **23**, 177–181.

Harrison, B. F., Glanges, E., and Sparkman, R. S. (1977) Gastric fistula following splenectomy. *Ann Surg.* **185**, 210–213.

Hashizume, M., Ohta, M., Ueno, K., Okadome, K., and Sugimachi, K. (1993) Laparoscopic ligation of splenic artery aneurysm. *Surgery* **113**, 352–354.

Hatley, R. M., Donaldson, J. S., and Raffensperger, J. G. (1989) Splenic microabscesses in the immune-compromised patient. *J. Pediatr. Surg.* **24**, 697–702.

Hays, D. M., Ternberg, J. L., Chen, T. T., Sullivan, M. P., Tefft, M., Fung, F., et al. (1986) Postsplenectomy sepsis and other complications after staging laparotomy for Hodgkin's disease in childhood. *J. Pediatr. Surg.* **21**, 628–632.

Helton, W. S., Carrico, C. J., Azveruha, P. A., and Schaller, R. (1986) The diagnosis and treatment of splenic fungal abscesses in the immunesuppressed patient. *Arch. Surg.* **121**, 580–586.

Heyman, M. R. and Walsh, T. J. (1987) Autoimmune neutropenia and Hodgkin's disease. *Cancer* **59**, 1903–1905.

Hicks, B. A., Thompson, W. R., Rogers, Z. R., and Guzzetta, P. C. (1996) Laparoscopic splenectomy in childhood hematologic disorders. *J. Laparoendosc. Surg.* **6(Suppl. 1)**, S31–S34.

Ho, H. S. and Wisner, D. H. (1993) Splenic abscess in the intensive care unit. *Arch. Surg.* **128**, 842–848.

Hobbs, J. R., Jones, K. H., Shaw, P. J., Lindsay, I., and Hancock, M. (1987) Beneficial effect of pretransplant splenectomy on displacement bone marrow transplantation for Gaucher's syndrome. *Lancet* **ii**, 1111–1115.

Hoefer, R. A., Scullin, D. C. Jr., Silver, L. F., and Weakley, S. D. (1991) Splenectomy for hematologic disorders: a 20 year experience. *J. KY Med. Assoc.* **89**, 446–449.

Hoeger, P. H., Helmke, K., and Winkler, K. (1995) Chronic consumption coagulopathy due to an occult splenic haemangioma: Kasabach-Merritt syndrome. *Eur. J. Pediatr.* **154**, 365–368.

Hoekstra, H. J., Tamminga, R. Y., and Timens, W. (1994) Partial splenectomy in children: an alternative for splenectomy in the pathological staging of Hodgkin's disease. *Ann. Surg. Oncol.* **1**, 480–486.

Hofer, B. O., Ryan, J. A., and Freeny, P. C. (1987) Surgical significance of vascular changes in chronic pancreatitis. *Surg. Gynecol. Obstet.* **164**, 499–505.

Hoffkes, H. G., Weber, F., Uppenkamp, M., Meusers, P., Teschendorf, C., Philipp, T., and Brittinger, G. (1995) Recovery by splenectomy in patients with relapsed thrombotic thrombocytopenic purpura and treatment failure to plasma exchange. *Semin. Thromb. Hemost.* **21**, 161–165.

Holcomb, G. W. III and Greene, H. L. (1993) Fatal hemorrhage caused by disease progression after partial splenectomy for type III Gaucher's disease. *J. Pediatr. Surg.* **28**, 1572–1574.

Holmes, F. F., Weyandt, T., Glazier, J., Cuppage, F. E., Moral, L. A., and Lindsey, N. J. (1981) Fulminant meningococcemia after splenectomy. *JAMA* **246**, 1119–1120.

Horowitz, J., Smith, J. L., Weber, T. K., Rodriguez-Bigas, M. A., and Petrelli, N. J. (1996) Postoperative complications after splenectomy for hematologic malignancies. *Ann. Surg.* **223**, 290–296.

Huang, P. P. and Urist, M. M. (1993) Evaluation of abdominal Hodgkin's disease. *Surg. Oncol. Clin. North Am.* **2**, 207–212.

Hunter, J. G. (1997) Advanced laparoscopic surgery. *Am. J. Surg.* **173**, 14–20.

Irving, M. (1985) Hodgkin's disease: is staging laparotomy necessary? *Br. J. Surg.* **72**, 589–590.

Irving, M. (1997) Postoperative complications after splenectomy for hematologic malignancies. *Ann. Surg.* **225**, 131–132.

Israel, D. M., Hassall, E., Culham, J. A., and Phillips, R. R. (1994) Partial splenic emolization in children with hypersplenism. *J. Pediatr.* **124**, 95–100.

Ivatury, R. R., Simon, R. J., Guignard, J., Kazigo, J., Gunduz, Y., and Stahl, W. M. (1993) The spleen at risk after penetrating trauma. *J. Trauma* **35**, 409–414.

Iwanaka, T., Nakanishi, H., Tsuchida, Y., Oka, T., Honna, T., and Shimizu, K. (1995) Familial multiple mesothelial cysts of the spleen. *J. Pediatr. Surg.* **30**, 1743–1745.

Jalovec, L. M., Boe, B. S., and Wyffels, P. L. (1993) The advantages of early operation with splenorrhaphy versus nonoperative management for the blunt splenic trauma patient. *Am. Surg.* **59**, 698–705.

Jameson, J. S., Thomas, W. M., Dawson, S., Wood, J. K., and Johnstone, J. M. (1996) Splenectomy for haematological disease. *J. R. Coll. Surg. Edinb.* **41**, 307–311.

Janu, P. G., Rogers, D. A., and Lobe, T. E. (1996) A comparison of laparoscopic and traditional open splenectomy in childhood. *J. Pediatr. Surg.* **31**, 109–114.

Jimmy, E. O., Bedu-Addo, G., Bates, I., Bevan, D., and Rutherford, T. R. (1996) Immunoglobulin gene polymerase chain reaction to distinguish hyperreactive malarial splenomegaly from 'African' chronic lymphocytic leukaemia and splenic lymphoma. *Trans. R. Soc. Trop. Med. Hyg.* **90**, 37–39.

Jockovich, M., Mendenhall, N. P., Sombeck, M. D., Talbert, J. L., Copeland, E. M. III, and Bland, K. I. (1994) Long-term complications of laparotomy in Hodgkin's disease. *Ann. Surg.* **219**, 615–624.

Jonasson, O., Spigos, D. G., and Mozes, M. F. (1985) Partial splenic embolisation: experience in 136 patients. *World J. Surg.* **9**, 461–467.

Kamel, R., Dunn, M. A., Skelly, R. R., Kamel, I. A., Zayed, M. G., Ramadan, M. R., et al. (1986) Clinical and immunological results of segmental splenectomy in schistosomiasis. *Br. J. Surg.* **73**, 544–547.

Kamelgard, J. and Trooskin, S. Z. (1996) Splenorrhaphy using oxidized regenerated cellulose in a case of adult blunt trauma. *Contemp. Surg.* **49**, 365–368.

Katkhouda, N., Waldrep, D. J., Feinstein, D., Soliman, H., Stain, S. C., Ortega, A. E., and Mouiel, J. (1996) Unresolved issues in laparoscopic splenectomy. *Am. J. Surg.* **172**, 585–590.

Keidl, C. M. and Chusid, M. J. (1989) Splenic abscesses in childhood. *Pediatr. Infect. Dis. J.* **8**, 368–373.

Keller, M. S. and Vane, D. W. (1995) Management of pediatric blunt splenic injury: comparison of pediatric and adult trauma surgeons. *J. Pediatr. Surg.* **30**, 221–225.

Khan, A. H., Bensoussan, A. L., Ouimet, A., Blanchard, H., Grignon, A., Ndoye, M. (1986) Partial splenectomy for benign cystic lesions of the spleen. *J. Pediatr. Surg.* **21**, 749–752.

Kidd, W. T., Lui, R. C., Khoo, R., and Nixon, J. (1987) The management of blunt splenic trauma. *J. Trauma* **27**, 977–979.

King, H. and Shumacker, H. B. (1952) Splenic studies: 1. Susceptibility to infection after splenectomy performed in infancy. *Ann. Surg.* **136**, 239–242.

Kizilcan, F., Tanyel, F. C., Buyukpamukcu, N., and Hicsonmez, A. (1993) Complications of typhoid fever requiring laparotomy during childhood. *J. Pediatr. Surg.* **28**, 1490–1493.

Klein, B., Stein, M., Kuten, A., Steiner, M., Barshalom, D., Robinson, E., and Gal, D. (1987) Splenomegaly and solitary spleen metastasis in solid tumors. *Cancer* **60**, 100–102.

Knudson, P., Coon, W., Schnitzer, B., and Liepman, M. (1982) Splenomegaly without an apparent cause. *Surg. Gynecol. Obstet.* **155**, 705–708.

Koehler, R. H., Smith, R. S., and Fry, W. R. (1994) Successful laparoscopic splenorrhaphy using absorbable mesh for grade III splenic injury: report of a case. *Surg. Laparosc. Endosc.* **4**, 311–315.

Kollias, J., Watson, D. I., Coventry, B. J., and Malycha, P. (1995) Laparoscopic splenectomy using the lateral position: an improved technique. *Aust. NZ J. Surg.* **65**, 746–748.

Kumar, P. V. (1995) Splenic hamartoma. A diagnostic problem on fine needle aspiration cytology. *Acta Cytol.* **39**, 391–395.

Kwon, S.J., Members of the Korean Gastric Cancer Study Group (1997) Prognostic impact of splenectomy on gastric cancer: results of the Korean Gastric Cancer Study Group. *World J. Surg.* **21**, 837–844.

Lally, K. P., Arnstein, M., Siegel, S., et al. (1986) A comparison of staging methods for Hodgkin's disease in children. *Arch. Surg.* **121**, 1125–1127.

Law, C., Marcaccio, M., Tam, P., Heddle, N., and Kelton, J. G. (1997) High-dose intravenous immune globulin and the response to splenectomy in patients with idiopathic thrombocytopenic purpura. *N. Engl. J. Med.* **336**, 1494–1498.

Lecomte, M. C., Garbarz, M., Gautero, H., Bournier, O., Galand, C., Boivin, P., and Dhermy, D. (1993) Molecular basis of clinical and morphological heterogeneity in hereditary elliptocytosis (HE) with spectrin alpha I variants. *Br. J. Haematol.* **85**, 584–595.

Lefor, A. T., Flowers, J. L., and Heyman, M. R. (1993) Laparoscopic staging of Hodgkin's disease. *Surg. Oncol.* **2**, 217–220.

Lefor, A. T., Melvin, W. S., Bailey, R. W., and Flowers, J. L. (1993) Laparoscopic splenectomy in the management of immune thrombocytopenia purpura. *Surgery* **114,** 613–618.

Lehman, H. A., Lehman, L. O., Rustagi, P. K., et al. (1987) Complement-mediated autoimmune thrombocytopenia. Monoclonal IgM antiplatelet antibody associated with lymphoreticular malignant disease. *N. Engl. J. Med.* **316,** 194–198.

Lerner, R. M. and Spataro, R. F. (1984) Splenic abscess: percutaneous drainage. *Radiology* **153,** 643–645.

Liew, S. C. and Storey, D. W. (1995) Laparoscopic splenectomy. *Aust. NZ J. Surg.* **65,** 743–745.

Linet, M. S., Nyren, O., Gridley, G., Adami, H. O., Buckland, J. D., McLaughlin, J. K., and Fraumeni, J. F. Jr. (1996) Causes of death among patients surviving at least one year following splenectomy. *Am. J. Surg.* **172,** 320–323.

Litzman, J., Jones, A., Hann, I., Chapel, H., Strobel, S., and Morgan, G. (1996) Intravenous immunoglobulin, splenectomy, and antibiotic prophylaxis in Wiskott-Aldrich syndrome. *Arch. Dis. Child.* **75,** 436–439.

Liu, E. T., Linker, C. A., and Shuman, M. A. (1986) Management of treatment failures in thrombotic thrombocytopenic purpura. *Am. J. Hematol.* **23,** 347–361.

Liu, D. L., Zia, S., Xu, W., Ye, Q., Gao, Y., and Qian, J. (1996) Anatomy of vasculature of 850 spleen specimens and its application in partial splenectomy. *Surgery* **119,** 27–33.

Livingstone, C. D., Levine, B. A., and Sirinek, K. R. (1983) Improved survival rate for intraperitoneal autotransplantation of the spleen after pneumococcal pneumonia. *Surg. Gynecol. Obstet.* **156,** 761–766.

Lortan, J. E. (1993) Management of asplenic patients. *Br. J. Haematol.* **84,** 566–569.

Lucas, C.E. (1991) Splenic trauma. Choice of management. *Ann. Surg.* **213,** 98–112.

Lum, L. G., Tubergen, D. G., Corash, L., and Blaese, R. M. (1980) Splenectomy in the management of the thrombocytopenia of the Wiskott-Aldrich syndrome. *N. Engl. J. Med.* **302,** 892–896.

Luna, G. K. and Dellinger, E. P. (1987) Nonoperative observation treatment for splenic injuries: a safe therapeutic option? *Am. J. Surg.* **153,** 462–468.

Lynch, A. M. and Kapila, R. (1996) Overwhelming postsplenectomy infection. *Infect. Dis. Clin. North Am.* **10,** 693–707.

Lynch, J. M., Ford, H., Gardner, M. J., and Weiner, E. S. (1993) Is early discharge following isolated splenic injury in the hemodynamically stable child possible? *J. Pediatr. Surg.* **28,** 1403–1407.

MacRae, H. M., Yakimets, W. W., and Reynolds, T. (1992) Perioperative complications of splenectomy for hematologic disease. *Can. J. Surg.* **35,** 432–436.

Malmaeus, J., Akre, T., Adami, H. O., and Hagberg, H. (1986) Early postoperative course following elective splenectomy in haematological diseases: a high complication rate in patients with myeloproliferative disorders. *Br. J. Surg.* **73,** 7203.

Mann, J. L., Hafez, G. R., and Longo, W. L. (1986) Role of the spleen in the transdiaphragmatic spread of Hodgkin's disease. *Am. J. Med.* **81,** 959–961.

Marmon, L. M., Vinocur, C. D., Wimmer, R. S., Konefal, S. H., and Weintraub, W. H. (1990) Fungal Splenic abscesses: management in childhood leukemia. *Pediatr. Surg.* **5,** 118–120.

Massey, M. D. and Stevens, J. S. (1991) Residual spleen found on denatured red blood cell scan following negative colloid scans. *J. Nucl. Med.* **32,** 2286–2287.

McAllister, E., Goode, S., Cordista, A. G., and Rosemurgy, A. (1995) Partial portal decompression alleviates thrombocytopenia of portal hypertension. *Am. Surg.* **61,** 129–131.

McDermott, V. G., Shlansky-Goldberg, R., and Cope, C. (1994) Endovascular management of splenic artery aneurysms and pseudoaneurysms. *Cardiovasc. Intervent. Radiol.* **17,** 179–184.

McGinley, K., Googe, P., Hanna, W., and Bell, J. (1995) Primary angiosarcoma of the spleen: a case report and review of the literature. *South. Med. J.* **88,** 873–875.

McNicholas, M. M., Mueller, P. R., Lee, M. J., et al. (1995) Percutaneous drainage of subphrenic fluid collections that occur after splenec-

tomy: efficacy and safety of transpleural versus extrapleural apporach. *Am. J.Radiol.* **165,** 355–359.

Meekes, I., van der Staak, F., and van Oostrom, C. (1995) *Eur. J. Pediatr. Surg.* **5,** 19–22.

Melikoglu, M., Colak, T., and Kavasoglu, T. (1995) Two unusual cases of wandering spleen requiring splenectomy. *Eur. J. Pediatr. Surg.* **5,** 48–49.

Mellemkjoer, L., Olsen, J. H., Linet, M. S., Gridley, G., and McLaughlin, J. K. (1995) Cancer risk after splenectomy. *Cancer* **75,** 577–583.

Mercan, S., Seven, R., and Erbil, Y. (1996) Laparoscopic treatment of accessory splenic tissue. *Surg. Laparosc. Endosc.* **6,** 330–331.

Mitchell, A. and Morris, P. J. (1985) Splenectomy for malignant lymphomas. *World J. Surg.* **9,** 444–448.

Moir, C., Guttman, F., Jequier, S., Sonnino, R., and Youssef, S. (1989) Splenic cysts: aspiration, sclerosis, or resection. *J. Pediatr. Surg.* **24,** 646–648.

Moll, S. and Orringer, E. P. (1996) Case report: splenomegaly and splenic sequestration in an adult with sickle cell anemia. *Am. J. Med. Sci.* **312,** 299–302.

Moores, D. C., McKee, M. A., Wang, H., Fischer, J. D., Smith, J. W., and Andrews, H. G. (1995) Pediatric laparoscopic splenectomy. *J. Pediatr. Surg.* **30,** 1201–1205.

Morgenstern, L., Rosenberg, J., and Geller, S. A. (1985) Tumors of the spleen. *World J. Surg.* **9,** 468–476.

Morgenstern, L., Verham, R., Weinstein, I., and Phillips, E. H. (1993) Subtotal splenectomy for Gaucher's disease: a follow-up study. *Am. Surg.* **59,** 860–865.

Morlat, P., Dequae, L., Dabis, F., Pellegrin, J. L., Lacoste, D., Chene, G., et al. (1996) Prognostic role of splenectomy in the progression of HIV infection: a retrospective cohort study. *Int. Conf. AIDS* **11,** 136 (Abstract).

Morrell, D. G., Chang, F. C., and Helmer, S. D. (1995) Changing trends in the management of splenic injury. *Am. J. Surg.* **170,** 686–690.

Mower, W. R., Hawkins, J. A., and Nelson, E. W. (1986) Postsplenectomy infection in patients with chronic leukemia. *Am. J. Surg.* **152,** 583–586.

Mozes, M. F., Spigos, D. G., Pollak, R., et al. (1984) Partial splenic embolization an alternative to splenectomy-results of a prospective randomized study. *Surgery* **96,** 694–702.

Mucha, P., Daly, R. C., and Farnell, M. B. (1986) Selective management of blunt splenic trauma. *J. Trauma* **26,** 970–979.

Mullen, C. A., Anderson, K. D., and Blaese, R. M. (1993) Splenectomy and/or bone marrow transplantation in the management of the Wiskott-Aldrich syndrome: long-term follow-up of 62 cases. *Blood* **82,** 61–66.

Mulligan, S. P., Matutes, E., Dearden, C., and Catovsky, D. (1991) Splenic lymphoma with villous lymphocytes: natural history and response to therapy in 50 cases. *Br. J. Haematol.* **78,** 206–209.

Musy, P. A., Roche, B., Belli, D., Bugmann, P., Nussle, D., and Le Coultre, C. (1992) Splenic cysts in pediatric patients: a report on 8 cases and review of the literature. *Eur. J. Pediatr. Surg.* **2,** 137–140.

Najean, Y., Dufour, V., Rain, J. D., and Toubert, M. D. (1991) The site of platelet destruction in thrombocytopenic purpura as a predictive index of the efficacy of splenectomy. *Br. J. Haematol.* **79,** 271–276.

Nallathambi, M. N., Ivatury, R. R., Lankin, D. H., Wapnir, I. L., and Stahl, W. M. (1987) Pyogenic splenic abscess in intravenous drug addiction. *Am. Surg.* **53,** 342–346.

Naouri, A., Feghali, B., Chabal, J., Boulez, J., Dechavanne, M., Viala, J. J., and Tissot, E. (1993) Results of splenectomy for idiopathic thrombocytopenic purpura. Review of 72 cases. *Acta Haematol.* **89,** 200–203.

Narasimharao, K. L., Venkateswarlu, K., Mitra, S. K., and Mehta, S. (1987) Hydatid disease of spleen treated by cyst enucleation and splenic salvage *J. Pediatr. Surg.* **22,** 138–139.

Neudorfer, O., Hadas-Halpern, I., Elstein, D., Abrahamov, A., and Zimran, A. (1997) Abdominal ultrasound findings mimicking hematological malignancies in a study of 218 Gaucher patients. *Am. J. Hematol.* **55,** 28–34.

Nicklin, J. L., Copeland, L. J., O'Toole, R. V., Lewandowski, G. S., Vaccarello, L., and Havenar, L. P. (1995) Splenectomy as part of cytoreductive surgery for ovarian carcinoma. *Gynecol. Oncol.* **58,** 244–247.

Nilsen, B. H., Naugstvedt, T., Odland, P., and Viste, A. (1995) Laparoscopic splenectomy in children: surgical technique. *Eur. J. Surg.* **161,** 199–201.

Nishiyama, T., Iwao, N., Myose, H., Okamoto, T., Fujitomi, Y., Chinen, M., Komichi Y., and Kobayashi, T. (1986) Splenic vein thrombosis as a consequence of chronic pancreatitis: a study of three cases. *Am. J. Gastroenterol.* **81,** 1193–1198.

Oguzkurt, P., Senocak, M. E., Akcoren, Z., Kale, G., and Hicsonmez, A. (1996) Splenic leiomyoma: an uncommon localization. *Eur. J. Pediatr. Surg.* **6,** 235–237.

O'Keefe, J. H. Jr., Holmes, D. R. Jr., Schaff, H. V., Sheedy P. F. II, and Edwards, W. D. (1986) Thromboembolic splenic infarction. *Mayo Clin. Proc.* **61,** 967–972.

Onundarson, P. T., Rowe, J. M., Heal, J. M., and Francis, C. W. (1992) Response to plasma exchange and splenectomy in thrombotic thrombocytopenic purpura. A 10-year experience at a single institution. *Arch. Int. Med.* **152,** 791–796.

Ooi, L. L. and Leong, S. S. (1997) Splenic abscesses from 1987 to 1995. *Am. J. Surg.* **174,** 87–93.

Ooi, L. L., Nambiar, R., Rauff, A., Mack, P. O., and Yap, T. L. (1992) Splenic abscess. *Aust. NZ J. Surg.* **62,** 780–784.

Pabst, R. and Kamran, D. (1986) Autotransplantation of splenic tissue. *J. Pediatr. Surg.* **21,** 120–124.

Pachter, H. L., Hofstetter, S. R., Elkowitz, A., Harris, L., and Liang, H. G. (1993) Traumatic cysts of the spleen: the role of cystectomy and splenic preservation: experience with seven consecutive patients. *J. Trauma* **35,** 430–436.

Paris, S., Weiss, S. M., Ayers, W. H. Jr., and Clarke, L. E. (1994) Splenic abscess. *Am. Surg.* **60,** 358–361.

Park, A., Gagner, M., and Pomp, A. (1997) The lateral approach to laparoscopic splenectomy. *Am. J. Surg.* **173,** 126–130.

Pegourie, B., Sotto, J. J., Hollard, D., Michallet, M., and Sotto, M. F. (1987) Splenectomy during chronic lymphocytic leukemia. *Cancer* **59,** 1626–1630.

Pereira, A., Monteagudo, J., Bono, A., Lopez-Guillermo, A., and Ordinas, A. (1993) Effect of splenectomy on von Willebrand factor multimeric structure in thrombotic thrombocytopenic purpura refractory to plasma exchange. *Blood Coagul Fibrinolysis* **4,** 783–786.

Peters, T. G., Lewis, J. D., Flip, D. J., and Morris, L. (1977) Antithrombin Ill deficiency causing postsplenectomy mesenteric venous thrombosis coincident with thrombocytopenia. *Ann. Surg.* **185,** 229–231.

Petit, P., Bret, P. M., Atri, M., Hreno, A., Casola, G., and Gianfelice, D. (1994) Splenic vein thrombosis after splenectomy: frequency and role of imaging. *Radiology* **190,** 65–68.

Petroianu, A. (1996a) Subtotal splenectomy in Gaucher's disease. *Eur. J. Surg.* **162,** 511–513.

Petroianu, A. (1996b) Subtotal splenectomy for treatment of patients with myelofibrosis and myeloid metaplasia. *Int. Surg.* **81,** 177–179.

Petroianu, A. and Barbosa, A. J. (1995) Splenic preservation based on preserved histology and phagocytic function using upper short gastric vessels. *Am. J. Surg.* **170,** 702.

Petroianu, A., Da Silva, R. G., Simal, C. J. R., De Carvalho, D. G., and Da Silva, R. A. P. (1997) Late postoperative follow-up of patients submitted to subtotal splenectomy. *Am. Surg.* **63,** 735–740.

Phyliky, R. L. and Fairbanks, V. F. (1997) Thromboembolic complication of splenectomy in unstable hemoglobin disorders: Hb Olmsted, Hb Koln. *Am. J. Hematol.* **55,** 53.

Picozzi, V. J., Roeske, W. R., and Creger, W. P. (1980) Fate of therapy failures in acute idiopathic thrombocytopenic purpura. *Am. J. Med.* **69,** 690–694.

Piomelli, S. (1995) The management of patients with Cooley's anemia: transfusions and splenectomy. *Semin. Hematol.* **32,** 262–268.

Platanias, L. C. and Golomb, H. M. (1993) Hairy cell leukaemia. *Baillieres Clin. Haematol.* **6,** 887–898.

Pohlson, E. C., Wilkinson, R. W., and Coel, M. N. (1994) Heat-damaged red cell scan for intraoperative localization of the accessory spleen. *J. Ped. Surg.* **29,** 604–608.

Politis, C., Spigos, D. G., Georgiopolou, P., et al. (1987) Partial splenic embolisation for hypersplenism of thalassaemia major: five year follow up. *Br. Med. J.* **294,** 665–667.

Posta, C. G. (1994) Laparoscopic management of a splenic cyst. *J. Laparoendosc. Surg.* **4,** 347–354.

Poulin, E. C. and Mamazza, J. (1998) Laparoscopic splenectomy: lessons from the learning curve. *Can. J. Surg.* **41,** 28–36.

Poulin, E. C. and Thibault, C. (1995) Laparoscopic splenectomy for massive splenomegaly: operative technique and case report. *Can. J. Surg.* **38,** 69–72.

Poulin, E. C. and Thibault, C. (1993) The anatomical basis for laparoscopic splenectomy. *Can. J. Surg.* **36,** 484–488.

Poulin, E. C., Thibault, C., DesCoteaux, J. G., and Cote, G. (1995) Partial laparoscopic splenectomy for trauma: technique and case report. *Surg. Laparosc. Endosc.* **5,** 306–310.

Pranikoff, T., Hirschl, R. B., Schlesinger, A. E., Polley, T. Z., and Coran, A. G. (1994) Resolution of splenic injury after nonoperative management. *J. Pediatr. Surg.* **29,** 1366–1369.

Pursnani, K. G., Sillin, L. F., and Kaplan, D. S. (1997) Effect of transjugular intrahepatic portosystemic shunt on secondary hypersplenism. *Am. J. Surg.* **173,** 169–173.

Putterman, C. and Polliack, A. (1992) Late cardiovascular and pulmonary complications of therapy in Hodgkin's disease: report of three unusual cases, with a review of relevant literature. *Leuk. Lymphoma* **7,** 109–115.

Rashba, E. J., Rowe, J. M., and Packman, C. H. (1996) Treatment of the neutropenia of Felty syndrome. *Blood Rev.* **10,** 177–184.

Ravikumar, T. S., Allen, J. D., Bothe, A. Jr., and Steele, G. Jr. (1989) Splenectomy. The treatment of choice for human immunodeficiency virus-related immune thrombocytopenia? *Arch. Surg.* **124,** 625–628.

Ravindranath, Y. and Beutler, E. (1987) Two new variants of glucose-6-phosphate dehydrogenase associated with hereditary non-spherocytic hemolytic anemia. *Am. J. Hematol.* **24,** 357–363.

Reese, J. C., Fairchild, R. B., Brems, J. J., and Kaminski, D. L. (1992) Splenopneumopexy to treat portal hypertension produced by venous occlusive disease. *Arch. Surg.* **127,** 1129–1132.

Rege, R. V., Merriam, L. T., and Joehl, R. J. (1996) Laparoscopic splenectomy. *Surg. Clin. North Am.* **76,** 459–468.

Rhodes, J., Rudd, M., O'Rourke, N., Nathanson, L., and Fielding, G. (1995) Laparoscopic splenectomy and lymph node biopsy for hematologic disorders. *Ann. Surg.* **222,** 43–46.

Rice, L. (1997) Splenectomy for relapsing thrombotic thrombocytopenic purpura. *Ann. Int. Med.* **126,** 915.

Robertson, D. A. F., Simpson, F. G., and Losowsky, M.S. (1981) Blood viscosity after splenectomy. *Br. Med. J.* **283,** 573–575.

Røder, O. C. (1984) Splenic vein thrombosis with bleeding gastroesophageal varices. *Acta Chir. Scand.* **150,** 265–268.

Rodgers, B. M., Tribble, C., and Joob, A. (1987) Partial splenectomy for Gaucher's disease. *Ann. Surg.* **205,** 693–699.

Rodkey, M. L. and Macknin, M. L. (1992) Pediatric wandering spleen: case report and review of literature. *Clin. Pediatr.* **31,** 289–294.

Rogers, F. B., Baumgartner, N. E., Robin, A. P., and Barrett, J. A. (1991) Absorbable mesh splenorrhaphy for severe splenic injuries: functional studies in an animal model and an additional patient series. *J. Trauma* **31,** 200–204.

Rose, M., Rowe, J. M., and Eldor, A. (1993) The changing course of thrombotic thrombocytopenic purpura and modern therapy. *Blood Rev.* **7,** 94–103.

Rowe, J. M., Francis, C. W., Cyran, E. M., and Marder, V. J. (1985) Thrombotic thrombocytopenic purpura recovery after splenectomy associated with persistence of abnormally large von Willebrand factor multimers. *Am. J. Hematol.* **20,** 161–168.

Rubin, M., Yampolski, I., Lambrozo, R., Zaizov, R., and Dintsman, M. (1986) Partial splenectomy in Gaucher's disease. *J. Pediatr. Surg.* **21,** 125–128.

Rutledge, R. (1996) The increasing frequency of nonoperative management of patients with liver and spleen injury. *Adv. Surg.* **30,** 385–415.

Saldinger, P. F., Matthews, J. B., Mowschenson, P. M., and Hodin, R. A. (1996) Stapled laparoscopic splenectomy: initial experience. *J. Am. Coll. Surg.* **182,** 459–461.

Sands, M., Page, D., and Brown, R. B. (1986) Splenic abscess after nonoperative management of splenic rupture. *J. Pediatr. Surg.* **21,** 900–901.

Sarkar, R., Coran, A. G., Cilley, R. E., Lindenauer, S. M., and Stanley, J. C. (1991) Arterial aneurysms in children: clinicopathologic classification. *J. Vasc. Surg.* **13,** 47–57.

Sasada, T., Maki, A., and Takabayashi, A. (1995) Recurrent splenic artery aneurysms developing after aneurysmectomy without splenectomy: report of a case. *Surg. Today* **25,** 168–171.

Savoiz, D., Froment, P., Chilcott, M., Aguilar, M., Savoiz, A., and Morel, P. (1997) Isolated blunt splenic trauma in adults. *Dig. Surg.* **14,** 277–281.

Saxe, J. M., Hayward, S. R., Lucas, C. E., et al. (1994) Splenic reimplantation does not affect outcome in chronic canine model. *Am. Surg.* **60,** 674–680.

Scher, K. S., Wroczynski, A. F., and Scott-Conner, C. E. H. (1985) Intraperitoneal splenic implants do not alter clearance of pneumococcal bacteremia. *Am. Surg.* **51,** 269–271.

Schilling, R. F. (1995) Estimating the risk for sepsis after splenectomy in hereditary spherocytosis. *Ann. Int. Med.* **122,** 187–188.

Schlinkert, R. T. and Mann, D. (1995) Laparoscopic splenectomy offers advantages in selected patients with immune thrombocytopenic purpura. *Am. J. Surg.* **170,** 624–627.

Schmidt, S. P., Andrews, H. G., and White J. J. (1992) The splenic snood: an improved approach for the management of the wandering spleen. *J. Pediatr. Surg.* **27,** 1043–1044.

Schneider, P. A., Rayner, A. A., Linker, C. A., Schuman, M. A., Liu, E. T., and Hohn, D. C. (1985) The role of splenectomy in the multimodality treatment of thrombotic thrombocytopenic purpura. *Ann. Surg.* **202,** 318–322.

Schneider, P. A., Abrams, D. I., Rayner, A. A., and Hohn, D. C. (1987) Immunodeficiency associated thrombocytopenic purpura (IDTP). *Arch. Surg.* **122,** 1175–1178.

Scholz, K. H., Herrmann, C., Tebbe, U., Chemnitius, J. M., Helmchen, U., and Kreuzer, H. (1993) Myocardial infarction in young patients with Hodgkin's disease: potential pathogenic role of radiotherapy, chemotherapy, and splenectomy. *Clin. Invest.* **71,** 57–64.

Schwalke, M. A., Crowley, J. P., Spencer, P., Metzger, J., Kawan, M., and Burchard, K. W. (1991) Splenic artery ligation for splenic salvage: clinical experience and immune function. *J. Trauma* **31,** 385–388.

Schwartz, S. I. (1985) Splenectomy for thrombocytopenia. *World J. Surg.* **9,** 419–421.

Schwartz, S. I. (1996) Role of splenectomy in hematologic disorders. *World J. Surg.* **20,** 1156–1159.

Schwerk, W. B., Gorg, C., Gorg, K., and Restrepo, I. (1994) Ultrasound-guided percutaneous drainage of pyogenic splenic abscesses. *J. Clin. Ultrasound* **22,** 161–166.

Seashore, J. H. and McIntosh, S. (1990) Elective splenopexy for wandering spleen. *J. Pediatr. Surg.* **25,** 270–272.

Seufert, R. and Mitrou, P. (1985) *The Surgery of the Spleen,* Theime, New York.

Seymour, J. F., Cusack, J. D., Lerner, S. A., Pollock, R. E., and Keating, M. J. (1997) Case/control study of the role of splenectomy in chronic lymphocytic leukemia. *J. Clin. Oncol.* **15,** 52–60.

Sharpe, R. W., Rector, J. T., Rushin, J. M., Garvin, D. F., and Cotelingam, J. D. (1993) Splenic metastasis in hairy cell leukemia, *Cancer* **71,** 2222–2226.

Shah, S. H., Hayes, P. C., Allan, P. L., Nicoll, J., and Finlayson, N. D. (1996) Measurement of spleen size and its relation to hypersplenism and portal hemodynamics in portal hypertension due to hepatic cirrhosis. *Am. J. Gastroenterol.* **91,** 2580–2583.

Shekhar, K. C. (1994) Tropical gastrointestinal disease: hepatosplenic schistosomiasis: pathological, clinical and treatment review. *Singapore Med. J.* **35,** 616–621.

Shiino, Y., Takahashi, N., Okamoto, T., Ishii, Y., Yanagisawa, A., Inagaki, Y., and Aoki, T. (1996) Surgical treatments of chronic idiopathic thrombocytopenic purpura and prognostic factors for splenectomy. *Int. Surg.* **81,** 140–143.

Sigueira-Batista, R. and Quintas, L. E. (1994) Tropical splenomegaly syndrome: a review from Brazil. *East Afr. Med. J.* **71,** 771–772.

Silverman, J. F., Geisinger, K. R., Raab, S. S., and Stanley, M. W. (1993) Fine needle aspiration biopsy of the spleen in the evaluation of neoplastic disorders. *Acta Cytol.* **37,** 158–162.

Silvestri, F., Russo, D., Fanin, R., et al. (1995) Laparoscopic splenectomy in the management of hematological diseases. *Haematologica* **80,** 47–49.

Skandalakis, P. N., Colborn, G. L., Skandalakis, L. J., and Richardson, D. D. (1993) Surgical anatomy of the spleen. *Surg. Clin. North Am.* **73,** 7477–7468.

Skootsky, S. A., Rosove, M. H., and Langley, M. B. (1986) Immune thrombocytopenia and response to splenectomy in chronic liver disease. *Arch. Intern. Med.* **146,** 555–557.

Slaiby, J. M., Crowley, J. P., and Amaral, J. F. (1996) Late recurrence of Hodgkin's disease after partial splenectomy. *J. Pediatr. Surg.* **31,** 731–732.

Smalley, R. V., Connors, J., Tuttle, R. L., Anderson, S., Robinson, W., and Whisnant, J. K. (1992) Splenectomy vs. alpha interferon: a randomized study in patients with previously untreated hairy cell leukemia. *Am. J. Hematol.* **41,** 13–18.

Smedley, J. C. and Bellingham, A. J. (1991) Current problems in haematology. **2,** Hereditary spherocytosis. *J. Clin. Pathol.* **44,** 441–444.

Smith, B. M., Schropp, K. P., Lobe, T. E., Rogers, D. A., Presbury, G. J., Wilimas, J. A., and Wong, W. C. (1994) Laparoscopic splenectomy in childhood. *J. Ped. Surg.* **29,** 975–977.

Smith, C. D., Meyer, T. A., Goretsky, M. J., Hyams, D., Luchette, F. A., Fegelman, E. J., and Nussbaum, M. S. (1996) Laparoscopic splenectomy by the lateral approach: a safe and effective alternative to open splenectomy for hematologic diseases. *Surgery* **120,** 789–794.

Smith, J. S. Jr., Cooney, R. N., and Mucha, P. Jr. (1996) Nonoperative management of the ruptured spleen: a revalidation of criteria. *Surgery* **120,** 745–751.

Solanki, D. L., Kletter, G. G., and Castro, O. (1986) Acute splenic sequestration crises in adults with sickle cell disease. *Am. J. Med.* **80,** 985–990.

Soper, N. J. and Rikkers, L. F. (1982) Effect of operations for variceal hemorrhage on hypersplenism. *Am. J. Surg.* **144,** 700–703.

Sow, M. L., Dia, A., and Ouedraogo, T. (1991) Anatomic basis for conservative surgery of the spleen. *Surg. Radiol. Anat.* **13,** 81–87.

Speck, B., Tichelli, A., Widmer, E., Harder, F., Kissling, M., Wursch, A., et al. (1996) Splenectomy as an adjuvant measure in the treatment of severe aplastic anaemia. *Br. J. Haematol.* **92,** 818–824.

Spier, C. M., Kjeldsberg, C. R., Eyre, H. J., and Behm, F. G. (1985) Malignant lymphoma with primary presentation in the spleen. *Arch. Pathol. Lab. Med.* **109,** 1076–1080.

Splenic Injury Study Group (1987) Splenic injury: a prospective multicentre study on non-operative and operative treatment. *Br. J. Surg.* **74,** 310–313.

Stein, R. S., Weikert, D., Reynolds, V., Greer, J. P., and Flexner, J. M. (1987) Splenectomy for end-stage chronic lymphocytic leukemia. *Cancer* **59,** 1815–1818.

Steinberg, J. J., Suhrland, M., and Valenski, Q. (1991) The spleen in the spleen syndrome: the association of splenoma with hematopoietic and neoplastic disease: compendium of cases since 1864. *J. Surg. Oncol.* **47,** 193–202.

Stiemer, B., Opri, F., Senger, D., Kreuser, E. D., Berdel, W., Hopp, H., et al. (1996) Successful emergency splenectomy during pregnancy in a patient with life-threatening idiopathic thrombocytopenia. Case report. *J. Perinat. Med.* **24,** 703–706.

Stringel, G., Soucy, P., and Mercer, S. (1982) Torsion of the wandering spleen: splenectomy or splenopexy. *J. Pediatr. Surg.* **17,** 373–375.

Studemeister, A. E., Beilke, M. A., and Kirmani, N. (1987) Splenic abscess due to *Clostridium difficile* and *Pseudomonas paucimobilis.* *Am. J. Gastroenterol.* **82,** 389–390.

Svarch, E., Vilorio, P., Nordet, I., et al. (1996) Partial splenectomy in children with sickle cell disease and repeated episodes of splenic sequestration. *Hemoglobin* **20,** 393–400.

Swerdlow, A. J., Douglas, A. J., Vaughan Hudson, G., Vaughan Hudson, B., and MacLennan, K. A. (1993) Risk of second primary cancer after Hodgkin's disease in patients in the British National Lymphoma Investigation: relationships to host factors, histology and stage of Hodgkin's disease, and splenectomy. *Br. J. Cancer* **68,** 1006–1011.

Talarico, L., Grapski, R., Lutz, C. K., and Weintraub, L. R. (1987) Late postsplenectomy recurrence of thrombotic thrombocytopenic purpura responding to removal of accessory spleen. *Am. J. Med.* **82,** 845–848.

Tarazov, P. G., Polysalov, V. N., and Ryzhkov, V. K. (1991) Transcatheter treatment of splenic artery aneurysms (SAA). Report of two cases. *J. Cardiovasc. Surg.* **32,** 128–131.

Targarona, E. M., Martinez, J., Ramos, C., Becerra, J. A., and Trias, M. (1995) Conservative laparoscopic treatment of a posttraumatic splenic cyst. *Surg. Endosc.* **9,** 71–72.

Taylor, M. A., Kaplan, H. S., and Nelsen, T. S. (1985) Staging laparotomy with splenectomy for Hodgkin's disease: the Stanford experience. *World J. Surg.* **9,** 449–460.

Tchernia G., Gauthier, F., Mielot, F., et al. (1993) Initial assessment of the beneficial effect of partial splenectomy in hereditary spherocytosis. *Blood* **81,** 2014–2020.

Teperman, S. H., Whitehouse, B. S., Sammartano, R. J., Rojas-Corona, R., Poulis, D., and Boley, S. J. (1994) Bloodless splenic surgery: the safe warm-ischemic time. *J. Pediatr. Surg.* **29,** 88–92.

Thanopoulos, B. D. and Frimas, C. A. (1982) Partial splenic embolization in the management of hypersplenism secondary to Gaucher disease. *J. Pediatr.* **101,** 740–743.

Thompson, C. E., Damon, L. E., Ries, C. A., and Linker, C. A. (1992) Thrombotic microangiopathies in the 1980s: clinical features, response to treatment, and the impact of the human immunodeficiency virus epidemic. *Blood* **80,** 1890–1895.

Touloukian, R. J. and Seashore, J. H. (1987) Partial splenic decapsulation: a simplified operation for splenic pseudocyst. *J. Pediatr. Surg.* **22,** 135–137.

Towell, B. L. and Levine, S. P. (1987) Massive hepatomegaly following splenectomy for myeloid metaplasia. *Am. J. Med.* **82,** 371–375.

Trastek, V. F., Pairolero, P. C., Joyce, J. W., Hollier, L. H., and Bernatz, P. E. (1982) Splenic artery aneurysms. *Surgery* **91,** 694–699.

Trias, M., Targarona, E. M., and Balague, C. (1996) Laparoscopic splenectomy: an evolving technique. A comparison between anterior and lateral approaches. *Surg. Endosc.* **10,** 389–392.

Tricarico, A., Tartaglia, A., Taddeo, F., Sessa, R., Sessa, E., and Minelli, S. (1994) Videolaparoscopic treatment of spleen injuries. Report of two cases. *Surg. Endosc.* **8,** 910–912.

Tsoukas, C. M., Bernard, N. F., Sampalis, J., et al. (1993) Effect of splenectomy on HIV infection. *Natl. Conf. Hum. Retroviruses Relat. Infect.* p. 172.

Tubbs, R. R., Thomas, F., Norris, D., and Firor, H. V. (1987) Is hemisplenectomy a satisfactory option to total splenectomy in abdominal staging of Hodgkin's disease? *J. Pediatr. Surg.* **22,** 727–729.

Tyler, D. S., Shaunak, S., Bartlett, J. A., and Iglehart, J. D. (1990) HIV-1-associated thrombocytopenia. The role of splenectomy. *Ann. Surg.* **211,** 211–217.

Ugochukwu, A. I. and Irving, M. (1985) Intraperitoneal low-pressure suction drainage following splenectomy. *Br. J. Surg.* **72,** 247–248.

Umlas, S. L. and Cronan, J. J. (1991) Splenic trauma: can CT grading systems enable prediction of successful nonsurgical treatment? *Radiology* **178,** 481–487.

Uranus, S., Kronberger, L., and Kraft-Kine, J. (1994) Partial splenic resection using the TA-stapler. *Am. J. Surg.* **168,** 49–53.

Uranus, S., Pfeifer, J., Schauer, C., Kronberger, L., Rabl, H., Ranftl, G., Hauser, H., and Bahadori, K. (1995) Laparoscopic partial splenic resection. *Surg. Laparosc. Endosc.* **5,** 133–136.

Uriarte, C., Pomares, N., Martin, M., Conde, A., Alonso, N., and Bueno, M. G. (1991) Splenic hydatidosis. *Am. J. Trop. Med. Hyg.* **44,** 420–423.

Van Norman, A. S., Nagorney, D. M., Martin, J. K., Phyliky, R. L., and Ilstrup, D. M. (1986) Splenectomy for hairy cell leukemia: a clinical review of 63 patients. *Cancer* **57,** 644–648.

Velanovich, V. (1995) Blunt splenic injury in adults: a decision analysis comparing options for treatment. *Eur. J. Surg.* **161,** 463–470.

Veltman, G. A., Brand, A., Leeksma, O. C., ten Bosch, G. J., van Krieken, J. H., and Briet, E. (1995) The role of splenectomy in the treatment of relapsing thrombotic thrombocytopenic purpura. *Ann. Hematol.* **70,** 231–236.

Wald, B. R., Ortega, J. A., Ross, L., Wald, P., Laug, W. E., and Williams, K. O. (1981) Candidal splenic abscesses complicating acute leukemia of childhood treated by splenectomy. *Pediatrics* **67,** 296–299.

Walsh, C., Krigel, R., Lennette, E., and Karpatkin, S. (1985) Thrombocytopenia in homosexual patients: prognosis, response to therapy, and prevalence of antibody to the retrovirus associated with the acquired immunodeficiency syndrome. *Ann. Intern. Med.* **103,** 542–545.

Wanebo, H. J., Kennedy, B. J., Winchester, D. P., Stewart, A. N., Fremgen, A.M. (1997) Role of splenectomy in gastric cancer surgery: adverse effect of elective splenectomy on longterm survival. *J. Am. Coll. Surg.* **185,** 177–184.

Wasvary, H., Howells, G., Villalba, M., et al. (1997) Nonoperative management of adult blunt splenic trauma: a 15-year experience. *Am. Surg.* **63,** 694–699.

Watson, D. I., Coventry, B. J., Gill, P. G., and Malycha, P. (1997) Laparoscopic versus open splenectomy for immune thrombocytopenic purpura. *Surgery* **121,** 18–22.

Weed, R. I. and Bowdler, A. J. (1966). Metabolic dependance of the critical hemolytic volume of human erythrocytes: relationship to osmotic fragility and autohemolysis in hereditary spherocytosis and normal red cells. *J. Clin. Invest.* **45,** 1137–1149.

Wells, A. D., Majumdar, G., Slater, N. G., and Young, A. E. (1991) Role of splenectomy as a salvage procedure in thrombotic thrombocytopenic purpura. *Br. J. Surg.* **78,** 1389–1390.

Wheeler, W. E. and Hardy, J. D. (1986) Splenectomy: acute infectious complications. *South. Med. J.* **79s,** 64.

Williams, D. N. and Kaur, B. (1996) Postsplenectomy care. Strategies to decrease the risk of infection. *Postgrad. Med.* **100,** 195–198, 201, 205.

Williams, R. J. and Glazer, G. (1993) Splenic cysts: changes in diagnosis, treatment and aetiological concepts. *Ann. R. Coll. Surg. Engl.* **75,** 87–89.

Williams, S. F. and Golomb, H. M. (1986) Perspective on staging approaches in the malignant lymphomas. *Surg. Gynecol. Obstet.* **163,** 193–201.

Willis, B. K., Deitch, E. A., and McDonald, J. C. (1986) The influence of trauma to the spleen on postoperative complications and mortality. *J. Trauma* **26,** 1073–1076.

Wilson, R. E., Rosenthal, D. S., Moloney, W. C., and Osteen, R. T. (1985) Splenectomy for myeloproliferative disorders. *World J. Surg.* **9,** 431–436.

Winde, G., Schmid, K. W., Lugering, N., et al. (1996) Results and prognostic factors of splenectomy in idiopathic thrombocytopenic purpura. *J. Am. Coll. Surg.* **183,** 565–574.

Winslow, G. A. and Nelson, E. W. (1995) Thrombotic thrombocytopenic purpura: indications for and results of splenectomy. *Am. J. Surg.* **170,** 558–563.

Wirbel, R. J., Uhlig, U., and Futtere, K. M. (1996) Case report: splenic hamartoma with hematologic disorders. *Am. J. Med. Sci.* **311,** 243–246.

Witte, C. L., Van Wyck, D. B., Witte M. H., Corrigan, J. J. Jr., Zukoski, C. F., Pond, G. D., and Woolfend, J. M. (1992) Ischaemia and partial resection for control of splenic hyperfunction. *Br. J. Surg.* **69,** 531–535.

Witte, C. L., Esser, M. J., and Rappaport, W. D. (1992) Updating the management of salvageable splenic injury. *Ann. Surg.* **215,** 261–265.

Wobbes, T., Van der Sluis, R. F., and Cubbers, E.-J. C.(1984) Removal of the massive spleen: a surgical risk? *Am. J. Surg.* **147,** 800–802.

Wolf, S. E., Ridgeway, C. A., Van Way, C. W., Reddy, B. A., Papasian, C. J., and Helling, T. S. (1996) Infectious sequelae in the use of polyglycolic acid mesh for splenic salvage with intraperitoneal contamination. *J. Surg. Res.* **61,** 433–436.

Yamashita, H., Ohuchida, J., Shimura, H., Aibe, H., Honda, H., Kuroki, S., Shijiiwa, K., and Tanaka, M. (1996) Laparoscopic splenectomy aided by balloon occlusion of the splenic artery: report of a case. *Surg. Laparosc. Endosc.* **6,** 326–329.

Yamataka, A., Fujiwara, T., Tsuchioka, T., Kurosu, Y., and Sunagawa, M. (1996) Heterotopic splenic autotransplantation in a neonate with splenic rupture, leading to normal splenic function. *J. Pediatr. Surg.* **31,** 239–240.

Yee, J. C. and Akpata, M. O. (1995) Laparoscoic splenectomy for congenital spherocytosis with splenomegaly: a case report. *Can. J. Surg.* **38,** 73–76.

Yeung, E., Hugh, T. B., and Rainer, S. (1996) Inflammatory pseudotumour of the spleen. *Aust. NZ J. Surg.* **66,** 492–493.

Yoshida, K., Yamazaki, Y., Mizuno, R., Yamadera, H., Hara, A., Yoshizawa, J., and Kanai, M. (1995) Laparoscopic splenectomy in children. Preliminary results and comparison with the open technique. *Surg. Endosc.* **9,** 1279–1282.

Yoshioka, H., Kuroda, C., Hori, S., Tokunaga, K., Tanaka, T., Nakamura, H., et al. 1985) Splenic embolization for hypersplenism using steel coils. *Am. J. Radiol.* **144,** 1269–1274.

Yuan, J., Bunyaratvej, A., Fucharoen, S., Fung, C., Shinar, E., and Schrier, S. L. (1995) The instability of the membrane skeleton in thalassemic red blood cells. *Blood* **86,** 3945–3950.

Zamir, O., Szold, A., Matzner, Y., Ben-Yehuda, D., Seror, D., Deutsch, I., and Freund, H. R. (1996) Laparoscopic splenectomy for immune thrombocytopenic purpura. *J. Laparoendosc. Surg.* **6,** 301–304.

Zamora, J. U. and Halpern, N. B. (1987) Splenectomy for metastatic neoplasms. *South. Med. J.* **80,** 80S.

Zer, M. and Freud, E. (1992) Subtotal splenectomy in Gaucher's disease: towards a definition of critical splenic mass. *Br. J. Surg.* **79,** 742–744.

Zimran, A., Elstein, D., Schiffmann, R., Abrahamov, A., Goldberg, M., Bar-Maor, J. A., et al. (1995) Outcome of partial splenectomy for type I Gaucher disease. *J. Pediatr.* **126,** 596–597.

Index*

*Page references in *italics* refer to figures and those in **bold** to tables. *CP(#)* = Color Plate.